MICROBIOLOGY
for the HEALTHCARE
PROFESSIONAL

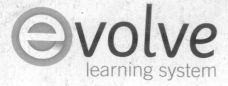
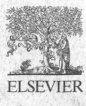

MICROBIOLOGY
for the HEALTHCARE PROFESSIONAL

Karin C. VanMeter, PhD
Lecturer
Iowa State University
Department of Biomedical Sciences
College of Veterinary Medicine
Ames, Iowa;
Lecturer
Gerontology Program
College of Human Sciences;
Adjunct Instructor
Des Moines Area Community College
Des Moines, Iowa

William G. VanMeter, PhD
(deceased)
Professor Emeritus
Iowa State University
Department of Biomedical Sciences
College of Veterinary Medicine
Ames, Iowa

Robert J. Hubert, BS
Laboratory Coordinator
Department of Animal Science
Microbiology Program
Iowa State University
Ames, Iowa

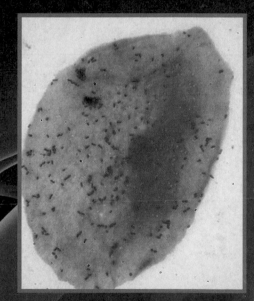

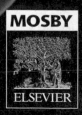
MOSBY
ELSEVIER

MOSBY
ELSEVIER

3251 Riverport Lane
Maryland Heights, Missouri 63043

Library of Congress Cataloging-in-Publication Data
VanMeter, Karin.
   Microbiology for the healthcare professional / Karin C. VanMeter, William G. VanMeter, Robert J. Hubert.
         p. ; cm.
   Includes bibliographical references.
   ISBN 978-0-323-04594-0 (pbk. : alk. paper)   1. Medical microbiology—Textbooks.   2. Microbiology—Textbooks.   3. Infection—Textbooks.   I. VanMeter, William G., 1933–2008.   II. Hubert, Robert J.   III. Title.
   [DNLM: 1. Microbiological Processes.   2. Infection—microbiology.   QW 4 V262m 2010]
   QR46.V347 2010
   616.9'041—dc22

                                                                    2009036074

Publisher: Jeanne Olson
Managing Editor: Billie Sharp
Developmental Editor: Kristen Mandava
Publishing Services Manager: Catherine Jackson
Senior Project Manager: Karen M. Rehwinkel
Cover/Text Designer: Amy Buxton

Printed in China

Last digit is the print number: 9 8 7 6 5 4 3 2

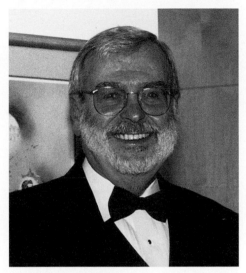

DEDICATED TO
William G. VanMeter
1933–2008

Preface

In preparation for writing this book the authors had two main goals: first, to produce a "user friendly" textbook for the student and second, to organize and write it in a way that effectively presents the material at different levels to accommodate different learning modalities and levels of understanding of basic science. To accomplish these goals we have organized the material to facilitate a progressive, building-block approach. The first chapters cover general concepts within the life sciences followed by chapters that apply these concepts toward a practical application in the life science/health field. Once the basic concepts were established, we presented each body system individually as they are impacted by microbial organisms. Finally, the closing chapters were designed to give the student a broader perspective of the field of microbiology and its impact on the world and society in general, including emerging fields. As we wrote the book it became apparent that it would be very easy to write volumes about microbiology and its impact on the health sciences, but a conscious effort was made to distill the material down to a level that is most useful to professionals who will be using this information on a very practical, everyday basis. Realizing that some students and instructors may want to study an area in more detail, we have included resource material at the end of each chapter. These sources include other texts, and more importantly, websites that can provide the most current, up-to-date information on the subject area.

In addition to creating a student-friendly text, we also organized and presented the material so it would be useful as a reference book that practicing healthcare professionals may want to retain and use as part of their professional library. Numerous tables that condense and organize some of the salient points in the text were designed to provide users with a quick, simple way to access information they frequently use in practicing their skills and developing their practical experience.

EVOLVE Resources

http://evolve.elsevier.com/VanMeter/microbiology/

Evolve is an interactive learning environment designed to work in coordination with this text. Instructors may use Evolve to provide an Internet-based course component that reinforces and expands the concepts presented in class. Evolve may be used to publish the class syllabus, outlines, and lecture notes; set up "virtual office hours" and e-mail communication; share important dates and information through the online class calendar; and encourage student participation through chat rooms and discussion boards. Evolve allows instructors to post examinations and manage their grade books online.

For the Instructor

For the instructor, Evolve offers valuable resources to help them prepare their courses, including:

- An image collection of figures from the book
- Instructor's manual with case studies and scenarios
- More than 1,200 Power Point slides
- Test bank of approximately 800 questions in ExamView
- Answers to Review Questions

Instructors also have access to Evolve student resources, including the Healthcare Application tables from the book.

For the Student

For the student, Evolve offers valuable resources to help them succeed in their courses, including:

- Healthcare Application Tables for quick reference and to assist in practical application of lessons and concepts
- Answers to Review Questions

For more information, visit http://evolve.elsevier.com/ VanMeter/microbiology/ or contact an Elsevier sales representative.

Acknowledgments

The authors would like to thank the editorial and production staff at Elsevier for all of their support and assistance throughout the whole process. A special thanks to Christina Pryor, Mindy Hutchinson, and Kristen Mandava. We also thank Jeanne Robertson, who illustrated the artwork.

Many thanks to all of the people who provided the outstanding photographs for this text, including the Rob Hubert Lab, Iowa State University: Lab Assistants Erin Richter, Tara Miller, Chelsea Clinton, Diana Karkow, Allison Schlapkohl, and Chris Mease, with support from Lab Technician Kay Christiansen. All electron micrographs were taken by Karin VanMeter.

I dedicate this book to my beloved husband Bill, who passed away during the final writings of the last few chapters of this book. He loved writing the "Why You Need to Know" boxes, and his excellent knowledge of science and the history of science provided a great contribution to the book. I also would like to thank my children, Christine and Andrew, for their constant support and understanding while we were writing the book and also their support during their father's final year of life. To my friend Rob Hubert—I can only say thank you for your professional and emotional support. Thank you for stepping in during a crucial time in the finishing of this great adventure; without you this project would not have been completed on time. Last but not least, thank you Dr. Peter Martin for providing me with a "safe haven" for writing this book and also for your wonderful support during difficult times.

Karin VanMeter

I would first like to thank Karin and Bill VanMeter for inviting me to become part of this team. I could not have asked for better co-authors and value not only the professional experience but the friendships that developed along the way. I would like to thank Dr. Joan Cunnick, along with the faculty and staff of the microbiology program at Iowa State University, for their support. I would also like to acknowledge and thank my parents, John and Ann Hubert, and my sister Donna for their constant love and unfailing support. I would like to offer my special thanks to Kristin Marshall, a doctoral candidate at the University of Wisconsin, Madison, for the incredible support she has given me both professionally and personally—she is a great colleague, friend, and my kindred spirit. Last, and most importantly, I thank God for the blessings and opportunities He has given to me.

Robert Hubert

Contents

1 Scope of Microbiology, *1*

2 Chemistry of Life, *18*

3 Cell Structure and Function, *40*

4 Microbiological Laboratory Techniques, *80*

5 Safety Issues, *98*

6 Bacteria and Archaea, *114*

7 Viruses, *135*

8 Eukaryotic Microorganisms, *158*

9 Infection and Disease, *180*

10 Infections of the Integumentary System, Soft Tissue, and Muscle, *200*

11 Infections of the Respiratory System, *216*

12 Infections of the Gastrointestinal System, *235*

13 Infections of the Nervous System and Senses, *256*

14 Infections of the Circulatory System, *275*

15 Infections of the Urinary System, *296*

16 Infections of the Reproductive System, *306*

17 Sexually Transmitted Infections/Diseases, *317*

18 Emerging Infectious Diseases, *331*

19 Physical and Chemical Methods of Control, *343*

20 The Immune System, *361*

21 Pharmacology, *390*

22 Antimicrobial Drugs, *404*

23 Human Age and Microorganisms, *423*

24 Microorganisms in the Environment and Environmental Safety, *435*

25 Biotechnology, *460*

Appendix   Bergey's Manual of Systematic Bacteriology, *476*

Glossary, *477*

MICROBIOLOGY
for the HEALTHCARE
PROFESSIONAL

Scope of Microbiology

OUTLINE

Origins of Microbiology and Microscopy
Microscopy and Its Founding Fathers
Types of Microscopes
Spontaneous Generation
Pasteurization
Germ Theory of Disease

Origin and Evolution of Microorganisms
Origin
Evolution

Classification of Microorganisms
Prokaryotes versus Eukaryotes
Bacteria, Archaea, and Eukaryotes
Viruses
Prions
Viroids
Taxonomy

Microorganisms in Health and Disease
Microbes in the Environment
Normal Flora
Pathogens

Applied Microbiology
Microorganisms in Food Production
Microorganisms in the Production of Alcoholic Beverages
Treatment of Water Supplies
Microbes and the Production of Pharmaceutical Agents
Microbes in Agriculture
Bioremediation
Microbes, Biomass, and Energy
Microbial Forensics

After reading this chapter, the student will be able to:
- Describe the achievements of scientists in the early years of microbiology
- Discuss the different types of microscopes and their use
- Explain the theory of spontaneous generation
- Discuss the germ theory of disease and its significance
- Name and describe Koch's postulates
- Discuss the origin and evolution of microorganisms
- Describe the differences between prokaryotes and eukaryotes
- Explain the role of taxonomy
- Describe the different ways of microbial transmission
- Name and briefly describe the different uses of microorganisms in everyday life

KEY TERMS

abiogenesis
algae
animalcules
archaea
aseptic
bacteria
binomial
biofilms
bioremediation
classification
commensalism
compound microscope
dissection microscopes
domains
electron microscopes

endospores
eukaryotic
foodborne diseases
fungi
genera
genus
identification
immunology
Koch's postulates
light microscopes
mutualism
nomenclature
normal flora
parasitism
pasteurization

pathogenic
phylogeny
phyla
prions
prokaryotes
protozoans
species
stereomicroscopes
sterilization
stromatolites
synergism
taxa
taxonomy
viroids
waterborne disease

WHY YOU NEED TO KNOW

HISTORY

To see where we're going from where we are, we must know where we've been. Measles, whooping cough, mumps, polio, cholera, influenza, rheumatic fever, pneumonia, diphtheria, tuberculosis, typhoid fever, meningitis, leprosy, syphilis, gonorrhea, tetanus, anthrax, the common cold, chicken pox, smallpox, rabies, encephalitis, malaria, dysentery, etc., etc., etc., numerous epidemics, pandemics, and too many others to list have been with humankind from approximately 4000 bce. to the present. Humankind has lived with diseases and been able to survive with varying degrees of success. Knowledge of the nature of disease has been slow and difficult to obtain. Rational use of this knowledge to alleviate the distress caused by disease has been even slower. Technological advances were and are needed to cope with the problems. For example, cholera—a killer of epidemic proportions—was linked to a public water source by John Snow, an English physician in the mid-1800s. He removed the pump handle, preventing access to the water, and the epidemic ended—ingenious, but serendipitous and of limited use.

IMPACT

The advancement of microbiology began with Robert Hooke's (1635–1703) observations utilizing the then new compound microscope that could magnify objects ×20 to ×30. Later, Antony van Leeuwenhoek (1632–1723), using his skills at lens grinding and the use of light, improved the resolving power of the microscope to ×200. His were among the first observations of bacteria and, arguably, the beginning of microbiology. Bacteria were eventually recognized as causative agents of disease. These observations and others led Pasteur and Koch in the late 1800s to develop the germ theory of disease, an understanding that boosted disease prevention and treatment significantly. For example, Robert Koch in 1883 microscopically identified the causative pathogen for cholera (*Vibrio cholerae*), which he had grown on a plate of agar. After acceptance of the germ theory of disease, new pathogens were reported on the average of every year and a half. Technological advancements in light microscopy and the development of electron microscopy permitted visualization of pathogens or their shadows,

Continued

allowing assessment of the effectiveness of treatment. Although it was deduced that the causative agent for the influenza pandemic of 1918 was a filterable agent, it was the advent of electron microscopy that allowed visualization of the virus in a rare lung sample from a victim. More recent advances in the biotechnology of genetic analysis have provided information on the nature of the functions of hemagglutinin and neuraminidase, viral coat proteins of the influenza virus. It is hoped that this information will direct investigations for methods of protection from another potential influenza pandemic.

THE FUTURE
Microbiology not only affords the detailed study of recognized pathogenic microorganisms but is invaluable in the identification of new pathogens in emerging diseases. Such studies are essential in monitoring the presence of microbes everywhere from water supplies to door knobs. Results from these studies are used to direct personal as well as public health and hygiene practices and policies. Technological advances in microscopy and biotechnology have provided a basis for the scientific discipline of microbiology and have stimulated the development of new concepts for research and vice versa. Meanwhile, hospital microorganisms such as *Staphylococcus aureus*, enterococci, and *Pseudomonas aeruginosa* are becoming resistant to the old tried and true antibiotics. Cephalosporins in many cases are the last line of defense. Clearly, much work lies ahead if we wish to bias the balance in favor of survival.

Origins of Microbiology and Microscopy

Microbiology is the study of microorganisms, using a variety of techniques for purposes of visualization, identification, and study of their function. The science of microbiology originated with the invention and development of the microscope. Microscopy allowed humans to magnify objects and microorganisms not detectable by the naked eye. Technological advances then have led to the improvement of microscopes, which became an essential investigative tool for biology in general and for the study of cells, tissues, and microorganisms (Figure 1.1) in particular.

Microscopy and Its Founding Fathers

The development of microscopes started in the sixteenth century and evolved through time into a sophisticated tool used routinely in many branches of science. To this day all different types of microscopes continue to be improved and new ones are being developed.

Zaccharias and **Hans Janssen,** a father-and-son team of Dutch eyeglass makers (around the year 1590) found that optical images could be enlarged and viewed using different lenses. The first microscope they produced was a **compound microscope** consisting of a simple tube with lenses at each end. Depending on the size of the diaphragm, the part of the microscope that regulates the amount of light striking the specimen, the magnification of objects under view ranged from three times (or ×3) to ×9.

Antony van Leeuwenhoek (1632–1723), another native of Holland, is considered to be the father of microscopy and is believed to be the first to observe live bacteria and protozoans. He was fascinated by the power of lenses, which made it possible to observe what the naked human eye could not see. The microscope he used contained only one convex objective lens

and is now called a *simple microscope*. His interest in science and his native curiosity led him to some of the most important observations of biology. Van Leeuwenhoek was able to see small life forms that he called **"animalcules"** (little animals). Throughout the years he observed bacteria, protozoans, blood cells, sperm cells, microscopic nematodes, rotifers, and more. Much of his inspiration came from Hooke's *Micrographia* (see later in this chapter). He published his observations in 1678 in a letter to the Royal Society of London. As a result of his findings, van Leeuwenhoek is referred to as the "father of microbiology." After some early skepticism, scientists in the late seventeenth century finally became convinced that microorganisms did, in fact, exist. Van Leeuwenhoek did not comment further on the origin of the microorganisms nor did he relate them to any diseases. The definitive relationship between microbes and disease was established later by Hooke, Pasteur, Koch, and others in what became known as the *"germ theory of disease."*

Robert Hooke (1635–1703), an English scientist with remarkable engineering abilities and an interest in many aspects of science, greatly improved the design and capabilities of the compound light microscope. With his microscope he observed insects, sponges, bryozoans, foraminifera, bird feathers, and plant cells. He published his observations with magnificent drawings in the book *Micrographia*. He was requested by the Royal Society of London to confirm van Leeuwenhoek's finding of animalcules and succeeded in doing so.

Table 1.1 lists some significant events in the history of microbiology.

Types of Microscopes

With advances in technology, continued development of microscopes for specific uses continues and many kinds of microscopes are now available to scientists. A brief overview and description of light and electron microscopes currently used in teaching, service, and research laboratories follows.

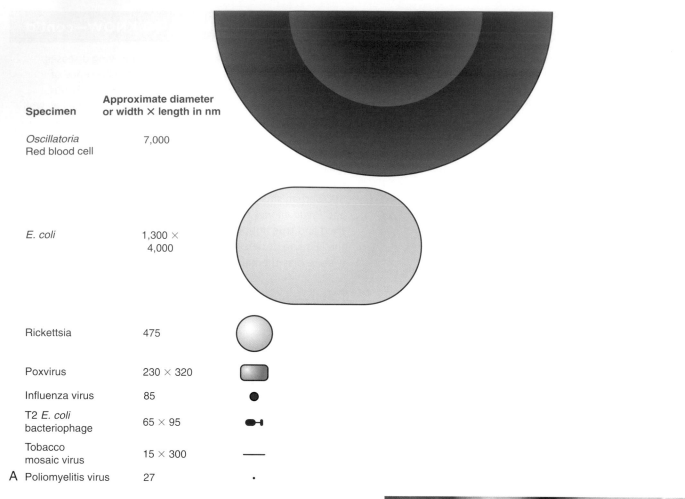

Specimen	Approximate diameter or width × length in nm
Oscillatoria Red blood cell	7,000
E. coli	1,300 × 4,000
Rickettsia	475
Poxvirus	230 × 320
Influenza virus	85
T2 *E. coli* bacteriophage	65 × 95
Tobacco mosaic virus	15 × 300
Poliomyelitis virus	27

A

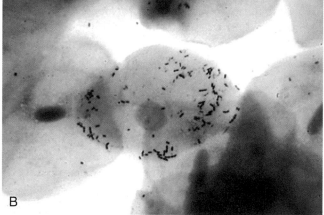

B

FIGURE 1.1 A, Comparison of cell sizes. This drawing shows relative size comparisons of bacteria, eukaryotic cells, and viruses. Although a few bacteria are actually larger than some eukaryotic cells, the vast majority are much smaller. **B,** Cheek cell with resident bacteria. This photo shows a human cheek cell with resident bacteria, which are stained and appear as small dark purple spheres or rods. Note that the bacteria are even much smaller than the nucleus in the center of the cell. (Approximate magnification: ×1000.)

All **light microscopes** use visible light to illuminate, and optical lenses to observe, enlarged images of specimens. They are classified as either simple or compound. A simple light microscope, such as van Leeuwenhoek's, has a single magnifying lens and a visible light source, and can magnify objects approximately ×266. A compound light microscope also uses visible light, usually provided by an electric source, but uses multiple lenses for magnification. The lens or lenses close to the eye are called *ocular lenses* and are located in the headpiece of the microscope. The lenses closer to the specimen are located in the body of the microscope and are referred to as *objective lenses*. Each lens has its own magnifying power, and the final magnification of a compound microscope is the product of the enlarging power of the ocular lens multiplied by the power of the objective lens. Most often the ocular lenses, either single (monocular) or in pairs (binocular), magnify by a power of 10

TABLE 1.1 Significant Events in Microbiology

Name	Year	Event
Zaccharias Janssen	1590	Invention of the first compound microscope
Robert Hooke	1660	Explores living and nonliving matter with a compound microscope
Francesco Redi	1668	Experiments to disprove spontaneous generation
Antony van Leeuwenhoek	1676	Observes bacteria and protozoan "animalcules" with simple microscope
Francesco Redi	1688	Published experiments on spontaneous generation of maggots
Lazzaro Spallanzani	1776	Conducts further experiments to disprove spontaneous generation
Edward Jenner	1796	Introduction of smallpox vaccination
Ignaz Semmelweis	1847–1850	First use of antiseptics to reduce hand-borne disease
Louis Pasteur	1857	Proves that fermentation is caused by microorganisms; introduces pasteurization
Louis Pasteur	1861	Completes experiments that show without doubt that spontaneous generation does not occur
Joseph Lister	1867	Antiseptic surgery—begins the trend toward modern aseptic techniques
Robert Koch	1876–1877	Studies anthrax in cattle and implicates *Bacillus anthracis* as causative agent
Louis Pasteur	1881	Develops anthrax vaccine for animals
Robert Koch	1882	Identifies causative agent of tuberculosis
Robert Koch	1884	Describes his postulates

(×10). The objective lenses are mounted on a revolving nose-piece and usually magnify ×4 or ×5, ×10, ×40, and ×100. In general, compound microscopes can magnify an object up to 1000 times (i.e., an ocular lens with a magnification of ×10 times the objective lens with a power of ×100 = ×1000). The specimens for compound light microscopy can either be visualized as whole (i.e., bacteria and other microorganisms) or are specially prepared for viewing with a given type of microscope. After specific dehydration procedures larger specimens are cut into 1.0- to 10-μm sections. Both smear preparations, for single cells, and sections are usually stained for better visual images (see Chapter 4, Microbiological Laboratory Techniques). Photographs taken through a microscope are referred to as *photomicrographs* or *micrographs*.

Dissection microscopes and **stereomicroscopes** are low-power microscopes designed for observing larger objects such as insects, worms, plants, or any objects that may have to be dissected for further observation. These microscopes provide three-dimensional images to determine surface structures and specific locations on a specimen.

Bright-field Microscopes

The bright-field microscope, a type of compound microscope, can be used to examine small specimens and some of their details. The microscope exhibits a background brighter than the observed specimen and is dependent on altering the light path (refraction) only. For this reason most specimens require staining for optimal observation. Bright-field microscopes are most commonly used to observe sectioned and stained tissues, organs, and microorganisms (Figure 1.2).

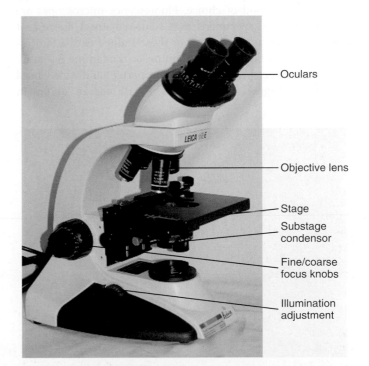

FIGURE 1.2 **Bright-field microscopy.** Bright-field microscopes vary somewhat in appearance based on brands, special features, or attached equipment, but they all have the same basic parts as labeled in the photo.

Dark-field Microscopes

Unfixed, unstained specimens such as living organisms (i.e., bacteria) can be observed with a dark-field microscope. Because of its design, the background of the microscope slide is dark, whereas the organism itself is bright (Figure 1.3). Some bacteria that are difficult to stain, including spirochetes (see Chapter 6, Bacteria and Archaea), can best be observed by dark-field microscopy. Bacterial capsules are also good candidates to be observed with dark-field microscopes.

Phase-contrast Microscopes

Phase-contrast microscopy, first described in 1934 by Frits Zernike, is done with a contrast-enhancing optical instrument that can be used for a wide variety of applications. It produces high-contrast images of transparent specimens such as:

- Living plant and animals cells
- Microorganisms
- Thin tissue slices, and more (Figure 1.4)

This type of instrument is ideally suited for the observation of cytoplasmic streaming, motility, and the dynamic states of cell organelles. Cell division and phagocytosis are examples of processes well suited for phase-contrast microscopy. The development of video technology enabled the recording and demonstration of these processes.

Fluorescence Microscopes

If a specimen can emit light (fluoresce) of one color when illuminated by ultraviolet radiation then fluorescence microscopy may be the method of choice. Fluorescence microscopes are used to visualize specimens that contain natural fluorescent substances such as chlorophyll or those stained with a fluorescent dye such as fluorescein, auramine, or rhodamine B (Figure 1.5). Fluorescence microscopy is an important and widely used tool in the diagnosis of infectious disease and in studies in microbial ecology. Fluorescence techniques are applied to identify specific antibodies, which are proteins produced in response to antigens (see Chapter 20, The Immune System). By attaching a fluorescent dye to these protein molecules, labeled antibodies are created that can be visualized, monitored, and studied.

Confocal Microscopes

In 1955 Marvin Minsky invented confocal microscopy, which was patented in 1957. Confocal microscopes have several advantages over the conventional optical microscopes, such as creating sharper images of specimens that would appear blurred with the use of a conventional compound microscope. In a confocal imaging system a single point of light focuses sequentially across a specimen, avoiding most of the unwanted scattered light that usually obscures an image when the entire

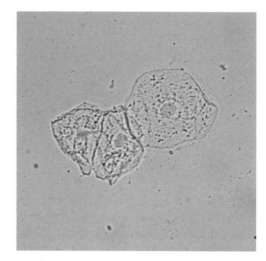

FIGURE 1.4 **Phase-contrast microscopy.** The phase-contrast microscope enhances the contrast of the image by shifting the phase of the light. These cheek cells are in a living state and did not require any staining. (Approximate magnification: ×400.)

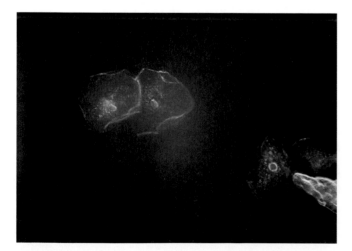

FIGURE 1.3 **Dark-field microscopy.** The dark-field microscope illuminates from the side rather than directly through the specimen. These cheek cells are in a living state and did not require any staining. (Approximate magnification: ×400.)

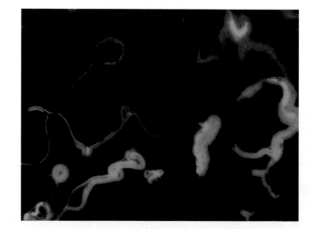

FIGURE 1.5 **Fluorescence microscopy.** The fluorescence microscope uses an ultraviolet lamp to illuminate specimens stained with fluorescent stain. This is a fluorescence microscopy photo of a modified strain of *Pseudomonas*. (Approximate magnification: ×1000.) Courtesy Dr. Larry Halverson, Iowa State University.

specimen is illuminated at one time. An image is built by visualizing different planes of the layers of the specimen as the stage of the microscope is moved up and down.

Electron Microscopes

Electron microscopes (EMs) are sophisticated instruments of the twentieth century that use a beam of electrons rather than light as the source of energy to visualize specimens. Magnetic fields instead of optical lenses are used to focus the electron beam. This allows much better resolution of the image than is possible with the light microscope. Specimens for EM studies require more extensive preparation, expensive laboratory equipment, and specially trained personnel than are required for the preparation of specimens used for light microscopy.

Bacteria can be visualized by light microscopy, but their detailed structure or specifics of their attachment to hosts are best seen by electron microscopy. Although most viruses are not visible by light microscopy, their effects on cells and tissues are. Investigations of specimen surfaces use scanning electron microscopy (SEM), whereas studies of the interior of cells and tissues use transmission electron microscopy (TEM).

Transmission Electron Microscopes

In a transmission electron microscope the electron beam travels through an ultrathin sectioned specimen (approximately 100 nm in thickness) and provides a two-dimensional image of the cell or other object. The resolving power of a TEM is approximately 0.002 μm, which is 100 times greater than can be achieved with a light microscope. The usual magnification of a TEM ranges from 500,000 to 1,000,000. Pictures taken of images created with an electron microscope are called *electron micrographs* (Figure 1.6).

Scanning Electron Microscopes

A scanning electron microscope also provides images of high resolution, but in contrast to the TEM, the SEM does not require ultrathin sections. It scans the surface of an object, producing a three-dimensional image (Figure 1.7). Moreover, the SEM has a large depth of field that allows the surface areas of large samples to be in focus at the same time. The usual magnification that can be achieved with an SEM ranges from ×10 to ×100,000.

Spontaneous Generation

Before microorganisms were discovered and described by Antony van Leeuwenhoek, life was hypothesized to develop from nonliving matter **(abiogenesis)**. Maggots, for example, were believed to arise spontaneously from rotting meat. The big question among scientists at that time was whether microbes were produced spontaneously by decay and fermentation, or whether they caused decay and fermentation—raising the basic dilemma of "which comes first, the chicken or the egg?"

One of the first serious attacks on this controversial spontaneous generation theory came in 1688 from **Francesco Redi,** an Italian physician. He believed that maggots developed from fly eggs. In his experiments he put meat into different flasks, kept some of them exposed to the atmosphere and flies, and the rest sealed. As he expected, maggots developed only in the open flasks where flies had access to the meat.

At about the same time, Antony van Leeuwenhoek's invention of the first microscope allowed him to observe small organisms, which he called *"animalcules."* He further showed that when hay was placed into a mixture of water and soil and allowed to incubate for a few days, new creatures in the hay infusion could be observed. Yet, these findings were interpreted by some scientists of the time as being additional proof of spontaneous generation.

This debate over the existence of spontaneous generation continued for centuries and in 1745 an English clergyman, **John Needham,** claimed victory for spontaneous generation with his experimental observations. He boiled chicken and corn broth, put it into a flask, and sealed it. After a few days cloudiness appeared in the broth, which is evidence of microbial growth. However, **Lazzaro Spallanzani,** an Italian priest, questioned Needham's interpretation and suggested that microorganisms could have entered the flask from the air before the tube was sealed. In his own experiments he also placed chicken broth in a flask, sealed it, and then drew off the air before boiling the broth. As a result no microorganisms grew, which he inter-

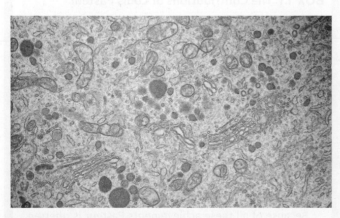

FIGURE 1.6 Transmission electron microscopy. This is a TEM image of a neuron.

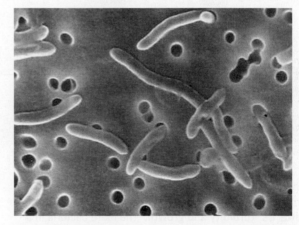

FIGURE 1.7 Scanning electron microscopy. Photo of an SEM image of the bacteria *Campylobacter* passing through the pores of a filter. (Approximate magnification: ×5000.) Courtesy Dr. James Dickson, Iowa State University.

preted as evidence that spontaneous generation did not exist. However, proponents of spontaneous generation held that Spallanzani only proved that spontaneous generation could not occur in the absence of air.

Louis Pasteur (1822–1895), a French chemist, finally ended the controversy. In 1861 he designed and conducted a definitive experiment in which he boiled meat broth in a flask and then heated the neck of the flask until it could be bent it into an S shape (swan-necked flask). Thus air could enter the flask but microorganisms trapped in the S-shaped neck were unable to reach the broth. There was no evidence of microbial growth. However, when he tilted the flask so that the broth could reach the organisms in the neck, the broth gradually became cloudy due to microbial growth (Figure 1.8).

In 1877 **John Tyndall** (1820–1893) demonstrated that microorganisms exist in dust. In a set of experiments similar to Pasteur's, but in the absence of dust, the broths remained sterile even when exposed to air. In addition, Tyndall provided evidence of the existence of heat-resistant bacteria. **Ferdinand Cohn** (1828–1898), independent of Tyndall's studies, also described heat-resistant bacterial **endospores** (see Chapter 3, Cell Structure and Function).

Pasteurization

In addition to his other findings Louis Pasteur invented the process we know as **pasteurization** (Box 1.1). The Emperor Napoleon III asked Pasteur to investigate the spoiling of wine that caused a negative impact in the production of wine, damaging the French wine industry. Pasteur discovered that wine spoilage (wine disease) is caused by microorganisms. He "pasteurized" the wine by heating it to 55° C for several minutes, which killed enough microorganisms to prevent the wine from spoiling. Pasteurization does not kill all microorganisms, but reduces the number of viable organisms so they are less likely to cause spoilage or disease. **Sterilization** (see Chapter 4, Micro-

biological Laboratory Techniques), on the other hand, kills all microorganisms including their endospores.

Germ Theory of Disease

During the time when the existence of spontaneous generation was being debated, several physicians began to suspect that microorganisms not only could cause spoilage and decay but might also play a role in infectious disease. Two physicians in different parts of the world, one in the United States and one in Vienna, significantly contributed to the concept that microorganisms had a role in infectious diseases. **Oliver Wendell Holmes** (1809–1894) in the United States showed that death following childbirth was often caused by material on the hands of midwives or physicians. **Ignaz Semmelweis** (1818–1865) in Vienna observed that women in the maternity ward became infected after being examined by physicians or students who came directly from the autopsy room or from examining infected patients. Semmelweis also noted that these students' and physicians' hands stunk from putrefaction and that they did not wash their hands before examining patients in the maternity wards. He also suspected that microorganisms were responsible for the odor. Consequently, he required everyone to wash their hands in a solution of chlorine before entering the maternity ward and examining patients. The result was a drastic decline in the death rate on the wards.

Joseph Lister (1827–1912) studied the observations of Semmelweis and hypothesized that airborne microbes might play a role in postsurgical infections as well. He discovered that applying carbolic acid to dressings and using an aerosol of carbolic acid on the surgical field significantly decreased the number of wound infections. He was the first physician to introduce the use of **aseptic** techniques.

The germ theory of disease proposed by Louis Pasteur and **Robert Koch** (1843–1910) is based on the existence of infectious microorganisms. Although Pasteur was convinced that microbes caused disease in humans he was never able to link a specific microbe with a particular disease. Koch's investigations focused on anthrax, an infectious disease that seriously affects

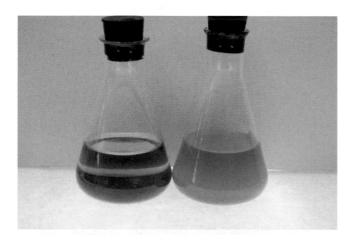

FIGURE 1.8 Turbidity and growth. The more bacteria in a container of broth, the cloudier or more turbid it is. The clear flask on the left is uninoculated and contains no bacteria. The turbid (cloudy) flask on the right contains a culture that has grown for 18 hours and contains an enormous number of bacteria.

BOX 1.1 The Contributions of Louis Pasteur

The contributions of Louis Pasteur to the emerging field of microbiology include the following:

- Different microorganisms produce different fermentation products
- Pasteurization
- Infectious agents cause disease
- Germ theory of disease, in contrast to spontaneous generation
- Minimization of the spread of pathogens
- Development of vaccines to prevent several diseases in chickens, sheep, cattle, and pigs

Because of all these achievements Pasteur is referred to as the father of *modern* microbiology.

animal herds and humans brought in contact with the microorganism. Koch also discovered that anthrax produced endospores that persist after the death of the exposed animals. Moreover, he proved that these spores can survive and later develop into the active anthrax microbe and infect other animals. This established that a specific organism caused a specific disease. After many years of experimentation he developed what we now know as **Koch's postulates** (Box 1.2), which set forth the conditions that should identify an organism as the specific cause of a specific disease.

Immunology begins with the work of **Edward Jenner** (1749–1823). Jenner observed that milkmaids who had contracted cowpox did not become infected with smallpox, a major killer during the eighteenth century. He applied material from cowpox lesions, containing the vaccinia virus, to small incisions or puncture wounds made in human arms. These human subjects did not develop smallpox but only occasionally showed a mild fever associated with the disease. With this procedure Jenner proved that immunity against smallpox could be achieved through vaccination.

Origin and Evolution of Microorganisms

Origin

Although earth formed about 4.5 billion years ago, life on earth probably has been present for most of the planet's history and likely began remarkably early, between 3.5 and 4.0 billion years ago. Although no one knows precisely how or when life began, scientists tend to agree on several things:

- In earliest times the earth was dominated by volcanoes, a lifeless ocean, and a very turbulent atmosphere.
- Intensive chemical activity occurred and the ocean received organic matter from land, atmosphere, and meteorites.
- Several elements formed key molecules such as sugars, amino acids, and nucleotides, all of which are building blocks for living organisms (see Chapter 2, Chemistry of Life).

The origin of microorganisms is described in geological time. The rich fossil record of prokaryotic life suggests that microbes were perhaps the first living things on earth. Microbes impact human life from birth to death and even to this day microbes are found in almost every environment on earth. **Stromatolites** (layered mound-shaped deposits along ancient seashores) represent some of the oldest microbial communities. Evolution of plants and animals as we know them has occurred in the last 550 million years.

Evolution

Evolution is an important concept that involves all living things including microorganisms. Evolution implies that living things gradually change over millions of years, resulting in structural and functional changes of organisms throughout generations. The millions of different species on earth and their successful adaptation to different habitats are indicators of the evolutionary process.

For the first three quarters of evolutionary history the only organisms on earth were microscopic and mostly unicellular. Fossils of **prokaryotes** go back to 3.5 to 4 billion years followed by **eukaryotic** life approximately 2.2 billion years ago. Eukaryotic cells are larger and more complex than prokaryotic cells and scientists believe that eukaryotes have evolved from prokaryotic symbiotic communities. It is estimated that there are about 5 to 100 million species of organisms living on earth today. The evolutionary relationship between organisms is the subject of **phylogeny.** Today, the phylogenetic relationship between organisms can be determined by nucleic acid and nucleotide sequencing. Results from ribosomal RNA (rRNA) sequencing identify three evolutionarily distinct cell lines that are classified as bacteria, archaea, and eukarya. These three distinct lineages, based on the origin of cell lines, are referred to as **domains** (Figure 1.9).

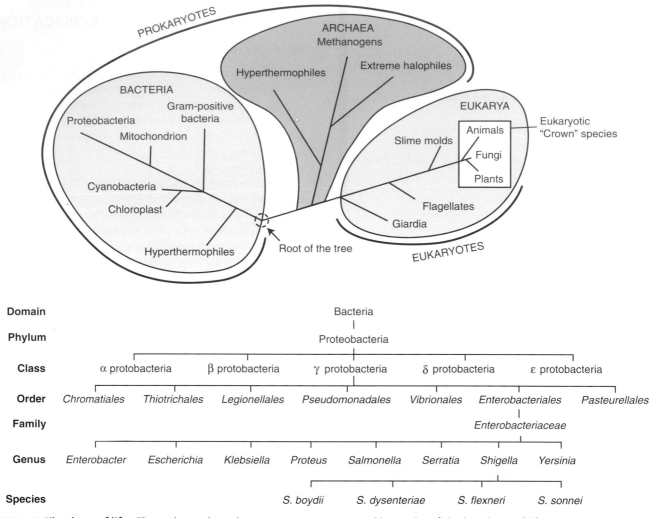

FIGURE 1.9 Kingdoms of life. These charts show the present organization and hierarchy of the kingdoms of life. The bacteria *Shigella sonnei* has been traced from kingdom to the level of species to illustrate its place in the overall scheme.

Classification of Microorganisms

To better understand the different types of microorganisms (microbes), they are grouped or classified in various ways. Microbes are diverse and in terms of numbers, most of the diversity of life on earth is represented by microbes. Further detailed description and discussion of the individual groups of microorganisms is provided in Chapter 6 (Bacteria and Archaea), Chapter 7 (Viruses), and Chapter 8 (Eukaryotic Microorganisms).

Prokaryotes versus Eukaryotes

Differentiation between prokaryotes (*pro*, before; *karyon*, nucleus) and eukaryotes (*eu*, good or with; *karyon*, nucleus) was greatly advanced as more sophisticated microscopes became available, allowing scientists to identify membrane-bound structures in unicellular organisms. Significantly, scientists discovered that some unicellular organisms contained membrane-bound organelles such as a nucleus, whereas others did not. The cells without membrane-bound organelles and therefore without a nucleus were classified as prokaryotes and the ones with membrane-bound organelles and a nucleus were designated eukaryotes. All bacterial cells are prokaryotic, whereas algae, fungi, and protozoans are eukaryotes (see Chapter 3, Cell Structure and Function).

Bacteria, Archaea, and Eukaryotes

Bacteria, archaea, and eukaryotes are examples of diversity and the root of microbial diversity is evolution. Within **bacteria** several evolutionary branches are present including some **pathogenic** (disease-causing) bacteria, occurring in soil and water, in animal digestive tracts and skin, as well as in many other environments. Also, different bacteria require different sources of energy such as light, organic chemicals, inorganic chemicals, or combinations thereof.

Archaea are a group of single-celled microorganisms, similar to bacteria because they are also prokaryotes, but evolutionarily different. They are characterized by their preference to live in extreme environments including hot springs, glaciers, or highly salty environments (see Chapter 6, Bacteria and Archaea).

Eukaryotic microorganisms include algae, fungi, and protozoans (see Chapter 8, Eukaryotic Microorganisms). **Algae** are a large and diverse group of simple organisms, ranging from unicellular to multicellular forms, containing chlorophyll that is needed for photosynthesis. They are common in aquatic bodies (both freshwater and saltwater) and in all types of soil, but have limited medical significance. **Fungi** include yeasts, molds, and mushrooms, which are not microbes. Their energy sources are organic compounds found in soil and water. Fungi play a major role in the breakdown of dead organic matter in a variety of environments. However, some fungi are pathogenic and can cause disease in humans and animals. **Protozoans** are colorless, mobile organisms feeding on other organisms for their energy source. In general, protozoans are free-living microorganisms and several of them are also pathogenic to humans and animals.

Viruses

Viruses are noncellular, submicroscopic particles (visible only by electron microscopy) and consist of nucleic acid surrounded by a protein coat. They are metabolically inert, incapable of carrying out biosynthetic functions, and they are dependent on host machinery for their multiplication. Viruses are classified according to the type of nucleic acid (RNA or DNA) they contain. Many viruses are pathogenic and can be classified on the basis of their host as animal viruses, plant viruses, and bacterial viruses (see Chapter 7, Viruses).

Prions

Prions (**pro**teinaceous **in**fectious particles) are not cellular organisms, nor are they viruses. Prions lack nucleic acids; they are normal proteins of animal tissues that can misfold during protein synthesis and become an infectious agent (see Chapter 7, Viruses).

Viroids

Viroids are plant pathogens that can cause serious economic problems. They are much smaller than viruses (15 to 100 nm) and exist of a small single-stranded, naked RNA circle. Viroids cannot produce proteins and do not have a protein coat (see Chapter 7, Viruses).

MEDICAL HIGHLIGHTS

Transmissible Spongiform Encephalopathies

Prions are associated with a group of diseases called *transmissible spongiform encephalopathies* (TSEs), for example, spongiform encephalopathy (BSE), also referred to as *"mad cow" disease.* A research group at the University of California led by Stanley B. Prusiner purified the infectious material, confirmed that the agent was a protein, and named it "prion." In 1997, Prusiner received the Nobel Prize for this research.

Taxonomy

The formal system of organizing, classifying, and naming of living organisms is called **taxonomy.** Taxonomy sorts organisms on the basis of mutual similarities into nonoverlapping groups called **taxa.** The goal of taxonomy is **classification, nomenclature,** and **identification** for clarification and ease of reference.

- Classification is the assignment of organisms into taxa based on similarities.
- Nomenclature deals with the rules for naming organisms.
- Identification is the process of specifying, identifying, and recording the traits of organisms.

The current system of taxonomy began with a Swedish botanist, Carolus Linnaeus (1707–1778). He provided a system that standardized the naming and classification of organisms on the basis of common characteristics. Linnaeus's system groups similar species into genera, genera sharing common features into families, similar families into orders, orders into classes, classes into **phyla,** and phyla into kingdoms (see Figure 1.9). In addition, in 1990, Carl Woese (1928–) and his colleagues introduced a three-domain system of taxonomy (archaea, bacteria and eukarya) based on genetic rather than morphological similarities (see Figure 1.9).

All these categories in the Linnaeus system are taxa, which are hierarchical, starting with the **species** and **genera,** followed by successive taxa, each with a broader description than the preceding one. All names in the taxa are Latin or Latinized.

Linnaeus assigned each species a descriptive name of its genus and a specific name for the species. This method of assigning the scientific name is called the **binomial** (two-name) system of nomenclature. A **genus** is the name of an organism and is often abbreviated by a single capital letter, whereas the species name is never abbreviated. For example, *Escherichia coli* can be abbreviated to *E. coli.* A genus typically contains several species, and a particular species can be further subdivided into different strains. For instance, there are several species in the genus *Bacillus,* such as *B. subtilis* or *B. cereus.*

The taxonomic resource for bacteria is the *Bergey's Manual of Systematic Bacteriology,* the second edition of which is being published in five volumes. In addition to the number of keys for bacterial identification, newer versions of the manual also contain some molecular sequencing information for various bacterial groups. An outline of *Bergey's Manual* can be found in Appendix A of this book.

Microorganisms in Health and Disease

Microbes form various mutualistic relationships with different organisms, and many of these are important to human well-being. *Microbial ecology* is the study of the interrelationship between microbes and their environment. Microbes are everywhere in the environment and generally have an impact in maintaining ecosystems.

Microbes in the Environment

Microorganisms in nature are often organized into complex communities of different organisms called **biofilms.** A biofilm consists of surface-associated microbial cells enclosed in an extracellular polymeric substance matrix. Antony van Leeuwenhoek observed and described layers of microorganisms on tooth surfaces, representing a microbial biofilm (see Chapter 3, Cell Structure and Function). However, detailed, high-magnification observations of microbial biofilms did not occur until electron microscopy became available. Biofilms are found on a variety of surfaces such as medical devices (Table 1.2), industrial water system piping, natural aquatic systems, foods, and also on living tissues. An established biofilm structure provides a perfect environment for the exchange of genetic material between different organisms in the biofilm community.

Free-living fungi and bacteria decompose organic matter and return minerals and other nutrients to the soil. Decomposition is dependent on microbes, as is the cycling of elements. Examples of nutrient cycling in nature that requires microorganisms are the nitrogen, carbon, oxygen, sulfur, and phosphorus cycles.

Ecological interactions between organisms in a community, including **mutualism, commensalism, synergism,** and **parasitism,** are classified according to the degree of benefit or harm they pose to one another. In mutualism both organisms benefit, in commensalism the waste product of a microbe provides useful nutrients for another organism, in synergism two organisms are dependent on each other to break down a nutrient that neither breaks down alone, and in parasitism one organism benefits and the other is harmed (see Chapter 9, Infection and Disease).

Normal Flora

Blood, lymph, cerebrospinal fluid, and internal organs are sterile. Before birth the entire healthy body is free of microbes. However, starting at birth microorganisms contaminate some of these previously sterile environments; for example, bacteria and other microorganisms colonize the mucous membranes of the upper respiratory tract, the digestive tract, and the surface of the skin. Microorganisms regularly found at any anatomical site in healthy humans and not causing infection or disease are referred to as the **normal flora.** The normal flora provides protection against pathogens by preventing attachment to the host tissue and by competing for the same nutrients. If successful, the pathogens cannot flourish or colonize and therefore are unable to reach sufficient numbers to cause infection (see Chapter 9, Infection and Disease).

Pathogens

The human body is in continual contact with microorganisms and if a particular microbe is pathogenic, colonizes, and is present in sufficient numbers, this interaction can lead to disease. Diseases caused by communicable microorganisms are referred to as *infectious diseases*. Control of these diseases can be achieved by application of the aseptic technique, the development and use of antimicrobial drugs, and immunization. These practices have drastically reduced the death rate from infectious diseases in the United States. However, death from infectious diseases in developing countries remains extremely high, due in large part to inadequate healthcare and poor sanitation. Infectious diseases may be transmitted by direct or indirect contact and can be acute, subacute, or chronic. Within communities they can be epidemic, pandemic, endemic, or sporadic (see Chapter 9, Infection and Disease).

Infectious diseases in economically important species, such as domestic animals, are of great concern to agriculture. Not only is there an economic impact, but also the possibility that the disease can become *zoonotic,* meaning transmissible from the primary animal host to humans. Some typical examples are rabies and yellow fever. Fortunately, many of these infectious diseases can be prevented by vaccination and compliance with regulated practices of public health and hygiene.

Foodborne diseases result from consuming food that is contaminated with different pathogenic species of bacteria, viruses, parasites, or microbial toxins. At greater risk are young children, the elderly population, pregnant women and their fetuses, and anyone with a weakened or compromised immune system. Treatments vary depending on the severity of the illness and they range from fluid and electrolyte replacement to hospitalization for severe conditions. In general, foodborne diseases can be prevented by:

- Washing hands with hot, soapy water before food preparation, after using the bathroom, or changing diapers

---

TABLE 1.2 Microorganisms Associated With Biofilms on Medical Devices

Device	Microorganisms
Hip prosthesis	Coagulase-negative staphylococci
	Enterococcus spp.
	Pseudomonas aeruginosa
	Staphylococcus aureus
Intrauterine device	*Candida albicans*
	Coagulase-negative staphylococci
	Enterococcus spp.
	Staphylococcus aureus
Prosthetic heart valve	Coagulase-negative staphylococci
	Enterococcus spp.
	Staphylococcus aureus
Urinary catheter	Coagulase-negative staphylococci
	Enterococcus spp.
	Klebsiella pneumoniae
	Pseudomonas aeruginosa
Venous catheter	*Candida albicans*
	Coagulase-negative staphylococci
	Enterococcus spp.
	Klebsiella pneumoniae
	Pseudomonas aeruginosa
	Staphylococcus aureus
Voice prosthesis	*Candida albicans*
	Coagulase-negative staphylococci

- Keeping raw meat, poultry, seafood, and their juices away from prepared, ready-to-eat foods
- Cooking foods thoroughly at high enough temperatures to kill harmful bacteria and their toxins
- Refrigerating foods within 2 hours of cooking. Cold temperatures will slow bacterial growth and multiplication
- Cleaning sufficiently all surfaces on which food is to be prepared

Waterborne disease is the general term used to describe diseases acquired from contaminated water supplies, resulting in four fifths of all illness in developing countries and a high infant death rate. Major floods contribute to large cholera epidemics, such as occurred in West Bengal, and have caused serious outbreaks in 1968, 1984, 1992, 1998, and 2000. Increased risk factors for waterborne diseases are multiple and include but are not limited to travel, living in rural areas, poverty, geographical location, the immediate environment (flooding, feces, overcrowding, and poor sanitation), inadequate personal health and hygiene, and poor water treatment practices and facilities. Floodwaters also often contain raw sewage, silt, oil, and chemical wastes. Parasites, viruses, and bacteria are readily transmitted by floodwaters. To reduce exposure to waterborne disease, the following recommendations should be practiced.

- Do not drink, swim, bathe, or play in floodwaters.
- Keep children away from floodwaters.
- Do not expose cuts or open wounds to floodwater.
- Monitor the quality of water supplies frequently.
- Keep the water clean and avoid using contaminated water.
- Drink water that has been purified by boiling or treatment with chlorine.
- Rinse fruits and vegetables with clean water.

Foodborne Diseases and Waterborne Diseases

Disease	Organism	Mode of Transmission	Symptoms
Cholera	*Vibrio cholerae*	Ingestion of contaminated water, raw or partially cooked fish or shellfish	Sudden onset of vomiting, watery diarrhea, rapid dehydration, acidosis, possible circulatory collapse and death
E. coli infection	*Escherichia coli*	Uncooked meat or other food contaminated by fecal material; swimming in contaminated water	Severe bloody diarrhea, abdominal cramps
Shigellosis	*Shigella* spp.	Hand-to-mouth contact with feces from infected people or animals; contaminated foods	Diarrhea, fever, stomach cramps
Salmonelloses	*Salmonella choleraesuis, S. enteritidis*	Contaminated poultry, eggs, and meat, fecal–oral route	Gastroenteritis, enteric fever, septicemia
Hepatitis (inflammation of the liver)	Hepatitis A virus	Contaminated food, water contaminated with human feces	Fever, anorexia, nausea, abdominal discomfort
Gastroenteritis	Norwalk virus	Ingestion of contaminated seafood, handling of contaminated food; person-to-person transmission by fecal–oral route	Watery diarrhea, vomiting
Dysentery	*Shigella*	Contaminated water, contaminated milk	Abdominal pain, watery diarrhea, fever, blood and mucus almost always present in stool
Leptospirosis	*Leptospira interrogans*	Exposure to urine, contaminated water from infected animals	High fever, severe headache, chills and vomiting; kidney and liver failure
Shigellosis or bacillary dysentery	*Shigella dysenteriae, S. sonnei*	Drinking contaminated water	Diarrhea, fever, stomach cramps
Typhoid fever (enteric fever)	*Salmonella typhi*	Water contaminated with feces and urine from carriers	Septicemia
Gastroenteritis	Norwalk virus	Water contaminated by infected individuals	Watery diarrhea, vomiting
Giardiasis	*Giardia lamblia*	Water contaminated by feces of infected person or animal	Diarrhea, abdominal cramps

Airborne Diseases

Disease	Organism	Mode of Transmission	Symptoms
Influenza	Influenza viruses	Aerosols	Fever, chills, headache, muscle aches
Tuberculosis	*Mycobacterium tuberculosis*	Aerosols	Range from asymptomatic to fever, cough, fatigue, lack of appetite, weight loss, pulmonary hemorrhage
Legionellosis	*Legionella pneumophila*	Aerosols from humidifiers, air conditioning equipment	Atypical pneumonia, fever, cough, difficulty in breathing, chest pain
Psittacosis	*Chlamydia psittaci*	Bird to human by aerosols	Headache, fever, nonproductive cough, occasional septicemia
Common cold	Rhinoviruses, adenoviruses, coronaviruses, and other viruses	Aerosols	Slight fever, headache, sore throat, coughing, sneezing, nasal discharge
Mumps	Paramyxovirus	Airborne droplets or contact with saliva of infected person	Swelling of parotid glands, fever, headache, generalized muscle aches

- Avoid swallowing water from lakes, rivers, or swimming pools.
- Clean food preparation areas with clean water before use.
- Wash hands if exposed.

The Centers for Disease Control and Prevention (CDC) estimates that approximately 900,000 people in the United States become ill each year from drinking contaminated water. Mortality from a lack of clean water and sanitary waste disposal, especially in underdeveloped countries, coupled with inadequate personal health and hygiene practices is likely responsible for over 12 million deaths per year.

Airborne diseases are transmitted from infected people by coughing, sneezing, or talking. Pathogens are in small mucous saliva particles suspended as aerosols. Movements and directions of air currents play an important role in the spread of airborne respiratory diseases such as tuberculosis, legionellosis, and influenza. The public healthcare issues related to travel and airborne diseases are also discussed in Chapter 18 (Emerging Infectious Diseases).

Applied Microbiology

Applied microbiology is the human use of microorganisms to improve certain aspects of life. Microbes are used in this capacity by the food, pharmaceutical, and agricultural industries, and in forensics and other endeavors. Application of new technologies in genetic engineering has further increased the industrial use of microbes.

Microorganisms in Food Production

Many nonpathogenic microorganisms occur naturally in food, are beneficial, and are used as starter cultures to produce foods

---

BOX 1.3 Some Food Products Produced With the Use of Microorganisms

- Bread
- Butter
- Buttermilk
- Cheese
- Cottage cheese
- Pickles
- Sauerkraut
- Sour cream
- Vinegar
- Yogurt

---

such as vinegar, sauerkraut, pickles, fermented milks, yogurt, cheese, and bread (Box 1.3). For example, vinegar is made from foods containing starch or smaller sugars. The production requires a two-way fermentation process that begins with apple juice or other raw materials, to which the yeast *Saccharomyces cerevisiae* is added to speed up the fermentation process. In the second stage, cultures of acetic acid bacteria such as *Acetobacter aceti* are added to this alcoholic liquid, converting the alcohol into acetic acid. In the United States most vinegar is produced from apples and is named apple cider vinegar.

Sauerkraut is another product made by fermentation of shredded cabbage in the presence of salt. The shredded cabbage is tightly packed in an anaerobic environment, where it becomes dehydrated. The addition of salt promotes the growth of lactic acid bacteria.

Dairy products such as butter, buttermilk, sour cream, cottage cheese, and yogurt are produced from fermented milk. Raw milk contains the fermentable sugar lactose in addition to several acid-producing microorganisms. The natural microflora of raw milk is often inefficient, uncontrollable, and can produce unpredictable results. Moreover, these organisms are destroyed during heat treatments needed to pasteurize milk. Therefore, starter cultures that can provide a more controlled and predictable fermentation process are added to produce the desired products. The function of the lactic acid starters is the production of lactic acid from lactose of the milk. Other starter cultures may provide flavor, aroma, and alcohol production.

Microorganisms in the Production of Alcoholic Beverages

Wine is produced by yeast fermentation of carbohydrates in freshly harvested grape juice, peaches, berries, pears, and other fruits or plants (even dandelions), and is marketed as such. In beer production barley or other grain is used as the source of fermentable carbohydrate. Beer and wine generally are limited to about 15% alcohol because yeast fails to ferment beyond this point. Beverages higher in alcohol content are produced through distillation and are called *spirits* or *liquor*.

Treatment of Water Supplies

Good health depends on a clean, drinkable water supply. It must be free of pathogens, toxins, odor, color, and bad taste to achieve these standards. The microbial content of drinking water should be constantly monitored to make sure the water is free of infectious agents. Most water purity assays are focused on the detection of fecal material, which would indicate the presence of pathogens. Wells, reservoirs, and other water resources can be analyzed for the presence of indicator bacteria that can be readily identified by routine laboratory procedures before selection of the appropriate water treatment.

Microbes and the Production of Pharmaceutical Agents

Louis Pasteur observed the inhibition of microorganisms by products formed by other microbes. This phenomenon is called *antibiosis*. The discovery of the penicillin-producing mold *Penicillium* by Alexander Fleming in the 1920s started the successful search for other antibiotic-producing microorganisms. Today, with the help of genetic engineering and recombinant DNA technology, not only antibiotics and semisynthetic antibiotics but also various hormones and other drugs are available on the market (see Chapter 22, Antimicrobial Drugs).

Microbes in Agriculture

Agricultural microbiology focuses on the relationships between microbes and domesticated plants and animals. Farmers use microbes and their products in a variety of ways, particularly for crop management via recombinant DNA biotechnology (see Chapter 25, Biotechnology). Plant microbiology involves the management of plant disease, soil fertility, and nutritional interactions. For example, the availability of nitrogen in the soil is essential for the growth of crops and bacteria involved in the nitrogen cycle of the soil are essential (see Soil Microbiology in Chapter 24, Microorganisms in the Environment and Environmental Safety). On the animal side, agricultural microbiology deals with the management and prevention of infectious diseases in farm animals as well as other associations animals have with microorganisms.

Bioremediation

Bioremediation is the process of using microorganisms to clean up toxic, hazardous, or unmanageable compounds by degrading them to harmless compounds. Some microbes performing these tasks have been genetically engineered to clean up specific wastes or pollutants. For example, genetically engineered petroleum-digesting bacteria assist in the cleanup of oil spills. Another form of bioremediation that has long been in use is the treatment of water and sewage. Reclamation procedures for treatment of polluted water to convert it to drinkable water are becoming more important worldwide because of the rapid dwindling of clean freshwater sources.

Microbes, Biomass, and Energy

By a process referred to as *bioconversion*, microorganisms can convert biomass such as organic matter and human, agricultural, and industrial wastewater into alternative fuels, including ethanol, methane, and hydrogen.

Ethanol produced during fermentation is one of the simplest alternative fuel sources to produce and can be mixed with gasoline to make gasohol. Although at present crops such as corn are used, it would be more economic to utilize crop wastes (i.e., corn stalks).

Some communities already use landfills as immense sources of methane, where methanogens anaerobically convert wastes into methane by the process of fermentation. Methane gas can be piped through natural gas lines and used as an energy source in common households.

The concept of using microbes to power fuel cells is not new; however, in 2003, scientists found a way to generate electricity by feeding bacteria common sugars and other carbohydrates. In this study bacteria were grown on graphite electrodes within a fuel cell. When the organisms were fed sugars, they generated electrons and transferred them to the graphite electrodes. This flow of electrons generated electricity that the battery could store. The generation of power by microbes has led many scientists to develop microbial fuel cells. In 2005, Pennsylvania State University environmental engineers and scientists at Ion Power Inc. (in New Castle, Delaware) published the first process that shows bacteria can retrieve four times the amount of hydrogen out of a biomass than would typically be generated by fermentation alone.

Microbial Forensics

Microbial forensics is a relatively new field applied to solving bioterrorism cases, medical negligence, and outbreaks of foodborne diseases. Use of microorganisms as weapons is not a new idea. They can be the weapon of choice in terrorists' activities such as in the anthrax attacks of 2001. Forensic cases also have been reported about HIV-infected people intentionally infecting others as well. Microbes are also of interest in cases of medical negligence, in which medical personnel are implicated in postsurgical or other hospital-acquired infections due to inadequate or relaxed hygiene practices. In the case of outbreaks of foodborne diseases or intentional food contamination, it is critical to trace the infecting microbe to the source, either the company or person(s) of origin. Microbial forensics is becoming an essential part of data collection and their interpretation. Inquiries should stand up to the review of scientists and healthcare professionals as well as to the scrutiny of judges and juries.

Summary

- The invention of microscopes made it possible to observe details of organisms and microorganisms that are invisible to the naked eye.
- Different types of microscopes developed over the years have been and continue to be specialized to perform different functions.
- Spontaneous generation was disproved and the germ theory of disease developed. This promoted vaccination and the use of aseptic techniques in surgery among other hygienic practices to reduce infection.
- The first life on earth is dated at 3.5 to 4 billion years ago, and is believed to be represented by prokaryotes, which are still found in every environment on earth today. Through evolution, eukaryotic life appeared approximately 2.2 billion years ago.
- Microorganisms include bacteria, viruses, prions, algae, fungi, and protozoans.
- Taxonomy is the classification, nomenclature, and identification of living organisms. Classification starts with domain, followed by kingdom, phylum, class, order, family, and genus.
- Microbes occur in every environment, may build relationships with other organisms, and often form biofilms. Biofilms represent problems for many industries including healthcare.
- Microorganisms are routinely found in and on humans without causing an infection or disease. These organisms are part of the normal flora.
- Transmission of infectious diseases can be airborne, waterborne, foodborne, or through direct contact.
- Microorganisms play a major role in the production of food, alcoholic beverages, and pharmaceuticals. They are also used in water treatment, agriculture, bioremediation, forensics, and as fuel cells.

Review Questions

1. One type of microscope that provides a three-dimensional image of a specimen is a:
   a. Phase-contrast microscope
   b. Transmission electron microscope
   c. Bright-field microscope
   d. Scanning electron microscope

2. One type of microscope capable of observing living microorganisms is the:
   a. Bright-field microscope
   b. Phase-contrast microscope
   c. Fluorescence microscope
   d. Electron microscope

3. Which scientist is most responsible for ending the controversy about spontaneous generation?
   a. John Needham
   b. Joseph Lister
   c. Louis Pasteur
   d. Robert Koch

4. Fossils of prokaryotes go back _____ billion years.
   a. 4.0 to 5.0
   b. 3.5 to 4.0
   c. 2.5 to 3.0
   d. 2.2 to 2.7

5. Which of the following is *not* a microorganism?
   a. Bacterium
   b. Algae
   c. Insect
   d. Fungus

6. The correct order of the taxonomic category is:
   a. Species, domain, phylum, kingdom, order, division, class, genus
   b. Domain, kingdom, phylum, class, family, order, genus, species
   c. Domain, kingdom, phylum, class, order, family, genus, species
   d. Kingdom, domain, phylum, order, class, family, genus, species

7. Complex communities of microorganisms on surfaces are called:
   a. Colonies
   b. Biofilms
   c. Biospheres
   d. Flora

8. A relationship between organisms in which the waste product of one provides nutrients for another is called:
   a. Mutualism
   b. Competition
   c. Synergism
   d. Commensalism

9. Which of the following sites of the human body does *not* have a normal flora?
   a. Intestine
   b. Skin
   c. Vagina
   d. Blood

10. Which of the following industries use(s) microorganisms?
    a. Chemical
    b. Wine
    c. Cheese
    d. All of the above

11. All bacteria are _____ cells.

12. Cells that contain a nucleus are _____ cells.

13. The taxonomic resource for bacteria is the _____.

14. The proteins implicated in spongiform encephalopathy are _____.

15. The cleanup of different industrial waste is referred to as _____.

16. Name and briefly describe the different types of microscopes.

17. Describe Koch's postulates.

18. Compare and contrast prokaryotic and eukaryotic cells.

19. Describe how foodborne diseases can be prevented.

20. Describe the role of microorganisms in food production.

Bibliography

Bauman R: *Microbiology: With Diseases by Taxonomy*, ed 2, 2007, Benjamin Cummings/Pearson Education, San Francisco.

Garrity G: Bergey's Manual of Systematic Bacteriology, Vols. 1–5, New York, 2005, Springer.

Madigan MT, Martinko JM, Dunlap PV, et al: *Brock Biology of Microorganisms*, ed 12, 2009, Benjamin Cummings/Pearson Education, San Francisco.

Mims C, Dockrell HM, Goering RV, et al: *Medical Microbiology*, ed 3, St. Louis, 2004, Mosby/Elsevier, St. Louis, MO.

Sur D, Sengupta PG, Mondal SK, et al: *A localized outbreak of Vibrio cholerae 0139 in Kolkata, West Bengal*, Indian J Med Res 115:149–152, 2002.

Talaro KP: *Foundations in Microbiology*, ed 6, 2008, McGraw-Hill, New York.

Woese CR, Kandler O, Wheelis ML: *Towards a natural system of organisms: proposal for the domains, archaea, bacteria, and eucarya*, Proc Natl Acad Sci USA, 87:4576–4579, 1990.

Internet Resources
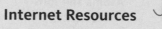

The Microbial World: A Look at All Things Small, http://www.bact.wisc.edu/Microtextbook/

National Digestive Diseases Information Clearinghouse (NDDIC), http://digestive.niddk.nih.gov

The INFO Project, Johns Hopkins Bloomberg School of Public Health, http://www.infoforhealth.org

Fact Sheet Series: Microbes in Drinking Water, http://www.waterbornediseases.org/FactSheets/microbes.htm

American Society for Microbiology, http://www.asm.org

U.S. Food and Drug Administration, Center for Food Safety and Applied Nutrition, Prions and Transmissible Spongiform Encephalopathies, http://www.cfsan.fda.gov/~mow/prion.html

USDA Agricultural Research Service, http://www.ars.usda.gov

Wikipedia, http://en.wikipedia.org/wiki/Main_Page

Nobelprize.org, http://nobelprize.org/nobel_prizes/medicine/laureates/1905/koch-bio.html

Museum der Wissenschaft von Kurt Paulus, http://www.amuseum.de/

Access Excellence @ The National Health Museum, http://www.accessexcellence.org/

Science Daily, http://www.sciencedaily.com/releases/2005/12/051214220432.htm

Genome News Network, http://www.genomenewsnetwork.org/articles/09_03/battery.shtml

University of Arizona, Cellular Imaging Facility Core, Microscopy & Imaging Resources on the WWW, http://swehsc.pharmacy.arizona.edu/exppath/micro/

Dairy Science and Food Technology, http://www.dairyscience.info/

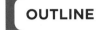

2

Chemistry of Life

OUTLINE

Atoms and Ions
Elements
Atomic Model
Ions

Chemical Bonds and Molecules
Formation and Classification of Chemical Bonds and Forces
Types of Chemical Reactions
Chemical Notations

Inorganic Compounds
Acids, Bases, and the pH Scale
Buffers
Salts
Water

Organic Molecules
Carbohydrates
Proteins
Lipids
Nucleic Acids

LEARNING OBJECTIVES

After reading this chapter, the student will be able to:
- Define/describe matter, element, atom, and ion
- Define/describe the atomic nucleus and define atomic weight, neutron, proton, electron, valence, and isotope
- Name, describe, and rank the different types of chemical bonds
- Describe the different types of chemical reactions
- Define the rules of chemical notation
- Discuss acid–base balance and the pH scale
- Discuss the properties of water and define solvent, solute, solution, hypertonic, hypotonic, isotonic, hydrophilic, and hydrophobic
- Describe the common properties of all organic molecules
- Name the monomers of carbohydrates and describe the structure and function of disaccharides and polysaccharides

- Describe the structures and functions of amino acids, peptides, and proteins
- Name and describe the structures and functions of the different lipids
- Describe the structures of nucleic acids and nucleotides; name and discuss the function of the different nucleic acids and explain complementary base pairing

KEY TERMS

adenosine triphosphate (ATP)
anabolism
anions
atoms
atomic nucleus
atomic number
atomic weight
bases
catabolism
cations
chemical bond
chemical compounds
chemical formula
cholesterol
covalent bonds
dehydration synthesis
deoxyribonucleic acid (DNA)
disaccharides

electrolyte
electrons
elements
endergonic
exchange reactions
exergonic
hydrogen bonds
hydrolysis
hydrophilic
hydrophobic
hypertonic
hypotonic
ions
ionic bonds
isotonic
isotopes
matter
molecules
monosaccharides
neutrons

nonpolar
oxidation
phospholipids
pH scale
polysaccharides
prostaglandins
protons
radioactivity
redox
reduction
ribonucleic acid (RNA)
shells
solutes
solution
solvent
steroids
synthesis
triglycerides
valence electrons
van der Waals forces

WHY YOU NEED TO KNOW

HISTORY

Before Aureolus Paracelsus (Philippus Theophrastus Bombastus von Hohenheim; 1493–1541 ce) the principles of Western medical practice evolved primarily from witchcraft, folk remedies, and religious mysticism. An organized step forward had occurred earlier with the Greek physician Hippocrates (460–377 bce), known as the *father of medicine,* and Galen (131–201 ce), another Greek physician who practiced during the Roman era. Hippocrates accepted some of the rational concepts of his predecessors and taught that the body has natural resources to respond to disease and injury. Moreover, he believed that recovery from injury or disease is best implemented by getting the body in a condition to heal itself by using fresh air, water, and healthy food from nature, with limited intervention in the form of massages, purges, enemas, therapies, or drugs. His concepts of medical practice were based on a balance of the so-called *"four humors"*: blood, phlegm, black bile, and yellow bile, to which Galen added the four *"elements"*: earth, air, fire, and water. In addition, Galen introduced numerous medicaments called *"galenicals,"* some of which are still in use today (i.e., Galen's cerate or cold cream) and an alcoholic extract called *tincture of opium* to alleviate pain.

Paracelsus in a much later era did not ascribe to these theories. Although he had studied medicine he didn't obtain a degree to practice and was more interested in chemistry and alchemy. He proposed that the body was made up of chemicals and that disease was an imbalance of these chemicals that could be treated and/or corrected by the use of chemicals. He favored simple chemicals rather than complex compound chemical mixtures. He also prepared alcohol extracts or tinctures. Furthermore, he understood that the dose of a chemical was an important factor in determining effects that ranged from therapeutic to lethal, writing "All things are poisons, for there is nothing without poisonous qualities. It is only the dose which makes a thing a poison." Successful, effective modern medical therapeutics stem from this chemical concept.

IMPACT

The realization and acceptance of the role of body chemistry in health and disease have impacted and shaped the understanding of current medical practice and of rational drug development. This understanding extends to the body's native physiological responses and to its responses to drugs. For example, according to the concept of chemical molecular structure (CMS), the configuration of specialized molecules on some cells complements or recognizes and fits the configuration of certain molecules (receptors) on other cells in a lock-and-key fashion. When this chemical recognition coupling occurs it may initiate or interfere

Continued

with a cascade of events that lead to a particular response. This chemical communication, modified by the genetic chemical directions given our cells, is the foundation for responses to our individual internal and external environments. If drugs such as antibiotics are administered, their degree of effectiveness is determined by how well the CMS of the antibiotic complements or fits the molecules of the receptor for that antibiotic. Thus the administration of an antibiotic, its distribution via the blood vascular system to its site of action, and the response are all understood through knowledge of chemistry. Microbiology is understood by understanding its chemistry within the network of the chemistry of life.

FUTURE

Improved technologies in chemistry coupled with investigative advances in other disciplines such as computer science have significantly improved the development of new antibiotics for existing and emerging infectious diseases. For example, the CMS of an antibiotic determines its microbiological activity. This CMS can then be modified and tested by specific pharmacological procedures to identify the microbiological characteristics and potencies of its action. Therapies for current, emerging, and future infectious diseases are not only possible but are forthcoming as new technologies yield insights into their chemistry and the chemistry of the body.

Atoms and Ions

All cells and organisms are made up of chemicals, and understanding the basic chemical principles is essential to understanding the structure and function of all organisms.

Elements

Knowledge of the chemistry of life begins with an understanding of those chemical principles that govern the processes occurring in **matter.** *Matter* is defined as anything that occupies space and has mass. It can be in liquid, gaseous, or solid form and is composed of **elements,** the smallest particles of which are **atoms.** Elements cannot be broken down further by natural forces. Oxygen, carbon, hydrogen, nitrogen, phosphorus, and sulfur are some of the elements most commonly found in living cells (Table 2.1). Although these chemical elements usually do not exist in free form, they do occur in combinations called **chemical compounds.** The shorthand expression of a chemical compound is its **chemical formula.** For example, the chemical formula of table salt or sodium chloride is NaCl (see Chemical Notations, below).

Atomic Model

All atoms have the same fundamental structure consisting of a center, or atomic nucleus, and surrounding shells (Figure 2.1), but because of the different numbers of subatomic particles, each element has its own characteristic atomic structure. Located in the center of the atom is the **atomic nucleus,** which consists of positively charged particles called **protons,** and particles without charge called **neutrons.** The **atomic weight** (atomic mass) of an atom is equal to the sum of protons and neutrons. The **atomic number** indicates the number of protons in the atomic nucleus. Surrounding the atomic nucleus in shells are negatively charged subatomic particles called **electrons.** Electrons travel around the nucleus at high speed and occupy positions in a volume of space called an *orbital* or *electron cloud.* These orbitals form an energy

TABLE 2.1 Common Elements in Living Organisms

Element	Symbol	Atomic Number	Atomic Weight
Hydrogen	H	1	1
Carbon	C	6	12
Nitrogen	N	7	14
Oxygen	O	8	16
Sodium	Na	11	23
Magnesium	Mg	12	24.3
Phosphorus	P	15	31
Sulfur	S	16	32.1
Chlorine	Cl	17	35.5
Potassium	K	19	39.1
Calcium	Ca	20	40.1
Iron	Fe	26	55.8
Cobalt	Co	27	58.9
Copper	Cu	29	63.5
Zinc	Zn	30	65.4
Iodine	I	53	126.9

level also referred to as **shells,** in which the electrons usually remain. Electrons fill the orbitals and shells in pairs, and each orbital within a shell can carry two electrons.

The nucleus of a given atom is surrounded by successive shells spaced further and further away from the nucleus. The energy level of electrons increases with the distance of their shells from the nucleus. The innermost (first) shell can be occupied by up to two electrons within one orbital, the second shell with up to eight within four orbitals, and each consecutive shell can potentially hold more electrons. However, most elements with biological significance need eight electrons to fill the out-

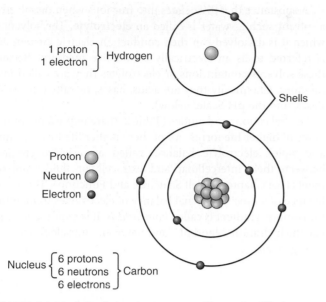

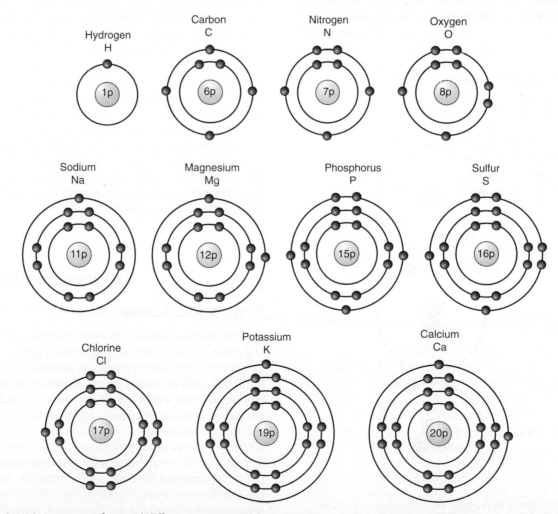

FIGURE 2.1 **Models of atomic structure.** These simplified diagrams of hydrogen and carbon atoms show the atomic nucleus containing protons and neutrons in the center of the atom, and the electrons in the surrounding shells.

ermost shell. The shells always fill sequentially from the inside out: two electrons in the first shell, eight in the next, and so on. For example, carbon with 6 electrons carries 2 electrons in the first shell and 4 in the second shell, and sodium with 11 electrons has 2 electrons in the first shell, 8 in the second, and 1 in the third shell (Figure 2.2).

In general, the number of protons and electrons of an atom are equal, making the atom an electrically neutral unit. The stability of an atom depends on the number of electrons in the outermost shell. For example, an atom is most stable if the outermost shell is filled to its capacity. Hydrogen is the simplest element, with the atomic number of 1, and therefore has one electron in the outermost shell. Helium, with the atomic number of 2, has two electrons in the outermost shell. This shell is fully occupied and is stable. Helium atoms will not react with each other and also cannot combine with atoms of other elements. Helium is therefore called an *inert gas*.

If the outermost shell is not complete, the atom can participate in a chemical reaction and form a **chemical bond.** Electrons in the outermost shell of an atom that are available for chemical bonding are called **valence electrons.** These electrons determine what kind of chemical bonds, if any, the atom can form.

FIGURE 2.2 **Atomic structure of several different atoms important in living systems.** The diagrams illustrate that the number of protons equals the number of electrons in each of these atoms, which are found in association with living systems.

Isotopes are atoms with the same number of protons but a different number of neutrons. The atomic number of isotopes is unchanged because the number of protons remains the same and only the atomic weight is different. For example, the element hydrogen has two isotopes (Figure 2.3):

- Hydrogen (one proton)
- Deuterium (one proton and one neutron)
- Tritium (one proton and two neutrons)

Radioisotopes are unstable because of their imbalance of energy within the nucleus. When the nucleus loses a neutron it gives off energy and is said to be radioactive. **Radioactivity** is the release of energy and matter that results from changes in the nucleus of an atom. Tritium is an example of a radioactive isotope that is used in research and clinical procedures.

Ions

Ions are electrically charged atoms, molecules, or subatomic particles that are formed when one or more valence electrons are transferred from one atom to another (see Formation and Classification of Chemical Bonds and Forces, below). If an atom loses one or more electrons to another atom, it becomes positive (+), whereas the atom that gains the electron becomes negative (−). Positively charged ions are called **cations,** and in an electric field move toward the negative pole, the cathode. Negatively charged ions, referred to as **anions,** move toward the positive pole, or anode, of an electric field.

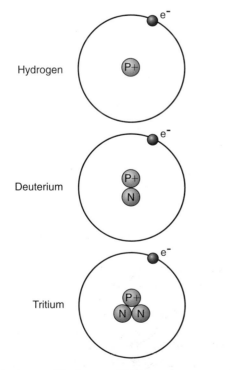

FIGURE 2.3 Isotopes of hydrogen. Hydrogen has one proton only, deuterium has one proton and one neutron, and tritium has one proton and two neutrons.

A substance that dissociates into free ions when dissolved in a solvent such as water is called an **electrolyte.** The solvent in which it is dissolved can then conduct an electric current and is referred to as an electrically conductive medium. Because these solvents contain ions or electrolytes they are called *ionic solutions.* Chemically they are acids, bases, or salts (see Acids, Bases, and the pH Scale, below).

Several cations and anions (Table 2.2) are important components of higher life forms. All of these higher life forms require a complex electrolyte balance, called an *osmotic gradient,* between their intercellular and extracellular fluid compartments (see Chapter 3, Cell Structure and Function). This maintenance of a precise internal balance of electrolytes to maintain the osmotic gradient is called *homeostasis.* It is required to regulate the hydration, blood pH, and nerve and muscle function of an organism.

TABLE 2.2 Common Ions in Living Organisms

Cations	Anions
Sodium (Na^+)	Chloride (Cl^-)
Potassium (K^+)	Bicarbonate (HCO_3^-)
Calcium (Ca^{2+})	Phosphate (PO_4^{3-})
Magnesium (Mg^{2+})	Sulfate (SO_4^{2-})

TABLE 2.3 Common Functional Groups in Living Organisms

Functional Group	Formula	Functional Group	Formula
Acetyl	CH_3	Ethyl	C_2H_5
Aldehyde	CHO	Hydroxyl	OH
Amino	NH_2	Keto	CO
Ammonium	NH_4	Methyl	CH_3
Bicarbonate	HCO_3	Nitrate	NO_3
Carbonate	CO_3	Phosphate	PO_4
Carboxyl	COOH	Sulfate	SO_4

Chemical Bonds and Molecules

Molecules are two or more atoms linked together by chemical bonds formed by their valence electrons. As stated above, atoms are most stable when their outermost shell is filled with eight electrons. This is the *octet principle*. The number of bonds a single atom can have is dependent on how many electrons are needed to complete the outermost shell. Hydrogen with one electron in the outermost shell can form one chemical bond; oxygen with eight electrons (2 + 6) (and therefore six in the outermost shell) can form two bonds; and carbon with six electrons (2 + 4) (four in the outermost shell) can form up to four chemical bonds to fill the outermost shell. When the outermost shell is not completely occupied with electrons, the atom has the tendency to interact with other atoms forming chemical bonds to achieve higher stability. These atoms then become stable and cannot react with others.

Formation and Classification of Chemical Bonds and Forces

Molecules made from atoms of different elements are called **compounds.** Compounds are new chemicals with properties that are different from those of the atoms of which they are composed. Groups of atoms that consistently form specific groups within compounds are referred to as *functional groups.* They have specific characteristics that are different from those of the individual participating atoms of that given group. Some molecules have more than one functional group, which may differ from one another. The most common functional groups found in molecules important to living organisms are shown in Table 2.3.

The principal types of chemical bonds formed by the interactions of atoms and/or molecules are covalent bonds, ionic bonds, hydrogen bonds, and those based on van der Waals forces. Covalent and hydrogen bonds occur between atoms to form a molecule, whereas hydrogen bonds and van der Waals forces are intermolecular connections. Chemical bonds vary in their strength but, in general, covalent bonds are considered the strongest bond, followed by ionic bonds, hydrogen bonds, and—with the weakest connection—the van der Waals forces.

Covalent bonds result from a sharing of electrons between two atoms of the same element or between atoms of different

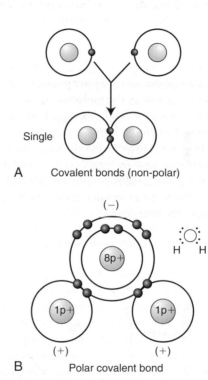

FIGURE 2.4 Covalent bonds: a sharing of electrons. A, Nonpolar covalent bond between two hydrogen atoms (H_2), formed by an equal sharing of electrons. **B,** Polar covalent bond between an oxygen atom and two hydrogen atoms (H_2O), formed by an unequal sharing of electrons.

elements. In bonds between identical atoms such as oxygen and hydrogen, the electrons are shared equally by each atom. Covalent bonds usually are the strongest chemical bonds. Because the electrons are equally distributed, the resulting molecule is nonpolar and the bond is called a **nonpolar** covalent bond (Figure 2.4, *A*). Carbon atoms play a significant role in large organic molecules because they form stable nonpolar covalent bonds with each other. This stable framework is the backbone of organic carbon-based molecules, providing the chemical foundation of organic chemistry and of life.

The covalent bonds between atoms of two different-sized elements are **polar** covalent bonds, in which the electrons are

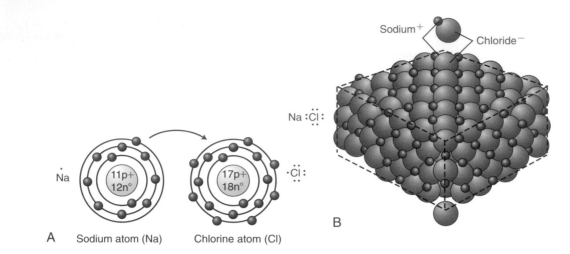

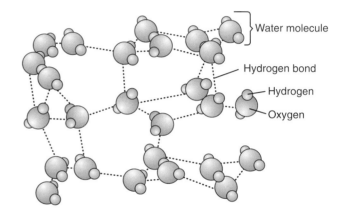

FIGURE 2.5 Ionic bond. A, The electron in the outermost shell of the sodium atom is transferred to the chlorine atom, resulting in a sodium (+) and a chloride (–) ion. **B,** Crystal of sodium chloride (table salt). The sodium and chloride ions alternate in a definite, regular, geometric pattern.

unequally distributed because they are pulled toward the larger atom. As a result, one end of the molecule becomes more negative compared with the other end (Figure 2.4, *B*). Oxygen, nitrogen, and phosphorus atoms have a tendency to form polar covalent bonds. Polar covalent bonds are somewhat weaker than nonpolar covalent bonds. Coordinate covalent bonds, such as occurs in the formation of the ammonium ion from ammonia, are formed when both electrons are from one atom. The molecule no living organism can exist without is water, in which the atoms hydrogen and oxygen are held together by polar covalent bonds. Some properties of water result from this type of bond.

Depending on the number of electrons shared, molecules can be formed from a single covalent bond by sharing one pair of electrons, such as the bond between hydrogen atoms. Single covalent bonds are indicated by one solid line (H—H). Double covalent bonds are formed by sharing two pairs of electrons, as seen between oxygen atoms. These bonds are indicated by two solid lines (O=O). Triple covalent bonds may occur through the sharing of three pairs of electrons, such as between nitrogen atoms. These bonds are identified by three solid lines (N≡N).

Ionic bonds are formed when one or more electrons from one atom are transferred to another. If an atom loses one electron in the process it will have a charge of +1; if two electrons are lost the charge will be +2, because the protons in the nucleus will be unbalanced by the remaining electrons. The resulting anions and cations in an ionic bond are held together by attraction of their opposite charges and form an ionic compound. Ionic bonds can easily dissociate (break down) in water to form electrolyte solutions. For example, in water metals such as Na^+, readily give up electrons, and nonmetals such as Cl^- readily take up electrons ($Na^+ + Cl^- \rightarrow NaCl$). If the water is evaporated, a solid crystal of NaCl, common table salt, is formed. Sodium with a total of 11 electrons (2 + 8 + 1) has only 1 electron in its outermost shell, whereas chlorine with a total of 17 electrons (2 + 8 + 7) only needs 1 electron to fill its outermost shell. The only electron in sodium's outermost shell is therefore attracted to chlorine's outermost shell and its transfer forms an ionic com-

FIGURE 2.6 Hydrogen bond between water molecules. The positively charged hydrogen portion of one water molecule is slightly attracted to the negatively charged oxygen portion of another water molecule. Hydrogen bonds are always indicated by dotted lines.

pound (Figure 2.5, *A*). The charged sodium chloride molecules and other salts form characteristic large crystal structures in which the atoms of the molecules alternate in a regular, geometric pattern (Figure 2.5, *B*). In water, NaCl readily dissociates to form an electrolyte.

Hydrogen bonds are weak chemical bonds with only about 5% of the strength of covalent bonds. However, when many hydrogen bonds are formed between two molecules, the resulting union can be strong enough to be stable. These bonds are formed by attraction forces between charged atoms within a large molecule or between adjacent molecules (Figure 2.6). Hydrogen bonds always involve a hydrogen atom with a slight positive charge and an oxygen or nitrogen atom with a slightly negative charge. Although hydrogen bonds do not form molecules they can alter the shapes of molecules or hold together different molecules. Examples of hydrogen bonds include bonds between water molecules, acetic acid molecules, amino acid molecules, and nucleic acid molecules. Hydrogen bonds are always indicated by dotted lines (---). The attraction created by hydrogen bonds keeps water in the liquid state over a wide range of temperatures.

Van der Waals forces are the weakest of the intermolecular forces in all chemical reactions. The van der Waals force of attraction is inversely proportional to the seventh power of the interatomic distance, whereas the force of an ionic bond diminishes as the square of the distance. Therefore a very slight increase in the interatomic distance between atoms markedly reduces the van der Waals force of attraction. In terms of the "lock and key" concept of reactants and their receptors, such as between antigens and antibodies and between drugs and their receptors, van der Waals forces determine the final molecular arrangements that define selectivity and specificity properties. In other words, if there is an interaction (selectivity), how well it fits (specificity) is a function of the van der Waals forces. Van der Waals forces explain how a spider can hang upside down from a ceiling and why a gecko can hang by one toe from a glass surface. For drug–receptor interactions, ionic bonds based on electrostatic attraction probably come into play as the drug approaches the immediate vicinity of the receptor, followed by additional attraction based on van der Waals forces. Covalent bonding is more of a factor in longer lasting drug actions.

Types of Chemical Reactions

Pathways of chemical reactions trace metabolic activities in living organisms. Within these pathways, several chemical reactions occur that are essential for the survival of living organisms, including microbes. These reactions are as follows:

- Dehydration synthesis (condensation)
- Hydrolysis (decomposition)
- Endergonic (energy-requiring) reactions
- Exergonic (energy-producing) reactions
- Oxidation and reduction (redox)
- Exchange reactions

Dehydration synthesis, or condensation, is the formation of a larger compound (polymer) from smaller ones (monomers). Monomers are the unit molecules (building blocks) of these larger molecules, called *polymers*. These reactions require specific enzymes and the removal of water from the reactants, that is, a hydroxyl group (OH) is removed from one monomer and combined with a hydrogen (H) from the other (Figure 2.7). Enzymes (see Chapter 3, Cell Structure and Function) are biological catalysts and function to speed up the rate of chemical reactions without changing themselves. The **synthesis** of new compounds within a cell occurs during **anabolism,** which utilizes energy provided by **catabolism** (see Cellular Metabolism in Chapter 3, Cell Structure and Function). An example of synthesis is the production of complex sugars from simple sugars (see Carbohydrates, below).

$$\text{Glucose} + \text{glucose} \rightarrow \text{maltose}$$

$$\text{Monomer} + \text{monomer} \rightarrow \text{polymer}$$

Hydrolysis (decomposition) breaks down large molecules (polymers) into their unit molecules (monomers). An example of hydrolysis is the breakdown of nutrient molecules such as carbohydrates, proteins, and lipids into smaller molecules during the digestive process. Hydrolysis is the reverse of dehydration synthesis and occurs during the metabolic process of catabolism. This complex reaction of breaking down polymers requires water and the resulting monomers can be used in cellular metabolism for the generation of energy.

Reactions that yield energy are called **exergonic** reactions. Reactions that utilize energy are **endergonic** reactions. Hydrolysis that occurs during catabolism is an exergonic reaction and it releases energy. Endergonic reactions require energy such as occurs in the dehydration synthesis of nutrient molecules during anabolism.

Redox (*red*uction–*ox*idation) reactions are chemical reactions in which atoms have their oxidation number (oxidation state) changed. An oxidation reaction does not occur without a reduction reaction happening at the same time. **Oxidation** is

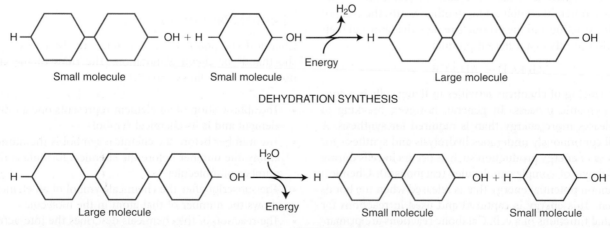

DEHYDRATION SYNTHESIS

HYDROLYSIS

FIGURE 2.7 Dehydration synthesis and hydrolysis. Dehydration synthesis is an anabolic reaction (requires energy) producing polymers (large molecules) from monomers (small molecules) by removing water. Hydrolysis is a catabolic reaction (releasing energy) in which polymers are broken down into monomers. These reactions require water.

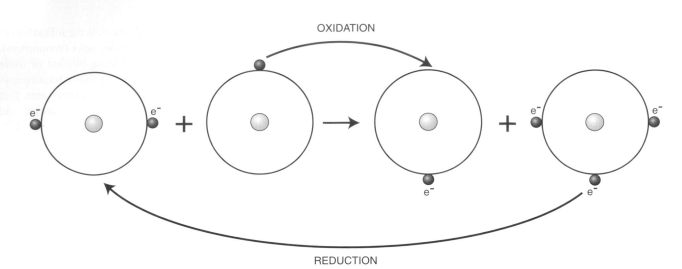

OXIDATION

REDUCTION

FIGURE 2.8 Oxidation–reduction (electron transfer) reactions. Oxidation refers to the loss of electrons, whereas reduction involves gaining electrons.

loss of electrons and is a common reaction in the production of cellular energy. The transfer of electrons is catalyzed by enzymes within the metabolic pathways. The electrical state of an atom is identified as the oxidation state or by its oxidation number. Atoms are neutral and their oxidation state is therefore zero. The oxidation state changes because of a loss or gain of electrons. Loss of electrons results in a positive oxidation state of an atom and a gain of electrons results in a negative oxidation state. Oxidation reactions are indicated as follows, using calcium as an example:

$$Ca \rightarrow Ca^{2+} + 2e^-$$

Oxidation–reduction (electron transfer) reactions are coupled. In other words, oxidation reactions occur with reduction reactions (Figure 2.8). **Reduction** is the gain of electrons. It is also catalyzed by enzymatic reactions and is written as follows:

$$O + 2e^- \rightarrow O^{2-}$$

Exchange reactions transfer the same molecules in a reaction but in a different combination. In other words, the components of the reaction and the products remain the same but their combination results in a different product.

$$AB + CD \rightarrow AD + CB$$

The balancing of chemical activities in living cells is a continuous, dynamic process. In general, however, breaking of bonds releases more energy than is required for synthesis. A living cell continuously undergoes hydrolysis and synthesis for the purpose of energy production such as occurs in cells during the breakdown of complex molecules (catabolism). Chemical bonds contain potential energy that is released when the bonds are broken. This energy is captured and used in reactions for the essential functions of a cell. Catabolic reactions are primarily oxidation reactions and are divided into different pathways, namely, glycolysis, the Krebs cycle (citric acid cycle), and the electron transport chain (see Chapter 3, Cell Structure and Function).

LIFE APPLICATION

Bleach

The decolorizing action of bleaching agents is partly due to their ability to remove the electrons that are activated by light to produce the various colors. Most chemical bleaches contain sodium hypochlorite (NaOCl) or hydrogen peroxide (H_2O_2), which are both oxidizing agents. Hypochlorite (OCl⁻) is reduced to chloride ions and hydroxyl ions.

$$OCl^- + 2e^- + HOH \rightarrow Cl^- + 2OH^-$$

Bleaches are sometimes combined with other compounds that are different from bleaches but are capable of absorbing wavelengths of ultraviolet light, which is invisible to the human eye. They convert these wavelengths to visible blue or blue-green light that is reflected, making the fabric appear brighter.

Chemical Notations

Chemical compounds and reactions are shown by "chemical shorthand" or chemical notation. The rules of the chemical notation are as follows (Box 2.1):

- The abbreviation of an element represents one atom of that element and is its chemical symbol.
- The number before the chemical symbol is the number of atoms; the number before the chemical formula is the number of molecules.
- The subscript after the chemical symbol of an element shows the number of that atom in the molecule.
- The reaction of the chemicals describes the interaction of the participants, called the *reactants*. Chemical reactions form one or more products. Arrows in the formula indicate the direction of the reaction, from reactant to product. Arrows in both directions indicate a reversible

Nitrogen Fixation

Nitrogen, the most abundant element in the atmosphere of the earth, is a vital element in many of the compounds essential to living systems. For example, in all green plants nitrogen is a primary nutrient. However, it must be modified by a process called *nitrogen fixation* before it can be used. Nitrogen fixation is a complex process that reduces nitrogen to nitrogen compounds such as ammonia, nitrate, and nitrogen dioxide. This process is performed by different nitrogen-fixing bacteria present in soil. Nitrogen fixation involves a number of oxidation–reduction reactions that occur sequentially to yield ammonium ions. Also, nitrogen in the form of ammonia is used by living systems in the synthesis of many organic compounds. Ammonia can be formed by the process of nitrification, during which nitrates and nitrites released by decaying organic matter are converted to ammonium ions by nitrifying bacteria, again present in the soil. This process can also be achieved by a series of oxidation–reduction reactions. Denitrifying bacteria, acting on ammonia and nitrates produced by decay, recycle these compounds to free nitrogen to complete what is called the *nitrogen cycle.*

BOX 2.1 Chemical Notation

Symbols

H: An atom of hydrogen   C: An atom of carbon
O: An atom of oxygen   N: An atom of nitrogen

Prefixes

2H: Two individual atoms of hydrogen
2O: Two individual atoms of oxygen
3C: Three individual atoms of carbon
4N: Four individual atoms of nitrogen

Number of Atoms in a Molecule

H_2: A molecule with two hydrogen atoms
O_2: A molecule with two oxygen atoms
C_6: A molecule with six carbon atoms
N_4: A molecule with four nitrogen atoms

Superscripts

Na^+: A sodium atom that has lost one electron, resulting in a positively charged ion
Cl^-: A chlorine atom that has gained one electron, resulting in a negatively charged ion
K^+: A potassium ion
$Ca2^+$: A calcium atom that has lost two electrons

Chemical Equation

Balanced: $2H + O \rightarrow H_2O$
$2H_2 + O_2 \rightarrow 2H_2O$
$NaOH + HCl \rightarrow NaCl + H_2O$
Unbalanced: $H_2O_2 \rightarrow H_2O$
$2NaOH + HCl \rightarrow NaCl + H_2O$

---

chemical reaction that can go in either direction. For example,

$$2H + O \rightarrow H_2O$$

The equation indicates that two atoms of hydrogen and one atom of oxygen combine to form water (H_2O). Another example:

$$NaOH + HCl \rightleftharpoons NaCl + H_2O$$

Here one molecule of sodium hydroxide (NaOH) and one molecule of hydrochloric acid (HCl) form salt (NaCl) and water (H_2O); the reaction is reversible.

- A superscript of plus or minus after the atomic symbol indicates an ion. A single plus or minus shows the charge of an ion. If more than one electron has been lost or gained the charge of the ions is shown with a number before the plus or minus sign.
- Chemical reactions do not form or destroy atoms; they just rearrange them into new combinations. In any given chemical equation the number of atoms of each element must be the same on both sides, resulting in a balanced equation.

Inorganic Compounds

Inorganic compounds consist of molecules that do not contain carbon with the exception of a few molecules that are classified as inorganic compounds although they contain carbon, such as carbon dioxide (CO_2) and carbon monoxide (CO).

Acids, Bases, and the pH Scale

Some chemical compounds dissociate in water as ions, carry an electric current, and display an electrical charge. Substances that release hydrogen ions (H^+) are **acids,** and those that release hydroxyl ions (OH^-) are **bases.** The strength of acids and bases is determined by the hydrogen ion concentration of the water in which they dissociate. The higher the hydrogen ion concentration in the solution the more acidic the solution is. A low hydrogen ion concentration of a solution indicates a basic solution (Box 2.2).

BOX 2.2 Definitions

Acid: A molecule that can release H^+ into a solution; it is called a *"proton donor"*
Base: A molecule that can combine with H^+ and removes it from the solution; it is called a *"proton acceptor"*
pH: The negative logarithm of the H^+ concentration of a solution, indicated in pH units on a pH scale that runs from 0 to 14 with pH 7 (pH of pure water at 25° C) as neutral
Buffer: A system of molecules and ions that stabilize the pH of a solution by resisting changes in the H^+ concentration of the solution

---

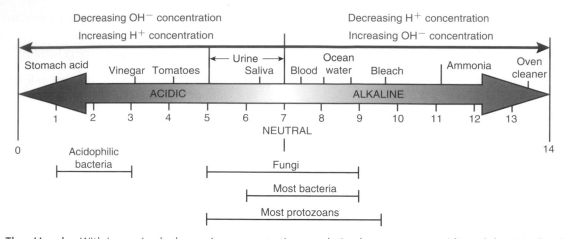

FIGURE 2.9 The pH scale. With increasing hydrogen ion concentrations a solution becomes more acidic and the pH value decreases. When the hydrogen ion concentration decreases the solution becomes more basic and the pH value increases.

This acidity or alkalinity of a solution is measured by the **pH scale** ("potential hydrogens"). It is a chemical symbol that ranges from 0 to 14 and is the negative logarithm of the hydrogen ion concentration (Figure 2.9). A solution that has a neutral pH is one in which the concentrations of H^+ and OH^- ions are equal (10^{-7} M), and the chemical symbol for this negative logarithm is pH 7. The point of neutrality is standardized as the pH of pure water at 25° C. As the H^+ concentration increases, the OH^- concentration decreases and vice versa. A change one of 1 unit on the pH scale (the negative logarithm scale) represents a 10-fold change in the hydrogen ion concentration. The higher the hydrogen ion concentration of a solution, the lower the number on the pH scale and the more acid the solution; the higher the number on the scale, the higher the hydroxyl ion concentration and the more basic (alkaline) the solution.

Chemical reactions in a living cell respond to slight changes in the pH of their environment. The majority of microbes as well as human cells survive better in a neutral or slightly basic environment. This sensitivity of microbes to changes in pH is used in the control of microbial growth and in food preservation (see Chapter 19, Physical and Chemical Methods of Control). However, as mentioned in Chapter 1, some microorganisms are found to exist successfully in all environments, such as sulfur-oxidizing bacteria, which prefer a very acidic environment, and yeast, which flourishes under slightly acidic conditions.

Buffers

Buffers are chemicals that can absorb hydrogen or hydroxyl ions and therefore resist changes in the pH of a solution. In a living organism buffers are essential to maintain the pH necessary for the survival of its cells. A common endogenous buffer in cells is the bicarbonate (HCO_3^-) ion. Bicarbonate picks up hydrogen ions (H^+), forming carbonic acid (H_2CO_3).

$$HCO_3^- + H^+ \rightleftarrows H_2CO_3$$

This reaction is readily reversible so that adjustments in the pH can be made to maintain the required pH in a given envi-

ronment. All biological fluids, both intracellular and extracellular, are heavily buffered.

Salts

Substances that dissociate in water and normally do not release hydrogen or hydroxyl ions are known as *normal salts*. Natron is a salt, composed of a mixture of sodium bicarbonate (common baking soda), sodium carbonate (soda ash), a small amount of sodium chloride (table salt), and sodium sulfate. Natron is called *impure salt* because it has lost its saltiness. Salts that contain a hydroxide ion are basic salts and salts that contain a hydrogen ion are acid salts. Salts are formed when acids and bases react. Solutions of salts in water are called *electrolytes* and they conduct electricity.

Salts are formed by chemical reactions between a base and an acid or between a metal and an acid. The name of a salt starts with the name of the cation (ammonium, magnesium, etc.) followed by the name of the anion (chloride, sulfate, etc.).

For example:

$$NH_3 + HCl \rightarrow NH_4Cl \text{ (ammonium chloride)}$$

$$Mg + H_2SO_4 \rightarrow MgSO_4 + H_2 \text{ (magnesium sulfate)}$$

Sometimes salts are referred to less specifically by the name of the cation (e.g., sodium salt, ammonium salt) or by the name of the anion (e.g., chloride, acetate). Common salt-forming cations and anions are shown in Table 2.4.

Salts are usually solid crystals but can exist as a liquid at room temperature and are called *ionic liquids*. Different salts can stimulate sensations of all five basic tastes: salty (sodium chloride), sweet (lead diacetate), sour (potassium bitartrate), bitter (magnesium sulfate), and umami (monosodium glutamate). Pure salts are odorless whereas impure salts may smell acidic (acetates) or basic (ammonium salts). Salts can be clear and transparent (sodium chloride), opaque (titanium dioxide), or metallic (iron disulfate). They also exist in different colors (Table 2.5). Most mineral, inorganic pigments and many synthetic organic dyes are salts.

TABLE 2.4 Common Salt-forming Anions and Cations

Salt-forming Anions*		Salt-forming Cations	
Name	Formula	Name	Formula
Acetate (acetic acid)	CH_3COO^-	Ammonium	NH_4^+
Carbonate (carbonic acid)	CO_3^{2-}	Calcium	Ca^{2+}
Chloride (hydrochloric acid)	Cl^-	Iron	Fe^{2+} and Fe^{3+}
Hydroxide	OH^-	Magnesium	Mg^{2+}
Nitrate (nitric acid)	NO_3^-	Potassium	K^+
Oxide	O_2^-	Pyridinium	$C_5H_5NH^+$
Phosphate (phosphoric acid)	PO_4^{3-}	Quaternary ammonium	$NR_4^{+\dagger}$
Sulfate (sulfuric acid)	SO_4^{2-}	Sodium	Na^+

*Parent acid in parentheses.
†A side chain/group.

TABLE 2.5 Colors of Salts

Name of Salt	Formula	Color
Sodium chloride	$NaCl$	Clear, transparent
Titanium dioxide	TiO_2	Opaque, white
Iron disulfide	FeS_2	Metallic
Sodium chromate	$Na_2Cr_2O_4 \cdot 2H_2O$	Yellow
Sodium dichromate	$Na_2Cr_2O_7 \cdot 2H_2O$	Orange
Mercury sulfide	HgS	Red
Cobalt dichloride hexahydrate	$CoCl_2 \cdot 6H_2O$	Mauve
Copper sulfate pentahydrate	$CuSO_4 \cdot 5H_2O$	Blue
Ferric hexacyanoferrate	$Fe_4[Fe(CN)_6]_3$	Blue
Nickel oxide	Ni_2O_3	Green
Magnesium sulfate	$MgSO_4$	Colorless
Manganese dioxide	MnO_2	Black

LIFE APPLICATION

Water Insects

Many insects can skate across the surface of water because of the water's high surface tension. One of the most common examples is the water strider, an insect that never breaks the surface as it skates on the water of streams, rivers, ponds, and even the ocean. Long-distance water movement is essential to the survival of land plants. On a dry, warm, sunny day a leaf may lose almost 100% of its water in a very short time. Therefore, the water evaporated from the leaves must be replaced by the uptake of water from the soil. This water transport can be explained by the cohesion–tension theory that states that the driving force of this transport is the evaporation (transpiration) of water from the leaf surfaces. The water molecules stick together (cohere) and are pulled up the plant by capillary action (tension) exerted by the evaporation at the leaf surface.

Water

Life on earth most likely exists because of the abundance of liquid water. Water is unique because it can exist in three different temperature-dependent states: gas (steam), liquid, and solid (ice). Water is a molecule that consists of hydrogen and oxygen at a ratio of 2 to 1 and is absolutely necessary for all life forms. The bond between the oxygen atom and the hydrogen atom is a polar covalent bond, resulting in the molecule having a slightly positive side and a slightly negative side. The water molecules in water are held together by hydrogen bonding. Water molecules can quickly break down and reform their hydrogen bonds, which results in the property of cohesion. Water's high level of cohesion, or "stickiness," allows things to float easily on its surface at the air–water interface, and also causes water to form beads when dispersed. It is the most abundant molecule in the human body and in microorganisms, which contain at least 70% water, and the earth's surface is 71% covered by water as well.

Water's freezing and boiling points at sea level are the baseline from which temperature is measured. Zero degrees Celsius (0° C) is water's freezing point and 100° C is its boiling point. The solid form of water (ice) is less dense than the liquid form and for that reason ice floats on water. Whereas most liquids contract as they become colder, water expands until it is solid.

Water is a contributor in most chemical reactions of cells and is essential to break down polymers into monomers by the process of hydrolysis. The amount of water needed for metabolic activities varies among different microorganisms. The availability of water influences microbial growth rates (see Chapter 6, Bacteria and Archaea). Some of the properties of water are shown in Box 2.3.

Water is a **solvent** and can dissolve many different substances, and is therefore often called the *"universal solvent."* The substances dissolved in water or another solvent are **solutes,** and the combination of a solvent and its solutes is referred to as a **solution** (Figure 2.10). The solubility of molecules is determined by their molecular structure. Molecules that exhibit local differences in electrical properties, or polar areas, are water soluble and those that do not are insoluble in water. The survival of living cells depends on the appropriate concentration of solutes in a solution. Most organisms do not tolerate environments where the concentration of solutes is much higher than that in their intracellular environment. Depending on the amount of solutes within or outside a cell, the environment can be:

- **Isotonic:** The solute concentration and hence the osmotic pressure within the cell (intracellular) is the same as it is

outside of the cell (extracellular). A cell placed in an isotonic solution will not change its cell volume.
- **Hypertonic:** The solute concentration in the cell is less than in the extracellular environment, which causes a net loss of water from the cell, resulting in cell shrinkage. The cell shape becomes notched or crenated.
- **Hypotonic:** The solute concentration in the extracellular environment is less than that inside the cell (intracellular), causing the uptake of water into the cell, resulting in the bursting of the cell (Figure 2.11)

Because of their polarity, ions attract the polar water molecules that surround the ions, which in turn attract other water molecules to form hydration spheres around each ion (Figure 2.12). Formations of hydration spheres are responsible for the solubility of ions in water. Organic molecules such as glucose, amino acids, and others are water soluble if the covalent bonding pattern permits the formation of hydration spheres around their atoms of oxygen, nitrogen, and phosphorus. These molecules are **hydrophilic** (water loving) water-soluble compounds. Molecules held together by nonpolar covalent bonds are **hydrophobic** (water repelling) and insoluble in water because of their inability to form hydration spheres. Parts of drug molecules may be hydrophilic, conferring water solubility properties on them, and vice versa for hydrophobic parts of drug molecules (see Chapter 21, Pharmacology).

Organic Molecules

All organic molecules contain atoms of carbon and hydrogen. Organic molecules have a backbone of chains or rings formed by the carbon and hydrogen atoms, referred to as a hydrocarbon

---

BOX 2.3 Properties of Water

- Water is colorless, tasteless, and odorless.
- Water feels wet.
- Water makes a distinctive sound when dripping or crashing as a wave.
- Water exists in three forms: liquid, solid, and gas.
- Water can absorb a large amount of heat.
- Water has cohesive properties and "sticks" together into drops.
- Water has surface tension (the tendency of water molecules to stick together at the surface due to cohesion) and capillary action (the tendency of water molecules to stick to another surface and to move along with it).
- Water is part of all living organisms.

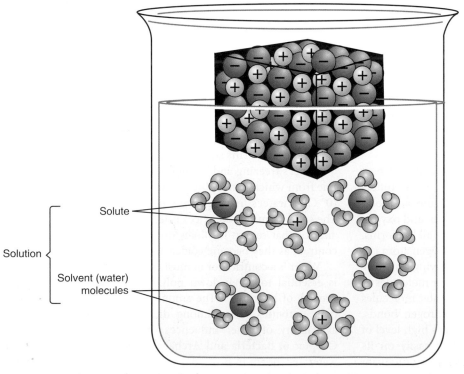

Solute

Solution

Solvent (water) molecules

FIGURE 2.10 Solvent, solutes, and solution. In this diagram water acts as the solvent, sodium and chloride ions are the solutes, and when solutes are dissolved (dissociated) in a solvent, a solution is formed.

backbone. Carbons commonly form covalent bonds not only with hydrogen, but also with oxygen, nitrogen, sulfur, and phosphorus. It is this covalent bonding of carbons with other carbons that yields the immense number and variety of organic molecules and allows different arrangements of chains or rings (Figure 2.13). The major organic molecules in living organisms are carbohydrates, proteins, lipids, and nucleic acids. Each of these compounds is composed of specific unit molecules or monomers (Table 2.6).

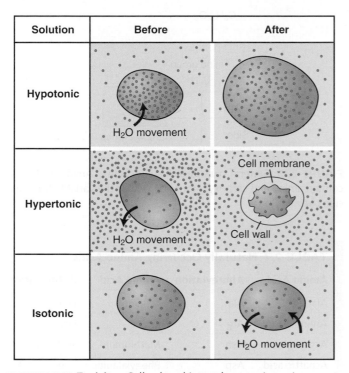

Solution	Before	After
Hypotonic	H$_2$O movement	
Hypertonic	H$_2$O movement	Cell membrane / Cell wall
Isotonic		H$_2$O movement

FIGURE 2.11 Tonicity. Cells placed into a hypotonic environment will take up water, swell, and may eventually burst. Cells placed into a hypertonic environment will lose water and shrink. Cells placed in an isotonic environment will remain unchanged.

Carbohydrates

Carbohydrates (sugars) include monosaccharides (monomer), disaccharides (two monosaccharides), and polysaccharides (many monosaccharides—polymer), all of which have a characteristic ratio (2:1:2) of carbon, hydrogen, and oxygen atoms. The name "carbohydrate" (hydrates [water] of carbon) is derived from this ratio. Sugars store carbon as well as large amounts of energy that are extracted during catabolism. Many microorganisms prefer sugars, when they are available, as their source of energy. Carbohydrates are also present in a large variety of cellular structures.

Monosaccharides are simple sugars that contain three to seven carbon atoms and an aldehyde group or a keto group. Monosaccharides represent the unit molecules (monomers) of carbohydrates. Monosaccharides include glucose ($C_6H_{12}O_6$), fructose, galactose, ribose ($C_5H_{10}O_5$), and deoxyribose ($C_5H_{10}O_4$).

Disaccharides (Figure 2.14, *A*) are compounds formed when two monosaccharides combine with the loss of a water molecule. Disaccharides include the following:

- Sucrose: Composed of glucose and fructose
- Lactose: Composed of glucose and galactose
- Maltose: Composed of two glucose molecules

TABLE 2.6 Organic Molecules and Their Monomers

Organic Molecule	Monomer
Carbohydrates	Monosaccharides
Proteins	Amino acids
Lipids	Glycerol and fatty acids
Nucleic acids	Nucleotides

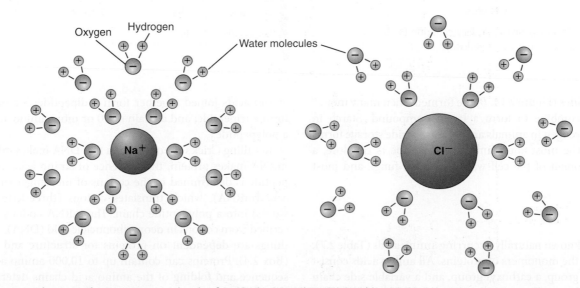

FIGURE 2.12 Hydration spheres. Water molecules form hydration spheres around ions.

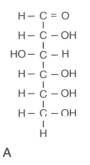

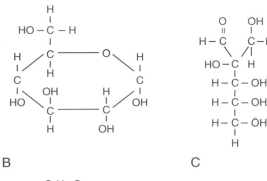

FIGURE 2.13 Carbon backbone of organic molecules. Carbon atoms can be arranged in **(A)** chains, **(B)** rings, or **(C)** branched chains.

A

B

C

$C_6H_{12}O_6$

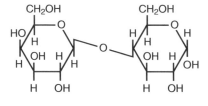

A   **Lactose (α form)**

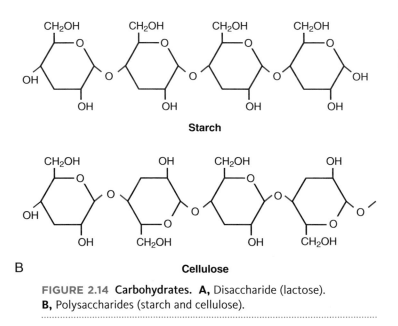

Starch

Cellulose

B

FIGURE 2.14 Carbohydrates. A, Disaccharide (lactose). **B,** Polysaccharides (starch and cellulose).

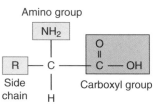

FIGURE 2.15 General structure of amino acids. Amino acids contain amino and carboxyl groups as well as the variable R group side chain.

TABLE 2.7 Naturally Occurring Amino Acids

Amino Acid	Abbreviation	Amino Acid	Abbreviation
Alanine	Ala	Leucine	Leu
Arginine	Arg	Lysine	Lys
Asparagine	Asn	Methionine	Met
Aspartic acid	Asp	Phenylalanine	Phe
Cysteine	Cys	Proline	Pro
Glutamic acid	Glu	Serine	Ser
Glutamine	Gln	Threonine	Thr
Glycine	Gly	Tryptophan	Trp
Histidine	His	Tyrosine	Tyr
Isoleucine	Ile	Valine	Val

Polysaccharides (Figure 2.14, *B*) are formed when many monosaccharides combine to form a larger compound. Starch in plants and glycogen in animals are polysaccharide storage forms of glucose. The most abundant polysaccharide is cellulose, a major component of the cell walls of plants, fungi, and most algae.

Proteins

There are 20 known naturally occurring amino acids (Table 2.7), and they are the monomers of proteins. All amino acids consist of an amino group, a carboxyl group, and a variable side chain designated chemically as R (the R group; Figure 2.15). Two amino acids joined together form a dipeptide; 3 amino acids form a tripeptide; and a chain of 10 or more amino acids form a polypeptide.

Recalling Crick's central dogma that DNA makes mRNA and mRNA makes protein, the sequence of amino acids in a polypeptide is determined in the codons of messenger ribonucleic acid (mRNA), which translates codons (three-letter genetic words) into a polypeptide chain. The mRNA codons are transcribed from codons in deoxyribonucleic acid (DNA). All living things are dependent on proteins for structure and function (Box 2.4). Proteins can contain up to 10,000 amino acids. The sequence and folding of the amino acid chains determine the shape, which in turn determines the function and specificity of a protein. Different combinations of amino acids yield an infinite variety of polypeptides, which provides the chemical basis for the incredible biological diversity in structure and function among living organisms.

Proteins occur in four different structural arrangements (Figure 2.16):

- A primary structure is represented by a single chain of amino acids. Examples of primary structure proteins are small hypothalamic hormones such as gonadotropin-releasing hormone (GnRH) and thyrotropin-releasing hormone (TRH).
- A secondary structure is made of polypeptide chains that are either folded into a β sheet (β conformation) or form an α helix. The right-handed helix makes a complete turn in a clockwise direction every 3.6 amino acids. The α helix is held together by hydrogen bonds. β Sheets consist of two or more polypeptide chains lying side by side and are also stabilized by hydrogen bonds. Examples of such helical proteins are keratin, myosin, and collagen; silk represents a β-pleated sheet.
- A tertiary structure has a globular shape because of the additional coiling of secondary structure proteins. This structure is stabilized by the formation of additional hydrogen, ionic, and disulfide bonds. Properties of solubility are determined by hydrophobic nonpolar chains, which are generally positioned on the inside of the protein, and by hydrophilic polar chains, which are positioned on the outside of protein molecules. Examples of tertiary structure proteins are enzymes and some peptide hormones such as insulin.
- A quaternary structure contains several polypeptides that form a functional unit. Such complexes can consist of several copies of the same polypeptide or different polypeptides. An example of a quaternary structure protein is the hemoglobin molecule.

Heat, pH, salts, radiation, and heavy metals can change the shape of a protein, causing protein denaturation. This process results in nonfunctioning protein compounds. Denatured enzymes (proteins) can no longer function as biological catalysts, and their metabolic reactions come to a stop. Denatured antibodies can no longer bind to an antigen and fail to produce the all-important antigen–antibody complex in immune reactions (see Chapter 20, The Immune System). Denatured hormones are no longer able to act on their target cells. And the denaturing of bacterial or viral proteins often will eliminate the microbe (see Chapter 22, Antimicrobial Drugs).

When proteins are combined with inorganic or organic nonprotein compounds they are called *conjugated proteins*. These compounds are named accordingly as glycoproteins, lipoproteins, nucleoproteins, and phosphoproteins.

BOX 2.4 Functions of Proteins

- Structural support
- Contractile elements in muscles
- Receptors
- Enzymes
- Hormones
- Integral (transmembrane) and peripheral membrane proteins
- Transcription factors
- Antigens (some but not all)
- Antibodies
- Histocompatibility molecules

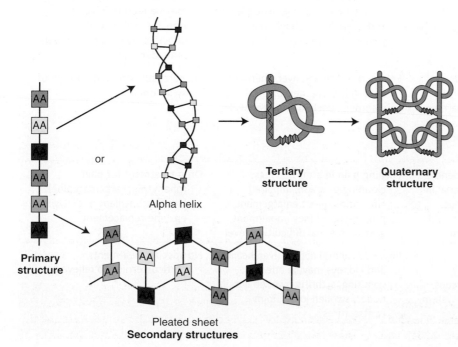

FIGURE 2.16 Structural arrangements of proteins. The primary structure consists of a chain of amino acids (AA), the secondary structure can be either an α helix or a β sheet, the tertiary structure has a globular shape, and the quaternary structure contains several different polypeptides forming a functional unit.

Lipids

Lipids are molecules that vary markedly in their chemical structures. With the exception of phospholipids they are hydrophobic and are soluble in organic solvents such as ether, acetone, chloroform, benzene, and alcohols. They consist of hydrocarbon chains and rings, as triglycerides, phospholipids, steroids, cholesterol, prostaglandins, or leukotrienes.

Triglycerides (fats and oils) consist of glycerol and fatty acid chains (neutral fats). At room temperature fats are solid whereas oils are liquid. Structurally a fatty acid has a tail portion, which is a long hydrocarbon chain, and a head portion that consists of a carboxyl group (COOH). The tails of the fatty acids are hydrophobic and the heads are hydrophilic. When the head portion of the fatty acid is attached to a glycerol molecule to form fat, the entire molecule becomes hydrophobic and therefore insoluble in water (Figure 2.17).

Depending on the absence or presence of double bonds between the carbon atoms of the fatty acid chains, the fats are called *saturated, monounsaturated,* or *polyunsaturated* (Figure 2.18). In animal fats the carbons of the fatty acid chains are all bonded by single covalent bonds, meaning that all carbons are bonded to the maximal number of hydrogens. Therefore, animal fats are saturated, closely packed together, and solid at room temperature. On the other hand, plant lipids are oils. They have some double bonds between the carbons, causing bends in the

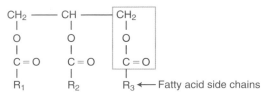

FIGURE 2.17 Triglycerides. The triglyceride molecule consists of glycerol and fatty acid side chains.

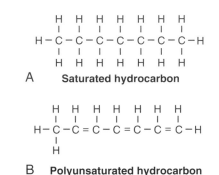

FIGURE 2.18 Saturated and unsaturated fats. A, Saturated fat with no double bonds within the carbon chain. **B,** Polyunsaturated fat with several double bonds within the carbon chain.

HEALTHCARE APPLICATION

Selected Lipid Storage Diseases

Disease	Cause	Symptoms	Treatment
Gaucher disease (three common clinical subtypes)	Glucocerebrosidase deficiency	Enlarged spleen and liver, liver malfunction, skeletal disorders, neurological complications, lymph node swelling, distended abdomen, low platelet count, yellow spots in eyes	Enzyme replacement; bone marrow transplant for nonneurological manifestations; splenectomy may be required; blood transfusion for anemia; no effective treatment for severe brain damage
Niemann-Pick disease (four categories)	Accumulation of fat and cholesterol in cells of the liver, spleen, bone marrow, lungs, and sometimes brain; inherited in an autosomal recessive pattern	Enlarged spleen and liver, cherry red spot in the eye, neurological disorders, decline of motor skills	No cure, supportive treatment of symptoms
Fabry disease	α-Galactosidase-A deficiency; buildup of fatty material in the autonomic nervous system, eyes, kidneys, and cardiovascular system	Burning pain in arms and legs, clouding of vision, impaired circulation, heart enlargement, progressive kidney impairment, gastrointestinal difficulties, fever	Drug treatment for pain (phenytoin, carbamazepine); kidney transplant or dialysis; enzyme replacement
Farber's disease	Ceramidase deficiency; accumulation of fatty material in joints, tissues, and central nervous system	Impaired mental ability; liver, heart, and kidneys may be affected; vomiting, arthritis, swollen lymph nodes, swollen joints, joint contractures	No specific treatment; corticosteroids to relieve pain

shape of the molecule. These oils are unsaturated fats and are liquid at room temperature.

Fats and oils are essential forms of energy storage. Animals convert excess sugars into fats if the glycogen storage capacity is reached. Although some seeds and fruits store energy as oil, most plants store excess sugars as starch. Fats can store over twice the amount of energy (9.3 kcal/g) than do carbohydrates (3.79 kcal/g).

Phospholipids consist of glycerol, two fatty acid chains, and a phosphate group at one end (Figure 2.19). These molecules are composed of polar (hydrophilic) heads and nonpolar (hydrophobic) tails. The fatty acid groups are hydrophobic whereas the phosphate group is hydrophilic. Phospholipids therefore have a water-soluble polar head and a nonpolar hydrophobic tail. Cell membranes, for example, are composed of a phospholipid bilayer with the tails facing toward each other and the heads facing outward, making their surfaces hydrophilic and their interior hydrophobic. This arrangement is the basis for their biological barrier properties.

Steroids (Figure 2.20) have a carbon skeleton consisting of four fused rings with various functional groups attached. Hundreds of different steroids have been found in plants, animals, and fungi. Categories are as follows:

- Anabolic steroids interact with androgen receptors to increase muscle and bone mass. Besides the naturally occurring anabolic steroids, synthetic ones exist that are used (sometimes illegally) by athletes in an attempt to enhance their performance.

- Sex steroids are responsible for the secondary sex characteristics of males and females. They include androgens, estrogens, and progesterones.
- Mineralocorticoids help maintain blood volume, electrolyte balance, and osmolarity by controlling the renal secretion of electrolytes.

LIFE APPLICATION

Hand Washing

Fatty acids are the main component of soap, an important emulsifying agent. An emulsifying agent is a substance that is soluble in both oil and water and enables both to mix. The tail portions of fatty acids are soluble in oil and their head portions are soluble in water. The heads emulsify the oil or oily dirt and wash it away.

Hand washing with soap and water is an essential hygiene practice to prevent the spread of disease. Dr. Ignaz Semmelweis first demonstrated in 1847 that routine hand washing can prevent the spread of hand-borne diseases (see Chapter 1, Scope of Microbiology). This was a landmark achievement in healthcare settings and for public health in general. Healthcare specialists now state that hand washing is the single most effective way to prevent the transmission of disease.

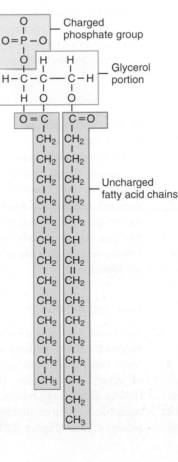

FIGURE 2.19 Phospholipid. A, Phospholipid bilayer as seen in plasma membranes. **B,** The phospholipid molecule is composed of a polar, hydrophilic head and a nonpolar, hydrophobic tail.

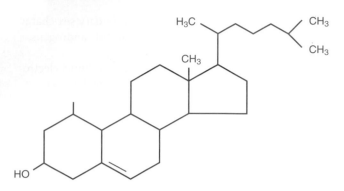

Cholesterol

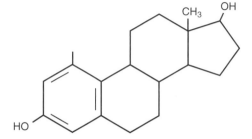

Estrogen

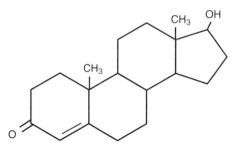

Testosterone

FIGURE 2.20 **Steroids.** Various steroid molecules are shown, all with four fused carbon rings but differing in their functional groups.

- Glucocorticoids play a role in many aspects of metabolism and in immune function. They are often prescribed to reduce inflammatory conditions.
- Phytosterols are a group of steroid alcohols that naturally occur in plants such as yeasts and fungi. Plants contain a wide range of phytosterols that are a structural component in their cell membrane and serve the same function as cholesterol does in animal cells. Ergosterol, a phytosterol, is also referred to as provitamin D_2. It is a biological precursor that is converted by ultraviolet irradiation into ergocalciferol, or vitamin D_2.

Cholesterol ($C_{27}H_{45}OH$) is a sterol, a combination of a steroid and an alcohol. Cholesterol plays a major role in many biochemical processes such as in the metabolism of fat-soluble vitamins (vitamins A, D, E, and K) and acts as a precursor for vitamin D. Cholesterol also is a precursor for the synthesis of

steroid hormones and is an important component of cell membranes.

Prostaglandins consist of a fatty acid and a cyclic hydrocarbon group. A variety of prostaglandins have been identified and all of them play different roles in a variety of tissues. Prostaglandins are called *local hormones* because they act as chemical messengers but do not move to other sites. They play a major role in a variety of body and cell regulatory processes, including involvement in defense mechanisms such as blood clotting and inflammation.

Nucleic Acids

The monomers of nucleic acids are nucleotides, containing the elements carbon, hydrogen, oxygen, nitrogen, and phosphorus. Main functions of nucleic acids include the following: storage of genetic information (DNA), directing protein synthesis (RNA), and energy transfers (ATP and NAD). Nucleotides are composed of three units: a pentose sugar, a phosphate, and nitrogen base (Figure 2.21). The nucleotide structure can be

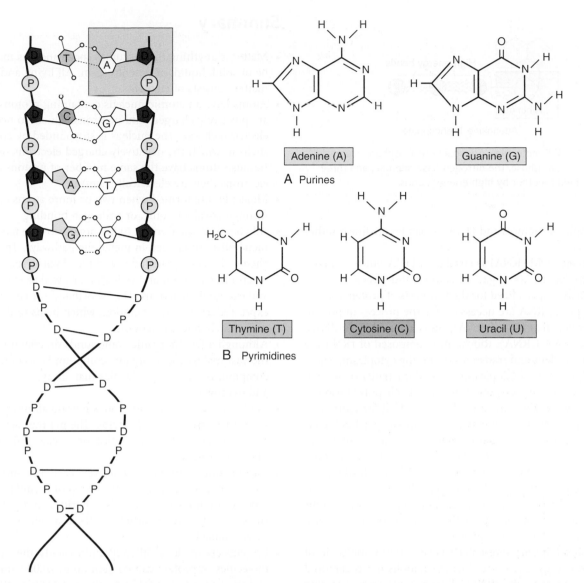

FIGURE 2.21 DNA molecule. Deoxyribonucleic acid (DNA) is composed of nucleotides, each of which consists of a phosphate, a pentose sugar (deoxyribose), and a nitrogen base (shaded area). The nitrogen bases of nucleic acids are either **(A)** purines or **(B)** pyrimidines.

broken down into two main functional parts: a sugar–phosphate backbone and the base. Individual nucleic acids are named according to the sugar they contain, a ribose (RNA) or a deoxyribose (DNA). Five possible nitrogen bases are subdivided into two main groups: purines with adenine (A) and guanine (G) that have a distinctive two-ring structure, and pyrimidines with cytosine (C), thymine (T), and uracil (U) with a single-ringed structure (see Figure 2.21). The bases in a nucleic acid polymer can form hydrogen bonds with the neighboring bases by a process called *complementary base pairing*. In DNA molecules, adenine always pairs with thymine and guanine with cytosine. In RNA molecules, thymine is replaced with uracil.

Deoxyribonucleic acid (DNA) is a nucleic acid with a double helix structure containing the sugar deoxyribose and 10 bases per turn (see Figure 2.21). DNA polymers can be thousands of bases long. DNA contains the genetic code and therefore serves for information storage. DNA is responsible for inherited characteristics, growth, and cell reproduction. It is

present in both prokaryotic and eukaryotic cells as well as in a group of viruses. DNA contains the information necessary for protein synthesis. The language of DNA, the genetic code, consists of four letters that represent the nitrogen bases, C, G, A, and T, used in three-letter "words" called *codons* to indicate the 20 naturally occurring amino acids. The combination of codons can create an infinite variety of "sentences." Each codon represents a specific amino acid and the combination of amino acids results in different polypeptides (see Table 3.6 in Chapter 3, Cell Structure and Function).

Chromosomes are the microscopic structures that carry DNA within the nucleus of cells. One chromosome represents a single molecule of DNA. In bacteria chromosomes with two types of DNA are present: the chromosomal DNA located in the nucleoid area and plasmids, which are simple circles of DNA floating feely in the organism. Plasmids are capable of autonomous replication and therefore can replicate independently of the chromosomal DNA. In eukaryotes the chromosomes are

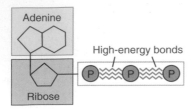

FIGURE 2.22 ATP molecule. Adenosine triphosphate is a nucleic acid with the sugar ribose, the nitrogen base adenine, and three phosphates held together by high-energy bonds.

highly complex structures and DNA molecules are linear rather than circular.

Ribonucleic acid (RNA) is similar to DNA but is a single-stranded molecule, its sugar is ribose, and uracil replaces thymine. RNA is specialized for the synthesis of proteins. Three different types of RNA are necessary for the process of protein synthesis: ribosomal RNA (rRNA), messenger RNA (mRNA), and transfer RNA (tRNA). Ribosomes composed of rRNA are made in the nucleus and transported into the cytoplasm, where they attach to rough endoplasmic reticulum (rER) or remain free in the cytoplasm as polyribosomes. Both polyribosomes and ribosomes on the rER (see Chapter 3, Cell Structure and Function) are sites of protein synthesis. Messenger RNA contains genetic information that encodes the sequence of amino acids in proteins. Base triplets, referred to as codons, direct the amino acid sequence in a polypeptide chain. The third type of RNA, tRNA, contains a triplet of nitrogen bases called the *anti-codon*. Anticodons contain complementary bases to the codons on mRNA, and are necessary for the synthesis of polypeptides (see Protein Synthesis in Chapter 3).

Adenosine triphosphate (ATP) is the energy molecule of cells. When energy is released during catabolism it is captured in the high-energy bonds of ATP (Figure 2-22). In transferring energy to other molecules, ATP loses one or two of its phosphate groups, resulting in adenosine diphosphate (ADP) or adenosine monophosphate (AMP). This is an exergonic reaction. Both ADP and AMP can be converted back to ATP by photosynthesis or through chemical energy during anabolism. Photosynthetic microorganisms use sunlight as an energy source during their anabolism. Microorganisms that need nutrient molecules for ATP production are called *chemotrophs* and the ones utilizing sunlight for energy are called *phototrophs* (see Chapter 6, Bacteria and Archaea).

Summary

- Matter is anything that occupies space and has mass. It can be in solid, liquid, or gaseous form. All living and nonliving matter consists of elements.
- Atoms have an atomic nucleus containing protons, which are positively charged, and neutrons, which do not have an electrical charge. The nucleus is surrounded by concentric shells in which the negatively charged electrons reside. Because atoms have the same number of protons and electrons they are electrically neutral.
- Molecules are formed when two or more atoms combine through covalent, ionic, or hydrogen bonding.
- All chemical reactions in living organisms are part of metabolism organized in metabolic pathways. These chemical reactions include synthesis, hydrolysis, exchange reactions, oxidation and reduction, as well as endergonic and exergonic reactions. The "shorthand" of chemistry is expressed as chemical notation, which helps to describe the different chemical reactions.
- Although a few inorganic compounds do contain carbon, the vast majority of inorganic compounds do not. Organic compounds are large molecules that always contain carbon and hydrogen.
- Acids, bases, buffers, salts, and water are all inorganic molecules essential to life forms. The pH measures the acidity or alkalinity of a solution on a scale of 0 to 14, with pH 7 set as neutral.
- Carbohydrates store carbon as well as energy and provide part of cellular structures. This group of organic molecules includes monosaccharides, disaccharides, and polysaccharides. Bacteria prefer carbohydrates as an energy source when available.
- Proteins are made of different amino acids, their unit molecules. A protein can contain up to 10,000 amino acids and its sequence and folding pattern determine the shape, which in turn determines the function of the protein.
- The categories of lipids are triglycerides, phospholipids, steroids, cholesterol, and prostaglandins. Functionally, fats provide and store energy, are part of the cell membrane, and play a regulatory role as hormones.
- The monomers of nucleic acids are nucleotides, which consist of a phosphate, a sugar, and a nitrogen base. The functions of nucleic acids include genetic information storage (DNA), protein synthesis (RNA), and energy transfers (ATP and NAD).

Review Questions

1. The atomic number equals the number of:
   a. Protons
   b. Neutrons
   c. Electrons
   d. Protons and neutrons

2. A chemical bond in which electrons are equally shared is a(n):
   a. Ionic bond
   b. Polar covalent bond
   c. Nonpolar covalent bond
   d. Hydrogen bond

3. The bond between water molecules is a(n):
   a. Ionic bond
   b. Polar covalent bond
   c. Nonpolar covalent bond
   d. Hydrogen bond

4. The outermost shell of an atom can hold up to _____ electrons.
   a. 2
   b. 6
   c. 8
   d. 10

5. The bond between sodium and chlorine atoms in sodium chloride is a(n):
   a. Hydrogen bond
   b. Ionic bond
   c. Polar covalent bond
   d. Nonpolar covalent bond

6. Sucrose is composed of:
   a. Glucose and galactose
   b. Glucose and fructose
   c. Fructose and maltose
   d. Glucose and maltose

7. The unit molecules (monomers) of carbohydrates are:
   a. Monosaccharides
   b. Amino acids
   c. Nucleic acids
   d. Fatty acids

8. The bond between amino acids is a(n):
   a. Ionic bond
   b. Peptide bond
   c. Hydrogen bond
   d. Covalent bond

9. The RNA nucleotide base that pairs with adenine of DNA is:
   a. Cytosine
   b. Guanine
   c. Thymine
   d. Uracil

10. Glucose and fructose are examples of:
    a. Monosaccharides
    b. Disaccharides
    c. Polysaccharides
    d. Lipids

11. Neutrons are particles with a(n) _____ charge.

12. An atom with the same number of protons but a different number of neutrons is called a(n) _____.

13. A positively charged ion is a(n) _____.

14. The breakdown of large molecules into smaller ones in the presence of water is called _____.

15. Molecules that can absorb hydrogen ions are _____.

16. From the strongest to weakest, name and describe the different types of chemical bonds.

17. Describe anabolism and catabolism.

18. Name and describe the functions of proteins.

19. Compare and contrast saturated and unsaturated fats.

20. Describe complementary base pairing and compare DNA and RNA.

Bibliography

Bauman R: *Microbiology: With Diseases by Taxonomy*, ed 2, 2007, Benjamin Cummings/Pearson Education, San Francisco.

Garrity G: Bergey's Manual of Systematic Bacteriology, Vols. 1–5, New York, 2005, Springer.

Madigan MT, Martinko JM, Dunlap PV, et al: *Brock Biology of Microorganisms*, ed 12, 2009, Benjamin Cummings/Pearson Education, San Francisco.

Fox SI: *Human Physiology*, 2005, McGraw-Hill, New York.

Meisenberg G, Simmons W: *Principles of Medical Biochemistry*, St. Louis, 2006, Mosby/Elsevier.

Talaro KP: *Foundations in Microbiology*, ed 6, 2006, McGraw-Hill, New York.

Thibodeau GA, Patton KT: *Anatomy and Physiology*, St. Louis, 2007, Mosby/Elsevier.

Internet Resources

Wikipedia, http://www.wikipedia.org/

National Gaucher Foundation, http://www.gaucherdisease.org/

National Institute of Neurologic Disorders and Stroke, Lipid Storage Diseases Fact Sheet, http://www.ninds.nih.gov/disorders/lipid_storage_diseases/detail_lipid_storage_diseases.htm

Fabry Support & Information Group (FSIG), http://www.fabry.org/FSIG.nsf/Pages/Fabry

3

Cell Structure and Function

OUTLINE

General Structure of Prokaryotic and Eukaryotic Cells
Plasma Membrane and Cell Wall
Surface Appendages
Biofilms
Cytoplasm, Cytoskeleton, Cell Organelles, and Inclusions

Fluid Compartments and Membrane Transport Mechanisms
Intracellular Fluid Compartment
Extracellular Fluid Compartment
Passive Transport
Active Transport

Cellular Metabolism
Enzymes
Cellular Respiration and Photosynthesis
Protein Synthesis

DNA Replication and Cell Division
DNA Replication
Cell Division

LEARNING OBJECTIVES

After reading this chapter, the student will be able to:
- Describe the structure of prokaryotic and eukaryotic cells, and identify their differences
- Describe the structure of gram-positive and gram-negative cell walls and explain their differences
- Explain the formation of biofilms and discuss their importance in healthcare
- Differentiate between the extracellular and intracellular fluid compartments
- Name and describe the different membrane transport mechanisms across a cell membrane
- Describe the structure and function of enzymes, and factors influencing enzyme activity
- Describe aerobic and anaerobic cellular respiration, fermentation, and photosynthesis
- Explain the processes of transcription and translation, and the role of RNA during protein synthesis

- Describe the mechanisms of DNA replication
- Describe the different stages of the cell cycle and list the events that occur in the different stages of mitosis
- Describe meiosis and discuss its importance in sexual reproduction

KEY TERMS

active site
active transport
aerobic cellular
    respiration
affinity
algae
allosteric site
amphitrichous
anabolism
anaerobic cellular
    respiration
anticodon
apoenzyme
archaea
binary fission
biofilm
catabolism
cell organelles
cellular respiration
central dogma
chemotrophs
chloroplast
coenzymes
cofactors
competition
competitive enzyme
    inhibition
cytoplasm
cytoskeleton
cytosol
diffusion
electron transport chain
endocytosis

endoenzymes
enzymes
exocytosis
exoenzymes
fermentation
fimbriae
first law of
    thermodynamics
flagella
fluid compartments
fluid-mosaic
fungi
G_1 phase
G_2 phase
glycocalyx
glycolysis
gram-negative bacteria
gram-positive bacteria
helicase
holoenzymes
hydrolases
inclusions
integral proteins
irreversible inhibition
isomerases
Krebs cycle
ligases
light-dependent reaction
light-independent
    reactions
lophotrichous
lyases
meiosis

mitosis
monotrichous
motility
noncompetitive
    inhibition
nuclear envelope
osmosis
oxidoreductases
passive transport
peptidoglycan
peripheral proteins
peritrichous
phagocytosis
phosphogluconate
    pathway
photosynthesis
phototrophs
pili
pinocytosis
plant
plasma membrane
primer RNA
promoter
receptor-mediated
    endocytosis
saturated
specific protein carrier
S phase
stroma
taxis
terminator sequence
thylakoid membranes
transferases

WHY YOU NEED TO KNOW

HISTORY

Aristotle (384–322 bce), Paracelsus (1493–1541), and other ancient scientists and philosophers realized the existence of a continuity in the macroscopic parts of plants and animals. They observed structures that kept repeating themselves from animal to animal, from plant to plant, and from generation to generation. Centuries later with the advent of magnifying lenses and compound microscopes built by Robert Hooke (1635–1703) and Jan Swammerdam (1637–1680), descriptions of objects magnified ×20–×30 were possible. Then van Leeuwenhoek (1632–1723), using his skills at lens grinding and the use of light, improved the resolving powers of the microscope to ×200. In his letters to the newly formed

Royal Society of London, he described "very little living animalcules very prettily a-moving" in samples taken from his own and other mouths. These are among the first descriptions of living bacteria. Other firsts for van Leeuwenhoek with his microscopic observations were the discovery of blood cells; the circulation in the capillaries of eels; and the first observations of living animal sperm cells, nematodes, and rotifers to mention a few. Later, Claude Bernard (1813–1878) described the cell as the primary representative of life. The cell is the basic unit of life, whether in single-unit organisms, as in protozoa, or in multicellular organisms, where cells group and differentiate into tissues and organs.

Continued

IMPACT

The arrival of the concept of functions for these microscopic structures marks the beginning of the study of the cell as an independent unit—cytology with its subsequent disciplines such as cytochemistry and cytogenetics. Moreover, the integrity of a cell as a functional unit becomes essential because if disease or physical disruption occurs to severely compromise or destroy it, the cell dies even though some of its functions such as enzyme activity remain. This persistence of cellular function allows the study of cellular contents from cell-free preparations in which cellular integrity is intentionally compromised. Moreover, the cell changes in response to its environment and the demands for its products. It is a chemical factory, the output or products of which are essential not only for the tissue and organism, but for the maintenance and repair of the cell itself. The cell doctrine—life exists in cellular form whether singular or multicellular; each cell can exist on its own; and all cells come from preexisting cells—guides scientific exploration of the role of cells in living organisms. Science is dependent on advances in technology to afford new ways of looking at new and at old persistent problems.

FUTURE

One of the recent developments in science focuses on progenitor pluripotent cells that differentiate to form the tissues of the human body. Embryonic stem cells form along the inside of blastocysts and create an inner cell mass during growth of the embryo. After being harvested, they grow on a layer of feeder cells in a culture medium. Potentially, these cells can develop into muscle, pancreatic, hepatic, nerve, and practically any other cell line. Uses of these new discoveries include replacement of tissues damaged, diseased, infected, maldeveloped, or otherwise undesirable and development of antimicrobial and other drugs. Because it is an entirely new and untested area of exploration, there is the potential for unknown consequences, which makes their use controversial. The understanding of cell structure and function is essential for human survival. Microorganisms, small though they are, can easily destroy human life. If science can proceed rationally with adequate suitable controls and limits, then as always, the future is bright. Without these qualifications the future, as always, may hold many problems.

General Structure of Prokaryotic and Eukaryotic Cells

Cells are the basic structural and functional unit of all living organisms. The name *cell* comes from the Latin word "cella," a small room. Robert Hooke (see Chapter 1, Scope of Microbiology) selected this term in 1655, when he discovered cells in a piece of cork with his microscope, and compared the cork cells with small rooms. In 1838, Schleiden and Schwann proposed a formal cell theory, or cell doctrine, that marked the start of modern cell biology. The current cell theory states:

- The cell is the smallest form of life.
- All life forms are composed of one or more cells.
- All cells come from preexisting cells.

The major events leading to the knowledge of cell biology today are shown in Table 3.1.

Two different types of cells exist, prokaryotes and eukaryotes, which are structurally and functionally different from one another (Table 3.2). However, both cell types share certain properties, and these are as follows:

- Methods of reproduction—cell division, **binary fission,** mitosis, or meiosis
- The presence of DNA and RNA for protein synthesis
- Cellular metabolism organized in specific metabolic pathways

- Response to external and internal stimuli (changes in temperature, pH, and nutrient levels)
- Plasma (cell) membranes

Plasma Membrane and Cell Wall

In order to survive, all living cells need to be protected from the continuous changes of their surrounding environment. This is achieved by the **plasma membrane** and in some types of cells by an additional structure, a cell wall.

Plasma Membrane

All living cells, both prokaryotes and eukaryotes, are surrounded by a plasma membrane, about 8 nm (nanometer) thick, creating an intracellular and extracellular environment/compartment. The intracellular and extracellular **fluid compartments** (ICF and ECF, respectively) are aqueous and the plasma membrane provides the barrier between them. The membrane is composed primarily of phospholipids and proteins. Phospholipids are polar molecules with a polar (hydrophilic) head and a nonpolar (hydrophobic) tail (see Chapter 2, Chemistry of Life). Because the environment on each side of the plasma membrane is aqueous, the hydrophobic tails face each other and the hydrophilic heads are exposed to water on both surfaces of the membrane. This results in the formation of a phospholipid bilayer, illustrated in Figure 3.1.

Embedded in the phospholipid bilayer are peripheral and integral (transmembrane) proteins and cholesterol. The **peripheral proteins** are partially embedded on one side of the membrane, whereas **integral proteins** extend from one side through the membrane to the other side. Although the specific lipid and

TABLE 3.1 Major Events in Cell Biology

Year	Name	Event
1655	Robert Hooke	Observes cells of a cork
1674	Antony van Leeuwenhoek	Discovers protozoans
1683	Antony van Leeuwenhoek	Discovers bacteria
1838	Schleiden and Schwann	Propose the cell theory
1855	Carl Naegeli and Carl Cramer	Describe the cell membrane as a barrier essential to explain osmosis
1857	Rudolph Albert von Kölliker	Discovers mitochondria in muscle cells and describes them as conspicuous granules aligned between the striated myofibrils of muscle
1890	Richard Altman	Develops mitochondrial stain and postulates genetic autonomy
1898	Carl Benda	Develops crystal violet as mitochondria-specific stain and coins the name
1882	Robert Koch	Identifies tuberculosis- and cholera-causing bacteria with aniline dyes
1898	Camillo Golgi	Discovers the Golgi apparatus with a silver nitrate stain (Golgi stain)
1931	Ernst Ruska	Builds the first transmission electron microscope
1965	Cambridge Instrument Company	First commercial scanning electron microscope
1997	Roslin Institute, Scotland	Sheep cloned

TABLE 3.2 Comparison of Prokaryotic and Eukaryotic Cells

Characteristic	Prokaryotic Cell	Human Eukaryotic Cell
Size	0.2–60 µm	5–100 µm
Chromosome	One	Multiple
Cell membrane	Yes	Yes
Cell wall	Yes	Yes (prokaryotes) No (eukaryotes)
Nucleus	No	Yes (except red blood cells)
Nucleoid area	Yes	No
Mitochondria	No	Yes
Endoplasmic reticulum	No	Yes
Golgi apparatus	No	Yes
Cytoskeleton	No	Yes
Ribosome	70S	80S
Mode of reproduction	Asexual	Asexual and sexual

protein components vary in different membranes, the basic structure and composition of the plasma membrane are the same, as are those membranes that surround cell organelles. Because the plasma membrane is not solid, its components are freely movable, presenting a constantly changing **fluid-mosaic** membrane structure (see Figure 3.1, *A*).

Whereas the phospholipids are the main lipid component of the cell membrane, cholesterol is another major cellular membrane lipid and the amount varies with the type of plasma membrane. For example, the plasma membrane of animal cells contains almost one cholesterol molecule per phospholipid molecule, plant cells contain much less, and prokaryotic cells have no cholesterol but instead contain sterol-like molecules called *hopanoids*. Cholesterol and hopanoids (pentacyclic sterol–like compounds) immobilize the first few hydrocarbon groups of the phospholipid molecules. This makes the lipid bilayer less elastic and decreases permeability to small water-soluble molecules.

Glycolipids, also a component of membranes, project into the extracellular space. Functionally, these may protect, insulate, and serve as receptor-binding sites. In addition, the outer membrane of gram-negative cell walls (see Chapter 6, Bacteria and Archaea) contains lipopolysaccharide bacterial endotoxins that are released on lysis of these cells.

The functions of membrane proteins differ depending on their composition and location in the plasma membrane. They can:

- Provide structural support
- Transport molecules across the membrane
- Act as enzyme regulators to control chemical reactions
- Act as specific receptors for hormones and other regulatory substances
- Act as surface antigens (see Chapter 20, The Immune System)

Glycocalyx

Many cells have a matrix formed outside the plasma membrane. This extracellular fabric is composed of polymeric material called a **glycocalyx,** produced by some bacteria, epithelia, and other cells. In general the glycocalyx is a network of polysaccharides that project from the cellular surface and functions in/as:

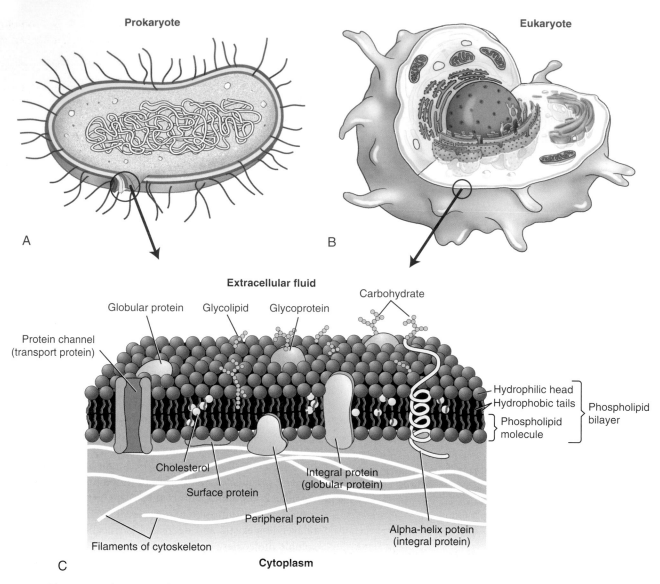

FIGURE 3.1 Plasma membrane. Both prokaryotic cells **(A)** and eukaryotic cells **(B)** are surrounded by a plasma membrane **(C)** composed of a phospholipid bilayer, cholesterol, proteins, and carbohydrates.

MEDICAL HIGHLIGHTS

Endotoxin Shock

Endotoxins located within the gram-negative cell wall are released when the cell lyses, either due to an immune response or due to the action of antibiotics. Endotoxin shock is generally associated with a systemic spread of gram-negative bacteria, in which the massive release of endotoxins acting as pyrogens (see the section on fever in Chapter 20, The Immune System) causes systemic inflammatory reactions that may have serious, life-threatening consequences.

- Cell-to-cell communication
- Interaction with other extracellular matrix
- Anchoring of cells to the extracellular matrix
- Protection from pathogens
- Modulation of the immune responses
- Attachment site for bacteria to inert surfaces (formation of biofilms)

In the case of bacteria the glycocalyx is a coating of macromolecules that protects the cell and sometimes helps the bacteria to adhere to its environment. The chemical composition, thickness, and organization of the glycocalyx differ among bacteria. One specialized function of the bacterial glycocalyx is the formation of capsules (Figure 3.2). Capsules protect pathogens, such as *Streptococcus pneumoniae* and *Bacillus anthracis,* from phagocytosis by white blood cells, thus adding to their pathogenicity.

Cell Wall

A cell wall is located immediately below the glycocalyx surrounding the plasma membranes. Bacteria, archaea, fungi, plants, and algae can all have cell walls of different chemical composition. The purpose of the cell wall is to maintain the shape of a cell and to protect the cell from any physical or chemical damage.

The bacterial cell wall is a unique rigid structure that maintains the shape of bacteria and protects them from hostile environments, including protection from the immune system of a host (see Chapter 20, The Immune System). The strength of the cell wall is due to the presence of **peptidoglycan** (mucopeptide or murein), a mixed polymer of hexose sugars (*N*-acetylglucosamine and *N*-acetylmuramic acid) cross-linked by short peptide fragments (Figure 3.3). The amount and composition of peptidoglycan vary among the major bacterial groups and provide

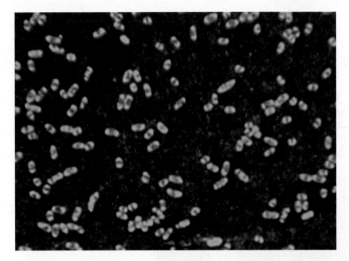

FIGURE 3.2 Glycocalyx. This micrograph shows the bacterial capsule surrounding *Klebsiella pneumoniae*.

the basis for Gram staining (see Chapter 4, Microbiological Laboratory Techniques), dividing bacteria into so-called *gram-positive* and *gram-negative* organisms.

However, some bacteria do not have a characteristic cell wall structure and some lack a cell wall altogether (i.e., *Mycobacterium;* see Chapter 6, Bacteria and Archaea). Differences in cell wall composition are an important consideration in the selection of antimicrobial drugs in treatment regimens of bacterial diseases. The cell wall structure is also important in choosing specific methods to control microbial growth in a variety of environments (see Chapter 19, Physical and Chemical Methods of Control).

Characteristics of cell walls in the different microorganisms are as follows:

Gram-positive bacteria have a thick peptidoglycan layer (20–80 nm) located external to the cell membrane (Figure 3.4, *A*). It also contains acidic polysaccharides such as teichoic acid and lipoteichoic acid, which aid in cell wall maintenance and contribute to an acidic cell surface. The small space between the plasma membrane and the cell wall is the periplasmic space, which can be minimal in some of the gram-positive bacteria.

Gram-negative bacteria have a thin (5- to 10-nm) peptidoglycan layer that is more complex because it has an outer membrane that provides a cover that is anchored to the lipoprotein molecules of the peptidoglycan layer (Figure 3.4, *B*). The outer membrane is similar in structure to the plasma membrane, but it contains lipopolysaccharides extending from its surface. These lipopolysaccharides can function as receptors or as antigens. In addition, the membrane contains porin proteins, which allow penetration only of small molecules. This serves as a defense mechanism against larger molecules such as antibiotics. The periplasmic space between the plasma membrane and the outer membrane may constitute up to 40% of the total cell volume. This space houses biochemical pathways for nutrient acquisition, peptidoglycan synthesis, electron transport, and detoxification of substances otherwise harmful to the cell.

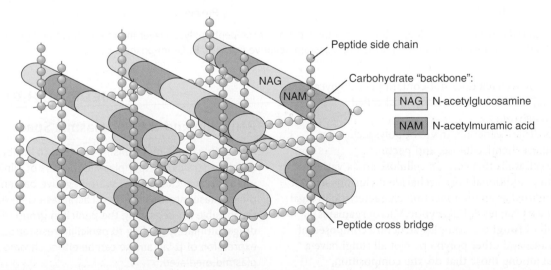

FIGURE 3.3 Structure of peptidoglycan. Peptidoglycan is composed of *N*-acetylglucosamine (NAG) and *N*-acetylmuramic acid (NAM) chains linked by peptide cross-bridges and peptide side chains to form a relatively rigid structure. The amount and exact composition of peptidoglycan vary among bacterial species.

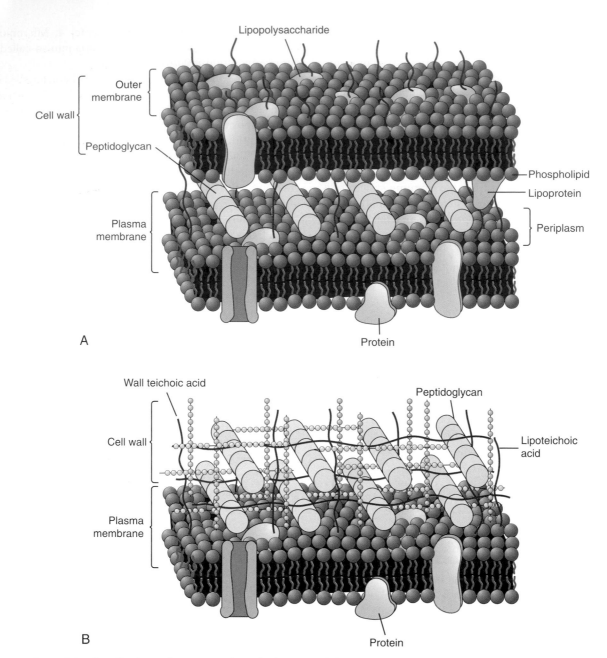

FIGURE 3.4 Bacterial cell wall. These illustrations show the location of the peptidoglycan layer in gram-positive and gram-negative cell walls along with other features unique to their structure. **A,** Gram-negative cell wall. **B,** Gram-positive cell wall.

- The cell wall of **archaea** does not contain peptidoglycan, but some may contain a similar chemical called *pseudopeptidoglycan*.
- **Plant** cell walls are generally made of polysaccharides, mostly cellulose, hemicellulose, and pectin.
- **Algae** have cell walls that contain cellulose and a variety of glycoproteins. Additional polysaccharide inclusions in their cell walls are used as an identification characteristic in algal taxonomy (see Chapter 8, Eukaryotic Microorganisms).
- The cell wall of **fungi** is a complex structure composed of chitin, glucans, and other polymers. Not all fungi have a cell wall but among those that do, the composition, properties, and form of it change during the cell cycle and during growth conditions (see Chapter 8, Eukaryotic Microorganisms).

MEDICAL HIGHLIGHTS

Penicillin and the Periplasmic Space

Although various mechanisms can lead to antibiotic-resistant strains, the periplasmic space is of clinical importance because some gram-negative bacteria secrete β-lactamase into this space. β-Lactamase is an enzyme responsible for degrading the penicillin group of antibiotic drugs, ultimately leading to penicillin resistance. The expression of β-lactamase can be either chromosomal or plasmid-mediated.

Surface Appendages

Surface appendages are present in both prokaryotic and eukaryotic cells. Prokaryotic cells can have pili (fimbriae) and **flagella,** whereas cilia, flagella, and microvilli are common in eukaryotic cells. The functions of surface appendages include motility, attachment, absorption, and sensory capacity (Table 3.3).

Bacterial Flagella

Bacterial flagella are long (3 to 12 micrometers [μm]) helical filaments about 12 to 30 nm in diameter, which they use for movement in their environment. The protein components are flagellins and are assembled to form a cylindrical structure with a hollow core. A flagellum consists of three parts (Figure 3.5):

- A long filament, which lies external to the cell surface
- A hook located at the end of the filament; and
- A basal body to which the hook is anchored; the basal body consists of a rod and one or two pairs of disks

Flagellins are immunogenic and represent a group of antigens called the *H antigens*. These antigens are characteristic of a species, strain, or variant of an organism. The species specificity of the flagellins is the result of differences in the primary structures of the proteins (see Chapter 2, Chemistry of Life). The flagella may be present at the poles of the cells as a single polar structure at one end of the bacterium (**monotrichous**), or at each end (**amphitrichous**). Flagella also may be present in tufts at one or both ends of the organism, in which case such

---

TABLE 3.3 Surface Appendages of Prokaryotic and Eukaryotic Cells

Surface Appendage	Cell Type	Composition	Function
Flagella	Eukaryotic cell	Nine pairs of peripheral microtubules made of protein tubulin + two central microtubules	Motility through whiplike action
	Prokaryotic cell	Single microtubule composed of flagellin subunits arranged in a helical formation around a hollow core	Motility through propeller-like rotation
Pili	Prokaryotic cell	Pilin proteins helically arranged around a hollow core. Similar to flagella but shorter and more rigid	Adhesion (fimbriae) Twitching motility across solid surface Conjugation (sex pili)
Cilia	Eukaryotic cell	Similar arrangement to flagella but much shorter	Motility Movement of fluid over cell surface Sensory
Microvilli	Eukaryotic cell	Extensions of the plasma membrane	Absorption Secretion Adhesion Motility

---

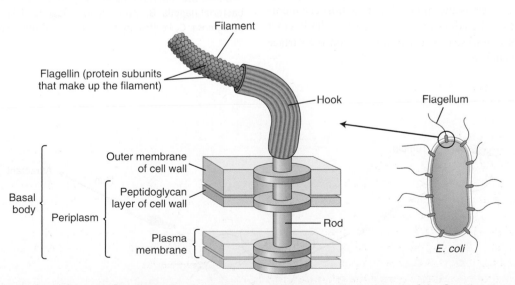

FIGURE 3.5 Structure of a prokaryotic flagellum. The illustration shows the parts and attachment of the flagellum in a gram-negative bacterium.

organisms are **lophotrichous.** If the flagella are distributed over the general cell surface, they are **peritrichous** (Figure 3.6).

Bacterial Mobility

The thrust by which the flagella propel the bacterial cell is produced by either clockwise or counterclockwise rotation of the basal body driven by energy from a proton-motive force rather than directly from adenosine-5′-triphosphate (ATP). Bacterial flagella do not rotate at a constant speed; the speed of rotation depends on the cell's generation of energy. Bacteria can change speed and direction of their flagellar movements and as a result are capable of various patterns of **motility.** Movements are referred to as runs (swims) or tumbles. A bacterium moving in one direction for a period of time is said to run, and when the direction changes the bacterium tumbles (Figure 3.7). Any movement of bacteria toward or away from a particular stimulus is called **taxis.** As bacteria run, they may show properties of chemotaxis (response to chemical stimuli) or phototaxis (response to light). Both require sophisticated sensory receptors located in the cell surface and periplasm.

Not all prokaryotes have flagella, but some are still capable of movement by the process of gliding. In general, gliding prokaryotes are filamentous or rod shaped in contact with a solid surface (e.g., filamentous cyanobacteria).

Pili

Pili (fimbriae) are another form of bacterial surface projection (Figure 3.8) and are more rigid than flagella. They are composed of pilin proteins. In some organisms, such as *Shigella* species and *Escherichia coli,* as many as 200 pili are distributed over a single cell surface. Pili come in two types: short, abundant common pili, and a smaller number (one to six) of very long sex pili. Sex pili attach male to female bacteria during conjugation. Pili of many enteric bacteria have adhesive properties that can attach to various epithelial surfaces and to surfaces of yeast and fungal cells. These adhesive properties of piliated bacteria play an important role as factors in the colonization of epithelial surfaces. Adhesion to host cells is dependent on specific interactions between the adhesins and molecules in the host cell membranes. For example, the adhesins of *E. coli* chemically interact with molecules of mannose (a sugar monomer) on the surface of intestinal epithelial cells.

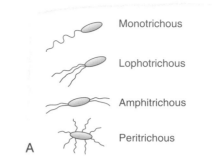

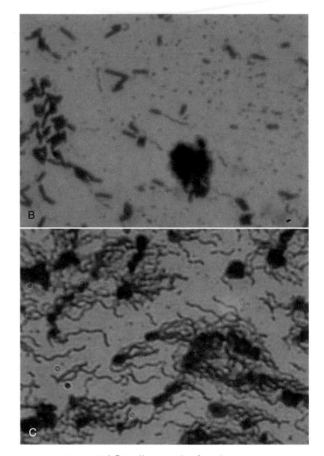

FIGURE 3.6 Bacterial flagella. A, The four basic arrangements of bacterial flagella. **B,** Monotrichous flagella of *Pseudomonas aeruginosa.* **C,** Peritrichous flagella of a *Proteus* sp.

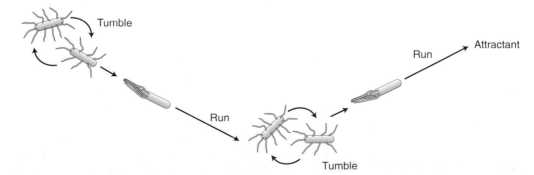

FIGURE 3.7 Bacterial movements. Bacteria can move toward or away from a stimulus by runs (swims) and tumbles.

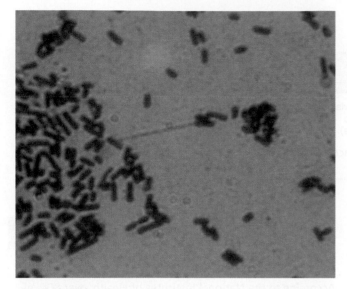

FIGURE 3.8 Pili. Conjugative pilus between two *Escherichia coli* bacteria.

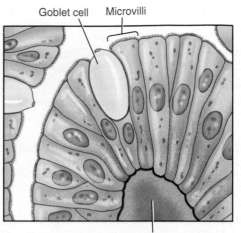

FIGURE 3.10 Microvilli. This drawing shows microvilli lining the apical surface of intestinal epithelial cells. Functionally these microvilli are responsible for absorption of materials from the intestinal lumen.

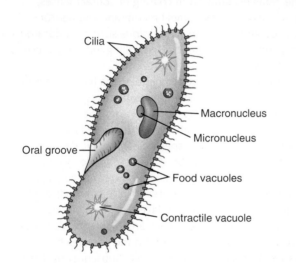

FIGURE 3.9 Eukaryotic flagella lining the plasma membrane of a paramecium.

Cilia

Cilia and eukaryotic flagella are structurally identical hairlike appendages, about 0.25 μm in diameter, made from microtubules (Figure 3.9). They are motile and either move the cell or move substances over or around the cell. Protozoans use cilia to collect food particles and for locomotion (see Chapter 8, Eukaryotic Microorganisms). The primary action of cilia in most animal species is to move fluid, mucus, or cells over their surface. The major difference between cilia and eukaryotic flagella is their length, which is much greater for flagella. Cilia can either be motile, constantly beating in one direction, or nonmotile, nonbeating sensors. Motile cilia rarely occur singly and they are usually present in large numbers on cell surfaces, beating in coordinated waves. Nonmotile cilia, on the other hand, generally are single structures per cell.

Microvilli

Microvilli are plasma membrane extensions on the surface of eukaryotic cells. Most often they occur in groups on the surface of absorptive and secretory epithelial cells such as in the kidney and intestine (Figure 3.10). They are approximately 0.08 μm in diameter, 1 μm long, and greatly increase the surface area of cells to facilitate absorption and secretion. Microvilli can also be found on the surface of white blood cells, where they aid in the migration of the cells.

Biofilms

A **biofilm** is a microbial community enclosed by an extracellular, mostly polysaccharide polymeric matrix (Figure 3.11). Noncellular materials such as mineral crystals, corrosive particles, blood, and other substances can also be found in the biofilm matrix. The kind of inclusions depends on the environment where a biofilm develops. Biofilms develop when free-floating microorganisms attach to a surface. The first colony initially adheres to a given surface by van der Waals forces (see Chapter 2, Chemistry of Life). If not immediately separated from that surface, the organisms can anchor themselves more permanently via adhesion molecules such as pili. Once adhered these microbes then provide various adhesion sites for other new incoming cells, resulting in the building of a matrix that holds the biofilm together. Microbial species that cannot attach to certain surfaces on their own can often attach to the biofilm matrix or to earlier colonized organisms. The biofilm then grows through a combination of cell division and recruitment. The cells on the surface of the biofilm are different from the ones within the matrix and the behavior of the embedded cells may change within the thickness of the biofilm.

Biofilms can form on a wide variety of surfaces including living tissues, indwelling medical devices and catheters, industrial or clean water system piping, natural aquatic systems, and

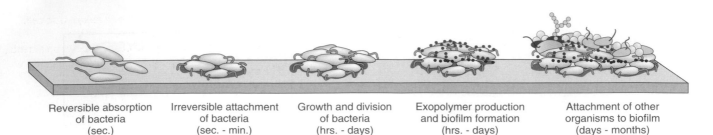

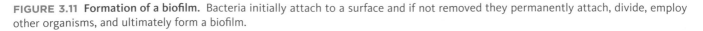

| Reversible absorption of bacteria (sec.) | Irreversible attachment of bacteria (sec. - min.) | Growth and division of bacteria (hrs. - days) | Exopolymer production and biofilm formation (hrs. - days) | Attachment of other organisms to biofilm (days - months) |

FIGURE 3.11 Formation of a biofilm. Bacteria initially attach to a surface and if not removed they permanently attach, divide, employ other organisms, and ultimately form a biofilm.

rocks and pebbles, and on the surface of stagnant pools of water. Moreover, biofilms are important components of the food chains formed by the living matter of rivers and streams.

Microbial biofilms can cause equipment damage and therefore can be the source of product contamination and microbial infections. They do represent a concern in the food industry because they can arise from raw materials, surfaces, people, animals, and even the air. Once food or a surface in a food-processing plant is contaminated, microbial colonies and eventually biofilms can form. Cleaning materials commercially used to clean countertops will kill planktonic or single cells of bacteria, but might be unable to penetrate a biofilm. For example, chlorination of a biofilm is often unsuccessful because the agent only affects the outer layers, whereas the inner layers of the biofilm remain healthy and are able to reestablish the biofilm.

Biofilms also provide an ideal environment for the exchange of plasmids (extrachromosomal bacterial DNA; see Chapter 6). Certain plasmids encode resistance to antimicrobial agents and their inclusion within a biofilm provides an opportunity to promote and spread bacterial resistance to antimicrobial agents. Repeated use of antimicrobial agents actually increases the possibility of resistance to biocides (see Chapter 19, Physical and Chemical Methods of Control).

On the other hand, microbial processes at the surface of the biofilms can give opportunities for positive industrial and environmental effects. Biofilms can be used in:

- Bioremediation of contaminated soil and water
- Vapor-phase biofilters to prevent industrial air pollution
- Wastewater treatment and other new developing uses

Research investigations exploring new uses for biofilm processes now include scientists from a variety of disciplines such as engineers, microbiologists, biochemists, computer scientists, statisticians, and physicists, to mention a few.

Cytoplasm, Cytoskeleton, Cell Organelles, and Inclusions

Other than a plasma membrane, cell wall, appendages, and glycocalyx, all of which play a specific role in the functioning and protection of cells, specific chemical processes (metabolism) occur within the cell. All metabolic processes in a cell are aided either by cell organelles or other structures and chemicals within the matrix of a cell.

Cytoplasm

The **cytoplasm** is a dense, gelatinous matrix composed of 70% to 80% water, located within the plasma membrane. It is the place for biochemical activities and therefore contains complex mixtures of sugars, amino acids, lipids, nucleic acids, and salts. The cytoplasm also holds a variety of **cell organelles** and different **inclusions** all embedded in the fluidlike **cytosol.** With the light microscope, the cytoplasm appears to be a homogeneous solution; however, electron microscopy reveals the cytoskele-

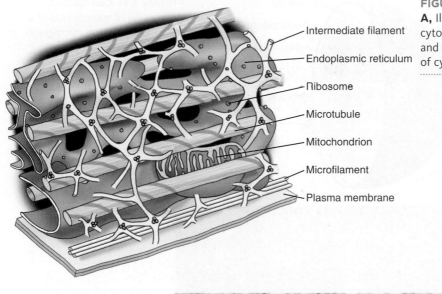

Intermediate filament
Endoplasmic reticulum
Ribosome
Microtubule
Mitochondrion
Microfilament
Plasma membrane

A

FIGURE 3.12 Cytoskeleton of a eukaryotic cell. **A,** Illustration of the components of the cytoskeleton, showing microtubules, microfilaments, and intermediate filaments. **B,** Electron micrograph of cytoskeletal components of a nerve cell.

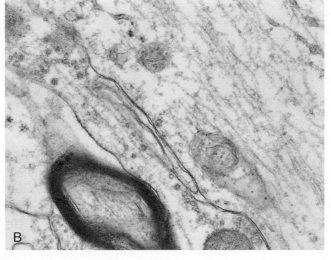

B

ton, a highly organized structure composed of microfilaments and microtubules arranged in a complex latticework.

Cytoskeleton

It was previously thought that the **cytoskeleton** was present only in eukaryotic cells, but more recent research shows that homologs of cytoskeletal proteins present in eukaryotic cells are also found in prokaryotes. Speculations indicate that constituents of today's eukaryotic skeleton (tubulin and actin) evolved from prokaryotic precursor proteins closely related to today's bacterial proteins. The studies indicate that the existence of a shape-preserving cytoskeleton is universally present in bacteria.

Structurally, the cytoskeleton (Figure 3.12) is not rigid but is dynamic and capable of rapid reorganization. This is essential for intracellular transport of vesicles and large molecules, as well as for the rearrangement of organelles. Furthermore, the cytoskeleton forms a spindle apparatus during cell division, which is discussed later in this chapter. The cytoskeleton is composed of actin filaments, intermediate filaments, and microtubules:

- Actin filaments (microfilaments) are made from the globular protein actin, which polymerizes in a helical fashion to form microfilaments. They are about 7 nm in diameter and provide mechanical support for the cell, determine the cell shape, and enable cell movements.
- Intermediate filaments are 8 to 11 nm in diameter and are the more stable components of the cytoskeleton. They organize the internal tridimensional structure of the cell. Intermediate filament proteins include keratins, vimentins, neurofilaments, and lamins.
- Microtubules are hollow cylinders with a diameter of about 24 nm and varying lengths, made of tubulin proteins. They serve as structural components within cells and take part in many cellular processes such as mitosis, cytokinesis, and vesicular transport.

Centrioles and centrosomes are also part of the cytoskeleton and are essential during cell division in eukaryotic cells. A centriole is a barrel-shaped microtubular structure present in most animal cells and cells of fungi and algae, but not frequent in plants. When two centrioles are arranged perpendicularly and

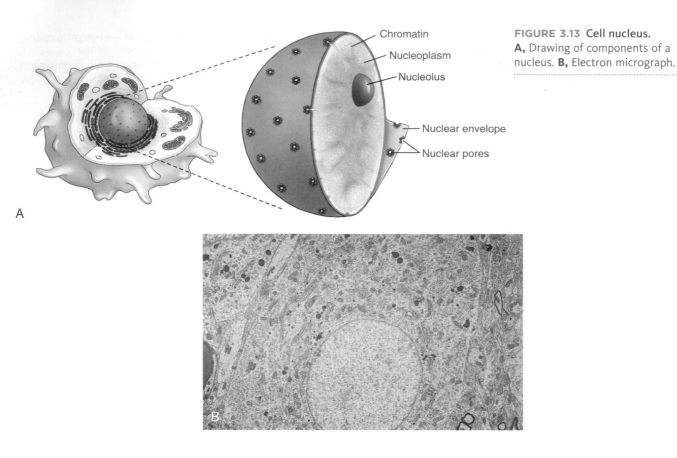

FIGURE 3.13 **Cell nucleus.**
A, Drawing of components of a
nucleus. **B,** Electron micrograph.

Chromatin

Nucleoplasm

Nucleolus

Nuclear envelope

Nuclear pores

A

B

are surrounded by additional proteins, they form the centrosome. The centrosome is known as the *microtubule-organizing center* and plays an important role in the microtubule organization of a cell. During the process of cell division centrioles form the mitotic spindle on which the chromosomes pull apart.

Cell Organelles

One of the main distinguishing factors between prokaryotic and eukaryotic cells is the presence of membrane-bound cell organelles in eukaryotic but not in prokaryotic cells.

Nucleus

The nucleus (Figure 3.13) is the control center of the eukaryotic cell, containing the DNA. A double membrane, the **nuclear envelope,** surrounds the nucleus, interrupted by nuclear pores. The nuclear envelope regulates molecular transport between the nucleus and the cytoplasm. The outer membrane of the nuclear envelope is continuous with the cell's endoplasmic reticulum (ER). Within the nucleus is a prominent structure, the nucleolus, that synthesizes ribosomal RNA (rRNA) and combines the rRNA with proteins to form the subunits of ribosomes.

Also visible in the nucleus is chromatin composed of DNA and its protein complex. Two different forms of chromatin exist in a eukaryotic cell: euchromatin and heterochromatin. Euchromatin is the least compact form of DNA and contains the genes expressed in a given cell (i.e., insulin gene in pancreatic cells). Heterochromatin is more tightly packed and it contains genes not expressed in that particular cell (i.e., thyroid hormone in pancreatic cells).

Endoplasmic Reticulum

The endoplasmic reticulum is part of the endomembrane system of eukaryotic cells. It consists of an elaborate network of membranous tubules and cisternae, continuous with the outer membrane of the nuclear envelope and held together by the cytoskeleton (Figure 3.14). The two forms of ER are rough ER (rER) and smooth ER (sER).

- rER is called *rough* because of the attachment of ribosomes on the cytoplasmic side of its membranes. The rER manufactures membranes and proteins, processes the proteins, and passes them to the Golgi apparatus. The secretory proteins produced by the rER are destined primarily for "export" into the extracellular fluid for use by other cells. Cells actively involved in the synthesis of secretory proteins have a very prominent rER.
- sER lacks attached ribosomes and functions in various metabolic processes such as lipid and carbohydrate synthesis as well as in detoxification of drugs and poisons.

Golgi Apparatus

The Golgi apparatus (also called the *Golgi complex*) consists of flattened, disc-shaped sacs called *cisternae* with somewhat dilated peripheries that give rise to various secretory vesicles and lysosomes (Figure 3.15). The Golgi apparatus is always closely associated with the ER, the production site of organic molecules. In preparation for export, the Golgi complex modifies and packages the proteins, carbohydrates, and lipids that it receives from the ER. In addition, the Golgi apparatus produces lysosomes for the use within the cell.

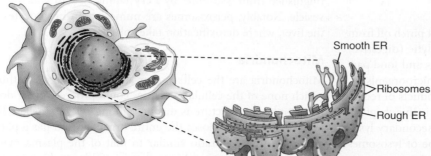

A

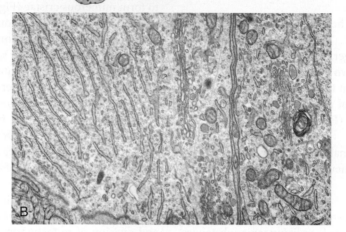

FIGURE 3.14 **Endoplasmic reticulum.** In both the drawing **(A)** and the electron micrograph **(B)** the rough endoplasmic reticulum (ER) can easily be identified by the presence of ribosomes on its cisternae.

Smooth ER

Ribosomes

Rough ER

B

Secretory vesicles

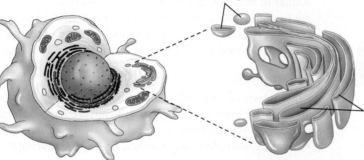

A

Cisternae

Golgi apparatus

FIGURE 3.15 **Golgi apparatus.** The drawing **(A)** and the electron micrograph **(B)** clearly show the cisternae of the Golgi apparatus and the pinched-off secretory vesicles.

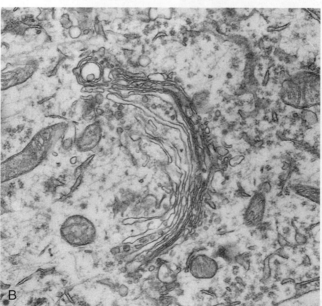

B

Lysosomes

Lysosomes are membrane-bound organelles that pinch off from the Golgi apparatus. Lysosomes contain hydrolytic (digestive) enzymes for intracellular digestion of cell debris and food particles, as well as for the breakdown of invading microorganisms. Another function of lysosomes is to process products of receptor-mediated endocytosis (see Endocytosis, later in this chapter). Lysosomes can be classified into primary and secondary lysosomes, and residual bodies. The size and shape of lysosomes vary with the degree of degradative activity.

- Primary lysosomes are small because they contain digestive enzymes only.
- Secondary lysosomes are larger, as they fuse with particles that require further breakdown (Figure 3.16, A).
- Residual bodies develop when the enzymes in the lysosome are insufficient or absent and cannot break down the material within the structure (Figure 3.16, B).

Whenever rupture of lysosomal membranes occurs, resulting in the subsequent release of their enzymes, cell death occurs.

Peroxisomes

Peroxisomes are self-replicating, small vesicular organelles that contain oxidative enzymes capable of oxidizing toxic substances such as hydrogen peroxide or other metabolites. They are distinguished from lysosomes by a crystalline structure inside the vesicle. Notably, peroxisomes are numerous in hepatocytes of the liver, where detoxification takes place.

Mitochondria

Mitochondria are the cell's power source for energy, without which none of the cellular activities could proceed. Their double-membrane structure is distinct among cell organelles. The outer membrane encloses the entire organelle and has a phospholipid-to-protein ratio similar to that of the plasma membrane and an inner membrane that has folds reaching inward to form numerous cristae (Figure 3.17). This organelle contains proteins for different functions, including those that carry out the reactions of the respiratory chain for ATP production. The mitochondrial matrix is the space enclosed by the inner membrane and contains a mixture of hundreds of enzymes, mitochondrial ribosomes, transfer RNA (tRNA), and several copies of the mitochondrial DNA genome. The mitochondrial genome encodes primarily proteins for oxidative phosphorylation, as well as rRNAs, tRNAs, and proteins involved in protein synthesis. Mitochondrial ribosomes are of the 70S type (also found in bacteria), distinct from the 80S ribosomes found elsewhere in the eukaryotic cell.

Mitochondria replicate their DNA and divide primarily in response to the energy demands of the cell. Therefore, growth and division of mitochondria depend on the energy needs of cells and not on the cell cycle. They divide by **binary fission** similar to bacterial cell division. Mitochondrial DNA is different from the DNA of nuclear genes. Mitochondrial DNA comes from the egg because the single mitochondrion of the sperm is usually destroyed as the sperm enters the egg at fertilization.

Chloroplasts

Chloroplasts are organelles found in algae and plant cells and are able to convert sun energy into chemical energy through the process of photosynthesis (see Photosynthesis later in this chapter). Chloroplasts are spherical or oval, measuring about 3

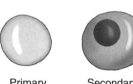

Primary lysosome   Secondary lysosome

A   Residual body

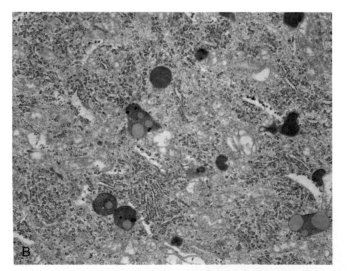

FIGURE 3.16 Lysosomes. A, The drawing illustrates the primary lysosome containing enzyme only, the secondary lysosome with material to be digested, and the residual body containing material that cannot be further broken down. **B,** Electron micrograph.

LIFE APPLICATION

Mitochondrial DNA and Maternal Lineage

Mitochondrial DNA (mtDNA) sequencing is a useful tool for forensic scientists, evolutionary biologists, genealogists, and anthropologists in the study of human migration patterns, evolution, maternally linked relationships and identification. Unlike nuclear DNA used in paternity testing, everyone inherits mtDNA from his or her biological mother. Therefore, mtDNA testing provides evidence of maternal inheritance features. In addition, these maternal lineage data may provide evidence in complicated paternity and inheritance questions as well as in cases when only small amounts of samples are available. Also, maternal lineage test data are useful in "chain of custody" evidence, which is a documentation process that makes the test data legally admissible by courts and other government agencies.

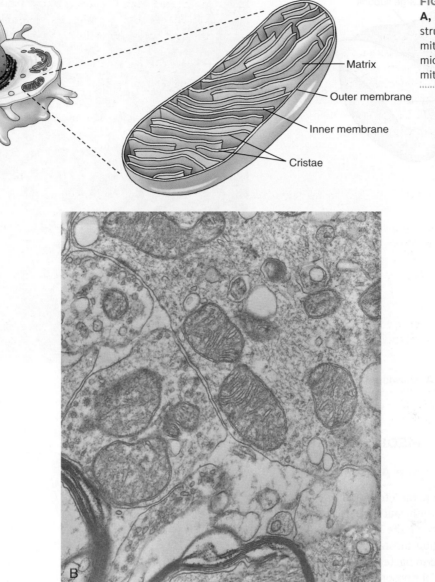

Matrix

Outer membrane

Inner membrane

Cristae

A

B

to 8 μm in diameter, surrounded by inner membrane system and outer membranes (Figure 3.18). The primary components of the inner membrane system are the thylakoids which consist of flattened disks stacked in parallel arrangements. They contain pigments such as chlorophyll and the enzymes necessary for photosynthesis. The **stroma** is the fluid within the chloroplast and contains small circular DNA, containing the chloroplast genome, and ribosomes. Chloroplast genes code for photosynthesis and autotrophy. Other genes in the chloroplast genome encode rRNA used in chloroplast ribosomes, tRNA used in translation, some proteins used in transcription and translation, and some other proteins. However, some proteins necessary for chloroplast function are encoded in the nuclear genes.

Ribosomes

Ribosomes are cell organelles common to both prokaryotic and eukaryotic cells. They consist of two subunits of ribosomal RNA and ribosomal proteins (Figure 3.19). The subunits fit together and operate in unison with tRNA to translate mRNA into a

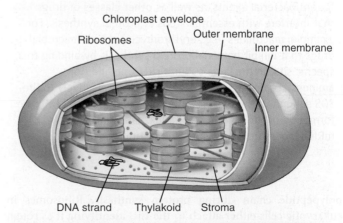

Chloroplast envelope

Ribosomes

Outer membrane

Inner membrane

DNA strand   Thylakoid   Stroma

FIGURE 3.18 Chloroplast. Photosynthesis takes place within chloroplasts. These organelles are surrounded by an envelope consisting of two membranes termed the *inner* and *outer* membranes, with a space between them. The stroma is the fluid within the chloroplast and the structures in which photosynthesis takes place are the thylakoids.

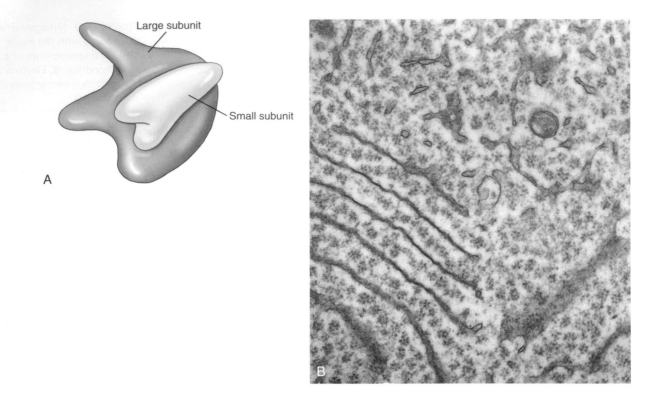

FIGURE 3.19 **Ribosomes. A,** Drawing showing the two ribosomal subunits. **B,** Electron micrograph.

Bacterial Ribosomes and Antimicrobials

All chemicals can be lethal; therefore treatment of bacterial infections must proceed with caution because of unwanted results (including lethality) to the host. The problem is one of selectivity, that is, to find substances that attack a metabolic pathway found in bacteria with minimal effects in the host. The 70S bacterial ribosome differs from the 80S eukaryotic ribosome, which qualifies it as a candidate target for antibacterial agents, as well as other classes of drugs that interfere with essential steps in protein synthesis. For example, macrolides (e.g., erythromycin) are antimicrobial drugs that inhibit bacterial protein synthesis by binding to a specific site on the large subunit rRNA. In addition, aminoglycosides (e.g., streptomycin) bind selectively to the 30S subunit of the bacterial ribosome and interfere with the formation of the initiation complex, causing misreading of mRNA (for more see Chapter 22, Antimicrobial Drugs).

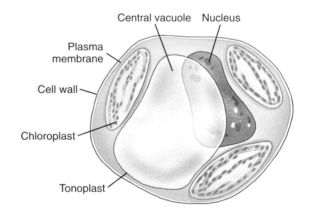

FIGURE 3.20 **Central vacuole of a plant cell.** The central vacuole of a plant cell is enclosed by a membrane called the *tonoplast*. As the cell matures the large vacuole slowly develops by fusion of smaller vacuoles.

Vacuoles

Vacuoles are membrane-bound structures in eukaryotic cells that serve a variety of functions. In general, vacuoles in animal cells are smaller than those of plants. Vacuoles store a variety of fluids, soluble materials, and ingested particles. Many freshwater protozoans contain contractive vacuoles that pump excess water out of the cell. Mature plant cells have a single central vacuole surrounded by a membrane called the *tonoplast* (Figure 3.20). Here the central vacuole often takes up more than 80% of the cell interior, leaving the rest of the cytoplasm confined in the space between the tonoplast and the plasma membrane. The

polypeptide chain during protein synthesis. Ribosomes in eukaryotic cells either attach to the ER, identifying it as rough ER, or float freely in the cytoplasm. Free ribosomes produce proteins for maintenance and repair within the cell or in the organelle in which they occur (i.e., mitochondria). The ribosomes in eukaryotic cells are of the 80S type, whereas prokaryotic cells have 70S ribosomes such as are found in mitochondria and chloroplasts.

vacuole plays a major role in the growth of plant cells, in that the cells elongate as the vacuole absorbs water to increase cell size with minimal increase in cytoplasm. Also, some vacuoles contain pigments that give color to the cells.

Vesicles

A vesicle is a relatively small (typically less than 1 μm), membrane-bound compartment used by the cell in the organization of metabolism, in transport, for enzyme storage, and as a chamber for chemical reactions. They can be formed by the Golgi apparatus, endoplasmic reticulum, or the plasma membrane. Examples are as follows:

- Transport vesicles, which move molecules between locations inside the cell (i.e., proteins from the rER to the Golgi apparatus)
- Secretory vesicles packaged by the Golgi apparatus with substances to be secreted (i.e., hormones)
- Synaptic vesicles, located in presynaptic terminals of axons, for storing neurotransmitters prior to release during chemical neurotransmission.

Inclusions

Inclusions, or inclusion bodies, are reserve deposits found in prokaryotic and eukaryotic cells. Inclusions in bacteria can be metachromatic granules (inorganic phosphate), polysaccharide granules (glycogen, starch), lipid inclusions, sulfur granules, carboxysomes, magnetosomes, or gas vacuoles. In contrast to vacuoles discussed earlier, gas vacuoles of bacteria are surrounded by a monolayer of a single protein, which is permeable to gases but not to water, and allows the bacterium to float at a desired depth in the water. Lipid inclusions and polysaccharide granules are found in eukaryotic cells as well.

Fluid Compartments and Membrane Transport Mechanisms

As previously stated, all living cells are separated from their external environment by plasma membranes and some organisms additionally by their cell walls. Prokaryotic cells and unicellular (single-cell) organisms are in direct contact with the external environment, whereas multicellular organisms form tissues, organs, and organ systems that are not in immediate contact with this environment. For a cell to survive, it must maintain a responsive, controllable, relatively stable, internal environment called *homeostasis*. In the human body cells are in contact with the extracellular fluid (ECF), which collectively is called the *extracellular fluid compartment,* or *ECF compartment.* The fluid inside the cell is the intracellular fluid (ICF), which collectively forms the intracellular fluid compartment or ICF compartment. In a 70-kg human under ideal conditions, the ideal ICF compartment volume is about 28 L and the ECF compartment is about 12 L. These are the volumes of fluid in which invading pathogens and antimicrobial drug treatments are distributed and in which effective concentration levels are reached to cause a disease or therapeutic levels for treatment are obtained. In order to understand the development of and the impact of infectious diseases on the body and drug treatments it is essential to have an understanding of the composition of the body's fluid compartments. Furthermore, it is essential to know the cellular transport mechanisms required to maintain a dynamic balanced distribution of fluids and electrolytes (homeostasis).

HEALTHCARE APPLICATION

Some Toxin-producing Bacteria That Cause Damage to Eukaryotic Cells

Organism/Toxin	Target	Damage	Disease
Aeromonas hydrophila/aerolysin	Glycophorin	Plasma membrane	Diarrhea
Clostridium perfringens/perfringolysin O	Cholesterol	Plasma membrane	Gas gangrene
Escherichia coli/hemolysins	Plasma membrane	Plasma membrane	Urinary tract infections
Staphylococcus aureus/α-toxin	Plasma membrane	Plasma membrane	Abscesses
Streptococcus pneumoniae/pneumolysin	Cholesterol	Plasma membrane	Pneumonia
Streptococcus pyogenes/streptolysin O	Cholesterol	Plasma membrane	Strep throat
Corynebacterium diphtheriae/diphtheria toxin	Elongation factor-2	Protein synthesis	Diphtheria
E. coli, Shigella dysenteriae/Shiga toxins	28S rRNA	Protein synthesis	Hemorrhagic colitis; hemolytic uremic syndrome

Intracellular Fluid Compartment

ICF, the largest compartment, encompasses two thirds of the human body's water. Normal values for body water, expressed as a percentage of total body weight, vary between 45% and 75%. These differences are due to age, fat content of the body, and gender. Adipose (fat) tissue contains the least amount of water among body tissues and therefore obese people have less body water per kilogram of weight than do slender ones. In contrast, muscle tissue contains the largest amount of water (65%). Old age is accompanied by loss of muscle mass and increases in body fat resulting in significant decreases in body water content, sometimes up to 45% of total body weight. The distribution of water in the body's compartments is shown in Figure 3.21. Intracellular fluid has high concentrations of potassium, phosphate, and magnesium ions, and lesser amounts of sodium, chloride, and bicarbonate ions.

Extracellular Fluid Compartment

The ECF consists of plasma, lymph, the interstitial fluid (fluid surrounding the cells), and the transcellular fluid such as cerebrospinal fluid (CSF), joint fluids, humors of the eye, digestive juices, and mucus, to mention a few. The extracellular fluids have high concentrations of sodium, chloride, and bicarbonate ions, with lesser amounts of potassium, calcium, magnesium, phosphate, and sulfate ions.

Osmotic pressure markedly influences the movement of water and electrolytes throughout the body's fluid compartments. Whereas the composition of the ECF and ICF differ, the total solute concentration and water amounts are normally equivalent. Thus, net gains of water or of solutes osmotically cause shifts affecting balances in the intracellular and extracellular fluids. These shifts can have a marked influence on uptake, redistribution, or removal of substances, including antibiotics or other drugs and chemicals (see Chapter 21, Pharmacology).

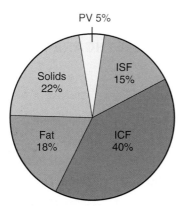

FIGURE 3.21 Distribution of water in the body's compartments of an adult. Forty percent is located in the intracellular fluid (ICF) compartment, 15% within the interstitial fluid (ISF), and 15% is plasma volume (PV). The ISF and the PV encompass the extracellular fluid (ECF) compartment. This distribution does change during the aging process because of the loss of muscle mass.

Passive Transport

In **passive transport,** molecules move from an area of higher concentration to an area of lower concentration without the use of cellular energy (ATP). The driving force of passive transport is atomic and molecular (Brownian) movement—the natural tendency of atoms and molecules to be in constant random movement. This motion can be demonstrated by the Brownian movement of small particles suspended in a liquid. For example, a few crystals of potassium permanganate put into a beaker of water and left undisturbed will slowly color the water in the entire beaker by the process of diffusion.

Diffusion

Diffusion, like other passive transport mechanisms, uses the concentration gradient to move molecules from an area of higher concentration to an area of lower concentration (Figure 3.22). Diffusion is an important mechanism by which cells can readily obtain diffusible materials such as oxygen and release carbon dioxide waste molecules into the external environment.

Facilitated Diffusion

Facilitated diffusion is a process necessary for molecules that cannot readily diffuse through cellular membrane barriers and require membrane transporters for movement across the membrane. As with diffusion, this type of transport does not require energy from ATP. The necessary transport molecules can either be specific membrane carriers or transmembrane channels. Carrier-mediated transport (Figure 3.23):

- Requires **specific** protein **carrier** molecules with binding sites for a particular molecule (i.e., glucose, sodium ion)
- Can become **saturated** because of limited numbers of carrier molecules, limiting the number of molecules that can be transported at a given time
- Can exhibit **competition** for binding sites on the carrier molecule when two similarly shaped molecules compete for the same binding site. Although the molecules with a better fit show a preference or **affinity** for the binding site, increases in concentration of the molecules with lesser affinity can facilitate their transport

Protein channel–mediated membrane transport provides selective pathways for specific ions or other small water-soluble molecules. For example, sodium ions can only pass through sodium channels and potassium can only pass through potassium channels. Furthermore, these channels are gated, that is, they are either open or closed. Gated channels can be triggered to open or close by voltage, light, mechanical, or chemical stimuli, and they are named according to the stimuli activating them (i.e., sodium channels, voltage-gated channels, pressure-gated channels, etc.)

Osmosis

Osmosis is the diffusion of water across a selectively permeable membrane. The plasma membrane of cells is selectively permeable to water molecules, allowing them to diffuse but excluding

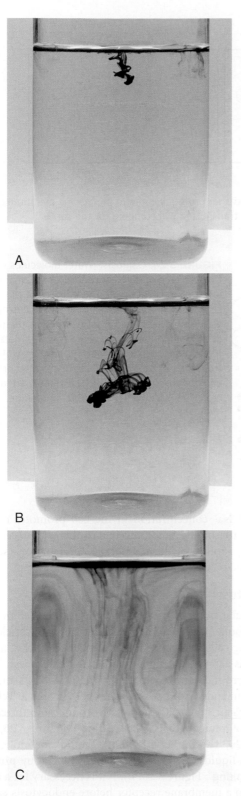

A

B

C

FIGURE 3.22 Diffusion. This sequence of three photos shows the diffusion of a single drop of dye in a container of water at room temperature.

substances dissolved in the water. When the concentration of water on one side of the plasma membrane is greater than that on the other side, water will follow its concentration gradient and diffuse to the area of lower water concentration (Figure 3.24). In living cells, however, isotonicity between the ICF and ECF avoids excessive movement of water either into or out of the cells (see Figure 2.11 in Chapter 2, Chemistry of Life). Although water is the solvent molecule that moves across the membrane during osmosis, the solute concentrations of the ECF and ICF dictate how much water is available for diffusion. For example, a 30% solution contains 30 parts of solute and 70 parts of water and a 3% solution contains 3 parts of solute and 97 parts of water. When these two solutions are placed on the opposite sides of a selectively permeable membrane, water will diffuse from an area of higher concentration of water molecules (the 3% solution) to an area of lower concentration of water molecules (the 30% solution).

Moreover, whereas isotonic conditions do not create stress on cells, hypotonic or hypertonic environments do. Some specific microbes adapt to different osmotic environments as illustrated by amoeba living in a freshwater pond, which is a hypotonic environment. In this case water continuously enters the cell through the plasma membrane. In order to prevent the eventual rupture of the cell, water is actively pumped out of the cell with the help of the contractile vacuole by the process of **active transport.**

Filtration

Filtration is the movement of molecules through a membrane along a concentration gradient from an area of high hydrostatic pressure to an area of lower hydrostatic pressure. The driving force for filtration can be gravity or, as exemplified in the human body, by the hydrostatic effects of blood pressure on blood plasma, filtering it from the blood capillaries into the ECF. Another important example is filtration from the capillaries of the kidneys into the collecting ducts during urine formation. In microbiology, filtration systems can eliminate microbes from liquid environments (see Chapter 4, Microbiological Laboratory Techniques).

Active Transport

The driving force for passive transport mechanisms is the concentration gradient. In active transport cellular energy (ATP) is required to move molecules uphill, against a concentration gradient. Active transport is also required when molecules need to be transported at a faster rate than is possible by diffusion, even if the molecules move with their concentration gradient. For example, some freshwater algae have an active transport system that is so efficient that nutrients are in much higher intracellular concentration than in the surrounding environment. Active transport mechanisms include transport by pumps or by vesicles such as occurs with endocytosis and exocytosis.

Pump Transport

Active transport of ions or molecules is due primarily to a pump transport mechanism working against a gradient. This work requires energy obtained by hydrolysis of ATP. Active transport

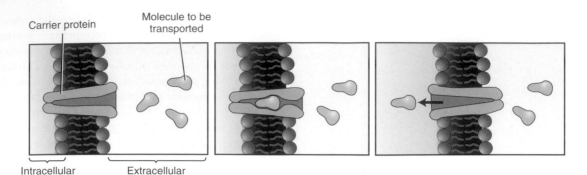

FIGURE 3.23 Carrier-mediated transport. This transport mechanism requires a carrier protein located in the plasma membrane. The carrier protein can transport only one molecule at a time and the molecules to be transported will compete for the carrier.

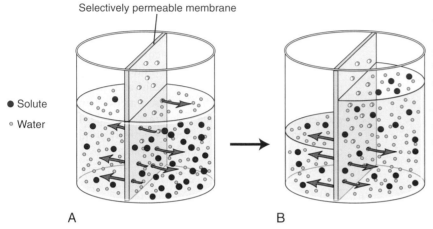

A   B

FIGURE 3.24 Osmosis. Water molecules will move from an area of high concentration to an area of lower concentration. **A,** The left side of the selectively permeable membrane contains more water molecules than solutes, whereas the right side of the membrane contains fewer water molecules and more solutes. Thus the water molecules will move from the left to the right side of the membrane until equilibrium is reached **(B).** The solutes are unable to cross the selectively permeable membrane.

carriers are composed of transmembrane proteins. The pump transport process requires:

- Binding of the ion or molecule to be transported to a specific recognition site or receptor on the carrier protein
- Initiation of ATP hydrolysis, which phosphorylates the carrier protein
- Changing of the carrier protein shape, which activates its transport function
- Carrying of the ion or molecule to the other side of the membrane, where it is released

Active pumping systems are important for cells because they allow the cells to move needed ions and other molecules to specific areas. The calcium pump, for example, moves calcium ions to specific areas within the muscle cell during muscle contraction and relaxation. The sodium–potassium pump removes three sodium ions (Na^+) out of a cell while it transports two potassium ions (K^+) into the cell. Both ions are transported against their chemical concentration gradient, which maintains an electrical charge on the cell membrane, referred to as membrane potential. Most cells contain many Na^+/K^+ pumps that are constantly active to maintain the membrane potential. The steep gradient of sodium and potassium ion concentration across cell membranes is essential for conduction and transmission of electrochemical impulses in nerve and muscle cells. If the active extrusion of Na^+ is blocked or markedly impeded, the increased Na^+ concentration in the cell promotes osmosis, a challenge to isotonic conditions that could result in cell damage, including rupture of the membrane or crenation (see Figure 2.11 in Chapter 2, Chemistry of Life).

Endocytosis

Extracellular material may be brought into the cell by **endocytosis,** a bulk transport mechanism that uses vesicles. Some eukaryotic cells transport large molecules, particles, liquids, or other cells across the cell membrane via this process. Typically, a cell surrounds and encloses a particle with its membrane, forming an endocytotic vesicle, and then engulfs it. Whole cells or large particles of solid matter are brought into the cell by the process of **phagocytosis** ("cell eating"; Figure 3.25, *A*) (see Chapter 20, The Immune System). Liquids, or molecules dissolved in liquids, are transported into the cell by **pinocytosis** ("cell drinking"; Figure 3.25, *B*). If it is necessary for a molecule to bind to a membrane receptor before endocytosis can occur, it is called **receptor-mediated endocytosis** (Figure 3.25, *C*).

Exocytosis

Large molecules, such as polypeptides, proteins, and others, may be excreted from the cell via the process of **exocytosis** (Figure 3.26). Unicellular organisms (i.e., protozoans) use exocytosis for the elimination of waste products. In multicellular organisms exocytosis has a signaling or regulatory function. Vesicles for exocytosis are produced by the Golgi apparatus,

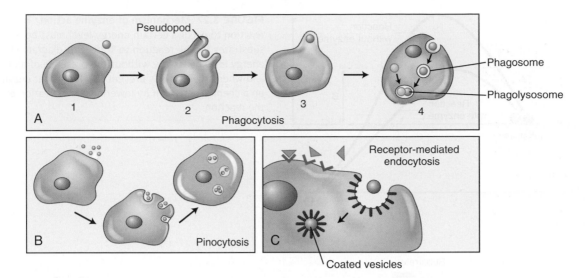

FIGURE 3.25 Endocytosis. A, *Phagocytosis*: Large particles (i.e., bacteria) *(1)*, are surrounded by pseudopods *(2)*, engulfed *(3)*, and form a phagosome *(4)*. The phagosome will merge with a lysosome, forming a phagolysosome and the digestion of the large particle can begin. **B,** *Pinocytosis*: Fluid is pinocytosed by small extensions of the cell membrane forming pinocytotic vesicles. **C,** *Receptor-mediated endocytosis*: Molecules in the extracellular space bind to membrane receptors, resulting in the plasma membrane being pulled inward by the cytoskeleton, forming a pocket around the substance to be transported into the cell. The edges of the pocket then fuse to form a coated vesicle.

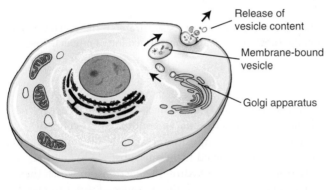

Exocytosis

FIGURE 3.26 Exocytosis. Proteins for export from the cell are sorted, modified, and packed by the Golgi apparatus. The membrane-bound vesicles then fuse with the plasma membrane and the contents of the vesicles are released into the extracellular environment.

from which they are transported to the cell membrane. Here the vesicles fuse with the cell membrane and their contents are emptied into the extracellular space or into a capillary. In addition to its transport function, exocytosis also adds material to the plasma membrane.

Cellular Metabolism

Cellular metabolism includes all chemical reactions within a cell, which are organized in sequences called *metabolic pathways*. Metabolic pathways that break down large molecules into smaller ones and release energy in the process are collectively part of **catabolism.** The pathways that produce larger molecules from smaller ones are part of **anabolism** and use energy released during catabolic reactions (also see Chapter 2, Chemistry of Life). Nutrients or sunlight supply the energy required to generate ATP molecules. Organisms that utilize energy from the breakdown of nutrient molecules are **chemotrophs;** those that use sunlight for photosynthesis are **phototrophs** and they release energy during the process. According to the **first law of thermodynamics,** energy is neither created nor destroyed; it is only transferred from one form into another. This includes energy for cellular metabolism and energy in general.

Enzymes

Enzymes are biological catalysts that initiate the chemical reactions necessary within the metabolic pathways of cells. All chemical reactions within a cell require enzymes. The mechanism of enzyme action is to lower the energy of activation needed to start a chemical reaction (Figure 3.27). Chemically, enzymes are proteins with a specific structure, usually in a tertiary or quaternary configuration (see Chapter 2, Chemistry of Life). The substances that enzymes act on are referred to as substrates, and the end result of the reaction is a product. Expressed in chemical notation:

$$E + S = P$$

(Enzyme + Substrate = Product)

The site to which substrates bind to an enzyme is called the **active site** and is specific for each substrate. After binding an enzyme–substrate complex is formed and the chemical reaction occurs resulting in a product. At the end of the reaction the enzyme itself is unchanged (Figure 3.28).

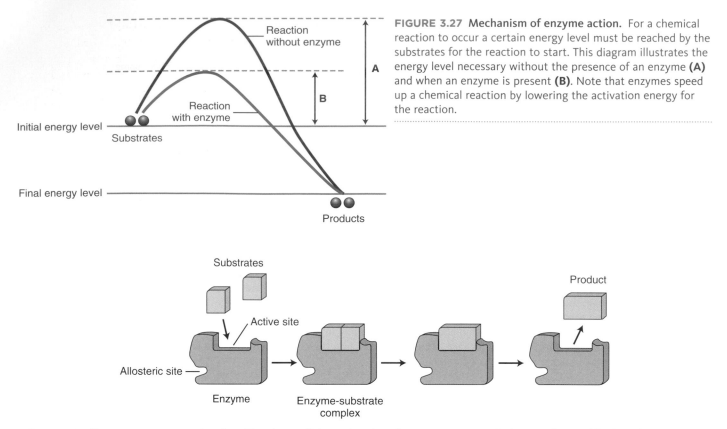

FIGURE 3.27 Mechanism of enzyme action. For a chemical reaction to occur a certain energy level must be reached by the substrates for the reaction to start. This diagram illustrates the energy level necessary without the presence of an enzyme **(A)** and when an enzyme is present **(B)**. Note that enzymes speed up a chemical reaction by lowering the activation energy for the reaction.

FIGURE 3.28 Enzyme structure and action. The shape of the active site of an enzyme is specific for its substrate(s). The substrate(s) bind with the active site of the enzyme to form an enzyme–substrate complex and the substrate(s) is/are transformed into a product. The enzyme remains the same after the chemical reaction.

Enzyme Specificity

The degree to which enzymes bind to specific binding sites on their substrates determines their specificity. The initial contact between the enzyme and substrate most likely occurs via attraction between electrostatic forces. How well the shape of the enzyme fits (complements) the binding site on the substrate defines specificity—like a key fitting into a lock. Some additional movement of the enzyme shape is often required, just like "jiggling" a key in a lock might be required to open it. This process between enzymes and their substrate(s) can be summed up and explained by:

- Differences in charge on the molecules
- Formation of weak bonds
- Attraction between closely spaced atoms/molecules (van der Waals forces)

Classification and Naming of Enzymes

Enzymes are classified according to the type of reaction they catalyze and all metabolic reactions are catalyzed by a specific class of enzyme. Thus, individual enzymes are typically named according to the type of reaction they catalyze, the name of the substrate they act on, and using the suffix *-ase*.

- **Oxidoreductases** catalyze the transfer of electrons in oxidation–reduction reactions.

- **Transferases** modify molecules and transfer energy-rich bonds from one molecule to another. This occurs in synthesis and decomposition reactions, in which functional groups are transferred from one substrate to another.
- **Hydrolases** catalyze hydrolysis reactions, in which they break chemical bonds in the presence of water to release energy.
- **Lyases** remove functional groups from a substrate without adding water, or add functional groups to a double bond.
- **Isomerases** rearrange atoms within molecules, changing the configuration of the atoms.
- **Ligases** form bonds between individual monomers to form polymers.

Exoenzymes and Endoenzymes

Enzymes may also be named according to the site in which they act. **Exoenzymes** are secreted by a cell into the extracellular environment, where they act to break down large molecules into smaller ones so that they can be taken up into the cell. The exoenzyme amylase produced by some microorganisms hydrolyzes starch into monosaccharides, which can then be transported across their plasma membrane. Other exoenzymes can be released into the intracellular environment for metabolic purposes within the cell. These include cellulase, caseinase, lipase, and nucleotidase. In contrast, **endoenzymes** work within specific biological membranes such as the enzymes used in **cellular respiration.**

Cofactors and Coenzymes

In many cases the enzymes require nonprotein **coenzymes** or **cofactors,** that is, other ions or molecules, in order to catalyze a reaction. The protein portion of an enzyme is the **apoenzyme** and the nonprotein portion is a coenzyme if it is an organic molecule (usually a derivative from water-soluble vitamins); if it is a metal ion, it is a cofactor. **Holoenzymes** are enzymes that may require one or more cofactors or coenzymes when combined (Figure 3.29).

Microorganisms require specific metal ions as trace elements and certain organic growth factors for survival (see Chapter 6, Bacteria and Archaea). The need for these substances occurs because of their roles as cofactors. Enzymes that require cofactors do not have an appropriate shape for the active site until they combine with the cofactor. Metals, therefore, activate enzymes by bringing the active site and the substrate closer together and then participate directly in the chemical reaction as a part of the enzyme–substrate complex. Coenzymes, on the other hand, remove a functional group from one substrate molecule and add it to another substrate. Coenzymes often function as intermediate carriers of hydrogen atoms, electrons, carbon dioxide, and amino groups. An example would be the role of nicotinamide adenine dinucleotide (NAD) in the transfer of electrons in coupled oxidation–reduction reactions (see Cellular Respiration, later in this chapter). Because coenzymes are vitamin derivatives, it might explain the importance of vitamins in our diet; a vitamin deficiency prevents the completion of the holoenzyme and the chemical reaction to be catalyzed fails to occur.

Regulation of Enzyme Activity

Rates at which enzyme reactions proceed within the metabolic pathways are influenced by temperature; pH; concentrations of substrate, enzyme, and product; and the presence or absence of cofactors and coenzymes.

- *Temperature:* Rates of most chemical reactions generally speed up at higher temperatures, and slow down at lower temperatures. However, high temperatures risk denaturing (changing the shape of) the protein portion of enzymes, causing them to lose specificity and functionality (see Chapter 2, Chemistry of Life).

- *pH:* Enzymes work best within an optimal pH range to promote the most rapid chemical reaction. For the majority of microbial enzymes, this is near pH 7 (neutral).
- *Substrate concentration:* If the amount of enzyme is fixed, then high concentrations of substrate speed the rate of reaction until the active sites on the enzymes saturate with substrate.
- *Enzyme concentration:* If the amount of substrate is constant, then the reaction rate initially rises but levels off as the substrate available for the reaction binds to the enzyme.
- *Product concentration:* Because many enzymes catalyze reactions in both forward and reverse directions, high concentrations may allow the enzymes to catalyze the reverse reaction. However, if the substrates are used in other reactions, then the direction of the first enzyme reaction remains forward.
- *Cofactors and coenzymes:* Depending on the presence (in sufficient numbers) or absence of cofactors and coenzymes, the rates of enzyme reactions will either increase or slow.

In addition, a variety of other substances such as drugs can either inhibit or reduce the rate of a reaction. The effectiveness of such an inhibitory substance depends on its reversible or irreversible binding properties with the enzyme. For example, in **irreversible inhibition,** the inhibitor competes with the substrate for the active site of the enzyme (Figure 3.30, *A*). The degree of inhibition is dependent on the relative concentrations of the inhibitor and the substrate; increasing the amount of substrate may result in reversible inhibition. **Competitive enzyme inhibition** is the basis for treatment of some infectious diseases by selectively inhibiting a specific metabolic pathway required for the pathogen but not necessary for the human. Antimetabolites function this way, and in so doing they provide an effective weapon against infectious diseases.

Another mechanism that influences the rate of enzyme reactions is **noncompetitive inhibition,** in which the substance binds to an **allosteric site** of an enzyme, causing a conformational change of the enzyme's active site (Figure 3.30, *B*). The process is irreversible and the degree of inhibition is dependent

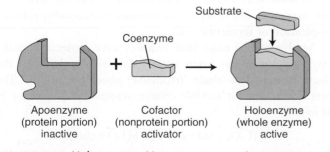

FIGURE 3.29 Holoenzyme. Many enzymes require coenzymes or cofactors to catalyze a reaction. The protein portion of such an enzyme is referred to as the *apoenzyme* and is inactive; the *coenzyme* or *cofactor* is the nonprotein portion. Together the apoenzyme and the coenzyme/cofactor produce the active holoenzyme.

Substrate

Coenzyme

Apoenzyme (protein portion) inactive + Cofactor (nonprotein portion) activator → Holoenzyme (whole enzyme) active

MEDICAL HIGHLIGHTS

Sulfa Drugs (Sulfonamides)

Sulfonamides are synthetic antimicrobial agents with a wide spectrum of activity (see Chapter 21 [Pharmacology] and Chapter 22 [Antimicrobial Drugs]) against both gram-positive and gram-negative bacteria. These drugs are an example of metabolic antagonism. All cells require folic acid for growth. Folic acid (vitamins in food) can be transported across human cells but cannot cross bacterial cell walls, and therefore must be synthesized by the bacteria. Sulfonamides are similar to and compete with *para*-aminobenzoic acid (PABA), a necessary intermediate in bacterial synthesis of folate—thereby killing bacteria.

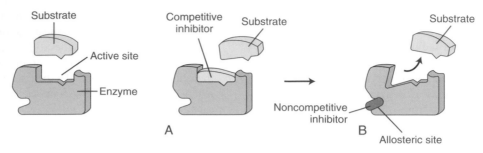

FIGURE 3.30 Enzyme inhibition. On the left side of the illustration an uninhibited enzyme and its substrate are shown. Enzyme action can be inhibited in two ways: **A,** by a competitive inhibitor that blocks the active site of the enzyme so that the substrate cannot bind; or **B,** by noncompetitive inhibition in which a substance binds to the allosteric site of an enzyme, resulting in a change of the shape of the active site so that the substrate cannot bind.

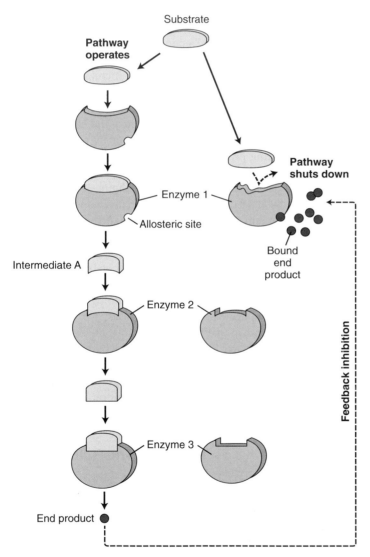

FIGURE 3.31 End product inhibition. The process of end-product inhibition is a negative feedback mechanism used to regulate the production of a given molecule.

on the concentration of the inhibitor. Also, enzyme activity is often regulated at specific points of the metabolic pathways by the process of end-product inhibition—when the amount of product formed is sufficient the reaction shuts down. This is

negative feedback inhibition and is an example of allosteric inhibition. In other words, in end-product inhibition, the inhibiting substance is the product formed by the initial enzyme activity. The amount of product formed then feeds back to slow down the reaction and prevent excessive accumulation of more final product (Figure 3.31).

Cellular Respiration and Photosynthesis

Prokaryotic and eukaryotic cells metabolize nutrients to generate ATP by respiration (cellular metabolic pathways), fermentation, and photosynthesis. Because ATP contains high-energy phosphate bonds for use in cellular respiration, it is a vital source of energy, and microorganisms utilize more than one process to produce it.

Cellular Respiration

Cellular respiration is the process by which the chemical energy of nutrient molecules is released and captured in the form of ATP. This energy transfer involves a series of oxidation–reduction reactions. In the breakdown of glucose and other nutrient molecules, some of the electrons originally present in these molecules are transferred to intermediate carriers and then to a final electron acceptor. When the breakdown is complete, with the end product being carbon dioxide and water, and oxygen the final electron acceptor, the pathway used is **aerobic cellular respiration.** If oxygen is not available cellular respiration continues with other inorganic molecules acting as the final electron acceptors, and this process is known as **anaerobic cellular respiration** or **fermentation.**

Aerobic cellular respiration requires three consecutive pathways: glycolysis, the Krebs cycle (citric acid cycle), and the electron transport chain (oxidative phosphorylation). The overall reaction for aerobic cellular respiration of glucose is as follows:

$$C_6H_{12}O_6 + 6O \rightarrow 6CO_2 + 6H_2O + energy$$

Glycolysis, the first pathway of the series, occurs in the cytoplasm and uses 10 enzyme reactions to break down glucose to produce a net yield of 2 molecules of pyruvic acid, 2 molecules of ATP, and 2 molecules of reduced NAD (Figure 3.32). The sequence of the principal steps of glycolysis that form ATP is as follows:

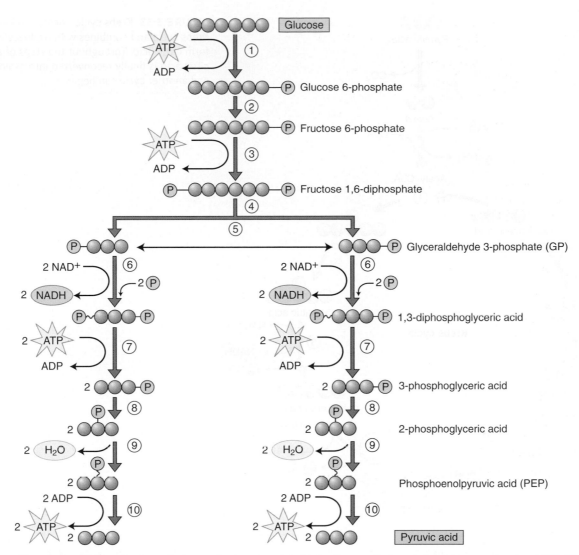

FIGURE 3.32 Glycolysis. *(1)* Once in the cell glucose is phosphorylated into glucose 6-phosphate, using a molecule of ATP. *(2)* Glucose 6-phosphate is converted into fructose 6-phosphate. *(3)* Using ATP, fructose 6-phosphate is phosphorylated into fructose 1,6-diphosphate. *(4)* This step represents the enzymatic conversion of fructose 1,6-diphosphate into two three-carbon molecules, dihydroxyacetone phosphate and glyceraldehyde 3-phosphate (GP). *(5)* Dihydroxyacetone phosphate is easily converted to glyceraldehyde 3-phosphate. *(6)* Each GP molecule is then converted to 1,3-diphosphoglyceric acid, with the formation of two NADH. *(7)* One phosphate is removed from each 1,3-diphosphoglyceric acid molecule, forming ATP and 3-phosphoglyceric acid. *(8)* The phosphate of the 3-phosphoglyceric acid is relocated by enzymatic action. *(9)* Water is removed from 3-phosphoglyceric acid to form phosphoenolpyruvic acid (PEP). *(10)* The phosphate is removed from PEP to form ATP and pyruvic acid.

1. Phosphorylation (addition of a phosphate group to a molecule) of glucose to yield glucose 6-phosphate. Phosphorylated organic molecules do not cross the plasma membrane and glucose now remains in the cell.
2. Conversion of glucose 6-phosphate into fructose 6-phosphate.
3. Use of another ATP molecule to phosphorylate fructose 6-phosphate into fructose 1,6-diphosphate.
4. Splitting of fructose 1,6-diphosphate into two three-carbon molecules of 3-phosphoglyceraldehyde.
5. Conversion of each molecule of 3-phosphoglyceraldehyde to 1,3-biphosphoglyceric acid (coenzyme NAD picks up hydrogen from each 3-phosphoglyceraldehyde molecule and forms NADH to which inorganic phosphate [P_i] is added).

6. Biphosphoglyceric acid donates a high-energy phosphate to ADP via substrate-level phosphorylation, forming an ATP molecule. The product of this reaction is 3-phosphoglyceric acid.
7. Isomerization (rearrangement of the chemicals in a given compound) of 3-phosphoglyceric acid produces 2-phosphoglyceric acid.
8. The removal of a water molecule from 2-phosphoglyceric acid produces phosphoenolpyruvic acid.
9. In the final step of glycolysis a phosphate group is removed from each phosphoenolpyruvic acid molecule and donated to ADP, forming another ATP molecule. The product of this reaction is pyruvic acid.

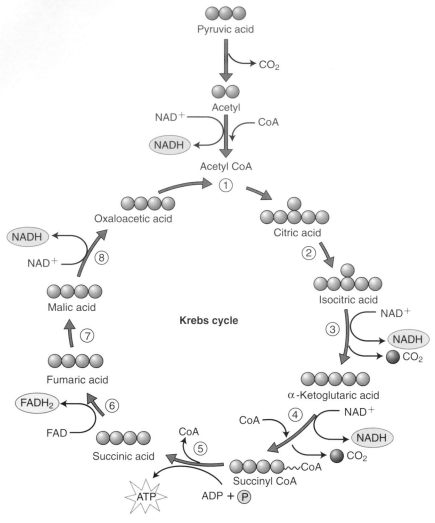

FIGURE 3.33 Krebs cycle. Acetyl-CoA enters the Krebs cycle and combines with oxaloacetic acid to form citric acid. Throughout the steps of the cycle citric acid is finally reconverted into oxaloacetic acid and another cycle can begin.

The overall equation for glycolysis is as follows:

$$\text{Glucose} + 2\text{NAD} + 2\text{ATP} + 2\text{P}_i \rightarrow 2 \text{ pyruvic acid} \\ + 2\text{NADH} + 2\text{ATP}$$

This is followed by:

$$\text{Pyruvic acid} \rightarrow \text{acetyl-CoA} + \text{CO}_2$$

Glycolysis is connected to the Krebs cycle by converting pyruvic acid into acetyl-coenzyme A (acetyl-CoA) and carbon dioxide (CO_2) while transferring two hydrogen ions to NADH. The NADH formed during this reaction will be sent to the electron transport chain. Each acetyl-CoA molecule will enter the Krebs cycle.

The **Krebs cycle** is the second pathway in aerobic cellular respiration. It occurs in the plasma membrane of prokaryotes and within the matrix of mitochondria in eukaryotes. After acetyl-CoA enters the Krebs cycle it combines with oxaloacetic acid to form citric acid. Through a series of reactions involving the elimination of two carbons and four oxygens (two CO_2 molecules) and the removal of hydrogens, citric acid is eventually converted to oxaloacetic acid to complete this metabolic cycle (Figure 3.33).

Steps in the Krebs cycle include the following:

- The production of a guanosine triphosphate (GTP) molecule in step 5, which donates a phosphate group to ADP to form one ATP molecule
- The release of CO_2 in steps 3 and 4 for use in endergonic pathways (excess CO_2 is released as a gas into the environment)
- The reduction of three molecules of NAD $\rightarrow$ NADH in steps 4, 5, and 8
- The reduction of one molecule of flavin adenine dinucleotide (FAD) $\rightarrow$ FADH$_2$ in step 6

For each glucose molecule entering aerobic respiration, the Krebs cycle runs twice because glycolysis produced two molecules of pyruvic acid. Molecules of NAD and FAD in glycolysis and the Krebs cycle are essential to pick up hydrogens and electrons. The reduced forms of these molecules then enter the electron transport chain, where they are oxidized in a series of reduction–oxidation reactions to regenerate coenzymes while producing ATP, oxygen, and water.

The **electron transport chain,** the last step in aerobic cellular respiration, takes place in the cristae of the inner mitochondrial

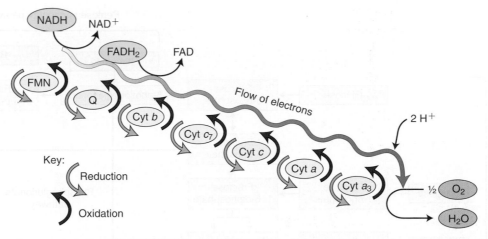

FIGURE 3.34 Electron transport chain. This is the final reaction in aerobic cellular respiration and consists of a series of carrier molecules capable of oxidation–reduction reactions. Electrons are passed down the chain and energy is released in this stepwise reaction and then used to form ATP. The final electron acceptor is oxygen.

TABLE 3.4 Summary of Aerobic Cellular Respiration per Glucose Molecule

Produced	Glycolysis	Krebs Cycle	Respiratory Chain	Net Total
ATP	4 (2 used)	2	34	38
NADH	2	8	0	10
FADH	0	2	0	2
CO_2	6	0	0	6
H_2O	2	2 used	6	6

membrane. In order to regenerate NAD^+ and FAD^+, electrons and hydrogen ions are transferred from reduced NAD and FAD molecules to carrier molecules in the electron transport chain. These molecules include flavoproteins, coenzyme Q, iron–sulfur enzymes, and cytochromes. The last carrier transfers the electrons to oxygen, the final electron acceptor of aerobic respiration. As the hydrogen ions and electrons are transferred in a stepwise fashion from NADH to the chain of carriers, energy is released. This energy is captured by ADP to generate many ATP molecules from each glucose molecule (Figure 3.34).

The breakdown of one glucose molecule in aerobic respiration is summarized in Table 3.4:

- NADH and FADH entering the respiratory chain produce an estimated 36 ATP molecules plus 4 ATP from glycolysis to create 40 molecules of ATP. But, 2 ATP are consumed during glycolysis, which leaves a maximum of 38 ATP molecules generated per glucose molecule.
- Six carbon dioxide molecules are generated during the Krebs cycle.
- Six oxygen molecules are used in the electron transport chain.
- A net six water molecules are produced in the electron transport chain. A total of eight water molecules are produced, including two in glycolysis, but two of this total

are used in the Krebs cycle. Thus, a net number of six water molecules is generated.

The total of 38 ATP molecules produced is theoretical, because the actual ATP yield is less in eukaryotic cells because of the energy expended in transporting NADH across the mitochondrial membrane. However, there are some aerobic bacteria that come close to achieving this theoretical total because they lack mitochondria and do not have to use ATP to transport NADH across the mitochondrial membrane.

The **phosphogluconate pathway** (also called the *pentose phosphate pathway* or *hexose monophosphate shunt*) is an alternative catabolic pathway followed by some bacteria (Figure 3.35). This pathway generates NADPH and synthesizes pentose sugars in two distinct phases. The first is the oxidative phase, which generates NADPH, and the second phase synthesizes pentose sugars. This is a common pathway for heterolactic fermentative bacteria. It yields various end products including lactic acid, ethanol, and carbon dioxide. In addition, this pathway is a significant source of pentose sugars during nucleic acid synthesis.

Anaerobic cellular respiration is a metabolic pathway by which glucose is converted to lactic acid if oxygen is not available. Some bacteria utilize anaerobic respiration (anaerobes) for energy production and the final electron acceptor is an inorganic molecule and not oxygen. Actually, oxygen is toxic to anaerobic microbes and exposure to it kills most of such bacteria. On the other hand, facultatively anaerobic bacteria can use anaerobic respiration when oxygen is absent or present in limited amounts only. The final electron acceptor of anaerobic bacteria can be CO_2, the ion SO_4^{2-}, or NO_3^-.

If the final electron acceptor is an organic molecule, then fermentation takes place. The process starts with glycolysis but the end product varies because of the variety of organic molecules that can act as final electron acceptor. Fermentative bacteria and yeast use specific enzymes to metabolize the end product of glycolysis, namely pyruvic acid, into the final product. In this process an electron transport system is not used and

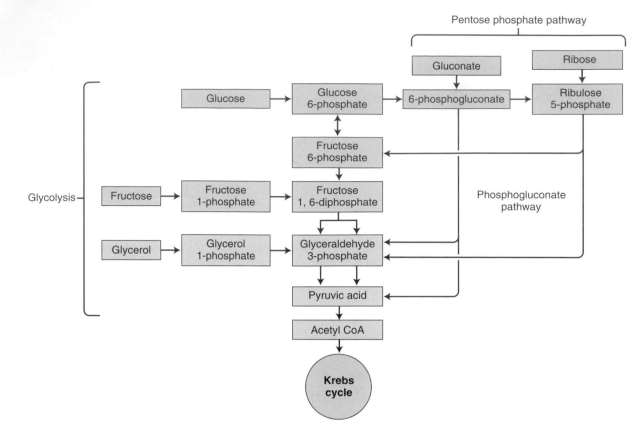

FIGURE 3.35 Phosphogluconate pathway. This pathway is an alternative pathway for glycolysis used by heterolactic fermentative bacteria. The diagram shows how different molecules can be utilized to produce NADPH.

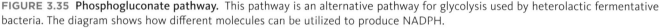

reduced NAD from glycolysis is oxidized by an organic molecule accepting electrons and hydrogens. With this pathway, the cell can catabolize sugar without oxygen, but this process is far less efficient than aerobic cellular respiration for the generation of ATP.

Fermentation end products produced by microorganisms can be beneficial to human life and various industries (i.e., dairy and brewing). Examples of bacteria and their fermentation end products are as follows:

- *Streptococcus* and *Lactobacillus*: Lactic acid, ethyl alcohol, and acidic acid
- *Escherichia coli*: Acetic acid, lactic acid, succinic acid, ethyl alcohol, CO_2, and H_2
- *Clostridium*: Butyric acid, butyl alcohol, acetone, acetic acid, isopropyl alcohol, CO_2, and H_2
- *Enterobacter*: Formic acid, ethyl alcohol, 2,3-butanediol, lactic acid, CO_2, and H_2
- *Actinomyces*: Formic acid, acetic acid, and ethyl alcohol
- *Saccharomyces* (yeast): Ethyl alcohol, acetaldehyde, and CO_2

Photosynthesis

Photosynthesis is a fundamental biochemical process by which plants, most algae, cyanobacteria, and some phototrophic bacteria convert light energy into chemical energy via ATP. Chlorophyll, a pigment found in chloroplasts (Figure 3.36, *A*) of

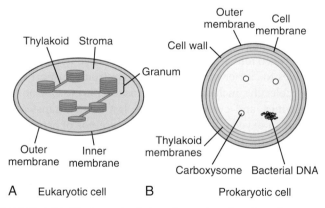

FIGURE 3.36 Photosynthesis in eukaryotic cells takes place within the thylakoid in chloroplasts, whereas prokaryotic cells use their thylakoid membranes located below the cell membrane.

plants and algae, is the site of photosynthesis. Photosynthetic bacteria do not have **chloroplasts** and photosynthesis takes place directly within the cell. Cyanobacteria contain **thylakoid membranes** (Figure 3.36, *B*) similar to those in chloroplasts and these are the only prokaryotes that perform oxygen-generating photosynthesis. Other photosynthetic bacteria contain a variety of different pigments, called *bacteriochlorophylls*, but they do not produce oxygen. Photosynthesis requires water for oxidation but some bacteria oxidize hydrogen sulfide instead and produce sulfur as a waste product. The rate of photosynthesis is affected by carbon dioxide, light intensity, and temperature.

Processes in photosynthesis are divided into two categories: reactions that require light, and reactions that occur in the dark and are light-independent. A simplified general equation for photosynthesis is as follows:

$$6CO_2 + 12H_2O + light \rightarrow C_6H_{12}O_6 + 6O_2 + 6H_2O$$

(Carbon dioxide + water + light energy → glucose + oxygen + water)

The first stage of photosynthesis is a **light-dependent reaction** that requires solar energy that is converted to chemical energy. Chlorophyll absorbs light and drives a transfer of electrons and hydrogen from water to an acceptor called $NADP^+$ *(nicotinamide adenine dinucleotide phosphate)*, which stores the energized electrons for a short period of time. During this process water is split and oxygen gas is given off. The process of producing ATP from sunlight is called *photophosphorylation*. There are two forms of photophosphorylation: noncyclic photophosphorylation (Figure 3.37, *A*) and cyclic photophosphorylation (Figure 3.37, *B*).

Noncyclic photophosphorylation, the predominant route, includes two sets of pigments called *photosystem I* (PSI) and *photosystem II* (PSII). These pigments are sensitive to or are excited by slightly different wavelengths of light. Wavelengths of about 700 nm excite the chlorophyll in PSI (P700) whereas the chlorophyll of PSII (P680) is excited by wavelengths under 680 nm. The stages of noncyclic photophosphorylation are as follows:

1. Oxidation of chlorophyll in PSII by light causes an electron to rise to a higher energy level. This electron is detained by the primary electron acceptor. This oxidized P680 chlorophyll now has a "hole" that needs filling.
2. Electrons are enzymatically removed from water and transferred to P680 to replace the electrons lost when light was absorbed by chlorophyll. A water molecule is then split into two hydrogen ions and an oxygen atom. The oxygen atom combines with another one to form O_2.
3. Each excited electron from the primary electron acceptor of PSII moves to PSI through the electron transport chain.
4. The energy released by electrons during the cascade down the electron transport chain is captured by the thylakoid membrane. This energy is used to produce ATP for synthesis of sugar during the second stage of photosynthesis—the Calvin cycle.
5. The electron "hole" in P700 of PSI, created by light energy driving an electron to the primary acceptor of PSI, is filled.

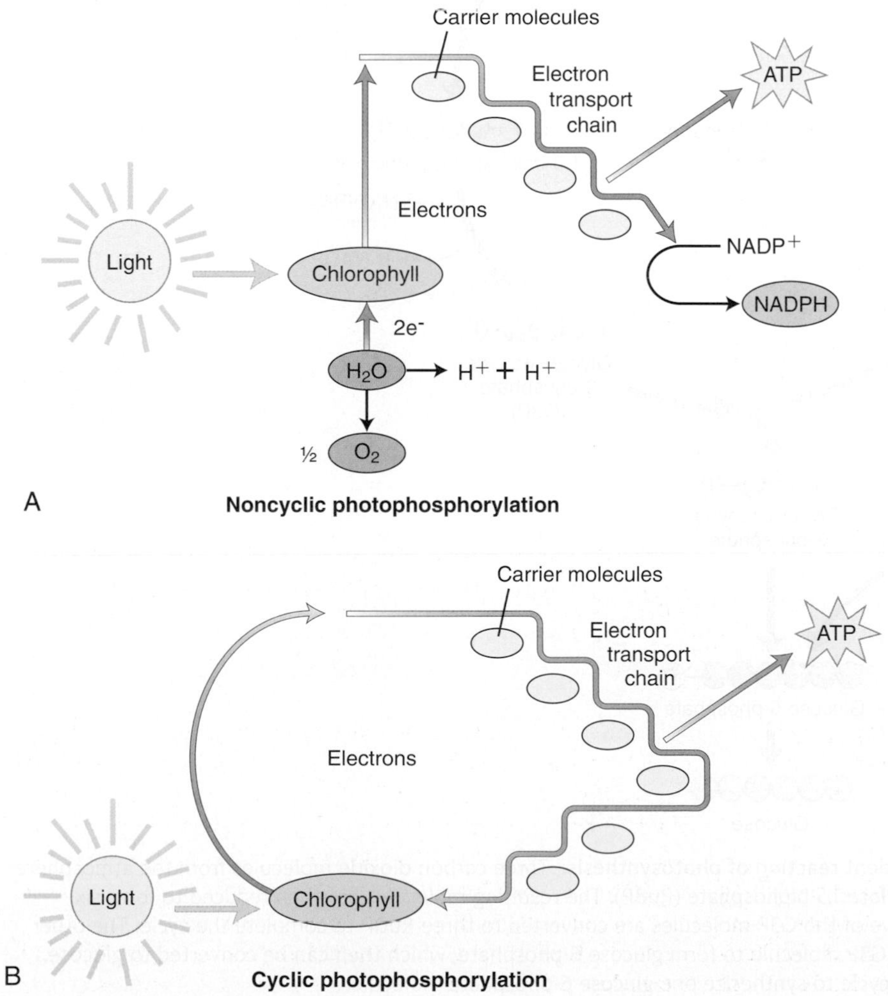

A

Noncyclic photophosphorylation

FIGURE 3.37 Light-dependent reaction of photosynthesis. A, Noncyclic photophosphorylation, the more common route by which the electrons released by chlorophyll are replaced by electrons from water. **B,** In cyclic photophosphorylation the released electrons return to the chlorophyll after going through the electron transport chain. Both pathways utilize the energy released through the electron transport chain to produce ATP molecules.

B

Cyclic photophosphorylation

6. Electrons are passed by the primary acceptor to the iron-containing protein ferredoxin (Fd) in a second electron transport chain. The enzyme NADP$^+$ reductase transfers the electrons from Fd to NADP$^+$. This reduction reaction stores the electrons in NADPH, which is the molecule that will also provide energy for the synthesis of sugar in the Calvin cycle.

Cyclic photophosphorylation occurs when the photo-excited electrons utilize photosystem I as an alternative path. The electrons cycle back from Fd to the cytochrome complex and then to the P700 chlorophyll. This cyclic system does generate ATP but not NADPH and no oxygen is released.

The second stage of photosynthesis, the **light-independent reactions** or dark reactions, takes place in the stroma within the chloroplast. The enzyme RuBisCO (ribulose-1,5-biphosphate carboxylase/oxygenase) captures CO_2 from the air and releases three-carbon sugars in a complex process called the *Calvin-Benson cycle*. The Calvin-Benson cycle is similar to the Krebs cycle because the starting material regenerates after molecules enter and leave the cycle. Carbon enters the cycle in the form of CO_2 and leaves in the form of sugar. The energy source for the cycle is ATP, and NADPH is the reducing power for adding high-energy electrons to make three-carbon sugars (glyceraldehyde 3-phosphate) that later combine to form glucose. The Calvin-Benson cycle is organized into three phases: carbon fixation, reduction, and regeneration of the CO_2 receptor (Figure 3.38).

Protein Synthesis

Cellular structure and function are dependent on proteins (see Chapter 2, Chemistry of Life). Amino acids are the monomers of proteins and 20 amino acids are the building blocks in the synthesis of the different polypeptide chains. The codes for the

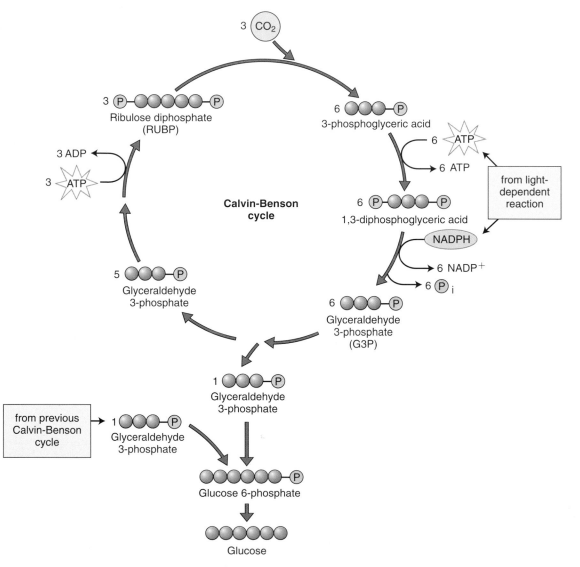

FIGURE 3.38 Calvin-Benson cycle, light-independent reaction of photosynthesis. Three carbon dioxide molecules from the atmosphere are fixed and combine with three molecules of ribulose 1,5-biphosphate (RuBP). The resulting molecules are then reduced to form six molecules of glyceraldehyde 3-phosphate (G3P). Five of the G3P molecules are converted to three RuBP to complete the cycle. The other G3P molecule remains and combines with another G3P molecule to form glucose 6-phosphate, which then can be converted to glucose. Therefore, it takes two turns of the Calvin-Benson cycle to synthesize one glucose 6-phosphate molecule.

amino acid sequence in polypeptides and proteins lie in the genes of DNA and must be copied to direct their synthesis. In order for a gene to be expressed a copy must be made from the DNA template. This copying process is called *transcription* and the subsequent production of a particular amino acid sequence in a polypeptide chain is called *translation*.

Transcription

Prokaryotic transcription occurs in the cytoplasm and eukaryotic transcription takes place in the nucleus. The description or **central dogma** of the flow of information from genetic material was first introduced by Francis Crick in 1958 (Figure 3.39). It states that DNA transfers information to RNA and RNA then controls protein synthesis. Or, DNA makes RNA and RNA makes protein. DNA also controls its own replication (see DNA Replication, later in this chapter). The structures of DNA and RNA are discussed in Chapter 2.

The initiation of transcription is controlled by the enzyme RNA polymerase, which recognizes the beginning of a gene so that it can start mRNA synthesis at a particular DNA sequence that appears at the beginning of genes. This sequence is called a **promoter.** The promoter is a unidirectional sequence on one strand of the DNA and tells the RNA polymerase where to start and in which direction to continue synthesis. RNA polymerase stretches open the double helix at that point and then begins the synthesis of mRNA. This synthesis of mRNA follows the principle of complementary base pairing (see Chapter 2). Termination of transcription occurs when the polymerase recognizes a DNA sequence known as a **terminator sequence.** In prokaryotic cells ribosomes can begin protein synthesis with the mRNA immediately, whereas in eukaryotic cells the mRNA must leave the nucleus before it combines with the ribosomes in the cytoplasm. As stated earlier in this chapter, eukaryotic ribosomes may be free in the cytoplasm, or attached to rER.

Each mRNA molecule contains several hundred or more nucleotides complementary to the DNA template. Every three bases form a base triplet or codon and each codon is the code for a specific amino acid. DNA triplets, RNA codons, and their amino acid translation are shown in Table 3.5. However, some amino acids can be translated by different codon sequences as indicated in Table 3.6. As mRNA moves through the ribosome,

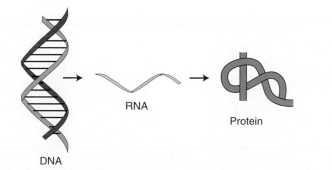

FIGURE 3.39 Central dogma. This drawing illustrates the basis of the flow of information in protein synthesis. The genetic information of the DNA is translated and transcribed by RNA to form the protein.

TABLE 3.5 DNA Base Triplets, mRNA Codons, and Their Amino Acids

DNA Triplet	mRNA Codon	Amino Acid
TAC	AUG	"Start" (methionine)
ATC	UAG	"Stop"
CGT	GCA	Alanine
GCT	CGA	Arginine
ACA	UGU	Cysteine
CCG	GGC	Glycine
CTC	GAG	Glutamic acid
GTG	CAC	Histidine
GAA	CUU	Leucine
AAA	UUU	Phenylalanine
GGG	CCC	Proline
AGG	UCC	Serine
ACC	UGG	Tryptophan

TABLE 3.6 Amino Acids Encoded by Multiple mRNA Codons

Amino Acid	mRNA Codons
Alanine	GCA GCC GCG GCU
Arginine	AGA AGG CGA CGC CGG CGU
Asparagine	AAC AAU
Aspartic acid	GAC GAU
Cysteine	UGC UGU
Glutamic acid	GAA GAG
Glutamine	CAA CAG
Glycine	GGA GGC GGG GGU
Histidine	CAC CAU
Isoleucine	AUA AUC AUU
Leucine	UUA UUG CUA CUC CUG CUU
Lysine	AAA AAG
Methionine	AUG
Phenylalanine	UUC UUU
Proline	CCA CCC CCG CCU
Serine	AGC AGU UCA UCC UCG UCU
Threonine	ACA ACC ACG ACU
Tryptophan	UGG
Tyrosine	UAC UAU
Valine	GUA GUC GUG GUU

the sequence of codons translates into a sequence of amino acids.

Translation

Specific enzymes and tRNA translate codons. Like other RNA molecules, tRNA is a single-stranded molecule; but it bends back in on itself to form a cloverleaf structure with an **anticodon** on one end (Figure 3.40). An anticodon consists of three nucleotides complementary to a specific codon on the mRNA molecule. Specific enzymes (aminoacyl-tRNA synthetase enzymes) in the cytoplasm bind specific amino acids to the ends of tRNA; and a tRNA molecule with a given anticodon can bind to a specific amino acid. Each tRNA molecule is therefore bound to one specific amino acid.

The binding of the tRNA anticodons to the codons of the mRNA, as it moves through the ribosome, forms a polypeptide chain. Translation occurs in three stages: initiation, elongation, and termination.

- *Initiation:* The ribosome assembles on the identified start codon (AUG—methionine) in mRNA and then each sequential base pair forms the next codon. The position of the start codon determines the open reading frame or order of codons that will be read to form a protein.
- *Elongation:* The first and second tRNAs bring the first and second amino acids close together. The first amino acid detaches from its tRNA and forms a peptide bond with the amino acid of the neighboring second tRNA, forming a dipeptide. When the third tRNA binds to the third codon, its amino acid binds to the second amino acid, which then detaches from its tRNA. The polypeptide chain grows as new amino acids are added to this tripeptide by the same process. This growing polypeptide chain remains attached by only one tRNA to the strand of mRNA (Figure 3.41).

- *Termination:* Elongation of the designated protein continues until a "stop" codon (UAA, UGA, or UAG) signals the end of the process. The building of the protein stops because there is no tRNA molecule that is complementary to the stop codon. A releasing enzyme frees the newly formed polypeptide chain from the last tRNA and the mRNA is released from the ribosome.

DNA Replication and Cell Division

DNA Replication

When a cell prepares to divide, the DNA duplicates, and therefore each cell after cell division contains identical DNA. This process is called *replication* or *DNA synthesis*. In eukaryotic cells it occurs during the S phase of the cell cycle and thus precedes mitosis and meiosis (see later in this chapter). The two resulting double strands are identical; each of them consists of one original strand and one newly synthesized strand of the genetic material. This process is called *semiconservative replication*.

The unwinding of DNA occurs through the action of the enzyme **helicase,** which separates the two strands of DNA. The site of separation is the replication fork (Figure 3.42). DNA synthesis begins when a short complementary strand of RNA **(primer RNA)** binds to each parent strand of DNA. The primer RNA serves as the point of attachment for the enzyme DNA polymerase III, which initiates the synthesis of complementary DNA. As the DNA chain lengthens, DNA polymerase I replaces the primer RNA. When the complementary nucleotides are in position opposite each of the nucleotides on the parent strand,

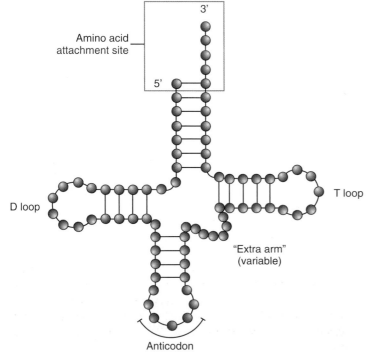

FIGURE 3.40 tRNA molecule. The transfer RNA (tRNA) is a small, cloverleaf-shaped RNA that is the transporting molecule for a particular amino acid. The molecule has an amino acid attachment site (acceptor stem) and a three-base region, the anticodon, that can base pair with the corresponding codon region of messenger RNA (mRNA).

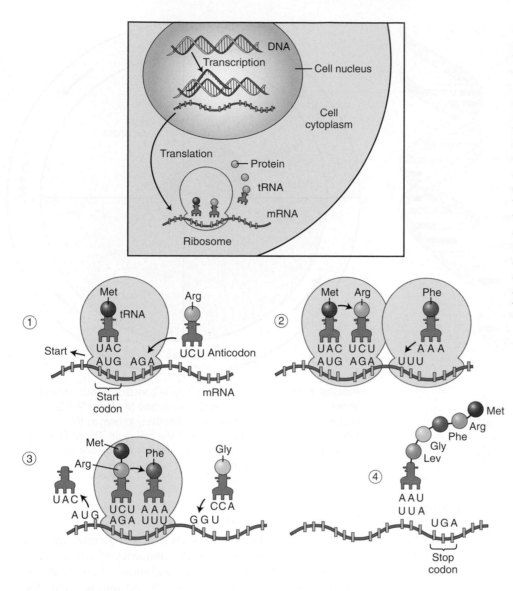

FIGURE 3.41 Translation. *(1)* On the ribosome a tRNA molecule carrying the first amino acid and the anticodon combine with the start codon on the mRNA. tRNA carrying the second amino acid is approaching its codon. *(2)* The ribosome moves along the mRNA so that the second tRNA can attach. When the second tRNA is attached a peptide bond is formed between the first two amino acids and a third tRNA is approaching. *(3)* Once the peptide bond has formed the first tRNA detaches, allowing the third tRNA to bind to its codon, the adjacent amino acids form another peptide bond, and a fourth tRNA is approaching. *(4)* This process of forming a peptide chain continues until the appearance of a stop codon.

covalent bonds are formed between the sugar and phosphate groups of adjacent deoxyribonucleotides on the new chain. Hydrogen bonds form, joining the complementary base pairs between the parental DNA strand and new DNA strand. DNA polymerase can synthesize DNA only in the $5' \rightarrow 3'$ direction. It is a bidirectional process during which one strand is copied continuously and the other discontinuously. The continuous strand of DNA is the leading strand and the discontinuous strand is the lagging strand. The lagging strand of DNA consists of short stretches of RNA primer plus newly synthesized DNA approximately 100 to 1000 bases long. These DNA fragments are Okazaki fragments that attach to the lagging strand by the action of the enzyme DNA ligase. Replication continues until the entire chromosome is duplicated, forming two identical DNA molecules.

Cell Division

The process by which a parental cell divides into two daughter cells is called *cell division*. It is the biological basis of life. For unicellular organisms such as protozoans, one cell division reproduces an entire organism. The different classes of cells use different processes for cell division. Prokaryotic cells, bacteria, divide by binary fission and eukaryotic cells divide by mitosis and meiosis.

Binary Fission

The form of asexual reproduction by which all bacteria and most protists reproduce is binary fission. A single cell separates into two identical daughter cells, each containing an identical copy of the parental DNA. This process occurs in a stepwise fashion starting with elongation of the bacterium. Next, the bacterial chromosomal DNA, which is a single circular molecule, replicates. After this, a central transverse septum forms that divides the cell into two daughter cells (Figure 3.43). This type of reproduction normally results in two identical cells. However, bacterial DNA has a relatively high mutation rate, which is a rapid rate of genetic change that is the underlying reason for the development of antibiotic-resistant bacterial strains.

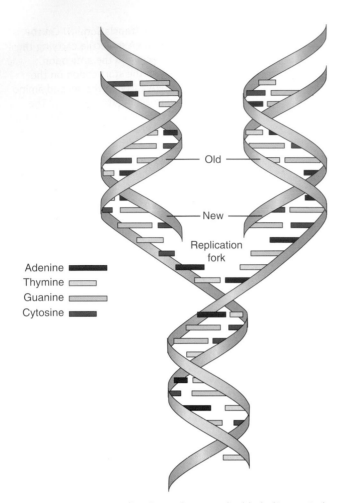

FIGURE 3.42 DNA replication. The DNA double helix unwinds, separating the two strands of DNA at the replication fork. New strands of DNA are formed on each old strand by complementary base pairing. Each new DNA molecule therefore contains an old strand and a new strand of DNA.

Old

New

Replication fork

Adenine
Thymine
Guanine
Cytosine

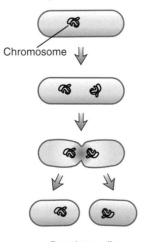

Binary fission in bacteria

Chromosome

Daughter cells

FIGURE 3.43 Binary fission. A single cell separates into two identical daughter cells, each with an identical copy of the parental DNA.

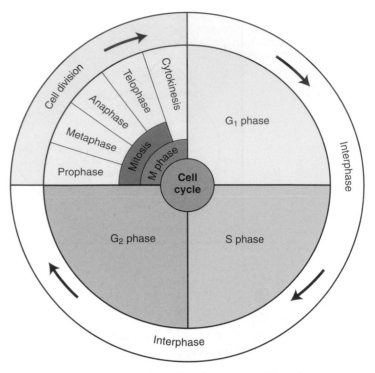

Cell division

Cytokinesis

Telophase

Anaphase

Metaphase

Prophase

Mitosis

M phase

Cell cycle

G_1 phase

Interphase

G_2 phase

S phase

Interphase

FIGURE 3.44 Cell cycle. The cell cycle consists of four distinct phases: the G_1 phase, S phase, G_2 phase, and M phase. The G_1 phase, S phase, and G_2 phase are collectively known as the *interphase* or the *nondividing stage* of the cell cycle. The M phase is composed of two coupled processes: mitosis and cytokinesis (division of the cytoplasm).

Cell Cycle and Mitosis

Eukaryotic cells undergo a cell cycle or a sequential series of events between cell divisions. The frequency of cell divisions varies between different cell types, and some cells never divide after they differentiate (i.e., nerve cells and muscle cells). The cell cycle consists of four distinct phases: the G_1 phase, S phase, G_2 phase, and M phase. The G_1 phase, S phase, and G_2 phase are collectively known as the *interphase* or the *nondividing* stage of the cell cycle (Figure 3.44). The M phase is composed of two tightly coupled processes: mitosis and cytokinesis.

- During the **G_1 phase,** cells carry out the metabolic activities characteristic of the tissue to which they belong. In preparation for cell division, a cell might increase the amount of cytoplasm and the number of cell organelles. Chromosomes are in their extended form, and their genes actively direct RNA synthesis. At the end of G_1, the cell commits to dividing and has reached the "point of no return." In yeast it is called *START* and in multicellular eukaryotes, it is the *restriction point*.
- During the **S phase** DNA duplicates.
- During the **G_2 phase** the cell continues to grow and its metabolic activities prepare for mitosis. The quantity of DNA increases and the chromatin condenses to form short, thick structures that indicate the end of the phase. Now, each chromosome consists of two strands called *chromatids* joined together by a centromere (Figure 3.45).

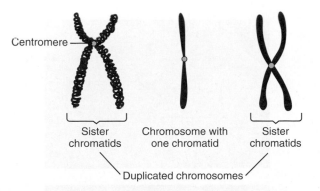

Centromere

Sister chromatids

Chromosome with one chromatid

Sister chromatids

Duplicated chromosomes

FIGURE 3.45 **Chromosome and sister chromatids.** During the G_2 phase the duplicated DNA condenses into chromosomes and each chromosome consists of two strands, called *chromatids*, held together by a centromere. After mitosis each chromatid becomes a separate chromosome.

The two chromatids contain identical DNA base sequences because each is produced by semiconservative replication of DNA. Each chromatid becomes a separate chromosome after mitotic cell division.

- During the **M phase**, mitosis and cytokinesis occur. **Mitosis** is divided into four stages: prophase, metaphase, anaphase, and telophase (Figure 3.46). The visible characteristics of these phases are as follows:
  - Prophase: The chromosomes become clearly visible by light microscopy. The centrioles migrate toward the opposite poles of the cell and each centrosome has spindle fibers extending from it. The nuclear membrane starts to disappear and the nucleolus is no longer visible.
  - Metaphase: The chromosomes line up at the equator of the cell. Spindle fibers from each centriole attach to the centromeres of the chromosomes. The nuclear membrane is now absent.
  - Anaphase: The centrosomes split and the sister chromatids separate as each is pulled to an opposite pole.
  - Telophase: The centrosomes become longer, thinner, and less distinct. New nuclear membranes form and the nucleolus reappears. The cell membrane develops a distinct furrowing at the cell midline. Two separate nuclei are now apparent within the same cell.
  - Cytokinesis: The cytoplasm divides to complete cell division.

Meiosis

Eukaryotic cells maintain a specific number of chromosomes characteristic for that species. The chromosome set exists either in a haploid state (single, unpaired) or in a diploid state (matched pair). Cells of most fungi, many algae, and some protozoans exist in the haploid state during most of their life cycle. Gametes of organisms that sexually reproduce are haploid. Cells of animals, plants, some protozoans, fungi, and algae are diploid throughout most of their life cycle. This state begins at fertilization when a female haploid gamete (egg) fuses with a male haploid gamete (sperm) to create a diploid offspring (haploid + haploid = diploid). Mitosis, however, maintains the normal chromosome number in all eukaryotic cells. Moreover, sexual

reproduction in diploid organisms requires haploid chromosome numbers to produce diploid offspring. The reduction of the diploid chromosome number to a haploid state in gametes occurs during reduction division or **meiosis.**

In meiosis, a single duplication of chromosomes occurs and two cell divisions follow. This type of cell division is diploid → haploid in nature, and occurs only during the production of gametes, that is, sex cells. The diploid cells in the sex organs undergo two cell divisions to produce haploid sex cells. The stages of meiosis subdivide depending on whether they occur in the first or in the second meiotic cell division. These stages are prophase I, metaphase I, anaphase I, and telophase I; and prophase II, metaphase II, anaphase II, and telophase II (Figure 3.47).

- During the first meiotic division in metaphase I, the pairs of homologous chromosomes of a diploid parent cell line up with each member facing a given pole of the cell. Maternal and paternal members of the homologous chromosomes randomly shuffle and each daughter cell obtains one complement from the homologous chromosome pair.
- During the second meiotic division, with each of the chromosomes containing duplicate strands (chromatids), the strands split and each daughter cell receives a haploid number of chromosomes.

It is important during meiosis that the genetic basis of the evolutionary process occurs. In other words, the significance of meiosis goes beyond the reduction of the chromosome number for sexual reproduction. First, during the lining up of the homologous pairs of chromosomes in metaphase I, each member of the pair comes from a different parent and randomly shuffles to end up in one of the daughter cells. Second, crossing-over or additional exchanges of parts of homologous chromosomes can occur in prophase I. In addition, this, together with the random lining up in metaphase I, results in genetic recombination to ensure that the gametes produced in meiosis are genetically unique. All of this provides the genetic diversity for sexually reproducing organisms that is needed to provide the characteristics that promote the survival of species over time—evolution.

Summary

- The cell is the basic structural and functional unit of all living organisms. Two main categories of cells exist: prokaryotes, the cells without a nucleus, and eukaryotes, cells with a membrane-bound nucleus.
- All cells are surrounded by a plasma membrane composed of a phospholipid bilayer and embedded proteins. Functionally, the plasma membrane is selectively permeable and controls the movement of particles in and out of the cell. Many cells have a matrix surrounding the plasma membrane, the multifunctional glycocalyx.
- A cell wall is present around the plasma membrane of many types of cells. The bacterial cell wall is a unique structure, which maintains the rigid shape of bacteria and protects

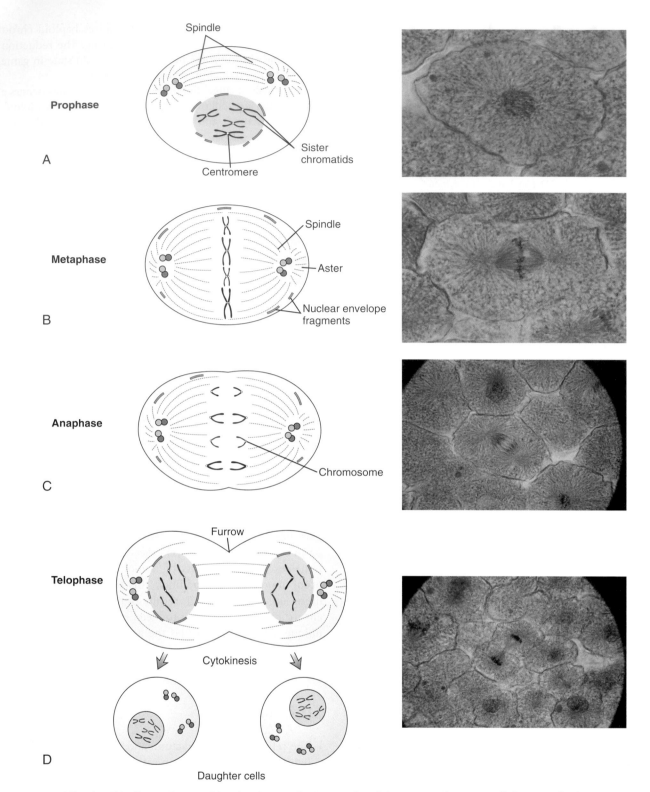

FIGURE 3.46 **Mitosis.** This illustration provides drawings and micrographs of the stages of mitotic cell division of eukaryotic cells. **A,** Prophase—chromosomes become clearly visible, centrioles migrate to the opposite poles of the cell, and spindle fibers form. **B,** Metaphase—the chromosomes line up at the equator of the cell, and the nuclear envelope is dissolved. **C,** Anaphase—the chromosomes split and the sister chromatids separate and are pulled to opposite poles. **D,** Telophase—the chromosomes are at the opposite poles, a nuclear membrane is formed around them, and the cell membrane forms a distinct furrowing at the cell midline just before cytokinesis.

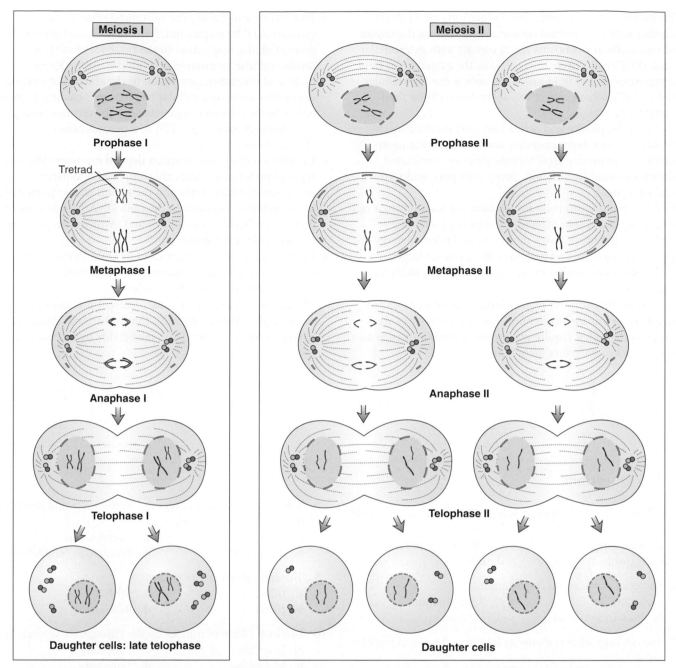

FIGURE 3.47 Meiosis. Meiosis occurs in a series of two divisions called *meiosis I* and *meiosis II*. During the first meiotic division in metaphase I, the pairs of homologous chromosomes of a diploid parent cell line up with each member facing a given pole of the cell. Maternal and paternal members of the homologous chromosomes randomly shuffle and each daughter cell obtains one complement from the homologous chromosome pair. During the second meiotic division, with each of the chromosomes containing duplicate strands (chromatids), the strands split and each daughter cell receives a haploid number of chromosomes. Note that each parental cell undergoing meiotic division produces four daughter cells.

them from hostile environments. On the basis of the composition of their cell wall, most bacteria when stained with the Gram stain, are either gram-positive or gram-negative. This classification provides a major tool for the identification of bacteria.

- Surface appendages are present in both prokaryotic and eukaryotic cells. Prokaryotic cells can have pili or flagella, whereas cilia, flagella, and microvilli are common in eukaryotic cells.

- Biofilms are collections of surface-associated microbes enclosed by an extracellular matrix. Biofilms can form on a wide variety of surfaces and can be the source of product contamination and microbial infections.
- Enclosed by the plasma membrane is the cytoplasm, a gelatinous matrix and the site for biochemical activities of a cell. Within the cytoplasm are the nucleus, other cell organelles, inclusions, and the supportive cytoskeleton.

- Prokaryotic cells and unicellular organisms are in direct contact with the external environment, whereas the tissues of multicellular organisms are in contact with extracellular fluid (ECF) collectively referred to as the extracellular fluid compartment. The fluid inside the cells is the intracellular fluid or ICF, which collectively is the intracellular fluid compartment.
- Cells exhibit passive and active transport mechanisms by which they can move materials across the plasma membrane. These mechanisms include diffusion, facilitated diffusion, osmosis, filtration, pump transport, endocytosis, and exocytosis.
- Cellular metabolism includes all chemical reactions in a cell and is organized into metabolic pathways. Metabolic pathways that break down molecules and release energy are part of catabolism, and pathways that produce larger molecules from smaller ones, using energy, are anabolic pathways.
- All metabolic pathways require biological catalysts, called *enzymes*, to initiate biochemical reactions. Enzymes are proteins that often require nonprotein compounds such as coenzymes or cofactors for action.

- Prokaryotic and eukaryotic cells metabolize nutrients to generate ATP by respiration, fermentation, and photosynthesis. Cellular respiration in the presence of oxygen is aerobic cellular respiration with glycolysis, the Krebs cycle, and the respiratory chain. In the absence of oxygen, cells utilize anaerobic cellular respiration including fermentation. Some cells and organisms can convert light energy into chemical energy via ATP, in a process called *photosynthesis*.
- Cellular structure and function depend on many different types of proteins. Proteins are composed of different sequences of amino acids and the amino acid sequence of a given protein is encoded in the cell's DNA. The process of protein synthesis requires RNA and involves two processes: transcription and translation.
- Before a cell divides, it duplicates its DNA to ensure that each cell after division contains identical DNA. This process is called *replication* or *DNA synthesis*.
- The different classes of cells use different processes for cell division. Prokaryotic cells, that is, bacteria, divide by binary fission and eukaryotic cells divide by mitosis and meiosis.

Review Questions

1. Which of the following is *not* found in *all* bacterial cells?
   a. Ribosomes
   b. Capsule
   c. Plasma membrane
   d. DNA

2. Bacterial capsules are important in:
   a. Storage
   b. Protein synthesis
   c. Reproduction
   d. Survival

3. The cell organelles responsible for the packaging of proteins are the:
   a. Ribosomes
   b. Golgi complexes
   c. rER
   d. Lysosomes

4. The cell organelle found only in algae and plant cells is the:
   a. Chloroplast
   b. Mitochondria
   c. Vacuole
   d. Vesicle

5. The intracellular fluid has a high concentration of:
   a. Sodium
   b. Potassium
   c. Bicarbonate
   d. Sulfate

6. Which of the following is an active transport mechanism?
   a. Osmosis
   b. Facilitated diffusion
   c. Filtration
   d. Pinocytosis

7. Which of the following is an enzyme?
   a. Fructose
   b. Ligase
   c. Dextrose
   d. Lactose

8. The compound that enters the Krebs cycle and combines with oxaloacetic acid is:
   a. Citric acid
   b. Pyruvic acid
   c. Acetyl-CoA
   d. Phosphoglyceraldehyde

9. The anticodons are located in:
   a. tRNA
   b. rRNA
   c. mRNA
   d. Ribosomes

10. In which phase of mitosis do the chromatids separate?
    a. Prophase
    b. Metaphase
    c. Anaphase
    d. Telophase

11. Cells without a nucleus are _____ cells.

12. The sterol-like molecules in bacterial plasma membranes are _____.

13. A cell organelle that contains digestive enzymes is a(n) _____.

14. The allosteric site is present in _____.

15. The organelle necessary for photosynthesis is a(n) _____.

16. Compare and contrast prokaryotic and eukaryotic cells.

17. Describe the cell wall of gram-positive and gram-negative cells.

18. Discuss the regulation of enzyme activity.

19. Name and describe the pathways of aerobic cellular respiration.

20. Describe the cell cycle and the phases of mitosis.

Bibliography

Donlan RM: *Biofilms and device-associated infections.* Emerg Infect Dis 7:277–281, 2001.

Donlan RM: *Biofilms: microbial life on surfaces.* Emerg Infect Dis 8:881–890, 2002.

Jabra-Rizk MA, Falkler WA, Meiller TF: *Fungal biofilms and drug resistance.* Emerg Infect Dis 10:14–19, 2004.

Mims C, Dockrell HM, Goering RV, et al: *Medical Microbiology,* ed 3, St. Louis, 2004, Mosby/Elsevier.

Thibodeau GA, Patton KT: *Anatomy and Physiology,* St. Louis, 2007, Mosby/Elsevier.

Internet Resources

University of Texas Medical Branch, Cell Biology Graduate Program, http://cellbio.utmb.edu/cellbio/

Nobelprize.org, http://nobelprize.virtual.museum/nobel_prizes/physics/laureates/1986/ruska-autobio.html

National Institutes of Health, Research on Microbial Biofilms, http://grants.nih.gov/grants/guide/pa-files/PA-03-047.html

Mayer F: Cytoskeletons in prokaryotes, Cell Biol Int 27(5):429–438, 2003. http://www.ncbi.nlm.nih.gov/pubmed/12758091?dopt=Abstract?

Northwestern University, Goldman Lab, http://www.goldmanlab.northwestern.edu/intro_lamins.htm

Schmitt CK, Meysick KC, O'Brien AD: Bacterial toxins: friends or foes? Emerg Infect Dis 5:224–234, 1999. http://www.cdc.gov/ncidod/eid/vol5no2/schmitt.htm

4

Microbiological Laboratory Techniques

[OUTLINE

Aseptic Technique in Laboratory Preparation and Analysis
Sterilization
Disinfection
Sanitization

Culture Techniques
Types of Culture Media
Live Media
Incubation and Isolation

Fixation and Staining
Negative and Simple Stains
Differential Stains
Special Stains
Fixation and Staining for Electron Microscopy

Identification Techniques
Morphology
Cultural Characteristics
Physiological/Biochemical Characteristics
Molecular Analysis

[LEARNING OBJECTIVES

After reading this chapter, the student will be able to:

- Describe the general concept of aseptic techniques used in laboratory preparation and analysis
- Explain and differentiate between sterilization, disinfection, and sanitization
- Describe the different types of culture media and their possible physical state
- Discuss inoculation, incubation, and isolation
- Describe the various fixation and staining techniques to identify microbes with the light microscope
- Describe the fixation and staining methods used in electron microscopy
- Classify the bacteria according to their shape for morphological identification
- Describe the different culture characteristics of microbes used for the purpose of identification
- Discuss the physiological, biochemical, and genetic characteristics used for microbial identification purposes

agar	enriched media	pleomorphic
antiseptics	filamentous	pour plate
aseptic technique	fomite	sanitization
bactericidal	fusiform	sediment
bacteriostatic	germicide	selective media
chemical defined media	hemolysins	semisolid media
complex media	incubated	solid media
contaminants	inoculation	spread plate
cultures	inoculum	sterile
culture media	isolation	sterilization
degermation	liquid media	streak plate
differential media	nonsynthetic media	synthetic media
disinfection	pellicle	the five "I's"
	peptone	turbid

WHY YOU NEED TO KNOW

HISTORY

To understand microbiology is to understand the laboratory; its basic equipment, how its equipment is used, the procedures carried out, and—importantly—the preparation of and meaning of test results.

In the 1600s, the newly created microscope yielded images of samples previously too small to be seen with the naked eye. Reports of interpretation of these early microbiological laboratory observations led to the realization that life could exist in a single cell, followed in the 1800s by the cell doctrine.

In addition, laboratory findings of Pasteur and Koch revealed pathogenic microorganisms to be causes and carriers of disease, from which evolved the germ theory of disease. In 1877, Pasteur and Joubert described microbial antagonism among bacteria and in 1899 the term "antibiotic" was coined. Present-day biotechnological methodologies have grown from laboratory findings that prompted the development of new technologies to drive further advances in microbiology as a scientific discipline.

IMPACT

Verification of the successes and failures of putative treatments for pathogenic diseases is performed under laboratory conditions in the search for new drug and antibiotic therapy. Moreover, results from the laboratory give basic understanding of microorganisms, their mechanisms of action, and their relationship with the environment.

The addition of clinical and laboratory experience permits a rational approach to the question of "what happens if?" and suggests pertinent experiments that can be carried out safely under carefully controlled laboratory conditions.

One of the beneficial outgrowths of microbiological investigations in the laboratory has been the need to use aseptic techniques for the growth and identification of specific microorganisms. Culture techniques were derived from the necessity to rapidly grow and accurately identify potential pathogens in order to treat individuals or take appropriate steps to prevent outbreaks of disease, epidemics, or pandemics.

FUTURE

The acknowledgment of threats to outbreaks of pathogenic disease has brought a public awareness to the importance of compliance with proven preventative procedures and therapies.

Aside from these ever-present battles against commonly confronted pathogens, another deadly issue has arisen—bacteriological warfare. Again, our most effective weapon against this potential disaster comes from the laboratory. Recently, the use of anthrax as a bioterrorism weapon was attempted in Washington, D.C. Through the prompt use of laboratory procedures, it was identified and safely disposed of, although weaponization of pathogens is and continues to be a bioterrorism threat.

Threats to human health via pathogenic organisms or via bioterrorism agents will be met by work done in laboratories. Laboratory work has been and continues to be the cornerstone of protection against disease, of microbiology, and of world health.

Aseptic Technique in Laboratory Preparation and Analysis

Medical and clinical laboratories test biological specimens to determine the health status of a patient and to identify the disease-causing pathogen for the purpose of appropriate treatment. Research laboratories include basic, clinical, and pharmaceutical laboratories, each dealing with a specific aspect of microbiological research.

Microorganisms are everywhere in the environment. In order to selectively identify specific microbes they must be grown in controlled laboratory environments. Beginning with pure sterile cultures, the key is to control the factors to which the cultures are subjected. In other words, when working with microbial **cultures,** it is necessary to ensure that organisms are selectively introduced into the culture and that other environmental organisms do not contaminate it. **Aseptic technique** is a procedure that is performed under sterile conditions, a method that prevents the introduction of unwanted organisms or **contaminants** into an environment. This process is characterized by strict adherence to details. The use of aseptic technique controls, limits, or prevents contamination by fomites. A **fomite** is any inanimate object or substance capable of transporting pathogens from one medium or individual to another. Aseptic technique is essential in the microbiology laboratory to prevent any contamination of laboratory personnel (see Chapter 5, Safety Issues), cultures, supplies, and equipment.

Air currents must be controlled by closing laboratory doors and windows to prevent microbes on surfaces from becoming airborne and entering the cultures. When handling cultures to prepare slides or to transfer organisms to another medium, the transfer loops and needles need to be sterilized by flame or incinerator before and after use (Figure 4.1). Furthermore, culture plates are held in a position that minimizes exposure of the medium to the environment. When removing lids/stoppers from test tubes, the lids should remain held in the hand and not placed on other surfaces such as countertops during the transfer of materials from one tube to another. Flaming is one of the physical methods of sterilization and must always be applied to the lips of test tubes and also of flasks whenever culture liquid is poured from one container to another, as in the case of pouring culture plates (Figure 4.2).

Sterilization and disinfection procedures are daily routines in microbiological laboratories. They are essential to ensure that cultures, containers, media, and equipment are handled in such a way that only the desired organism will grow and others will be eliminated or excluded.

Sterilization

Sterilization is the destruction or removal of all microorganisms, including bacteria and their endospores, viruses, fungi, and prions. This can be accomplished by physical methods such as heat, radiation, and filtration, or by chemical methods. The

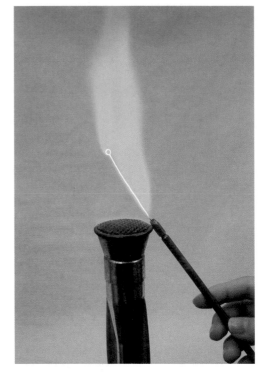

FIGURE 4.1 Sterilization of a loop. One of the primary inoculation tools in the microbiology laboratory is the loop. Metal loops must be sterilized in the flame of a Bunsen burner by heating the wire until it glows. Presterilized, disposable plastic loops are also available for inoculation.

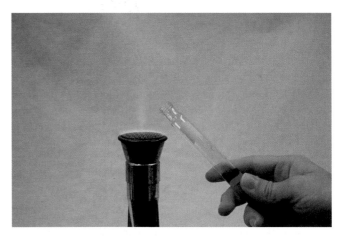

FIGURE 4.2 Aseptic technique and media containers. Bacteria and fungi are everywhere in the environment, including the air. The mouth of a tube or bottle opening is a potential point of contamination and flaming of the opening in direct flame immediately after opening and before closing is an effective technique to prevent potential contamination on this exposed surface.

wide application of sterilization processes makes it necessary to impose strict control measures to validate the results. When using dry heat or moist heat sterilization, physical, chemical, or biological indicators can be used to validate the desired results (Table 4.1). The general resistance of microbes to methods of sterilization ranges from bacterial endospores, with the highest

TABLE 4.1 Methods for Validating Dry or Moist Heat Sterilization

	Physical Methods	Chemical Methods	Biological Test Organism
Dry heat	Temperature-recording charts	Color change indicator	*Bacillus subtilis* var. *niger*
Moist heat	Temperature-recording charts	Color change indicator	*Bacillus stearothermophilus*

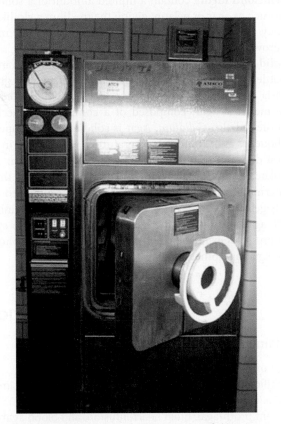

FIGURE 4.3 Autoclave. The autoclave is one of the primary tools for sterilization of equipment, containers, media, and biohazardous wastes. It is essentially a large pressure cooker that raises the temperature of steam to about 121° C under 15–20 psi pressure. The size and configuration of autoclaves vary but the basic operation is same.

resistance to sterilization, to vegetative cells, with moderate to least resistance.

Physical and chemical methods of sterilization are applied in the microbiological laboratory to ensure that equipment and materials are free of microorganisms. Aseptic technique is the first and most important step in ensuring that manipulation of specimens during investigative procedures does not infect laboratory personnel or contaminate cultures or the laboratory environment (see Chapter 5, Safety Issues). Bacteria are found practically everywhere including fingertips and bench tops and therefore it is essential to minimize contact with these surfaces. Only **sterile** items are free of potentially contaminating microorganisms and once a sterile object comes in contact with a nonsterile surface, the object can no longer be considered sterile. The most commonly used instrument in the microbiology laboratory for the sterilization of media and glassware is the autoclave (Figure 4.3). A detailed discussion of the different

types of physical and chemical methods of sterilization is provided in Chapter 19 (Physical and Chemical Methods of Control; for overviews see Tables 19.3 and 19.5).

Disinfection

Disinfectants are applied to inanimate surfaces, medical equipment, and other man-made objects whereas **antiseptics** are used to disinfect skin. The term **disinfection** refers to the use of a physical process or the use of a chemical agent to destroy vegetative microbes and viruses. This does not include bacterial endospores. The ideal disinfectant would result in complete sterilization without harming other forms of life. Unfortunately, ideal disinfectants as such do not exist and most of them only partially sterilize. In addition to the most resistant pathogens, endospores, other bacteria, and viruses are also highly resistant to many disinfectants.

Substances that kill bacteria are **bactericidal** and those that interfere with cell growth and reproduction are **bacteriostatic.** Disinfectants and antiseptics are bactericidal and bacteriostatic depending on the concentration applied. All disinfectants are by their nature potentially harmful, even toxic, to humans and animals. They should be handled with appropriate care to avoid harm to the handler or recipient. The type of disinfectant to be used depends on the surface or material to be disinfected. Specifics on the different types of disinfectants and their particular effectiveness are described in Chapter 19, with an overview in Table 19.5 (Chemicals Used in the Control of Microbes).

Sanitization

Several applications in everyday life and medicine do not require sterilization, disinfection, or antisepsis but need to reduce microorganisms in order to control possible infections or spoilage of substances. **Sanitization** achieves this by using any cleansing technique that mechanically removes microorganisms and other debris to reduce contamination to safe levels. Often the sanitizer used is a compound such as soap or detergent. Restaurants, dairies, breweries, and other food industries handle soiled utensils on a daily basis and must take appropriate measures to sanitize them for prevention of infection, spoilage, and contamination. This includes controlling microbes to a minimal level during preparation and processing.

Degermation is the process by which the numbers of microbes on the human skin are reduced by scrubbing, immersion in chemicals, or both. Some examples of degermation include the process of presurgical scrubbing of the hands with sterile brushes and germicidal soap before putting on sterile surgical gloves, the application of alcohol wipes to the skin, and the cleansing of a wound with germicidal soap and water.

Culture Techniques

Microbiologists use five basic procedures to examine and characterize microbes: Inoculation, Incubation, Isolation, Inspection (observation), and Identification—**the five "I's."** To culture a microorganism a small sample, the **inoculum,** is introduced into a culture medium usually with a platinum wire probe streaked across its surface. This process is called **inoculation** and the growth that appears on or in the medium is the culture. A culture can be pure—containing one type of organism, or mixed—containing two or more species.

Types of Culture Media

Nutritional requirements of particular microorganisms range from a few simple inorganic compounds to a complex list of specific inorganic and organic chemicals (Table 4.2). Access to carbon, the essential component required for molecular life, is obtained in different ways by microorganisms. Autotrophs acquire carbon from carbon dioxide in the atmosphere and heterotrophs obtain their carbon from organic compounds. This diversity is seen in the different types of media needed to ensure the growth of the organism for investigation. Media vary in nutrient content and consistency and can be classified according to their physical state, chemical composition, and functional type.

Physical State of Media

Liquid media are water-based solutions that do not solidify at temperatures above freezing and flow freely in the containers when tilted. Most commonly, liquid media are supplied in tubes or bottles and are called *broths*, *milks*, or *infusions*. A common laboratory medium is nutrient broth, which contains beef extract and **peptone** (partially digested protein) dissolved in water. Methylene blue milk and litmus milk are opaque liquids prepared from skim milk powder and dyes. After inoculation, growth occurs throughout the container. Enriched broths are used to grow bacteria that are present in few numbers such as in small specimen samples obtained from patients.

Semisolid media contain a limited amount of a solidifying agent such as agar or gelatin, giving the medium a clotlike consistency. Semisolid media are often used to determine motility and growth patterns of bacteria.

Solid media are dispensed in Petri plates or slanted in tubes or bottles to provide firm and maximal surfaces for growing bacteria or fungi. By far the most widely used and effective of these media is **agar,** composed of a complex polysaccharide from the red alga *Gelidium*. Agar is solid at room temperature and liquefies at the boiling temperature of water. Once in liquid form it does not solidify until it cools to 42° C. It then can be inoculated and poured in liquid form at temperatures that will not harm the microbes or the handlers. Agar added to media simply gels them into a solid form. Any medium containing 1% to 5% agar usually has the agar in the name of the specific medium as, for example, nutrient agar, phenylethyl alcohol agar, blood agar, and others.

TABLE 4.2 Nutritional Requirements for Microorganisms*

Macronutrients	Growth Factors (Vitamins)	Micronutrients (Trace Elements)
Carbon	p-Aminobenzoic acid	Boron
Hydrogen	Folic acid	Chromium
Oxygen	Biotin	Cobalt
Nitrogen	Cobalamin (B$_{12}$)	Copper
Phosphorus	Lipoic acid	Iron
Sulfur	Nicotinic acid (niacin)	Manganese
Potassium	Pantothenic acid	Molybdenum
Magnesium	Riboflavin	Nickel
Sodium	Thiamine	Selenium
Calcium	Vitamin B$_6$	Tungsten
Iron	Vitamin K group	Vanadium
	Hydroxamates	Zinc

*Not all microbes need all of the nutrients listed; therefore, for optimal growth environments media with specific nutrients are necessary for specific microorganisms.

LIFE APPLICATION

Raising Bacteria: A Labor of Love

Most of the bacteria raised in laboratories for testing, identification, or experimentation grow on relatively simple media. Complex media such as tryptic soy broth/agar, nutrient broth/agar, brain heart infusion, and blood agar are useful for growing a wide range of bacteria. The conditions that most organisms are grown under vary from anaerobic to microaerophilic (5% oxygen) to capnophilic ("carbon dioxide loving") to simply aerobic and in temperatures ranging from 4° C to about 60° C. These medium types and incubation conditions can be found and maintained in most microbiology/clinical laboratories. There are, however, some bacteria that are very picky eaters and require some extraordinary medium concoctions to raise them in the laboratory. The normal growth conditions of other bacteria, such as extremophiles, may be challenging to reproduce in the average laboratory. Some pathogenic bacteria such as those in the genera *Spiroplasma* and *Mycoplasma* need specialized media for culturing. Spiroplasma medium is a broth that contains more than 80 ingredients including various types of nutrients as well as antibiotics to suppress other possible competitors. Extremophiles, whose natural growth environment is at the vent holes at the bottom of the ocean, present some significant challenges for culturing. The extreme pressures and temperatures required as well as the unique nutritional requirements of these bacteria make their cultivation possible only in laboratories with sophisticated equipment to meet the organisms' needs.

Chemical Classification of Media

Depending on their chemical content media can be classified as complex or nonsynthetic media and as chemically defined or synthetic media.

- **Chemically defined media** or **synthetic media** are media with a defined, exact chemical composition. They are prepared by means of an exact formula, adding precise amounts of inorganic and/or organic chemicals to distilled water. Some of these media contain minimal amounts of chemicals such as some salts and a source of carbon; others are special media containing a variety of precisely measured substances.
- **Complex media** or **nonsynthetic media** contain at least one component that cannot be chemically defined and thus the medium cannot be represented by an exact chemical formula. Complex media contain extracts from animals, plants, or yeast. They may include blood, serum, meat extracts, milk, yeast extracts, soybean digests, and peptone.

Functional Types of Media

General-purpose media are designed to grow a broad spectrum of microbes that do not have any special growth requirements. Other media are available for special growth conditions of selected organisms. These include enriched, selective, and differential media.

- **Enriched media** contain complex organic substances such as blood, serum, hemoglobin, or growth factors for the growth needs of specific species. An example is blood agar, made by adding sterile sheep, horse, or rabbit blood to a sterile agar base. It is widely used to grow certain streptococci and other pathogens. Another enriched medium is chocolate agar. Chocolate agar is enriched with heat-treated blood, which turns brown and gives the medium the color and thus its name.
- **Selective media** inhibit the growth of selected organisms while allowing the growth of others. These media are useful in isolating bacteria or fungi from specimens that contain several different organisms. For example, mannitol salt agar contains 7.5% NaCl, inhibitory to most human pathogens with the exception of the genus *Staphylococcus*, which thrives in mannitol salt agar and consequently its growth can be amplified in mixed samples.
- **Differential media** can grow several different organisms that show visible differences. These differences can be variations in colony size or color, a change in medium color, or the formation of gas bubbles and precipitates. Dyes can be used as differential agents because many of them are pH indicators that change color in response to acid or base production by a specific microbe. For example, MacConkey agar contains neutral red, which is a dye that is yellow when neutral and pink or red when acidic. *Escherichia coli,* a bacterium common to the intestinal tract, produces acid when it metabolizes the lactose in the medium and develops red or pink colonies. In contrast, *Salmonella* does not give off acid and therefore remains in a natural off-white color. A comparison of general, selective, and differential media is shown in Figure 4.4.

Live Media

Viruses and certain bacteria that cannot grow on artificial media require cell cultures or host animals to grow. In the early times of microbiology animals were used to confirm the pathogenicity of bacteria isolated from cases of human infections (see Koch's postulates in Chapter 1, Scope of Microbiology). Today, animal inoculations are rarely used in diagnostic laboratories. Fluid or tissue suspensions from patients suspected to have viral, fungal, or protozoal infections are occasionally injected intraperitone-

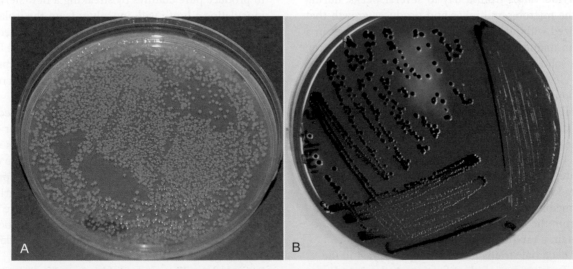

FIGURE 4.4 Types of media. Pictured are **(A)** tryptic soy agar—a complex medium used as an all-purpose growth medium, and **(B)** xylose lysine deoxycholate agar—a chemically defined agar that is both selective and differential and used primarily in selecting for and differentiating gram-negative enteric bacilli, especially *Shigella, Salmonella,* and *Providencia.* Yellow indicates the organism is utilizing the carbohydrate xylose and the black colonies indicate the production of hydrogen sulfide.

Growth Requirements of Selected Bacteria

Bacterium	Medium	Atmospheric Conditions
Pseudomonas aeruginosa	Simple nutritional requirements	Aerobic
Streptococcus pneumoniae	Blood agar	Anaerobic 5% CO_2
Mycobacterium tuberculosis	Middlebrook medium; Lowenstein-Jensen medium	Obligate aerobic
Escherichia coli	Glucose–salts medium MacConkey agar Eosin methylene blue (EMB) agar	Aerobic and anaerobic
Staphylococcus aureus	Heart infusion broth	Facultative anaerobic

ally into mice or hamsters; however, there are few pathogens that will not grow on some artificial medium. Of note is *Mycobacterium leprae,* the causative agent for leprosy, which can be cultured only in the footpads of mice or a species of armadillo.

Incubation and Isolation

After inoculation, the media are **incubated** by placing their containers in a temperature-controlled chamber or incubator, to facilitate the growth process. The incubator temperature in the laboratory is generally between 20° C and 40° C. The concentration of atmospheric gases may also be controlled in some incubators if required for the growth of a certain microbe. The incubation period varies from a day to several weeks, during which time the microbe multiplies and produces growth that can be visualized without a microscope. Microbial growth in a liquid medium manifests itself as cloudiness, sediment, scum, or color. On solid media the growth appears as colonies of various sizes, shapes, color, and texture.

Identification of bacterial cultures depends on isolating colonies that contain an uncontaminated single species of an organism—a pure culture. A pure culture can be obtained by three different techniques: streak plate, pour plate, or spread plate.

- **Streak plate:** The procedure of streaking a plate with an inoculating loop spreads millions of cells over the surface of a solid medium, and then separates individual cells at a distance from the others. Usually samples, such as lake water, contain a mixture of bacteria and isolation of individual bacterial strains needs to be performed in the laboratory for purposes of identification. A classic technique used for this purpose is the streak plate procedure by which bacteria from a sample are spread over the surface of an agar plate, using a series of strikes, basically

Vaccine Development in Eggs

Fighting influenza is a major annual undertaking that requires the resources of the Department of Health and Human Services, the World Health Organization, vaccine and drug companies, state and local health authorities, as well as the medical community at large. Each year, isolates of influenza viruses from laboratories in the United States and overseas are sent to the Centers for Disease Control and Prevention (CDC) in Atlanta, Georgia. These are tested and the results of the antigenic and molecular characteristics of the viruses are used in the production of appropriate vaccines for distribution to relevant medical facilities.

However, because viruses are dependent on a host cell for reproduction they cannot be grown on artificial media. To meet the annual demands for influenza (flu) vaccines, they are produced in fertilized chicken eggs. After fertilization, the egg is injected with the virus, which multiplies in the host. The virus is then harvested, purified, and chemically inactivated to produce the vaccine. Between one and two eggs are needed to produce one dose of vaccine and the entire production process takes at least 6 months—a slow process. In order to produce 300 million doses of vaccine, egg-based production requires approximately 900 million eggs. Alternative methods of flu vaccine production with cell and tissue cultures are currently being explored to facilitate and speed up production.

"thinning" the inoculum. After spreading, bacteria are separated at a distance from one another and can multiply to form isolated colonies. These colonies can then be used to produce pure cultures by streaking a new sterile plate or inoculating a broth with inoculum from the isolated colony. The isolated cultures are usually subjected to the streak plate procedure a few times until a single bacterial strain exists on the Petri plate. There are a number of different methods for mechanically diluting microorganisms on a streak plate, as shown in Figure 4.5.

- **Pour plate:** The pour plate technique can be used to determine the number of microbes per milliliter or the number of microbes per gram in a specimen, as well as to suspend isolated cells for culture. The advantage of this technique is that it does not require previously prepared plates and is often used to assay foods for bacterial contamination. With this technique, bacteria are inoculated into a tube of melted agar that has been cooled to 45° C to 47° C, mixed, and then poured into a sterile Petri plate (Figure 4.6).
- **Spread plate:** The number of bacteria in a solution can be quantified by using the spread plate technique. With this technique a small amount of a liquid inoculum is placed in the center of an agar medium plate and spread evenly over

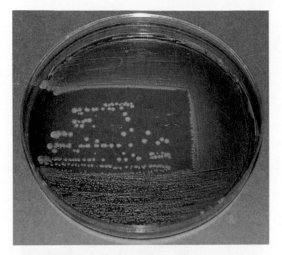

FIGURE 4.5 **Streak plate.** The streak plate is used primarily to produce isolated colonies from the inoculum. These isolated colonies represent pure cultures of the organism and can be used to produce additional pure cultures, to perform biochemical testing, or both. The plate shows the quadrant streaking pattern applied with a sterile loop.

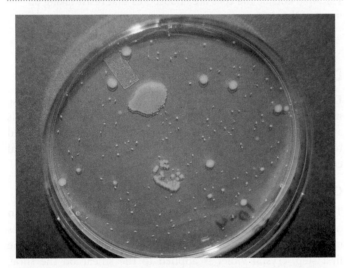

FIGURE 4.6 **Pour plate.** The pour plate can be used to produce isolated colonies as well as to perform plate counts. The technique involves adding the inoculum to warm liquid agar in a Petri plate and allowing the agar to cool and solidify. The colonies will grow on the surface as well as throughout the thickness of the agar. The smaller, oval-shaped colonies on the pour plate in this photo are actually embedded in the agar.

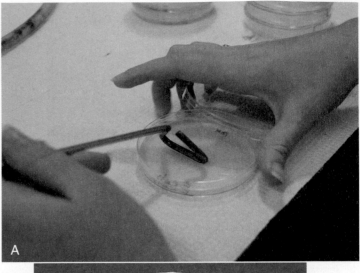

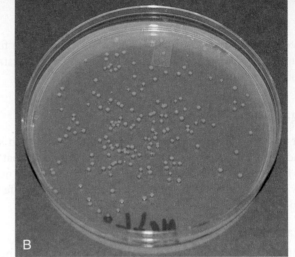

FIGURE 4.7 **Spread plate.** The spread plate is used primarily to perform cell counts on a sample. The original sample is serially diluted, a measured amount of inoculum is then spread over the surface of the agar, and the colonies are counted after incubation. **A,** Sterilization of the spreader stick and observance of aseptic technique are critical as any contamination will be spread over the plate and prevent an accurate count of the colonies of interest. The stick is sterilized by immersing it in alcohol, igniting it, and allowing it to burn off before and after use. **B,** This photo shows a spread plate after 24 hours of incubation. The colonies are evenly distributed over the agar surface and can easily be counted in order to calculate the original cell density of the sample.

the surface with a bent sterile glass, metal, or plastic (disposable) rod (Figure 4.7). Plates are then allowed to absorb the inoculum before being inverted for incubation. After the colonies are grown, they are counted and the number of bacteria in the original sample is calculated.

In the laboratory environment a mixed culture can contain two or more easily identifiable and differentiated microorganisms, using differential media. On the other hand, a contaminated culture is a culture that once was pure or mixed but was contaminated unintentionally with unwanted organisms.

Fixation and Staining

In order to observe microorganisms under the microscope the specimens must be specially prepared. Some organisms can be observed in the living state, but most often the specimens are dead or killed by chemical fixatives such as glutaraldehyde. Materials that have been dried on glass slides are called *smears* and are fixed to the slide with chemicals or heat (heat-fixed). Preparation of samples for electron microscopy requires differ-

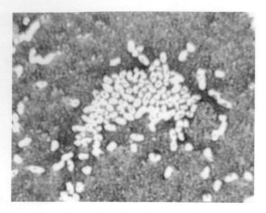

FIGURE 4.8 **Negative stain.** This micrograph shows a negative stain of *Klebsiella pneumoniae*, using India ink as the negatively charged stain. Note how the stain is repelled by the cell, producing a clear halo around the organism.

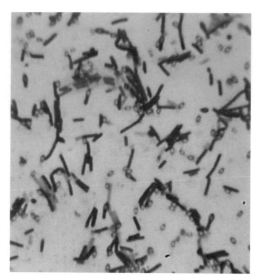

FIGURE 4.9 **Simple stain.** This micrograph illustrates a simple stain of *Bacillus cereus*, using crystal violet as the positively charged stain. The positively charged stain is attracted to the negatively charged cell wall. The clear egg-shaped voids inside some cells and scattered outside the cells are endospores that resist taking up much of the stain.

ent techniques, which are discussed separately. In order for fixed organisms to become visible under the light microscope, staining of the specimens is required.

Negative and Simple Stains

Most biological materials provide little contrast from their surroundings and must be stained for visualization. Dyes that are used to enhance the contrast of a cell can be positively or negatively charged, which allows the dye to attach itself to different components of the cell or to be repelled by the cell.

Negative Stain

Negative staining is an indirect staining process by which negatively charged dyes stain the background of the slide. Acidic stains such as India ink or nigrosin, when applied to bacteria, produce a dark background against the organisms. The organisms appear colorless because they do not pick up the stain, the result of the presence in their cell wall of negatively charged proteins that repel the stain (Figure 4.8). Negative stain techniques do not require fixation of the smear. This staining procedure is extremely valuable for identifying spirochetes, yeast capsules, and some other bacterial capsules.

Simple Stain

In simple staining, a single stain is applied to the specimen after fixation onto the slide. Simple stains are positively charged and are attracted to the negatively charged bacteria.

The most commonly used simple stains in microbiology include the methylene blue, crystal violet, and safranin stains. A drop of stain is put on the slide containing the specimen and allowed to react with the smear (specimen) for 30 to 60 seconds. The stain is then rinsed off with water, blotted or air dried, and the slide is ready for microscopic examination. Simple staining allows observation of the shape, size, and groupings of bacteria (Figure 4.9). Sometimes endospores can be identified because they do not take up stain and therefore appear colorless. However, endospores can be stained by special procedures (see Special Stains, later in this chapter).

Differential Stains

Differential stains are more complex than simple stains and use more than one stain to differentiate cellular components. This application of more than one stain to a fixed smear is often used to demonstrate different staining characteristics of bacterial cells and allows the differentiation between bacterial species.

Gram Stain

The Gram stain is the most widely used differential stain in microbiology. It is a four-step staining process that differentiates bacteria into gram-negative and gram-positive groups. In the first step, crystal violet is applied to the smear on the slide, which is then rinsed with water. Next, Gram's iodine, a mordant (a chemical that fixes the dye to intensify a staining reaction) is applied and the slide is again rinsed with water. At this point all bacteria appear purple. Now a decolorizing agent, a mixture of acetone and ethyl alcohol or just 95% ethyl alcohol, is applied to the slide. Gram-positive bacteria with their thick peptidoglycan layer will retain some of the crystal violet, but gram-negative bacteria with their thin peptidoglycan layer will not retain crystal violet and will be colorless after this step. The slide is then rinsed again with water. In the final step safranin, a counterstain, is applied followed by a last rinse with water (Box 4.1). Bacteria that retain crystal violet, the primary stain, along with the safranin, are called *gram-positive bacteria* and appear purple/blue. Gram-negative bacteria appear red due to the safranin counterstain because the crystal violet was lost during the decolorizing step (Figure 4.10).

The Gram staining procedure is most reliable with young bacterial cultures. However, as cultures age, some gram-positive bacteria may appear gram negative because they lose their ability to retain crystal violet. The Gram staining properties of

1. Stain with crystal violet for 1 minute.
2. Rinse with tap water.
3. Stain with Gram's iodine for 1 minute.
4. Rinse with tap water.
5. Decolorize with 95% ethyl alcohol or ethanol–acetone.
6. Rinse with tap water.
7. Stain with safranin for 1 minute.
8. Wash with tap water and blot dry.

1. Stain slide with basic carbolfuchsin while heating it slowly to the steaming point.
2. Continue steaming gently for 5 to 10 minutes, replacing stain when necessary.
3. Allow slide to cool and wash with water.
4. Decolorize with acid alcohol.
5. Wash with water.
6. Counterstain with methylene blue.
7. Wash with water and blot dry.

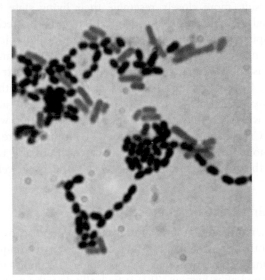

FIGURE 4.10 **Gram stain.** The Gram stain involves a four-step process in which the results will indicate whether the cells have a thick peptidoglycan layer in the cell wall (gram positive) or a thin layer (gram negative). This photo shows a mix of gram-positive cocci (dark purple/blue spheres), and gram-negative bacilli (red/pink rods).

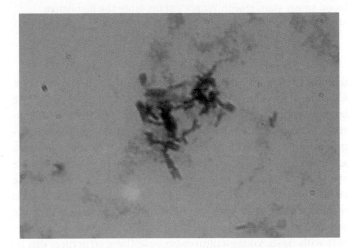

FIGURE 4.11 **Acid-fast stain.** Certain bacteria have mycolic acid in the cell wall, which resists conventional chemical staining. By means of either heat or chemicals, the acid-fast stain can be "driven" into the cell where it will resist decolorization. This micrograph is of *Mycobacterium smegmatis* (an acid-fast bacillus shown in red) and *Staphylococcus aureus* (a non–acid-fast coccus shown in blue). *S. aureus* was used as a negative control.

the bacteria are due to the composition and structure of their cell walls. Gram-positive bacteria contain a much larger amount of peptidoglycan (see Chapter 3, Cell Structure and Function) in their cell wall than do gram-negative bacteria. Because of the different composition of their cell walls, the bacteria can also react differently to antimicrobial drugs.

Acid-fast Stain

Acid-fast staining is used primarily for the diagnosis of tuberculosis, nocardiosis, and cryptosporidiosis, a disease commonly found in patients with AIDS. Acid-fast organisms contain mycolic acid in their cell wall, which resists simple stains. The primary stain in this procedure is basic carbolfuchsin followed by counterstaining with acid alcohol (Box 4.2), a more powerful decolorizer than the ethyl alcohol used in Gram staining. Acid-fast organisms retain the primary stain whereas others are decolorized and become counterstained (Figure 4.11).

The two main acid-fast staining procedures are the Ziehl-Neelson procedure and the Kinyoun procedure. The Ziehl-Neelson technique requires heating the slide during the basic carbolfuchsin step, but the other steps are performed on cooled slides. The Kinyoun technique is an alternative procedure that does not require heat. The lipid-rich wall of acid-fast bacteria makes them resistant to some dyes, antimicrobial drugs, and disinfectants.

Other Differential Stains

Wright's stain is the most widely used differential stain in clinical hematology laboratories. It is used to stain and differentiate the various types of blood cells (Figure 4.12), and it can also be used to examine spirochetes, intracellular bacteria, and some infectious protozoans and can identify malaria-causing protozoans. Protozoans and fungi are stained by a variety of other procedures as well.

Special Stains

Special staining procedures are necessary for the demonstration of structures such as bacterial flagella, capsules, and endospores. The endospore stain is similar to the acid-fast stain in that it requires heat or chemicals to enter the endospores. The stain

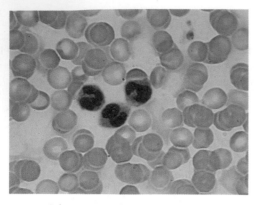

FIGURE 4.12 Wright's stain. The micrograph shows a human blood smear stained with Wright's stain. Note the distinctive staining of the nucleus of the different types of white blood cells.

distinguishes the spores from the cells in their vegetative state. Capsule stains allow visualization of an unstructured protective layer surrounding some bacteria and fungi—the microbial capsules. Capsules do not react with most stains, but the background of the slide can be stained with a stain such as India ink, and the cell itself with the capsule can be stained with a simple stain. The capsule will appear as a clear halo, surrounding the cell with a stained background. Flagellar staining reveals flagella too small to be seen with the light microscope unless they are coated on the outside and then stained. Flagellar staining works best with fresh, young cultures because these structures can be damaged or lost in older cells.

Fixation and Staining for Electron Microscopy

Transmission Electron Microscopy

Transmission electron microscopy (TEM) in biological science yields higher resolution than light microscopy for studying cells/ultrastructure, macromolecules, bacteria, and viruses. Transmission electron microscopy in microbiology generally is used for the observation and identification of microorganisms within cells and tissues, for observation of organisms attached to cells, and for details of cellular structures. The operating environment of a TEM dictates the use of special preparation techniques. Whereas light microscopy uses stains that color the microorganisms to differentiate them, EM staining uses metals to block the transmission of some of the electron beam through the sample and increase contrast.

Tissue samples or culture specimens are prepared by immersion in a special chemical fixative such as glutaraldehyde for a specific amount of time, usually between 12 and 24 hours. After the initial fixation period, the specimens are postfixed in 1% osmium tetroxide (OsO_4) for approximately 1 hour. This procedure is followed by staining of the entire specimen with a solution of uranyl acetate, a specific stain for transmission electron microscopy. The samples or specimens are then dehydrated through a series of increasing concentrations of ethanol. After dehydration, the samples are embedded in liquid epoxy resin, which infiltrates the specimens. After embedding at room temperature, the samples are poured into special dishes and placed

in an incubator held at a specific temperature for a specified period of time, during which the epoxy resin polymerizes into hard plastic blocks. These hard plastic specimen blocks are ready for the preparation of ultrathin sections with an ultramicrotome equipped with glass or diamond knives. The ultrathin sections are between 260 angströms (Å) and 640 Å thick and float on top of the water in the boat of the knife (an angström is equal to 0.1 nanometer [nm] or 1×10^{-10} meter [m]). The sections are then picked up with a small metallic grid and stained before examination with the electron microscope.

Another fixation technique for TEM is cryofixation, which provides structural and biochemical preservation of cells that, as a result, more closely resemble their living state than is obtained by preparation via chemical fixation. This technique uses rapid cooling rates during which the intracellular ice crystals formed within the cells on freezing are smaller than 5 nm, which is the minimal resolution required for ultrastructural studies. Before freezing, the specimens are coated with cryoprotective materials. After freezing, the specimens are sectioned with a cryoultramicrotome before observation with the TEM. Cryofixation is a useful tool in immunofluorescence. Immunofluorescence and ultrathin cryosections are used to reveal the presence and localization of antigens in cells and tissues.

Scanning Electron Microscopy

Specimen preparation for scanning electron microscopy (SEM) uses both chemical fixation and cryofixation techniques. In addition, hydrated materials such as biological samples must be dehydrated after fixation. This is typically done by passing the specimens through a graded series of ethanol treatments (see the previous description of sample preparation for TEM). The samples for SEM observation must then be completely dried by the critical-point drying method. This complicated process involves the replacement of liquid in the cells with gas to create a completely dry specimen with minimal or no cellular distortion. Freeze-fixed samples may also be freeze-dried. The completely dried sample is then mounted on an aluminum stub with special silver conductive glue. In the next step, if it is a nonmetallic sample (hair, insect, or biological tissue) the mounted specimen is sputter coated with gold to make it electrically conductive, after which it can be examined by SEM. If it is a metallic specimen, then it can be directly mounted and scanned.

Identification Techniques

To identify unknown microorganisms, it is essential to use their morphological, physiological, and chemical characteristics. This is readily done in the laboratory with differentially stained slides prepared from organisms grown on or in various media, recording observations of growth characteristics, and observing biochemical reactions. Microscopy in the microbiological laboratory is generally used for the detection and preliminary identification of microorganisms and, together with other laboratory techniques, more positive accurate identification of microorganisms can be achieved.

Scanning Tunneling Electron Microscope: Gazing at the Atom!

With the invention of the transmission electron microscope (TEM) and scanning electron microscope (SEM) scientists have been able to observe even more details of bacteria and viruses. The TEM is capable of magnifications up to approximately ×1,000,000 and the SEM is capable of magnifications up to ×100,000. The SEM uses a relatively simple concept as the specimen is covered with a very thin layer of a metallic substance and then the specimen is showered with a beam of electrons. Secondary electrons are bounced back to a receiver that collects them, amplifies the energy, and then displays an image on a screen. This concept has been expanded even further with the invention of the scanning tunneling electron microscope (STEM). The beam of electrons (a "tunnel") striking the surface of the specimen is emitted from a probe whose point has been refined down to essentially a single atom. The probe is maintained at a fixed distance from the surface as the probe scans over the specimen, and thus detects any peaks or troughs in the specimen surface. The STEM is capable of observing molecules and individual atoms! Using the STEM biologists can now actually see a DNA molecule with its double helix configuration and the nucleotides stretching across like rungs on a ladder.

Morphology

The morphological characteristics of cells and organisms are the major data components used for their identification and classification. On the basis of their morphological characteristics, cellular organisms are divided into prokaryotes and eukaryotes (see Chapter 3, Cell Structure and Function). Morphological characteristics are also the basis for determining whether eukaryotes are plant or animal cells. In other words, morphological characteristics are used for the preliminary identification of many bacteria and the definite identification of most fungi and parasites.

Bacteria grown in **culture media** vary according to their shape, size, and arrangements. According to their shape, bacteria are classified as bacilli, cocci, spirilla, vibrios, spirochetes, or coccobacilli (see Chapter 6, Bacteria and Archaea). Some bacteria show variation in size and shape as a result of environmental conditions and age of the organisms; these are called **pleomorphic** bacteria. During cell division, the different types of bacteria produce cultures of varied appearance. These characteristics can be used for purposes of identification. Whereas size, shape, and arrangement of bacteria are the first step in identification, many bacteria may look similar and require additional laboratory methods other than microscopy for more specific identification.

Cultural Characteristics

Growth behavioral patterns exhibited by unknown bacteria in various types of culture media are important characteristics that can be observed on solid medium plates or slants, or in broths. For example, selective **isolation** of individual species enables the examiner to observe the shape and texture of the colony, its pigmentation and odor. As stated earlier, some bacterial species exhibit a pleomorphic appearance under different environmental conditions (such as a temperature change) and at different ages. It is therefore important to incubate replicate plates at more than one temperature. For purposes of continuity, descriptive terms, illustrated in *Bergey's Manual of Systematic Bacteriology*, should be used in describing and recording cultural characteristics.

Growth requirements for fungi vary among species and also among strains. In general, fungi grow best on media that are formulated from the natural material from which they were isolated. Laboratory media include but are not limited to Sabouraud agar, hay infusion agar, and potato dextrose agar. More specific information about the growth requirements of fungi cultures is provided in Chapter 8 (Eukaryotic Microorganisms).

Growing algae in the laboratory also depends on the requirements of the specific algae and on the research interests of the scientists working with the selected species. Requirements for growth of algae cultures are also discussed in Chapter 8.

Culture Plates

Solid, agar-based media in sterile Petri dishes are routinely used to grow and subsequently identify colony characteristics such as shape, size, elevation, and margin type in particular. Inoculants from media on culture plates are used to select particular bacterial groups and to differentiate between two or more different species.

- **Nutrient agar** plates are the most commonly used general medium plates in the laboratory. This medium is safe for use in high school and college teaching laboratories because it does not selectively grow pathogenic bacteria.
- **Tryptic (Trypticase) soy agar** (TSA) is a general-purpose medium frequently used as the base medium of other agar plate types, for example, blood agar plates, which are made by enriching TSA plates with blood.
- **Phenylethyl alcohol agar** (PEA) is selective for gram-positive bacteria because it inhibits the growth of gram-negative bacteria. It is often used to isolate *Staphylococcus* and *Streptococcus* from specimens also containing gram-negative organisms.
- **Blood agar** plates (BAPs) are used both as enriched media and to differentiate between individual species on the basis of their ability to produce **hemolysins** (enzymes that lyse red blood cells).
- **Chocolate agar** (CHOC), a type of blood agar in which the blood cells have been lysed by heating the cells to 56° C, is used to grow fastidious respiratory bacteria. It should be noted that no chocolate is contained in the medium; it is named for the coloration only.

- **Thayer-Martin agar** (TM) is a chocolate agar designed to isolate *Neisseria gonorrhoeae* and *N. meningitidis*.
- **MacConkey agar** (MAC) is a selective and differential medium that differentiates between gram-negative bacteria, while inhibiting the growth of gram-positive bacteria. The addition of bile salts and crystal violet to the agar inhibits the growth of most gram-positive bacteria, making MAC selective. Lactose and neutral red are added to differentiate the lactose fermenters (pink colonies) from those not fermenting lactose (clear colonies).
- **Xylose lysine deoxycholate** (XLD) agar is used for the culture of stool samples, and is formulated to inhibit gram-positive bacteria, whereas the growth of gram-negative bacilli is facilitated. The colonies of lactose fermenters appear yellow.
- **Mannitol salt agar** (MSA) is a selective and differential medium that differentiates organisms that ferment mannitol. When mannitol fermentation occurs, lactic acid is produced and the pH will drop, causing the MSA plate to turn yellow. The salt component of the medium is selective for halophiles such as staphylococci. Organisms that cannot withstand a high salt content fail to grow.

Slants

An agar slant consists of agar-based medium in a culture tube. It is called a *slant* because the tube is placed at an angle during cooling to provide a large slanted surface for inoculation. After incubation the amount of growth is determined as:

- None
- Slight
- Moderate
- Abundant

Any pigments produced by the bacteria are associated with the colony or, if soluble, they diffuse into the growth medium. However, most bacteria do not produce pigments and their colonies are white or buff colored. The degrees of opacity of the growth can be classified as opaque, transparent, and partially transparent. The gross appearances of the different types of growth are illustrated in Figure 4.13 and are described as follows:

- *Filiform:* This type of growth is characterized by uniform growth along the line of inoculation.
- *Echinulate:* The margins of growth have a jagged, toothed appearance.
- *Beaded:* Separate or semiconfluent colonies appear along the line of inoculation.
- *Effuse:* The growth appears thin, veil-like, and usually spreading.
- *Arborescent:* The growth appears branched and treelike.
- *Rhizoid:* This type of growth has a rootlike appearance.

Gelatin Stabs

The gelatin stab method uses deep tubes containing 12% nutrient gelatin. Gelatin causes liquids to solidify at temperatures below 28° C, but at temperatures above 28° C it remains liquid. Some bacteria produce gelatinase, an enzyme that hydrolyzes gelatin. In the presence of gelatinase, gelatin is hydrolyzed and can no longer gel; it remains liquid even below 28° C. A heavy inoculum from a pure culture of the test organism is stabbed into the medium (Figure 4.14) and incubated for at least 48 hours followed by refrigeration for about 30 minutes. If the organism has produced enough gelatinase, the contents of the tube will remain liquid or partially liquid and not solidify in the refrigerator. If liquefaction has occurred the appearance can be:

- *Crateriform:* A saucer-shaped liquefaction
- *Napiform:* A turnip-like appearance
- *Infundibular:* A funnel-like or inverted cone
- *Saccate:* A tubular or cylindrical elongate sac
- *Stratiform:* Liquefaction to the walls of the tube in the upper region of the tube

The configuration of the liquefaction is not as significant as the fact that liquefaction takes place. It should be noted that some organisms produce the gelatinase at a very slow rate and need to be incubated for longer periods of time to determine whether or not liquefaction takes place. Pathogens that produce gelatinase often can cause extensive tissue damage in an infected patient.

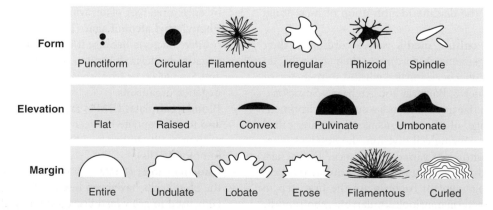

FIGURE 4.13 Colony growth on agar. This drawing shows the different types of colony morphology that organisms can display as they grow on the surface or agar, whether in a slant or on a Petri plate.

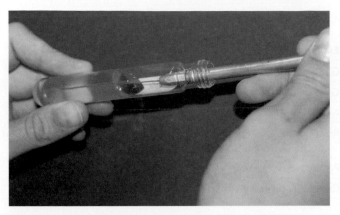

FIGURE 4.14 Gelatin stabs. This photo shows a gelatin stab being made with a sterile needle. The needle is stuck down through the center of the agar to the bottom of the tube. This technique is often used in performing the gelatinase and oxidation–fermentation tests.

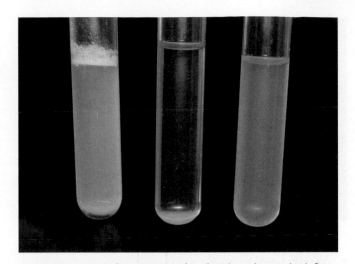

FIGURE 4.15 Growth patterns in broth. The tube on the left shows a pellicle growing at the surface of the broth, the center tube shows a sediment at the bottom of the tube, and the tube on the right shows turbid growth distributed throughout the broth.

Broths

When bacteria are grown in broths they may exhibit patterns of growth ranging from **sediment** at the bottom of the tube, **turbid** growth throughout the tube, or a **pellicle**—a thick growth at the top of the tube (Figure 4.15). Pellicle formation is sometimes due to an affinity for oxygen. It also may be the result of hydrophobic compounds present in the cell walls or the general formation of dry, light colonies. If an organism produces and releases soluble pigments, they will spread into the broth and change its color.

Physiological/Biochemical Characteristics

Specific biochemical patterns are blueprints for microbiologists to use in identifying microorganisms. Several biochemical tests can be used to identify their physiological characteristics. These tests include but are not limited to tests for hydrogen sulfide production, citrate use, phenylalanine deamination, litmus milk reactions, and the triple sugar iron test. These are just a few representative tests out of the many that can be used.

Hydrogen Sulfide Production

Certain bacteria such as *Proteus vulgaris* and *Salmonella* species produce hydrogen sulfide from the amino acid cysteine. The hydrogen sulfide production test is useful for the identification and differentiation of *Salmonella* species from other species of Enterobacteriaceae. Kligler's iron agar and SIM (sulfur reduction, *i*ndole production, and *m*otility) medium are used to detect the presence of sulfide. These media contain iron, which forms a dark precipitate when it reacts with hydrogen sulfide.

Citrate Use

The purpose of the citrate use test is to determine whether an organism, such as *Enterobacter aerogenes* and *Salmonella typhimurium,* is capable of using citrate as its sole carbon source for metabolism, with resulting alkalinity. This is a useful characteristic when differentiating species among enteric bacteria.

The synthetic Koser's citrate medium and Simmons citrate agar are used to detect citrate use by bacteria.

Phenylalanine Deamination

Bacteria that produce phenylalanine deaminase include *Proteus, Morganella,* and *Providencia.* They deaminate the amino acid phenylalanine to produce phenylpyruvic acid, which differentiates these genera from other Enterobacteriaceae.

IMViC Tests

Enterobacteriaceae (enterics) are gram-negative bacteria that are common in the intestinal florae of humans and other animals. The IMViC tests are commonly used for the identification and differentiation of these bacteria including *Klebsiella, Enterobacter, Proteus,* and *Escherichia coli.* IMViC is an acronym that stands for indole, methyl red, Voges-Proskauer, and citrate. To obtain results of these tests, three test tubes are inoculated: tryptone broth or SIM agar (indole test), methyl red–Voges-Proskauer broth (MR-VP broth), and citrate slants.

Litmus Milk Reactions

Litmus milk reactions are used to determine the action of a microorganism on milk, which contains lactose, glucose, proteins, fats, minerals, and vitamins. Litmus milk containing 10% powdered skim milk and a small amount of litmus as a pH indicator is used. After incubation, different reactions can be observed depending on the biochemical reactions of a species within litmus milk. The various possible reactions are shown in Table 4.3.

Rapid Identification Tests

The identification of bacteria and fungi can be facilitated by the use of packaged kit systems, manufactured for the rapid identification of medically important bacteria and fungi. Rapid identification and reporting are becoming increasingly important because of newly emerging pathogens (see Chapter 18, Emerg-

TABLE 4.3 Changes That Can Occur in Litmus Milk

Reaction	Condition of Medium	Explanation
Slight acid production	Pale pink indicator	Glucose but not lactose utilization
Acid reaction	Pink indicator	Glucose and lactose fermentation
Alkaline reaction	Blue or purple indicator	Amines or ammonia released from proteolytic bacteria
Litmus reaction	Culture becomes white	Result of rapidly reproducing bacteria, lowering the oxygen content at the bottom of the tube
Coagulation	Medium clotted, curd formation	Protein coagulation
Peptonization	Medium translucent	Caused by proteolytic bacteria

HEALTHCARE APPLICATION

Examples of Manual and Automated Systems for Microbial Identification

Name	Manufacturer	Organism(s) Identified
API/bioMérieux Vitek	bioMérieux Clinical Diagnostics	Enterobacteriaceae, other gram-negative bacilli, *Staphylococcus, Streptococcus, Enterococcus, Neisseria*, gram-positive bacilli, yeast, anaerobes
BactiCard	Remel	*Neisseria/Moraxella, Escherichia coli, Streptococcus*, yeast
Biolog MicroPlate	Biolog	Gram-positive and gram-negative organisms, yeast, anaerobes
BBL Crystal E/NF*	Becton Dickinson Microbiology Systems	Enterobacteriaceae, other gram-negative bacilli, *Neisseria, Haemophilus*, gram-positive cocci and bacilli
Enterotube II	Becton Dickinson Diagnostic Systems	Enterobacteriaceae, other gram-negative bacilli
Gonochek	EY Laboratories	*Neisseria/Moraxella*
Micro-ID (Rapid ID)	Remel	Enterobacteriaceae, other gram-negative bacilli, *Neisseria, Haemophilus, Streptococcus, Enterococcus*, yeast, anaerobes, gram-positive bacilli
MicroScan (TouchScan)	Siemens Healthcare Diagnostics	Gram-positive and gram-negative organisms, *Haemophilus, Neisseria*
Oxi/Ferm	Becton Dickinson Microbiology Systems	Nonfermenter gram-negative bacteria
Uni-Yeast Tek	Remel	Nonfermenters, yeast

*E/NF, Enteric/nonfermenter.

ing Infectious Diseases), the recognition of old pathogens in different settings, increasing nosocomial infections, world travel, and the increase in multidrug-resistant organisms.

The term *rapid method* includes a wide variety of procedures and applies to all procedures that provide faster results than conventional methods. Rapid identification methods are available for microscopy, biochemical identification, as well as antigen and antibody detection. Commercially available kits for rapid identification include both manual and automated systems. Kits designed to perform several biochemical tests at the same time can identify bacteria within 4 to 24 hours. Hospital microbiology laboratories typically use fully automated computerized systems for the identification and classification of enteric bacterial species, with the final identification report available in as little as 6 hours. Miniaturized multimedia systems

for bacterial identification also have been developed and are used when speed and cost-effective identification are needed. Some rapid identification methods for enteric bacteria are the Enterotube II, a tube with 12 compartments for different biochemical tests, the API 20 series with 20 tests, the BBL Crystal system with 30 tests, and the Biolog and VITEK systems with more than 90 tests.

Molecular Analysis

Serologic Analysis/Diagnosis

Immunologic techniques are used to detect, identify, and quantify antigens in clinical samples. Antibodies are sensitive and specific tools used to accomplish the detection of antigens from a virus, bacterium, fungus, or parasite. In addition, these techniques can evaluate the antibody response to infections (see Chapter 20, The Immune System). The specificity of the antibody–antigen interaction represents a powerful tool in the microbiology laboratory. In general, serological assays are designed to give negative or positive results; however, the antibody strength can be determined by a titer. A titer is a test that measures the presence and amount of antibodies in the blood in response to invasion by a particular antigen (see Chapter 20). In other words, the antibody level in the blood is a reflection of the body's past exposure to an antigen, a foreign substance.

Genetic Analysis

Given the rapid changes in technologies, laboratory procedures in general, and genetic analysis in particular, the abbreviated presentation on genetic analysis that follows will soon require updating as a result of advancements made in the future.

Identification of a specific microbe from within a microbial community is difficult because of their enormous diversity in environmental samples, and growing cultures of microbes to identify species is slow and often error prone. The most precise method of classifying and identifying microorganisms is genetic analysis. Today's technology allows the sequencing of entire genomes, which yields highly specific and informative data. This process is costly and labor intensive. As a result, scientists have been searching for ways to identify key segments of the genetic code that are short enough to be sequenced rapidly and can readily distinguish between species.

Whereas initially organisms were classified by their ratio of guanine to cytosine nucleotides, this method has been largely replaced by more discriminating methods. Genome structure and genetic sequence are major distinguishing characteristics of any organism. Specific strains of a microorganism can be differentiated on the basis of their DNA or RNA, or on the basis of DNA fragments produced by restriction enzymes—molecular scissors. Different restriction enzymes recognize specific DNA sites and cut the DNA at these sites. Depending on the restriction enzyme, the DNA is cleaved at different places, resulting in smaller fragments of different lengths. DNA or RNA fragments can be produced by different restriction enzymes, resulting in fragments of different lengths. The fragments of different sizes or structure can be distinguished by their rate of movement through an electrophoresis gel, which separates them, creating a specific profile (see Chapter 25, Biotechnology). Comparison of the patterns of DNA or RNA fragments generated by the restriction enzymes allows the identification of different strains of a species.

DNA probes can be chemically synthesized or generated by the cloning of specific genomic fragments. DNA probes are sensitive tools with which to detect, locate, and quantitate specific nucleic acid sequences of species that are difficult to grow. Rapid identification techniques have been developed by the use of DNA probes. If a probe binds to an organism's DNA the organism can be identified. This technique is a valuable tool for the rapid identification of slow-growing microorganisms such as mycobacteria, fungi, and organisms that currently cannot be cultured in the laboratory environment.

LIFE APPLICATION

Genetic Sensors

Detection of biological and potentially pathogenic organisms has been an important issue for scientists all over the world. Uncovering food and water contamination by pathogenic, toxin-producing bacteria as well as the threat of biological weapons requires rapid and precise identification of the microorganism involved. Genetic technologies are useful in the detection of these potential threats. Hand-held polymerase chain reaction (PCR) detectors have been used by United Nations inspectors in Iraq during their weapons inspection for the detection of *Bacillus anthracis*. DNA technology now allows for the rapid detection and identification of food and water contaminants as well as biological weapons (see Chapter 24, Microorganisms in the Environment and Environmental Safety).

Another genotypic method is nucleic acid sequence analysis. With this method, probes are used to localize specific nucleic acid sequences unique to a genus, species, or subspecies. The sequences are then amplified by the polymerase chain reaction (see the section on PCR in Chapter 25) and the amplified material is sequenced to define the identity of the isolates.

Most commonly used is the analysis of ribosomal DNA sequences because of their high species and subspecies specificity. This technique has also been used to determine the evolutionary relationship between organisms. Other molecular techniques used for identification are plasmid analysis, ribotyping, and analysis of chromosomal DNA fragments. Ribotyping is the use of universal probes that target specific ribosomal RNA coding sequences to detect band patterns. These methods have now been sufficiently modified so that they can be used for microbial identification in most clinical laboratories.

Summary

- Aseptic technique is essential in the microbiology laboratory to prevent contamination of cultures, laboratory personnel, specimens, and the environment.
- A variety of physical and chemical methods are applied to achieve sterilization, disinfection, and sanitation:
  1. Sterilization destroys or removes all microorganisms and their endospores.
  2. Disinfection destroys vegetative microbes and viruses but not endospores.
  3. Sanitation is the mechanical removal of microorganisms and debris to reduce contamination to safe levels.
- In order to gather data about a particular microbe, a variety of tools, techniques, and media are used to grow microbes in the laboratory environment.
- Various types of media are available to meet the different nutrient requirements for the growth of different microorganisms.

- Culture media are inoculated, followed by incubation and isolation, in order to identify and study particular microbes.
- In order to observe microorganisms with the help of a light or electron microscope, the specimens require special preparation and the use of stains to identify the bacteria.
- Morphological characteristics of microorganisms are a major component for their initial identification and classification. Bacteria are classified according to their variability in shape and size.

- The cultural characteristics organisms exhibit when growing in a variety of media are also used for identification of unknown bacteria.
- Bacteria can also be identified by their physical and biochemical characteristics when growing in or on differential and selective media.
- The ultimate indicator for classification is via analysis at the DNA test level.

Review Questions

1. The destruction of all microorganisms and their endospores is referred to as:
   a. Disinfection
   b. Degermation
   c. Sanitization
   d. Sterilization

2. The process by which the number of microbes on the human skin is reduced by scrubbing is called:
   a. Degermation
   b. Sanitization
   c. Disinfection
   d. Sterilization

3. Chemically, agar is a:
   a. Protein
   b. Lipid
   c. Carbohydrate
   d. Nucleic acid

4. Media that contain complex organic substances such as blood for the growth of specific bacteria are referred to as:
   a. Enriched media
   b. General-purpose media
   c. Differential media
   d. Reducing media

5. Which of the following media are used to determine motility and growth patterns of bacteria?
   a. Reducing media
   b. Liquid media
   c. Semisolid media
   d. Complex media

6. Nigrosin is a stain used in:
   a. Simple staining
   b. Gram staining
   c. Negative staining
   d. Acid-fast staining

7. The stain used to identify bacteria with a large amount of peptidoglycan in their cell walls is the:
   a. Acid-fast stain
   b. Methylene blue stain
   c. Gram stain
   d. Negative stain

8. The medium selective for the growth of *Staphylococcus* species is:
   a. Phenylethyl alcohol agar
   b. Tryptic soy agar
   c. Thayer-Martin agar
   d. Nutrient agar

9. A growth that appears separate or semiconfluent is referred to as:
   a. Filiform
   b. Echinulate
   c. Beaded
   d. Effuse

10. Which of the following media is *not* a differential medium based on fermentation?
    a. Blood agar
    b. MacConkey agar
    c. Xylose-lysine-deoxycholate agar
    d. Mannitol salt agar

11. A saucer-shaped liquefaction of gelatin stabs is said to have a(n) _____ appearance.

12. A culture that contains a single species of an organism is a(n) _____ culture.

13. A disinfectant is designed to be used only on _____ surfaces.

14. Bacteria that show variation in size and shape as a result of environmental conditions or age of the organisms are referred to as _____ bacteria.

15. Bacteria that appear red after Gram staining are said to be gram _____.

16. In correct order, describe the steps necessary in the Gram-staining procedure.

17. Compare and contrast differential and selective media.

18. Name and describe the action of three chemicals used for sterilization.

19. Name and describe the action of five commonly used disinfectants.

20. Describe the three different techniques that can be used to obtain organisms to produce pure cultures.

Bibliography

Bauman R: *Microbiology with Diseases by Taxonomy*, ed 2, 2007, Benjamin Cummings/Pearson Education, San Francisco.

Garrity G: *Bergey's Manual of Systematic Bacteriology*, Vols. 1–5, New York, 2005, Springer.

Madigan MT, Martinko JM, Dunlap PV, et al: *Biology of Microorganisms*, ed 12, 2009, Benjamin Cummings/Pearson Education, San Francisco.

Mahon CR, Lehman DC, Manuselis G: *Textbook of Diagnostic Microbiology*, ed 3, St. Louis, 2007, Saunders/Elsevier.

Mims C, Dockrell HM, Goering RV, et al: *Medical Microbiology*, ed 3, St. Louis, 2004, Mosby/Elsevier.

Murray PR, Rosenthal KS, Pfaller MA: *Medical Microbiology*, ed 5, St. Louis, 2005, Mosby/Elsevier.

Talaro KP: *Foundations in Microbiology*, ed 6, 2005, McGraw-Hill, New York.

Totora GJ, Funke BR, Case CL: *Microbiology: An Introduction*, ed 9, 2007, Benjamin Cummings/Pearson Education, San Francisco.

Internet Resources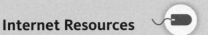

Centers for Disease Control and Prevention (CDC), http://www.cdc.gov/

National Institutes of Health, http://www.nih.gov/

U.S. Department of Health and Human Services, http://www.hhs.gov/

Wikipedia, http://en.wikipedia.org/wiki/Main_Page

The Microbial World (online book), http://www.bact.wisc.edu/Microtextbook/

CDC: Food Irradiation, http://www.cdc.gov/ncidod/dbmd/diseaseinfo/foodirradiation.htm

Sigma Aldrich: Microbiology, http://www.sigmaaldrich.com/Area_of_Interest/Analytical__Chromatography/Microbiology.html

Todar's Online Textbook of Bacteriology, http://www.textbookofbacteriology.net/

PandemicFlu.gov: Vaccine Production in Cells, http://www.pandemicflu.gov/vaccine/vproductioncells.html

5

Safety Issues

OUTLINE

Laboratory Safety
Biosafety
Chemicals
Equipment
Protective Gear

Safety in Healthcare Facilities
Physicians' Offices and Clinics
Hospitals
Nursing Homes and Personal Care Facilities

Emergency Response

Safety in Homes

LEARNING OBJECTIVES

After reading this chapter, the student will be able to:
- Define the various safety issues and safety precautions laboratory workers and administrators need to consider
- Identify the agencies involved in the development, control, and oversight of safety issues in the laboratory environment
- Name and explain the different levels of biosafety
- Give examples of organisms handled in the different biosafety levels
- Describe the different equipment used in a laboratory setting and explain the role of each
- Explain the role of protective gear used in the laboratory and discuss the use of each
- Discuss the safety regulations and concerns in healthcare facilities
- Specify the regulatory and safety issues in physicians' offices and clinics
- Describe the general safety requirements for hospitals, nursing homes, and personal care facilities
- Name the agencies involved in the surveillance, regulations, and support of the emergency response

American Society for
   Microbiology (ASM)
Association of
   Professionals in
   Infection Control and
   Epidemiology (APIC)
Centers for Disease
   Control and
   Prevention (CDC)
Chemical Abstracts
   Service (CAS) registry
   number
Healthcare Infection
   Control Practices
   Advisory Committee
   (HICPAC)
Infectious Disease
   Society of America
   (IDSA)

laboratory safety
   equipment
Lawrence Berkeley
   National Laboratory
   (LBNL)
manufacturer's material
   safety data sheets
   (MSDSs)
National Institute of
   Allergy and
   Infectious Diseases
   (NIAID)
National Institute for
   Occupational
   Safety and Health
   (NIOSH)
National Institutes of
   Health (NIH)
occupational hazard

Occupational Safety and
   Health Administration
   (OSHA)
protective gear
Registry of Toxic Effects
   of Chemical
   Substances (RTECS)
Society for Healthcare
   Epidemiology of
   America (SHEA)
U.S. Department of
   Health and Human
   Services (HHS)
U.S. Department of
   Transportation (DOT)
World Health Organiza-
   tion (WHO)

WHY YOU NEED TO KNOW

HISTORY

Personnel working with hazardous materials need safety guidelines for their personal protection and guidelines to prevent exposing those not working directly with these hazardous materials. Strict adherence to these guidelines is of particular importance for those working with microorganisms in order to control contamination and infection. To achieve these goals, it is essential to develop and have in place simple and direct protocols that are routinely reviewed, updated, and practiced. The key words are "current," "awareness," and "knowledgeable." Three organizations that illustrate efforts to facilitate acceptable, rational guidelines for safety are the **Occupational Safety and Health Administration (OSHA),** the **Centers for Disease Control and Prevention (CDC),** and the **World Health Organization (WHO).**

OSHA was established in 1971 as a result of the Occupational Safety and Health Act of 1970. Its objective is to provide a safe workplace. The CDC was created in 1946 as a major operating component of the **U.S. Department of Health and Human Services (HHS).** It is the lead agency of the federal government charged with protecting the health and safety of all Americans as well as providing essential human services for those in need. The WHO grew from the HO (Health Organization), an agency of the League of Nations, and was established by the United Nations (UN) in 1948. It functions as a coordinating authority on international public health.

IMPACT

Because of the implementation of OSHA regulations after its establishment in 1971, workplace fatalities have decreased by more than 60% and injuries and sickness incidences on the job have declined by 40% while the workforce has increased

from about 56 million to 115 million. The CDC, although initially charged to control malaria, since 1946 has led public health efforts in the prevention and control of infectious and chronic diseases, injuries, workplace hazards, disabilities, and environmental health emergencies. Its efforts are action oriented toward improving the quality of people's daily lives and alerting them in response to health emergencies. The WHO, in fulfilling its task of combating infectious disease while promoting the general health of the peoples of the world, coordinates and monitors outbreaks such as severe acute respiratory syndrome (SARS), malaria, and AIDS in addition to developing and distributing vaccines. In 1979, the WHO declared the viral disease smallpox to be eradicated, with polio the next disease expected to be eradicated.

FUTURE

OSHA will continue to monitor the workplace to identify hazards to the health and safety of the public in the workplace environment. The CDC will continue to study and develop contingencies against outbreaks of disease through vaccines, development of new drugs, and implementation programs, while monitoring possible epidemics and pandemics. Evaluation of pandemic flu resources, traveler's health, outbreaks of *Escherichia coli*, environmental health in general, emergency preparedness, and response to health and disease threats will continue to be at the forefront of their efforts. Additional local, national, and international agencies may be formed to meet needs for safety guidelines. Furthermore, the WHO has reversed its previous policy on the spraying of dichlorodiphenyltrichloroethane (DDT) to prevent the spread of malaria. This reversal has restored a useful tool in the fight against malaria.

Laboratory Safety

Work in any type of laboratory involves a variety of possible hazards that are not found in most workplaces and therefore special precautions are necessary in that type of environment. Although this textbook focuses on microbiology issues, a medical or clinical laboratory is an environment involved in testing of biological specimens to obtain information about the health of patients. In general, clinical laboratories deal with the following:

- Microbiology
- Hematology
- Urinalysis
- Biochemistry
- Immunology
- Serology
- Histology
- Cytology
- Cytogenetics
- Virology

Other laboratory environments require strict regulations for safety as well. Workers in laboratory environments are surrounded by physical, chemical, and biological hazards that present the potential for accidents and injury. The **Occupational Safety and Health Administration (OSHA),** a division of the U.S. Department of Labor, provides regulations, specific standards, and guidelines that, if followed, ensure the safety of workers in the laboratory environment.

Biosafety

Starting in the early days of microbiological research, people working in the laboratories recognized that acquiring infections from the agents they manipulated and worked with represented an **occupational hazard.** Biological agents include bacteria, viruses, fungi, other microorganisms, and their toxins. Biological agents have the capability to adversely affect human health, ranging from mild allergic reactions to serious medical conditions, and even death.

The most commonly acquired laboratory infections are caused by bacteria. As microbiologists learned how to culture animal viruses, it became evident that there is a potential for becoming infected by these agents also, as exemplified by the laboratory studies on yellow fever among others.

Guidelines and standards for the protection of personnel working in microbiological laboratories evolved on the basis of data and the understanding of the risks associated with various manipulations of virulent agents transmissible by different routes. These guidelines for protection include a combination of engineering controls, management policies, work practices and procedures, and medical interventions if necessary with records of compliance and updates noted. The simplest, yet most effective method of control to prevent the spread of infectious diseases is the proper washing of hands. Hand hygiene guidelines were developed by the CDC's **Health-**

The Miracle Cure: Soap and Water!

Throughout the first half of the nineteenth century the death rate for women in childbirth was high. Almost 25% of the women delivering their babies in hospitals and clinics were dying from a disease called *"childbed fever"* (puerperal sepsis) that was subsequently found to be caused by the bacterium *Streptococcus pyogenes*. In 1843, Dr. Oliver Wendell Holmes introduced the simple practice of proper hand washing as a primary means of preventing childbed fever. He believed and tried to convince the medical establishment at the time that the disease was in fact being passed on to pregnant women by the hands of their doctors. For the most part his ideas were viewed with skepticism and were rejected by many physicians at the time. In the late 1840s, Dr. Ignaz Semmelweis observed while working in a maternity ward in Vienna that the mortality rate among delivering mothers was much greater in patients treated by medical students than those treated by midwives. Semmelweis observed that the medical students were going from classes in the autopsy room to the delivery ward without washing their hands. When the students were ordered to wash their hands with a chlorine solution before touching the patients in the delivery process the mortality rate eventually dropped to less than 1%! Even after these results, the medical community still did not widely accept the importance of this simple procedure. It wasn't until the late 1800s and early 1900s that the support of people like Pasteur and Dr. Josephine Baker convinced the medical profession and the public as a whole that the simple act of hand washing was (and still is) one of the best tools available for preventing/controlling the spread of disease.

care Infection Control Practices Advisory Committee (HICPAC) together with the **Society for Healthcare Epidemiology of America (SHEA),** the **Association of Professionals in Infection Control and Epidemiology (APIC),** and the **Infectious Disease Society of America (IDSA).** In summary, the hand hygiene guidelines are a major part of the overall CDC strategy to reduce the spread of infections, especially in the healthcare settings.

In 1992, OSHA published a rule that deals with the occupational health risk caused by exposure to human blood and other potentially infectious materials. A Biosafety Program was developed as an information management system to provide a process and tools to assess the safety, needs, and precautions in the planning, initiation, and termination of activities involving biological materials. The program is intended to protect personnel from exposure to infectious agents and to comply with federal, state, and local requirements. At present the program includes four major components (Box 5.1):

- **Lawrence Berkeley National Laboratory (LBNL)** Biosafety Manual, which provides guidelines, policies, and

Hand-washing Guidelines

Person-to-person transmission of pathogens can play a significant role in the spread of infectious disease. Therefore, the Centers for Disease Control and Prevention (CDC) has developed Outbreak and Response Protocol (OPRP) guidelines to include hand-washing guidelines. Steps for proper hand washing are as follows:

1. Hands should be washed with soap and warm, running water.
2. Hands should be rubbed vigorously during washing for at least 20 seconds, with special attention paid to the backs of the hands, wrists, between the fingers, and under the fingernails.
3. Hands should be rinsed well under running water.
4. With the water running, hands should be dried with a single-use towel.
5. Water should be turned off with a paper towel, covering washed hands to prevent recontamination.

BOX 5.1 OSHA's Biosafety Program

LBNL Biosafety Manual:
    http://www.lbl.gov/ehs/biosafety/Biosafety_Manual/biosafety_manual.shtml

"On-line" Exposure Control Plan:
    http://www.lbl.gov/ehs/biosafety/Export_Control_Plan/export_control_plan.shtml

Bloodborne Pathogens Training Program:
    http://www.lbl.gov/ehs/biosafety/BBP_Training/bbp_training.shtml

Biosafety Training Program:
    http://www.lbl.gov/ehs/biosafety/Biosafety_Training/biosafety_training.shtml

TABLE 5.1 Summary of Recommended Biosafety Levels for Infectious Agents

Risk Group 1 (RG1)	Agents not associated with disease in healthy adult humans
Risk Group 2 (RG2)	Agents associated with human disease but generally not serious and for which preventive and therapeutic interventions are available
Risk Group 3 (RG3)	Agents associated with serious or lethal human disease. Preventive or therapeutic interventions may be available
Risk Group 4 (RG4)	Agents likely to cause serious or lethal human disease. Preventive or therapeutic interventions are not usually available

BOX 5.2 Examples of Organisms for Biosafety Level 1

- *Bacillus subtilis*
- *Naegleria gruberi*
- *Escherichia coli*
- *Lactobacillus* spp.
- *Micrococcus luteus*
- *Serratia marcescens*
- *Pseudomonas* spp.
- Varicella
- Canine hepatitis virus
- Bovine leukemia virus
- Guinea pig herpesvirus

procedures for the management of hazardous and potentially hazardous biological materials
- "On-line" Exposure Control Plan development tool to assist principal investigators in the preparation of the Exposure Control Plan required by OSHA for research involving human source material
- Blood-borne training program for the initial OSHA training requirements for individuals who are at risk of occupational exposure to blood and other bodily fluids
- Biosafety training program, which is designed to provide information about safe procedures and practices in biological/biomedical research

Different biosafety levels were developed for microbiological and medical laboratories for personal and environmental protection. Specifically, four levels of containment have been defined and these are termed biosafety levels (BSL-1 to BSL-4),

depending on the agent to be handled. The **National Institutes of Health (NIH)** has introduced the concept of "risk groups," in which agents are classified into four risk groups (RGs) on the basis of their relative pathogenicity (Table 5.1). The description of biosafety levels and procedures are presented as introductions and are not intended to be an in-depth treatise. In addition, they are being continuously updated by the NIH, and the NIH websites should be consulted for the most recent information (http://www.cdc.gov/OD/ohs/biosfty/bmbl5/bmbl5toc.htm).

Biosafety Level 1 (BSL-1)

BSL-1 applies to working with microorganisms that are generally not disease causing in healthy humans and therefore are of minimal potential hazard to laboratory personnel and the environment (Box 5.2). This safety level is used in municipal water-testing laboratories, high school laboratories, and in some community colleges teaching introductory microbiology classes with organisms that are not considered to be pathogenic and/or hazardous. These laboratories typically include a sink for hand washing, benchtops, sturdy furniture, windows with fly

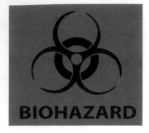

FIGURE 5.1 Biohazard symbol. This universal symbol indicates some form of a biological hazard. It may be found in different colors but is most often seen with a black logo against a red/orange background or a red/orange logo against a white background.

BOX 5.3 Examples of Organisms for Biosafety Level 2

BOX 5.3 Examples of Organisms for Biosafety Level 2

- *Acinetobacter baumannii*
- *Borrelia* spp.
- *Campylobacter coli*
- *Campylobacter jejuni*
- *Klebsiella* spp.
- *Salmonella* spp.
- *Staphylococcus aureus*
- *Streptococcus pyogenes*
- *Toxoplasma* spp.
- *Treponema pallidum*
- Adenoviruses: human, all types
- Coronaviruses
- Influenza viruses
- Measles virus
- Hepatitis A, B, and C viruses
- HIV
- Mumps virus

BOX 5.4 Some Examples of Organisms for Biosafety Level 3

- *Bacillus anthracis*
- *Brucella* spp.
- *Coxiella burnetii*
- *Francisella tularensis*
- *Mycobacterium tuberculosis*
- *Rickettsia* spp.
- *Yersinia pestis* (antibiotic-resistant strains)
- Arboviruses
- SARS
- Yellow fever virus
- St. Louis encephalitis virus

screens if they can be opened, and readily available disinfectants and antiseptics. The laboratory should be easily cleaned, decontaminated, and have procedures posted for the safe disposal of materials being used.

The laboratory at this safety level does not have to be isolated from other parts of the building; however, a door that can be closed while work with agents is in progress is highly desirable. Hazard warning signs (Figure 5.1) should be posted on doors, indicating any hazards that may be present. A sink for hand washing needs to be available because hand washing is one of the simplest yet most important procedures used by laboratory personnel to remove unwanted microbial agents or chemicals used in the laboratory.

Standard microbiological practices at BSL-1 include the use of mechanical pipetting devices and prohibition of eating, drinking, and smoking. People working in the laboratory should be wearing laboratory coats and gloves when working with biological agents. Adequate, efficient methods and procedures for disposal of materials used are also established.

The laboratory supervisor of a BSL-1 laboratory needs to have general training in microbiology or a related science and is responsible for establishing the general laboratory safety procedures, for training laboratory personnel, and for the updating of these procedures.

Biosafety Level 2 (BSL-2)

BSL-2 is similar to BSL-1 regarding the agents that are being handled. However, for BSL-2 work, the facility, containment devices, administrative controls, practices and procedural standards, and guidelines are designed to maximize safe working conditions for laboratories working with agents of moderate risk to personnel and the environment. Agents manipulated at BSL-2 are considered a moderate risk. They often include pathogens to which personnel have previously been exposed and to which they have had an immune response (e.g., childhood diseases) or against which they have received immunization (Box 5.3). Immunization is recommended before working with certain agents, for example, immunization against the hepatitis B virus which is recommended by OSHA for people at high risk of exposure to blood and blood products. In addition to procedures established in the BSL-1 level laboratory, the BSL-2 laboratory requires that:

- Laboratory personnel receive specific training in handling pathogenic agents and be directed by trained competent scientists
- Access to the laboratory be limited while work is in progress
- Extreme precautions be taken with contaminated sharp items and their disposal
- Specific procedures for dealing with infectious aerosols or splashes be developed for work carried out in biological safety cabinets, hoods, or other physical containment equipment

Biosafety Level 3 (BSL-3)

BSL-3 applies to clinical, diagnostic, teaching, research, or production laboratories using original or exotic agents (Box 5.4). Such agents can potentially cause serious disease or even lethality if exposure occurs. In addition to the laboratory procedures described in BSL-1 and BSL-2, laboratory personnel require specific training in handling pathogenic and potentially lethal agents with on-site supervision by scientists experienced and qualified in working with such agents. Many additional standards are necessary to qualify as a BSL-3 laboratory. Some of the additional procedures include but are not limited to:

- Control of access to the laboratory. This is the responsibility of the laboratory director, who restricts access to personnel required for program conduct or support purposes. Other personnel at risk of acquiring infection, such as those who are immunocompromised or immunosuppressed, should not have access. No minors are allowed in the laboratory.
- All laboratory personnel are required to receive appropriate immunizations and/or tests for sensitivities to the presence of the agents that will be handled or would potentially be present in the laboratory. Periodic testing is recommended and current records of all data kept.
- All procedures involving the manipulation of infectious material are done in biological safety cabinets or other physical containment devices, or by personnel with appropriate protective clothing and equipment.
- The laboratory should have specially engineered design features for BSL-3 laboratory work, for example, special exhaust air ventilation systems. (Please refer to the NIH guidelines for specifics: http://www.cdc.gov/OD/ohs/biosfty/bmbl5/bmbl5toc.htm).
- The laboratory is located separate from areas that are open and accessible to unrestricted traffic flow within the building.
- All windows in the laboratory are closed and sealed.
- Emergency treatment equipment must be readily accessible and kept updated.
- A change-of-clothes room may be included in entrance/exit passageways with appropriate disposal containers for lab-used clothing.
- The Biosafety Level 3 facility design and operational procedures must be documented and tested for appropriate design and parameters before, during, and after use. Data on all operations are kept current and all facilities should be reverified at least annually.

The **National Institute of Allergy and Infectious Diseases (NIAID)** in partnership with the **American Society of Microbiology (ASM)** conducted a brief survey of academic, biotechnology, and pharmaceutical facilities in the United States to provide the NIAID with information about the location, capacity, and status of existing and operating facilities capable of BSL-3 containment. This information can be viewed at http://www.asm.org/Policy/index.asp?bid=37789.

Biosafety Level 4 (BSL-4)

BSL-4 is required for working with dangerous and exotic agents that present a high risk of aerosol-transmitted laboratory infections and life-threatening disease (Box 5.5). All laboratory staff is required to have specific training in handling extremely hazardous infectious agents. The facility is located either in a separate building or in a controlled area within a building that is

---

> **BOX 5.5 Some Examples of Organisms for Biosafety Level 4**
>
> - Smallpox virus
> - Central European encephalitis viruses
> - Ebola viruses
> - Marburg virus
> - Hantavirus
> - Lassa virus
> - Hemorrhagic fever agents and viruses as yet undefined

---

completely isolated from all other areas of that building. In addition to all other laboratory procedures described previously, additional protocols and procedures are necessary for BSL-4. Some of these include but are not limited to the following:

- Personnel enter and leave the laboratory only through clothing-change and personal shower rooms. They are required to take a decontamination shower each time they leave the laboratory.
- All personal clothing is removed and replaced with completely decontaminated laboratory clothing before entering the laboratory. This laboratory clothing is removed and placed in appropriate containers before showering at the time of leaving the laboratory.
- All supplies and materials (laboratory and other) needed in the BSL-4 facility enter via a double-doored autoclave, fumigation chamber, or airlock device.
- A daily inspection of all containment parameters and life support systems will be completed and recorded before laboratory work is initiated. Data on all safety procedures will be kept current.

It is important to note that the description of the different biosafety levels (BSL-1 to BSL-4) in this chapter is an introduction only and does not reflect complete, more detailed, and specific governmental suggestions, standards, and regulations. Information about BSL-4 laboratories in the United States is summarized in Table 5.2.

Chemicals

As with biological agents, standards for the safe use and handling of chemicals also have been developed by the **National Institute for Occupational Safety and Health (NIOSH)** in connection with OSHA. The NIOSH Pocket Guide to Chemical Hazards contains key information and data for chemicals or substance groupings that can be found in the work environment. The following information is included for registered chemicals:

- Chemical name: First name of a drug and a precise description of its chemical composition
- Structural formula: A precise description of the atomic groups or arrangements of atoms

TABLE 5.2 BSL-4 Laboratories in the United States

Institution	Name of the Laboratory	Status	Other Information
Centers for Disease Control and Prevention (Atlanta, GA)	CDC Special Pathogens Branch, Emerging Infectious Diseases Laboratory http://www.cdc.gov/ncidod/dvrd/spb/mnpages/whoweare.htm#what	New facility opened in 2005; prior laboratory opened in 1988	
USAMRIID (Ft. Detrick, MD)	http://www.usamriid.army.mil/	1969; estimated completion for upgrades is 2012	
Southwest Foundation for Biomedical Research (San Antonio, TX)	BSL-4 Laboratory, Department of Virology and Immunology http://www.sfbr.org	Glove boxes since the 1970s, full biocontainment in 1999, opened in March 2000	Conducts classified research; has a national primate research center. Serves as part of the BSL-4 Core of the NIAID Western Regional Center of Excellence in Biodefense
University of Texas Medical Branch (Galveston, TX)	UTMB Robert E. Shope, MD, BSL-4 Laboratory http://www.utmb.edu/CBEID/safety.shtml	June 2004	Serves as part of the BSL-4 Core of the NIAID Western Regional Center of Excellence in Biodefense
Georgia State University (Atlanta, GA)	Viral Immunology Center http://www2.gsu.edu/~wwwvir/	Operational	
Virginia Commonwealth University (Richmond, VA)	Virginia Division of Consolidated Laboratory Services (DCLS) http://www.dgs.virginia.gov/DCLS.aspx	Operational	
Department of Homeland Security (Ft. Detrick, MD)	National Biodefense Analysis and Countermeasures Center (NBACC) http://www.dhs.gov/xres/labs/gc_1166211221830.shtm	Broke ground June 2005; planned opening in 2009	Governed by DHS Science and Technology Directorate; will conduct bioforensics and biological threat characterization. The NBACC facility will provide biocontainment laboratory space for the National Bioforensic Analysis Center (NBFAC) and the Biological Threat Characterization Center (BTCC)
National Institute of Allergy and Infectious Diseases (Hamilton, MT)	Rocky Mountain Laboratories (RML) Integrated Research Facility http://www3.niaid.nih.gov/about/organization/dir/rml/integratedResearchFacility.htm	Occupancy in 2007	
National Institute of Allergy and Infectious Diseases and University of Texas Medical Branch (Galveston, TX)	Galveston National Biocontainment Laboratory http://www.utmb.edu/GNL/	Completed in November 2008	Study of anthrax, plague, hemorrhagic fevers, typhus, West Nile virus, influenza, drug-resistant TB, etc.
NIAID and Boston University (Boston, MA)	Boston University Medical Center National Emerging Infectious Diseases Laboratories http://www.bu.edu/neidl/ http://www.bu.edu/dbin/neidl/en/	Expected construction completion date: 2009	
National Institute of Allergy and Infectious Diseases (Ft. Detrick, MD)	NIAID Integrated Research Facility at Fort Detrick http://www.niaid.nih.gov/factsheets/detrick_qa.htm	Estimated completion date: early 2009	

From Gronvall GK, Fitzgerald J, Chamberlain A, et al: High-containment biodefense research laboratories: meeting report and center recommendations, Biosecurity and Bioterrorism 5(1), 75–85, 2007 (accessed November 15, 2008). © Mary Ann Liebert, Inc. Reprinted with permission. DOI: 10.1089/bsp.2007.0902. Available at http://www.liebertonline.com/toc/bsp/5/1

BSL, Biosafety Level; *CDC,* Centers for Disease Control and Prevention; *DHS,* Department of Homeland Security; *NIAID,* National Institute of Allergy and Infectious Diseases; *TB,* tuberculosis; *USAMRIID,* United States Army Medical Research Institute for infectious diseases; *UTMB,* University of Texas Medical Branch.

- CAS number: The **Chemical Abstracts Service (CAS) registry number** is a unique number assigned to each chemical to aid in searching on computerized databases
- RTECS number: Likewise, the **Registry of Toxic Effects of Chemical Substances (RTECS)** is a unique number that aids in finding additional toxicological information about a specific substance
- DOT ID and guide number: This is a listing of the **U.S. Department of Transportation (DOT)** identification numbers of the chemicals regulated by the DOT and serves a similar purpose as the numbers listed previously
- Synonyms: Names with similar meanings
- Trade names: Also called a *proprietary* name; it is selected by the pharmaceutical company and may reflect its use. For example, the "-caines" in general are local anesthetics such as procaine in the United States, which is reflected by at least by 24 different "-caines" in worldwide trade names
- Conversion factors
- Exposure limits: These are the recommended exposure limits (RELs) established by NIOSH
- IDLH: This lists the concentrations of chemicals that are immediately dangerous to life or health
- Physical description: Provides brief information about the appearance and odor of a given substance
- Chemical and physical properties
- Incompatibilities and reactivities
- Measurement methods
- Personal protection and sanitation: This is a summary of recommended practices for safe handling of each substance
- First aid
- Recommendations for respirator selections
- Exposure route, symptoms, and target organs

Proper storage of chemicals in the laboratory is needed to minimize the hazards associated with accidental mixing of incompatible chemicals or simply procedures to avoiding the spilling of the chemicals. Again, OSHA provides employers with guidelines dealing with the occupational exposure to hazardous chemicals in the laboratory as well as guidelines for the appropriate storage and disposal of the chemicals used. In general, chemicals should be stored separately and labeled according to the following categories:

- Solvents
- Inorganic mineral acids
- Bases
- Oxidizers
- Poisons
- Explosives or unstable reactives

Furthermore, each laboratory should have a chemical hygiene plan, including guidelines on labeling of chemical containers and **manufacturer's material safety data sheets (MSDSs)** for each chemical used in that particular laboratory (Figure 5.2). An MSDS form contains data regarding the property of a particular substance intended to provide workers and emergency personnel with procedures for handling that particular substance in a safe manner. Sections on an MSDS data sheet usually include but are not limited to:

- Name of the substance
- Name, address, and telephone number of the manufacturer
- Hazardous ingredients
- Physical and chemical properties
- Toxicity
- Health effects and first aid
- Fire and explosion data
- Stability and reactivity
- Spill, leak, and disposal procedures
- Protective equipment
- Handling and storage
- Shipping data

A searchable MSDS database of chemicals and chemical compounds is available at http://hazard.com/msds/.

Equipment

Laboratory safety equipment is an integral component in all laboratories. Federal, state, and local laws and regulations are designed and intended to protect the health and safety of all laboratory personnel. In this section some of the most common items are described but many more are usually present in laboratories, depending on the levels of sophistication and needs of the individual laboratories.

Fire Extinguishers

In addition to fire alarms, fire extinguishers are required in all laboratories. They are classified and assigned a letter or symbol for that classification to a particular fire type they are designed to extinguish (Figure 5.3). However, multipurpose extinguishers are often recommended because they are effective against different types of fires. Extinguishers are located at specified places in a laboratory. They should be inspected at least every 12 months and records kept readily visible and easily accessible by appropriately trained persons in a given institution, usually safety officers. Fire extinguishers are classified as:

- *Type A:* For use on fires from combustibles such as wood, cloth, paper, rubber, and plastics
- *Type B:* For use on fires from flammable liquids such as grease, gasoline, oil, and paint thinners
- *Type C:* For use on electrically energized fires (electrical equipment such as electrophoresis units)
- *Type D:* For use on fires from flammable metals such as magnesium, titanium, sodium, lithium, and potassium
- *Type K:* For use against fires involving grease fire associated with cooking equipment
- *Multipurpose fire extinguishers:* These work effectively against type A, B, and C fires. Multipurpose fire extinguishers are recommended for home use

All laboratory workers should be appropriately trained by safety personnel in the proper use of fire extinguishers. These training procedures should be published, records kept, and the

ACC# 96151

Section 1 - Chemical Product and Company Identification

MSDS Name: Hydrobromic Acid, P.A.
Catalog Numbers: AC223320000, AC223325000
Synonyms: Hydrogen Bromide
Company Identification:
     Acros Organics N.V.
     One Reagent Lane
     Fair Lawn, NJ 07410
For information in North America, call: 800-ACROS-01
For emergencies in the US, call CHEMTREC: 800-424-9300

Section 2 - Composition, Information on Ingredients			
CAS#	Chemical Name	Percent	EINECS/ELINCS
7732-18-5	Water	51-53	231-791-2
10035-10-6	Hydrogen bromide	47-49	233-113-0

Hazard Symbols: C
Risk Phrases: 34 37

Section 3 - Hazards Identification

EMERGENCY OVERVIEW

Appearance: Clear colorless to faint yellow. **Danger!** Corrosive. Material is light sensitive. Air sensitive. Causes eye and skin burns. Causes digestive and respiratory tract burns.
Target Organs: None.

Potential Health Effects

Eye: May result in corneal injury. Causes severe eye irritation and burns.
Skin: Causes severe skin irritation. May be absorbed through the skin. Contact with liquid is corrosive and causes severe burns and ulceration.
Ingestion: Causes gastrointestinal tract burns. May cause respiratory failure. May cause corrosion and permanent tissue destruction of the esophagus and digestive tract.
Inhalation: Irritation may lead to chemical pneumonitis and pulmonary edema. Causes chemical burns to the respiratory tract. May cause effects similar to those described for ingestion.
Chronic: Chronic inhalation and ingestion may cause effects similar to those of acute inhalation and ingestion.

Section 4 - First Aid Measures

FIGURE 5.2 MSDS data sheet. This illustration shows the cover page of a typical MSDS data sheet. In all laboratories these sheets will be kept in a dedicated binder for quick reference by laboratory workers and emergency personnel.

current status of testing of laboratory personnel maintained under the direction of the laboratory supervisor. Some laboratories will also have sand or absorbent material available to extinguish small fires. These materials are generally stored in highly visible dispensers labeled for use according to the type of fire.

Fume Hoods

Fume hoods are the primary control method for exposure to noxious or poisonous vapors in the laboratory environment. They act by drawing ambient air from the laboratory, past the laboratory operator (who is located in front of the hood), and into the hood. The ability of a hood to provide adequate protection depends on a variety of factors including, but not limited

LIFE APPLICATION

How to Use a Fire Extinguisher: P A S S

P ull: Pull the pin at the top of the extinguisher (unlocks the handle and activates the unit).
A im: Point the nozzle of the hose at the base of the fire.
S queeze: Squeeze the handle to release the fire-fighting agent.
S weep: Sweep the nozzle back and forth at the base of the fire.

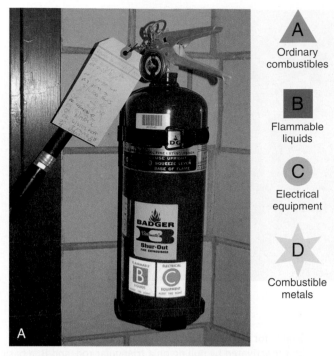

FIGURE 5.3 **Fire extinguishers.** This photo shows a typical multipurpose fire extinguisher used in many laboratories. Note the easy access location near the laboratory door, the inspection tag indicating regular inspections/maintenance, and the letters on the extinguisher indicating the class of fires it is designed to extinguish. All the classes and symbols are listed next to the photo.

A
Ordinary combustibles

B
Flammable liquids

C
Electrical equipment

D
Combustible metals

to, the control of the velocity of the ambient air at the hood face, air movement and flow patterns in the room, and turbulence within the hood. All laboratory workers with access to a fume hood should be familiar with its particular use, capabilities, and limitations. The various hoods found in different laboratories include the following:

- *General-purpose hoods:* These include standard fume hoods, bypass hoods, constant volume hoods, variable air volume hoods, and auxiliary air supply hoods.
- *Radioisotope hoods:* These are tested and authorized by radiation safety personnel for use with volatile radioactive materials.
- *Biosafety cabinets:* These are specialized hoods to prevent or minimize the exposure of humans or the environment to biohazardous agents or materials.
- *Perchloric acid hoods:* These must be used when performing any laboratory procedure that requires the use of perchloric acid.

Fume hoods should always be in good condition and capable for routine use, which requires regular inspections and current records. An emergency plan should be posted on or near the hood in case of ventilation malfunction.

Autoclave

An autoclave (see Figure 4.3 in Chapter 4, Microbiological Laboratory Techniques) is a common, routinely used piece of equipment in biological laboratories. It is a device that uses superheated steam under pressure to sterilize equipment and other objects. Sterilization is the elimination of all transmissible agents (see Chapter 4, Microbiological Laboratory Techniques) and autoclaves are widely used for this purpose. However, as an exception, it has been shown that certain archaea (strain 121) and prions have the capacity to survive autoclaving.

Autoclaves, if not operated properly, pose many hazards including physical (heat, steam, and pressure) and biological hazards. Each autoclave has its unique characteristics and therefore operators need to be trained appropriately and regularly performed maintenance recorded to ensure proper functioning. Before using any autoclave, it is necessary to review and understand the manual on instructions for use in order to prevent possible injuries. Autoclave maintenance is an important aspect of proper function and safety and should be performed periodically in accordance with the manufacturer's recommendations.

Eyewashes and Safety Showers

Eyewashes and safety showers are emergency units present in both public and private industry to protect employees from injury in case of contact with hazardous materials. Employees must be instructed and trained in the proper use of eyewashes and safety showers regardless of their previous experience background. The first seconds after exposure to hazardous materials are critical and decontamination equipment must be in reach for the exposed individual within 10 or fewer seconds after exposure. Therefore, eyewashes and safety showers should be in a clearly marked, accessible location within a laboratory. They provide effective protective treatment in the event of contact from a chemical or biological spill onto the skin or clothing. Many OSHA standards address problems that potentially can occur in the laboratory environment and protocols have been developed for the emergency eyewash and shower equipment (ANSI [American National Standards Institute] Z358.1-2004). The types of equipment addressed by the ANSI standard are listed below and in Figure 5.4.

- *Emergency shower:* Provides a continuous water flow and is operated by grasping a ring chain or triangular rod
- *Plumbed and self-contained eyewash units:* Includes devices permanently connected to a source of potable water, and those not permanently installed, but requiring refilling or replacement after use
- *Personal eyewash:* Used on site for immediate flushing. It has less of a water supply than the plumbed self-contained unit and is used until the victim reaches another unit
- *Hand-held drench hose:* A flexible hose connected to a water supply for use to irrigate and flush eyes, face, and body areas
- *Eye/face wash:* Used to irrigate and flush both the face and the eyes
- *Combination unit:* A shower combined with an eyewash or eye/face wash

Refrigerators/Freezers

Laboratory refrigerators, freezers, and ultralow freezers (down to −85° C) need to be carefully selected for specific chemical or

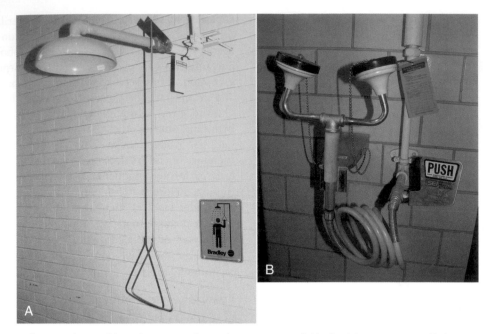

FIGURE 5.4 Showers and eyewashes. Although many styles and types are available for laboratory use, all showers and eyewashes have the same function and basic features. These photos show **A,** a basic plumbed shower activated by pulling on a triangular rod, and **B,** a basic plumbed eyewash activated by a push paddle.

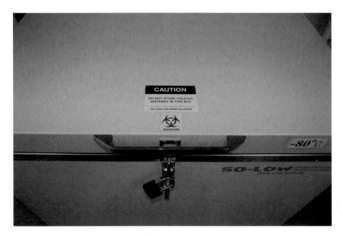

FIGURE 5.5 Freezers. This photo shows a chest-type ultralow temperature freezer with appropriate safety labeling such as temperature, a biohazard label, and a warning not to store volatile liquids in the box. If the gases from volatile liquids should accidentally ignite in the freezer, the tight seal of the box could cause a powerful explosion.

biological needs and records of routine, periodical inspections as well as removal of contents noted. The laboratory refrigerator, freezer, cooling unit, or ultralow freezer should be labeled as such with appropriate hazard signs posted on them (Figure 5.5). Containers placed in a given unit should be completely sealed or capped, securely placed, and have readily visible permanent labels.

Disposal of Hazardous Waste

Materials used in any laboratory environment must be disposed of in designated containers. Broken glass is placed in cartons labeled for broken glass and plastics in plasticware containers (Figure 5.6). Biohazardous wastes are disposed of in autoclave

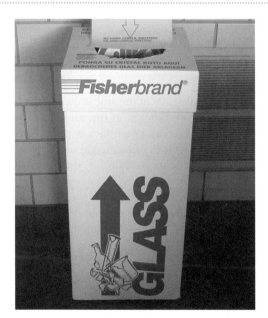

FIGURE 5.6 Glass containers. The size and shape of these containers may vary but certain features are common, such as a heavy-duty plastic liner contained in a sturdy cardboard box.

bags (Figure 5.7) and used sharps are placed in biohazard sharps containers (Figure 5.8).

Protective Gear

Personal protective equipment or gear is used to protect the wearer from specific hazards. While it does not eliminate the hazard or protect the immediate environment, it is used when other controls are insufficient or not feasible. **Protective gear** includes gloves, respiratory protection, eye protection, protective clothing, and any other protective gear as needed. The need for protective equipment depends on the nature, material, quantity, volatility, and (in the case of microbiological laboratories) pathogenicity of the agent (BSL-1 to BSL-4). All laboratory personnel using the protective gear must be instructed in and understand the proper use and function of the equipment, its limitations, and proper disposal procedures.

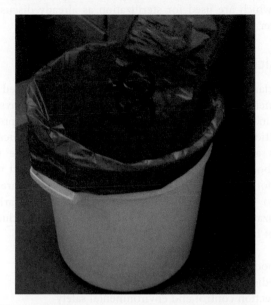

FIGURE 5.7 Autoclave bags. Autoclave bag come in many shapes and sizes but all have some common features: the color of the bags is red or orange, and they have the biohazard symbol printed on the bag. Some bags also incorporate a heat sensitive ink on the bag which will indicate when a bag has been autoclaved.

Gloves

Hand protection is a necessity in many laboratory settings and the selection of appropriate protection depends on the type of materials to be handled. In the microbiological and healthcare environment, gloves are used to ensure protection from exposure to potentially harmful infectious agents. Traditionally, medical and laboratory gloves are made of latex and powdered with cornstarch; however, because of an increase in occurrence of latex allergies in the general population and among health professionals, nonlatex materials such as vinyl or nitrile rubber are becoming useful alternatives. In addition, powder-free gloves are also available for individuals allergic to powder or in environments where powder is not desirable (e.g., medical clean rooms or electronic clean rooms). Special needs, such as for heavy insulated gloves for protection against burns from ultralow temperatures encountered during transfer or removal of materials from ultralow freezers or while removing hot items from an autoclave, should be identified and personnel trained in their use and limitations.

Respiratory Protection

Various types of respiratory protection are used in laboratory:

- Simple surgical masks for the filtration of large particles
- Nose and mouth masks with filtration canisters
- Full face masks covering the eyes, nose, and mouth with filtration canisters
- Full face mask with hood to cover head
- Self-contained breathing equipment with tanks or oxygen supply

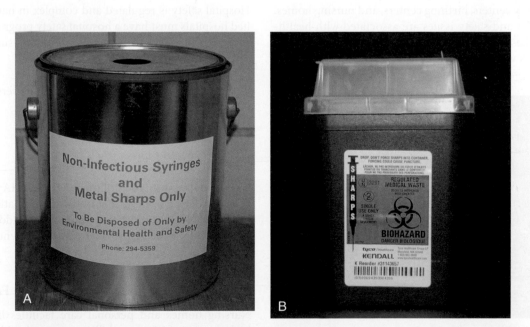

FIGURE 5.8 Sharps containers. All waste items that have the potential to puncture or cause any break in the skin are considered "sharps" and must be disposed of in a container that is puncture proof. As these photos show, these containers come in many shapes and sizes and are usually made of hard plastic or metal. Sharps containers that may contain sharps contaminated with biological waste must also be labeled with a biohazard symbol.

Clothing

Laboratory coats should be worn at all times in laboratory areas, but not outside the laboratory because of possible absorption and accumulation of contaminants on the material of the coat. In the presence of infectious material laboratory coats must be worn closed. Shoes need to be worn at all times in the laboratory but should not be sandals or any type of open-toed shoes to avoid exposure to potential spills. In addition, Kevlar-reinforced toe shoes may be required and their use enforced. The selection of the type of protective clothing is the responsibility of the laboratory director in accordance with the procedures manual. For some laboratory procedures additional aprons, either rubber or plastic, might be required. All clothing worn in laboratories handling infectious substances must be disposed of in a safe manner.

Eye Protection

Eye protection is mandatory in many laboratories where a potential for injury exists. The type of eye protection required depends on the hazard present in a given environment. For most situations safety glasses with side shields are adequate, but when there is danger of splashing of any kind goggles are required. The wearing of corrective lenses is no substitute for wearing protective eye equipment such as goggles or transparent face shields as required (Figure 5.9).

Safety in Healthcare Facilities

Healthcare facilities include hospitals, clinics, dental offices, outpatient surgery centers, birthing centers, and nursing homes. Numerous health and safety issues are associated with healthcare facilities. These include, among others, blood-borne pathogen exposures as well as biological hazards, potential chemical

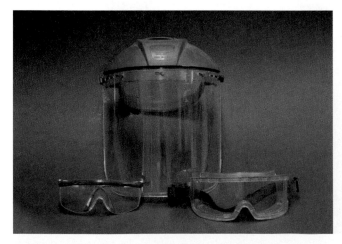

FIGURE 5.9 Eye protection. Pictured are various types of eye protection used in a typical laboratory. The complexity and level of the protection depends on the type of chemicals/agents being used.

and drug exposures, waste anesthetic gas exposures, respiratory hazards, ergonomic hazards from lifting and repetitive tasks, laser hazards, hazards associated with laboratories, radioactive material, x-ray hazards, and other special circumstances.

Some potential chemical hazards include exposure to formaldehyde, a fixative used for the preservation of specimens for pathology; and ethylene oxide, glutaraldehyde, and peracetic acid, which are used for sterilization as already discussed in Chapter 4 (Microbiological Laboratory Techniques).

Physicians' Offices and Clinics

Physicians' offices and clinics should have posted well-documented management procedures designed for physicians, office managers, and clinical personnel to provide appropriate protection for patients and workers. Physicians' offices and clinics are also regulated by OSHA, including the OSHA Bloodborne Pathogens Standard, which requires strict regulations for training healthcare workers. Safety guides are available to physicians' offices and clinics through a variety of organizations, and via the Internet. These guides include but are not limited to:

- Blood-borne pathogen training
- Medical device safety and management
- Infection control and environmental safety
- Patient safety
- Facility and worker safety and security
- Regulatory and governmental agency requirements
- Record-keeping issues
- Prescription medication safety

Hospital

Hospital safety is regulated and complex in nature. All accredited hospitals must have a hospital safety program, policies, and procedures in place, which will cover issues such as:

- Industrial hygiene
- Hazard communication and training of personnel
- Hazardous waste disposal procedures
- Disaster preparation procedures
- Risk management procedures
- Other special topics

Hospitals must also follow all the OSHA regulations for general safety, biosafety, chemical safety, radiation safety, asbestos safety, and hazardous material safety. In addition, education and training must be provided and documented on a regular basis for all employees.

Nursing Homes and Personal Care Facilities

Nursing homes and personal care facilities have one of the highest rates of injury and illness among healthcare industries. OSHA has issued ergonomic guidelines for the nursing home industry for the prevention of musculoskeletal disorders of nursing home personnel.

Blood-borne Pathogens in Healthcare Settings

Disease	Cause	Symptoms	Treatment
Hepatitis B	Hepatitis B virus (HBV)	Lifelong liver infection; cirrhosis of the liver; liver cancer; liver failure; death	Hepatitis B vaccine for prevention; symptomatic treatment and eventually liver transplant
Hepatitis C	Hepatitis C virus (HCV)	No initial symptoms until cirrhosis occurs	Interferon-α, ribavirin; no cure; liver transplant
AIDS	Human immunodeficiency virus (HIV)	Early symptoms of infection include fever, headache, tiredness, enlarged lymph nodes; later: lack of energy, weight loss, frequent fevers and sweats, persistent or frequent yeast infections, skin rashes, short-term memory loss, and many others. Symptoms of opportunistic infections in later stages of disease	Several drug treatments have been approved by the FDA but no cure has been found to this date
Viral hemorrhagic fever (VHF)	Ebola and Marburg viruses	Symptoms vary; initial signs include fever, fatigue, dizziness, muscle aches, loss of strength, exhaustion. Severe cases show signs of bleeding under the skin, internal organs, or from body orifices such as the mouth, eyes, or ears. Can be followed by shock, nervous system malfunction, coma, delirium, seizures, and death	Supportive therapy; no other treatment or established cure

FDA, U.S. Food and Drug Administration.

Transmission of both bacterial and viral infections in nursing homes is of great concern to both the staff and the occupants and is discussed in Chapter 9 (Infection and Disease).

Emergency Response

All laboratory workers should know the laboratory procedures at their institutions and the specific emergency procedures. In addition, OSHA and its State Plan partners set and implement national safety and health standards for emergency responders. Among these standards is the Hazardous Waste Operations and Emergency Response standard. Other special topics include chemical, biological, bioterrorism, radiation, and personal protective equipment; training and education; as well as safety equipment.

Safety in Homes

Physical, chemical, and biological safety not only applies to laboratories, healthcare facilities, and other public facilities, but also to the home environment.

Housing conditions can significantly impact public health. This is of concern with the increase in home-based hospice care. An opportune time to address these issues is when remodeling

Staphylococcus aureus in Healthcare Facilities and Nursing Homes

Dangerous drug-resistant *Staphylococcus* infections are appearing at alarming rates in nursing homes. Methicillin-resistant *Staphylococcus aureus* (MRSA) includes strains that are resistant to treatment with the usual antibiotics. MRSA most frequently occurs in patients who undergo invasive medical procedures or have a weakened immune system and are being treated in hospitals and healthcare facilities such as nursing homes. In these settings MRSA infections are potentially life-threatening. The spread of the infection often occurs when an asymptomatic patient transmits the disease to a healthcare worker, who then can inadvertently transmit the disease to another patient. To prevent the transmission of this disease from one patient to another appropriate hand-washing techniques and adherence to safety protocols are necessary. The Centers for Disease Control and Prevention, state and local health departments, and their nationwide partners are collaborating to prevent MRSA infections in the healthcare setting through a variety of surveillance systems/programs.

(wheelchair and walker access may be required). Healthy People 2010 goals published by the HHS identified major problems and the CDC developed the Healthy Homes Initiative, which is a coordinated, comprehensive, and holistic approach to prevent diseases and injuries related to housing hazards and deficiencies. The program focuses on the identification of health, safety, and quality-of-life issues in the home environment and actions to eliminate or alleviate the problems.

Summary

- All laboratory environments are governed by regulations to ensure the safety of the laboratory personnel and the general environment.
- Microbiological and clinical laboratories are regulated by biosafety level standards, depending on the organisms handled or manipulated in the particular laboratory.
- Standards for the safe use and handling of chemicals apply to all laboratory settings.
- Laboratory safety equipment, an important component in all laboratory settings, is designed to protect the health and safety of all laboratory personnel.
- Safety equipment includes, but is not limited to, fire extinguishers, fume hoods, autoclaves, eyewash and safety showers, and refrigerators/freezers.
- Personal protective gear is used to protect the wearer from specific hazards, but does not protect the immediate environment.
- Safety regulations mandated by federal and state agencies apply to all healthcare facilities, nursing homes, personal care facilities, as well as public institutions.
- All personnel in laboratory facilities and in healthcare and other public facilities should be aware of the specific emergency procedures required for their environment.

Review Questions

1. OSHA is a division of the:
   a. National Institutes of Health
   b. Centers for Disease Control and Prevention
   c. U.S. Department of Labor
   d. World Health Organization

2. There are _____ levels of biosafety depending on the organisms handled.
   a. 1
   b. 2
   c. 3
   d. 4

3. The biosafety level necessary in water-testing facilities is level:
   a. 1
   b. 2
   c. 3
   d. 4

4. Which of the following bacteria should be handled in a Biosafety Level 2 facility?
   a. *Micrococcus luteus*
   b. *Bacillus subtilis*
   c. *Salmonella*
   d. *Staphylococcus epidermidis*

5. Agents associated with human disease, but generally not a serious health risk, are classified in which of the following risk groups?
   a. RG1
   b. RG2
   c. RG3
   d. RG4

6. Ebola viruses need to be handled in which of the following biosafety levels?
   a. BSL-1
   b. BSL-2
   c. BSL-3
   d. BSL-4

7. Fires from flammable metals require type _____ fire extinguishers.
   a. A
   b. B
   c. C
   d. D

8. Bypass fume hoods belong to the group of:
   a. General-purpose hoods
   b. Radioisotope hoods
   c. Perchloric acid hoods
   d. Biosafety cabinets

9. Which of the following eyewash/safety showers should be used for immediate flushing only, until the victim reaches another safety unit?
   a. Emergency shower
   b. Personal eyewash
   c. Hand-held drench hose
   d. Combination unit

10. All of the following are blood-borne pathogens in the healthcare setting *except*:
    a. Hepatitis A
    b. Hepatitis B
    c. Hepatitis C
    d. HIV

11. Ergonomic guidelines for nursing homes are issued by _____.

12. PASS stands for pull, aim, squeeze, and _____.

13. CDC stands for the Centers for Disease Control and _____.

14. Dangerous and exotic agents need to be handled in a BSL _____ environment.

15. The type of fire extinguisher used on fires from flammable liquids such as gasoline would be a type _____ extinguisher.

16. List five specific areas for which clinical laboratories are responsible.

17. Name the types of personal protective equipment/gear.

18. Describe the different eyewash and safety showers found in laboratories.

19. Name five pieces of information provided by the NIOSH Pocket Guide to Chemical Hazards.

20. Name the different blood-borne pathogens that can be a hazard in healthcare settings.

Bibliography

Forbes BA, Sahm DF, Weissfeld AS: *Bailey & Scott's Diagnostic Microbiology*, ed 12, St. Louis, 2007, Mosby/Elsevier.

Mahon CR, Lehman DC, Mansuelis G: *Textbook of Diagnostic Microbiology*, ed 3, St. Louis, 2007, Saunders/Elsevier.

Internet Resources

CDC Office of Health and Safety, Biosafety in Microbiological and Biomedical Laboratories (BMBL), ed 5, http://www.cdc.gov/OD/ohs/biosfty/bmbl5/bmbl5toc.htm

CDC, OPRP (Outbreak Prevention and Response Protocol)—Handwashing Guidelines, http://www.cdc.gov/nceh/vsp/cruiselines/handwashing_guidelines.htm

Centers for Disease Control and Prevention, http://www.cdc.gov/

Occupational Safety and Health Administration, www.osha.gov/

National Institute for Occupational Safety and Health, NIOSH Pocket Guide to Chemical Hazards, http://www.cdc.gov/niosh/npg/

Oklahoma State University, Online Safety Library, Laboratory and Chemical Safety, http://ehs.okstate.edu/LINKS/Index.htm

U.S. Department of Energy, Office of Health, Safety and Security, http://www.hss.energy.gov/index.cfm

Hanford Fire Department (fire extinguisher information), http://www.hanford.gov/fire/safety/extingrs.htm

National Science Foundation, Office of Legislative and Public Affairs, Microbe from Depths Takes Life to Hottest Known Limit, http://www.nsf.gov/od/lpa/news/03/pr0384.htm

Decker FH: Nursing Homes 1977–99: What Has Changed, What Has Not? http://www.cdc.gov/nchs/data/nnhsd/nursinghomes1977_99.pdf

Siegel JD, Rhinehart E, Jackson M, et al: Management of Multidrug-resistant Organisms in Healthcare Settings, 2006, CDC, http://www.cdc.gov/ncidod/dhqp/pdf/ar/mdroGuideline2006.pdf

CDC, Guideline for Hand Hygiene in Healthcare Settings—2002, http://www.cdc.gov/handhygiene/

OSHA Bloodbourne Pathogens Standard, http://www.osha.gov/pls/oshaweb/owadisp.show_document?p_table=STANDARDS&p_id=10051

Hazardous Waste Operations and Emergency Response Standard, http://www.osha.gov/pls/oshaweb/owadisp.show_document?p_table=standards&p_id=9765?

Healthy Homes Initiative, http://www.cdc.gov/healthyplaces/healthyhomes.htm

Bacteria and Archaea

6

[OUTLINE

Bacterial Structure
  Shapes
  Arrangements
Bacterial Growth
  Basis of Bacterial Growth: Binary Fission
  Population Growth Curve
  Measuring Growth
Factors Influencing Microbial Growth
  Nutritional Requirements
  Temperature
  Osmotic Pressure
  Hydrostatic Pressure
  Atmospheric Conditions
  pH
Genetics
  Genotype and Phenotype
  Mutations
  Genetic Transfer in Prokaryotes
Classification of Bacteria and Archaea
  Criteria
  Classification According to *Bergey's Manual of Systematic Bacteriology*

[LEARNING OBJECTIVES

After reading this chapter, the student will be able to:
- Identify bacterial shapes and arrangements
- Discuss the basis of bacterial growth
- Explain the bacterial population growth curve
- Discuss factors that influence microbial growth
- Describe methods for measuring microbial growth
- Discuss the nutritional requirements for bacterial growth
- Discuss replication and expression of bacterial DNA
- Describe bacterial mutations and genetic transfer
- Describe the criteria used in the classification of bacteria
- Discuss medically important bacteria and their classification according to *Bergey's Manual*

KEY TERMS

aerotolerant anaerobes
autotrophs
bacilli
barophiles
barotolerant
binomial system
capneic
carbon
chemoautotrophs
chemoheterotrophs
chemotrophs
chromosome
cocci
conjugation
cryophiles
death phase
diplococci
episome
exponential growth
  phase
facultative anaerobes
facultative halophiles
frameshift mutations

gene
genotype
growth factors
heterotrophs
inversions
lag phase
logarithmic growth phase
macrolesion
mesophiles
microaerophiles
microlesion
minerals
mutations
nitrogen
nucleoid area
obligate aerobes
obligate anaerobes
obligate halophiles
osmophiles
phenotype
photoautotrophs
photoheterotrophs
phototrophs

plasmid
pleomorphic
point mutations
prototype
psychrophiles
psychrotrophs
reversions
sarcina
species
spirals
spirilla
spirochetes
staphylococci
stationary phase
strain
streptococci
sulfur
tetrads
thermophiles
transduction
transformation
transposons
vibrios

WHY YOU NEED TO KNOW

HISTORY

Bacteria have been present from the beginning. These unicellular organisms exist in water, soil, and all phases of our environment. The existence of nonvisible matter was considered early on and this reality was confirmed after van Leeuwenhoek observed "animalcules" through a microscope (see Chapter 1, Scope of Microbiology). Van Leeuwenhoek's descriptions of his microscopic observations of dental scrapings suggest he was observing what are currently called bacteria. The term "bacteria" comes from the Greek word meaning little rod or stick, which is one of the shapes (bacillus) that aids in the morphological description of bacteria. Pasteur, in his eloquent discourses on extensions of the germ theory, refers to "bacteridium," a term that we have shortened to bacteria (plural) or bacterium (singular).

IMPACT

Pure and simple, pathogenic bacteria and the germ theory are founded on the association of certain bacteria, that is, pathogens, with disease. Antibiotics, drug and chemical treatments for disease, the foundations of health and hygiene practice, the potential causes of bacterial disease outbreaks, and the steps necessary to keep them under control are all based on the growth of knowledge about bacteria, which has led to its development as the scientific discipline of bacteriology. In addition, Pasteur's studies on fermentation led to the demise of spontaneous generation (see Chapter 1) as a source for bacteria. Useful roles for bacteria have emerged as well, such as nitrogen fixation and the role of bacteria in food preparation.

FUTURE

There are three areas for concern regarding bacteria that need to be addressed: emerging bacterial infectious diseases, reemerging pathogenic diseases that may or may not be resistant to current antibacterial drugs, and bacteria with bioterrorism potential (see Chapter 18, Emerging Infectious Diseases, and Chapter 24, Microorganisms in the Environment and Environmental Safety). Some examples of emerging bacterial infectious diseases include, but are not limited to, *Staphylococcus aureus* inducing toxic shock syndrome, *Escherichia coli* O157:H7 hemorrhagic colitis and hemolytic uremic syndrome, and *Vibrio cholerae* O139, a new strain of cholera. Some reemerging bacterial diseases such as plague *(Yersinia pestis)* also will be a problem to deal with by healthcare professionals. In addition, the threat of bioterrorism by intentional release or contamination of areas, food, water, and other environments by biological agents including bacteria, viruses, or their toxins represents a real threat for the future of humankind (see Chapter 24).

On the other hand, bacteria are also being used in a variety of industries and research continues to explore the use of bacteria as a food source, in food production, in the production of a variety of pharmaceutical agents, in agriculture, and as microbial fuel cells, to just name a few (see Chapter 1).

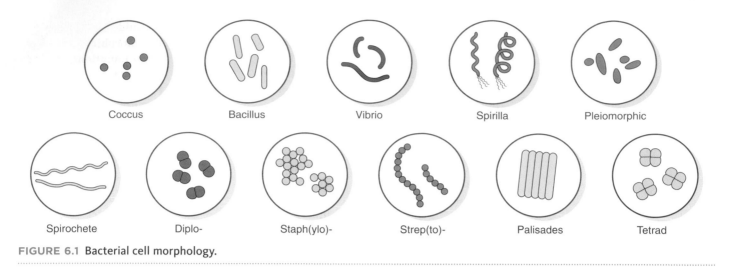

Coccus   Bacillus   Vibrio   Spirilla   Pleiomorphic

Spirochete   Diplo-   Staph(ylo)-   Strep(to)-   Palisades   Tetrad

FIGURE 6.1 Bacterial cell morphology.

Bacterial Structure

Bacteria are prokaryotic unicellular (single-celled) independent organisms that can live as an individual cell or attached to others, forming colonies or groupings, such as biofilms. Each of the cells in such a colony is capable of carrying out all essential activities for survival, such as regular cellular metabolism and reproduction.

Shapes

Bacterial cell morphology displays a variety of different shapes and sizes (Figure 6.1), and the cells are generally much smaller than eukaryotic cells. According to their morphological characteristics most bacteria are classified into different basic shapes: coccus, bacillus, spirochetes (spiral or helical), and pleomorphic (see Chapter 4, Microbiological Laboratory Techniques).

- **Cocci** (singular, coccus) are bacteria whose overall shape is spherical or nearly spherical (Figure 6.2). Several cocci are human pathogens causing, for example, urinary tract infections, food poisoning, toxic shock syndrome, gonorrhea, some forms of meningitis, throat infections, pneumonias, and sinusitis.
- **Bacilli** (singular, bacillus) are rod-shaped bacteria, some of which are endospore forming (Figure 6.3). Diseases caused by bacilli include anthrax, botulism, and tetanus, and gastrointestinal infections caused by bacilli such as *Escherichia coli* and *Salmonella*.
- **Pleomorphic** bacteria are bacterial species that are morphologically indistinct, depending on environmental conditions. This group includes *Coccobacillus* (coccobacilli), which are bacilli that are elongated as well as spherical in shape (Figure 6.4).
- **Spirals** occur as vibrios, spirilla, or spirochetes.
  - **Vibrios** are curved or comma-shaped rods (Figure 6.5) and several species are human pathogens associated with gastroenteritis, cholera, food poisoning, and septicemia. *Vibrio fischeri* and *V. harveyi* are symbiotes

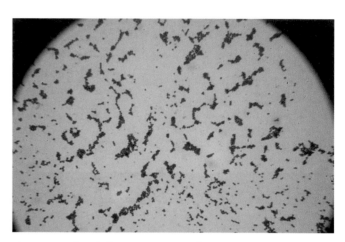

FIGURE 6.2 *Staphylococcus aureus.* This gram-positive coccus, appearing as grapelike clusters, is one of the most common causes of staph infections.

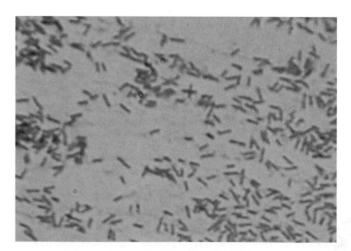

FIGURE 6.3 *Escherichia coli.* This micrograph shows a Gram stain of *E. coli*, a typical gram-negative bacillus.

of marine organisms such as jellyfish and produce light via bioluminescence.

- A **spirillum** (plural, spirilla) is a thick, rigid, spiral organism (Figure 6.6) that can cause rat bite fever, an uncommon but worldwide condition caused by rodent

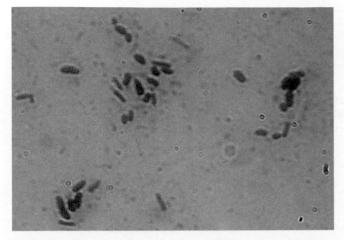

FIGURE 6.4 Coccobacilli. This micrograph illustrates a Gram stain of an organism from the genus *Corynebacterium*. The cells are variable in shape, from spheres to short rods, and therefore are considered pleomorphic (cells with a variable or indistinct shape).

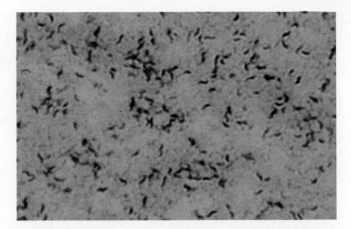

FIGURE 6.6 Spirillum. This micrograph is taken from a Gram stain of the genus *Campylobacter*, showing the corkscrew or "snakelike" shape referred to as *spirilla*. Although a spirilla and a spirochete may appear very similar in overall shape, the spirilla often have flagella as a means of locomotion, whereas the spirochetes have a structure called an *axial filament* that facilitates movement and lack flagella.

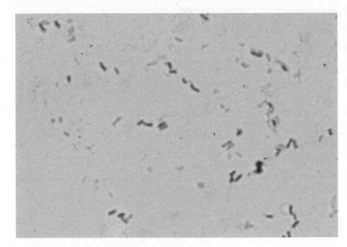

FIGURE 6.5 Vibrio. The micrograph shows a Gram stain of *Vibrio natriegens*, demonstrating the vibrioid shape, a simple curved rod. Note that not all cells appear curved, due to the viewing of the cells on the side with the convex/concave faces of the cell pointing directly at or away from the viewer.

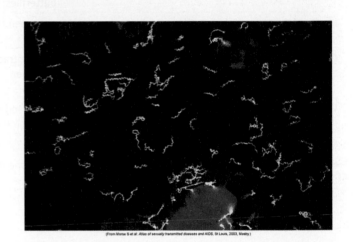

(From Morse S et al: *Atlas of sexually transmitted diseases and AIDS*, St Louis, 2003, Mosby.)

FIGURE 6.7 Spirochete. This micrograph shows *Treponema pallidum*, the causative agent of syphilis. From Murray PR, Rosenthal KS, Pfaller MA: *Medical Microbiology*, ed 5, St. Louis, Mosby, 2005.

bites. These bacteria are present in the oropharyngeal flora of approximately 50% of healthy wild and laboratory rats, as well as in other rodents.

- **Spirochetes** are thin, flexible spirals (Figure 6.7) and can cause leptospirosis, Lyme disease, and syphilis.

Arrangements

In addition to their shape, bacteria can also be categorized according to their arrangement or their style of grouping after cell division.

- Aggregations of cocci occur after cell division and can be classified as the following (Figure 6.8):
  - *Diplo-* is a prefix typically describing cells that occur in pairs of two, joined in one plane only. Examples of

diplococci are *Streptococcus pneumoniae, Neisseria gonorrhoeae,* and *Neisseria meningitidis.*
  - *Strepto-* is a prefix used to indicate an arrangement of cells in beadlike chains, because cell division occurs along a single axis, in contrast to **staphylococci,** which divide along multiple axes. Individual species of *Streptococcus* are identified primarily on the basis of their hemolytic properties on blood agar. The species *Streptococcus pyogenes* is responsible for strep throat, many cases of meningitis, bacterial pneumonia, endocarditis, erysipelas (acute skin infection), and necrotizing fasciitis ("flesh-eating" infections).
  - **Tetrads** are produced by division within two planes, with the cocci arranged in squares of four in irregular clusters. *Micrococcus luteus,* which can be

Examples of Pathogens and Opportunistic Pathogens by Shape

Organism	Shape	Reservoir	Disease(s)
Staphylococcus aureus	Coccus	Common on skin, nose, gastrointestinal and urogenital tracts of humans	Toxin mediated: Food poisoning, scaled skin syndrome, toxic shock syndrome, folliculitis, carbuncles, impetigo, wound infections, bacteremia, and more
Staphylococcus epidermidis	Coccus	Common on human skin	Bacteremia, endocarditis, urinary tract infections, opportunistic infections of catheters, shunts, prosthetic devises, and more
Enterococcus faecalis	Coccus	Common in human gastrointestinal tract	Bacteremia, endocarditis, urinary tract infections, wound infections
Bacillus anthracis	Bacillus	Soil organism	Anthrax
Bacillus cereus	Bacillus	Soil organism	Toxin mediated: Gastroenteritis (emetic, diarrheal), ocular infections, opportunistic infections
Bacillus thuringiensis	Bacillus	None (soil, gut of caterpillars, butterflies, moths)	Gastroenteritis, opportunistic infections
Haemophilus influenzae	Pleomorphic	Mucous membranes of humans	Meningitis, epiglottitis, pneumonia, bacteremia, opportunistic infections
Chlamydia trachomatis	Pleomorphic	Obligate intracellular human pathogen	Sexually transmitted: Prostatitis, epididymitis, cervicitis, pelvic inflammatory disease, urethritis, and more
Vibrio cholerae	Spiral (vibrio)	Estuarine and marine environments	Toxin mediated: Acute diarrheal illness
Spirillum minus	Spiral (spirillum)	Rodents	Rat bite fever
Borrelia burgdorferi	Spiral (spirochete)	Vector-borne, transmitted by ticks	Lyme disease

found in many areas including the human skin, water, dust, and soil, shows this growth pattern. It is considered to be a harmless bacterium but some cases of *Micrococcus* infections have been reported in people with a compromised immune system (e.g., HIV patients).

- **Sarcinae** are cocci arranged in cubes of eight as a result of division in three planes. This coccal grouping occurs when any cocci fail to separate after they divide and the resultant daughter cells remain attached.
- *Staphylo-* is a prefix indicating arrangements in grape-like clusters formed by cell division in random planes. Most members of the genus *Staphylococcus* are harmless and are part of the normal flora of the skin and mucous membranes in humans. A small percentage of staphylococci are also part of the soil microbial flora. The organism can cause an array of diseases in humans and other animals by invasion and also by toxin production. The toxins of *Staphylococcus* are a common cause of food poisoning because the bacteria can grow in improperly stored food. Although the organism is killed

by the cooking process, the enterotoxin is heat resistant and can survive boiling for several minutes.
- Bacilli divide in one plane, producing diplobacilli and streptobacilli (Figure 6.9).
  - Diplobacilli are paired rods that remain in pairs after division.
  - Streptobacilli fail to separate after they divide and remain in chains of cells.

Bacterial Growth

Growth is an increase in the quantity of cellular material and depends on the ability of the cell to form new protoplasm from available nutrients. Bacterial growth requires a source of energy for protein synthesis and to maintain bacterial metabolism. Bacteria must obtain or synthesize nucleic acids, carbohydrates, and lipids that are used as building blocks of cells. The minimal requirements for growth are a source of carbon and nitrogen, an energy source, water, and a variety of ions and minerals.

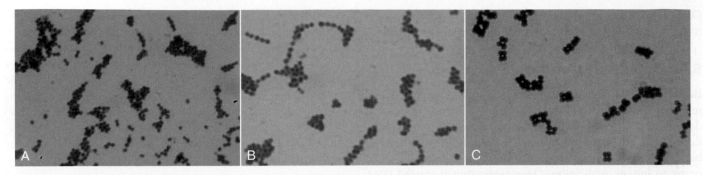

FIGURE 6.8 Arrangements of cocci. Cocci occur in five basic arrangements: diplo, in pairs; staph(ylo), in grapelike irregular clusters; strep(to), in chains; tetrads, in squares of four; and sarcinae, three-dimensional cubes. **A,** *Staphylococcus;* **B,** *Streptococcus;* **C,** *Micrococcus* in tetrads.

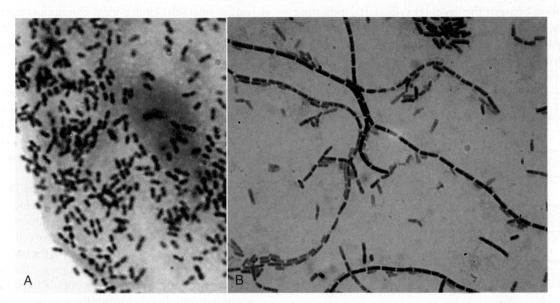

FIGURE 6.9 Arrangements of bacilli. Bacilli can be found in three basic arrangements: **A,** diplo, in pairs; **B,** strep(to), in chains; or palisades, lying next to each other along their long sides.

Fusobacterium: Dental Freeloaders

Bacteria of the genus *Fusobacterium* have a distinct shape—that of a rod with pointed ends or a spindle shape. This is, however, not the only interesting feature about these organisms. *Fusobacterium nucleatum* is a human pathogen that is typically found in the oral cavity, part of the oral flora that is responsible for plaque formation and tooth decay. One of the unique features about this spindle-shaped bacterium is its ability to adhere to other plaque-forming gram-negative

bacteria that have already established a biofilm on the surface of the teeth or mucous membranes. Once added to the existing biofilm, *F. nucleatum* shares the same environmental advantages that the original builders of the biofilm enjoy and their acidic metabolic by-products contribute to tooth decay and periodontal disease. Although linked primarily with the oral cavity, this pathogen has also been associated with infections in the digestive tract, lungs, and liver.

Oxygen is necessary for some bacteria but can be lethal for many others (see Atmospheric Conditions, later in this chapter).

Basis of Bacterial Growth: Binary Fission

Bacterial replication is a coordinated process accomplished primarily by binary fission. Binary fission results in two identical daughter cells (Figure 6.10). In order for growth to occur sufficient metabolites are necessary to support the synthesis of bacterial components. A cascade of regulatory events must occur to initiate replication. Once replication is started DNA synthesis must run to completion. Chromosome replication starts at the plasma membrane and each daughter chromosome is anchored to a different portion of the membrane. Membrane, peptidoglycan synthesis, and cell division are linked together and as the bacterial membrane grows, the daughter chromosomes are pulled apart. At the end of chromosome replication septum formation between the daughter cells starts, indicating cell division (see Chapter 3, Cell Structure and Function). New initiation may begin even before chromosome duplication and cell division are complete.

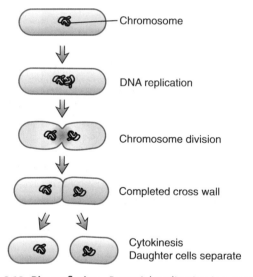

Chromosome

DNA replication

Chromosome division

Completed cross wall

Cytokinesis
Daughter cells separate

FIGURE 6.10 Binary fission. Bacterial replication is a coordinated process accomplished primarily by binary fission. The circular DNA molecule is replicated, the bacterial cell elongates, and the cell splits into two identical cells, each containing an exact copy of the original DNA.

At the point at which metabolites are depleted or toxic by-products build up, chemical alarmones are produced, which stops synthesis. Degradative processes and DNA synthesis continue until all initiated chromosomes are completed. Ribosomes are broken down during the degradative process to provide deoxyribonucleotide precursors. Peptidoglycan and proteins are degraded for metabolites and the cell may shrink in response. Complete cell division may not occur and the cell may ultimately die. Under degradative processes sporulation may occur in species capable of this process.

Population Growth Curve

To produce a bacterial culture in a laboratory environment, the organism must be added to a medium (see Types of Culture Media in Chapter 4, Microbiological Laboratory Techniques). Under favorable conditions a growing bacterial culture doubles at regular intervals. Under ideal conditions, bacterial growth can be described by four different phases: the lag phase, the exponential or logarithmic growth phase, the stationary phase, and the death phase (Figure 6.11).

- **Lag phase:** Bacteria must adapt to the medium before cell division starts. This period of time is referred to as the lag phase of the bacterial growth curve. During this phase the cells are metabolically active, producing molecules necessary for cell division; the individual bacteria are maturing, yet they are not able to divide at this time.
- **Logarithmic** or **exponential growth phase:** The rate of growth increases with time in the so-called *logarithmic* or *exponential growth* phase. Each cell introduced to the medium divides by binary fission into two cells. With each subsequent binary fission a doubling of the bacterial cells occurs as long as the growth conditions are favorable. The time required for doubling of the population is called the *generation time*. In other words the number of new bacteria per unit of time is proportional to the present population, and the actual rate of growth depends on the growth conditions, which directly affect the frequency of cell division.
- **Stationary phase:** A stationary phase occurs when essential nutrients are depleted or by-products of metabolism accumulate. A depletion of nutrients causes cells to decrease in size and toxic metabolic by-products limit the ability to undergo cell division. During this phase the total

FIGURE 6.11 Bacterial growth curve. Bacterial growth can be described by four different phases: the lag phase, the exponential or logarithmic growth phase, the stationary phase, and the death phase.

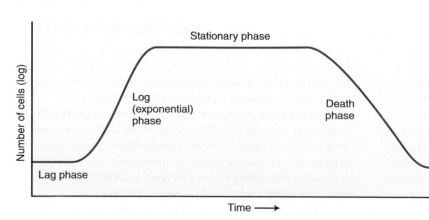

number of viable cells remains constant. This phase of population growth can last for a few hours to several days, depending on the environmental conditions.

- **Death phase:** Finally, the death phase begins when growth stops and the number of dead cells is larger than the number of viable cells.

Measuring Growth

The number and types of microbes present in a variety of samples can be measured by various techniques. This is important to identify the numbers and types of microorganism present in milk, food, water, and soil, and in clinical samples such as urine. Bacterial growth can be measured as an increase in cell mass or cell numbers.

Measurement of Cell Mass

Measurement of the cell mass can be achieved by determining dry or wet weight or by measuring the turbidity (visible cloudiness) of a liquid medium. Cell mass measurements cannot differentiate between living and dead cells.

- Dry weight measurements allow a more accurate estimation of cell masses but are more time consuming and only useful when dealing with massive populations of cells. With this procedure the cells need to be washed thoroughly and then dried before weighing. The dry weight of cells is roughly 20% to 25% of their wet weight.
- Microbial growth in liquid media causes turbidity and can be measured with a spectrophotometer. The turbidity is measured in optical density (OD) units, which is the logarithm of the ratio of intensity of light striking the suspension to the amount that is transmitted. The greater the cell mass the less light will pass through the spectrophotometer, an instrument that can measure light intensity. Measurement of very large populations will require dilution in order to obtain accurate estimates of cell mass.

Measurement of Cell Number

Determination of the number of cells in a sample plays an important role in the microbiological laboratory. Direct counts of cells in a microbial population can be estimated by microscopy or electronic devices, while viable cell counts are determined by a specific culture technique. Indirect counts involve the measurement of a particular end product or the amount of dye reduction, providing quantitative or semiquantitative information.

- Direct (total) cell counts can be obtained microscopically in counting chambers known as *Petroff-Hauser chambers* (Figure 6.12). Such a chamber consists of a slide with a grid of 25 small squares etched within 1 mm^2 under a coverslip.
- Viable counts only count the viable cells in a culture and can be accomplished by:
  - Pour plating
  - Spread plating
  - Most probable number method

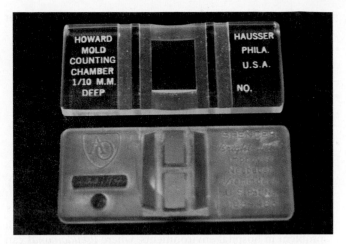

FIGURE 6.12 Slide counting chamber. Several different slide counting chambers are available including the Petroff-Hausser chamber, the Sedgwick-Rafter chamber, and the Neubauer chamber (pictured).

Factors Influencing Microbial Growth

Prokaryotes exist under a wide range of physical conditions. These environmental conditions include nutritional requirements, temperature, osmotic pressure and other atmospheric conditions, all of which greatly influence the growth of microbes. The type of microbial life present reflects the physical and chemical conditions of a given environment. Some microbes can tolerate extreme temperatures, high osmotic pressure, and other extreme chemical and atmospheric conditions, whereas others can grow and reproduce only in a limited range of environmental conditions. These conditions may support the growth of one organism, while inhibiting the growth of other microbes.

Nutritional Requirements

The nutritional requirements for different microbes vary significantly from one to another. Microorganisms that acquire energy from light are called **phototrophs,** and those that require chemical compounds for energy are called **chemotrophs.** The pathways for the generation of cellular energy are photosynthesis, fermentation, and respiration (see Chapter 3, Cell Structure and Function).

Carbon atoms provide the backbone for all organic compounds and are essential for all life forms. Microorganisms called **autotrophs** can obtain carbon from atmospheric carbon dioxide, and **heterotrophs** are organisms that use carbon from organic compounds. Depending on the source of carbon and energy, bacteria are classified as photoautotrophs, chemoautotrophs, photoheterotrophs, and chemoheterotrophs.

- **Photoautotrophs** use sunlight as the energy source and atmospheric carbon dioxide as their carbon source. Photoautotrophs include photosynthetic bacteria, algae, and green plants. They transform carbon dioxide and water into carbohydrates and oxygen by way of photosynthesis.

- **Chemoautotrophs** use inorganic chemical compounds as the source of energy and carbon dioxide as the carbon source.
- **Photoheterotrophs** use sunlight for energy, but cannot convert carbon dioxide into energy; instead, they use organic compounds as the source for carbon.
- **Chemoheterotrophs** use organic compounds for both the source of energy and a carbon source. Some chemohetero-trophs such as *Pseudomonas* can use many different organic compounds as energy and carbon source, and therefore can grow in many different environments such as in soap dispensers. This makes this organism a particular problem in hospital environments, where *Pseudomonas* can also grow in respiratory equipment.

Nitrogen is another essential element for all life forms because nitrogen is an element in many organic molecules such as amino acids and nucleic acids. Many bacteria produce enzymes for the breakdown of proteins into amino acids. Some bacteria can obtain nitrogen from inorganic compounds such as nitrites, nitrates, and ammonium. Few bacteria can reduce atmospheric nitrogen independently or in association with plants. This process is known as *nitrogen fixation*, an important occurrence in agriculture.

Sulfur and phosphorus requirements can be met by organic compounds, inorganic salts of sulfates, sulfides, and thiosulfates. If soluble phosphate salts are not available in the environment they can be a limiting factor for microbial growth in nature.

Minerals required in trace amounts by microorganisms include potassium, magnesium, calcium, iron, trivalent iron, molybdenum, manganese, and zinc. Small organic compounds are **growth factors** that are either not synthesized by a bacterium or synthesized in insufficient amounts. These growth factors include vitamins, amino acids, purines, pyrimidines, and porphyrins.

Temperature

Most microorganisms can grow in a wide range of temperatures, but optimal growth occurs within a narrow range. The minimal growth temperature is the lowest temperature that supports the growth of an organism, and the maximal growth temperature is the highest temperature that allows growth. The optimal growth temperature is the range of temperature that provides ideal conditions for the growth of a particular microbe. Depending on the range of temperature in which a microbe will grow, they are classified as mesophiles, thermophiles, psychrophiles, and psychrotrophs (Table 6.1).

- **Mesophiles:** Mesophiles are microorganisms that have optimal growth in moderate temperature, generally between 25° C and 40° C. The habitats of these organisms include soil, the human body, and animals. They also play an important role in food preparations such as the production of cheese and yogurt, as well as beer and wine production. Most medically important bacteria are

TABLE 6.1 Examples of Bacteria Growing at Different Temperatures

	Pathogens	Nonpathogens
Mesophiles	*Salmonella typhi*	*Micrococcus luteus*
Thermophiles	*Campylobacter* spp.	*Bacillus thermophilus*
Psychrophiles	*Yersinia enterocolitica*	*Pseudomonas* spp.
Psychrotrophs	*Listeria monocytogenes*	*Bacillus* spp.

mesophiles, and pathogenic organisms generally grow best at temperatures that are optimal for the cells of the host. In the laboratory environment these microbes are generally grown in incubators set at 37° C (human body temperature). Bacteria of the normal human flora are mesophiles.

- **Thermophiles:** These heat-loving organisms grow best at temperatures of 45° C or higher. Examples of such environments include hot springs, deep sea hydrothermal vents, tropical soil composts, and decomposing hay stacks. Some bacteria grow in water-boiling environments up to 110° C. Most photosynthetic prokaryotes are limited to environments of 70° C to 73° C, and most eukaryotic microbes cannot grow above 60° C.
- **Psychrophiles (cryophiles):** These bacteria are cold-loving and can grow at 0° C or lower, with an optimal growth around 15° C. They are usually found in Arctic and Antarctic regions and in streams that are fed by glaciers.
- **Psychrotrophs:** These organisms grow very slowly at 0° C but have an optimal growth range of 25° C to 30° C. Psychrotrophs are not considered to be psychrophiles. They are abundant in nature and can cause food spoilage at refrigerator temperatures.

Osmotic Pressure

Microorganisms with a cell wall can withstand some osmotic pressure, but most microorganisms do not tolerate environments in which the concentration of solutes is higher outside of the cell (hypertonic). Osmotolerant microorganisms can grow in the pressure of a hypertonic environment, and **osmophiles** are microbes that require a high solute concentration in the environment for optimal growth.

As stated previously, most microorganisms do not tolerate hypertonic concentrations of sodium chloride (NaCl), but some of them require it for optimal growth. The genera *Halobacterium* and *Halococcus* are present in saline lakes and basins where NaCl levels are close to the saturation level. Other **obligate halophiles** (salt lovers) found in oceans show optimal growth in about 3.5% NaCl. **Facultative halophiles** are salt tolerating and can live in NaCl concentrations up to 10%. Examples are *Staphylococcus aureus* and *Enterococcus faecalis*.

Hydrostatic Pressure

The hydrostatic pressure is a type of environmental pressure that a fluid exerts in a confined space. This pressure is applied to aquatic microorganisms because of the weight of water.

- **Barotolerant** microorganisms can survive under conditions of increased hydrostatic pressure, whereas most organisms are inhibited in growth by hydrostatic pressures of 200 to 600 atmospheres.
- **Barophiles** grow best under high hydrostatic pressures and occur only in the deepest parts of the oceans.

Atmospheric Conditions

Prokaryotes exist in nature under various physical conditions including different oxygen concentrations in the atmosphere (Table 6.2). It is necessary to know the atmospheric requirement of microorganisms when obtaining, transporting, and culturing microbes. Metabolic pathways or organisms often require oxygen to generate ATP molecules, but some pathways can produce energy without the presence of oxygen, and some organisms will be killed in the presence of oxygen.

- **Obligate aerobes** are organisms that grow only in the presence of oxygen and therefore they obtain their energy through aerobic respiration.
- **Obligate anaerobes** grow only in the absence of oxygen and are often inhibited or killed by the presence of oxygen. They obtain their energy through anaerobic respiration or fermentation.
- **Aerotolerant anaerobes** cannot use oxygen for energy requirements but can grow in the presence of oxygen. They can transform energy by fermentation only and are also called *obligate fermenters*.
- **Facultative anaerobes** can grow either in the absence or presence of oxygen. They use aerobic respiration in the presence of oxygen, and anaerobic respiration or fermentation in the absence of oxygen.
- **Microaerophiles** are organisms that require a low concentration of oxygen, about 2% to 10% (much less than atmospheric oxygen at 21%); a higher oxygen concentration will inhibit their growth. They acquire their energy through aerobic cellular respiration.
- **Capneic** bacteria (capnophiles) require more carbon dioxide than is present in earth's surface atmosphere.

pH

The pH of the natural environments ranges from about 0.5 in acidic soils to approximately 10.5 in alkaline lakes. The pH range of bacteria ranges from the minimal pH at which they can grow to the maximal pH above which the organism cannot grow. Microorganisms can be placed into groups based on their optimal pH requirements: neutrophiles (pH range of 5 to 8), acidophiles (grow best at pH below 5.5), and alkaliphiles (grow best at pH above 8.5). Most microorganisms tolerate alkaline environments, but grow best around pH 7. Some species, however, prefer an acidic environment for optimal growth. For example, *Helicobacter pylori* grows in the epithelial lining of the stomach despite the high acidity present in the lumen. Thermoacidophiles grow at high temperatures and low pH. Several groups of archaea belong in this category. Some bacteria such as *Vibrio cholerae* grow at pH 8.5 or higher. Fungi are generally more tolerant of acidic environments and grow best at pH 5 or 6.

MEDICAL HIGHLIGHTS

Peptic Ulcers: *Helicobacter pylori*

Peptic ulcers are open sores that develop in the lining of the stomach or duodenum. Peptic ulcers are common and for a long time have been believed to be caused by stress or by the eating of spicy food. Although these can make the ulcers worse, the real cause of the majority of peptic ulcers is *Helicobacter pylori*. *H. pylori* infections are common in the United States; however, most infected people do not develop ulcers. The bacterium potentially weakens the mucosa of the stomach and duodenum, allowing acids to penetrate the tissue and together with the bacterium causing a sore or ulcer. *H. pylori* infections are diagnosed by blood, stool, and tissue samples as well as urea breath tests. Treatment of these ulcers usually involves a combination of antibiotics, acid suppressors, and stomach protectors.

TABLE 6.2 Examples of Bacteria Growing Under Different Atmospheric Conditions

	Pathogens	Nonpathogens
Obligate aerobes	*Mycobacterium leprae*	*Pseudomonas fluorescens*
Obligate anaerobes	*Clostridium botulinum*	*Clostridium sporogenes*
Aerotolerant anaerobes	*Fusobacterium* spp.	*Bifidobacterium* spp.
Facultative anaerobes	*Escherichia coli*	*Staphylococcus epidermidis*
Microaerophiles	*Campylobacter jejunae*	*Thiovuhlum majus*
Capnophiles	*Neisseria gonorrhoeae*	*Mannheimia succiniciproducens*

Genetics

The genome of an organism is the sum of the genetic material of a cell and generally exists in the form of chromosomes but also can occur in nonchromosomal sites, such as in plasmids of bacteria and mitochondria and chloroplasts in eukaryotic cells. Characteristics of bacteria such as morphology, metabolism, antibiotic resistance, and other characteristics are determined by inherited information, which is encoded by genes in the DNA molecules.

- A **gene** is a unit that codes for particular information located on a DNA molecule. The total number of genes in an organism is called the *genome*. Bacteria and archaea have a smaller genome compared with eukaryotes.
- A **chromosome** is a single DNA molecule that includes proteins called *histones* in eukaryotes, but prokaryotic cells do not have a nucleus and their DNA is not associated with histones. In general, bacteria and archaea store their genomes in a single large circular chromosomal DNA molecule to be found in an area that is non-membrane bound and called the **nucleoid area.** In addition, many bacteria contain small extrachromosomal (nonchromosomal) DNA molecules called *plasmids*. Linear chromosomes and plasmids previously unknown have now been found in some species of gram-positive and gram-negative bacteria.
- A **plasmid** is independent from the chromosomal DNA of the organism; it is generally circular, self-replicating, and usually carries between 5 and 100 genes. Plasmids are not essential for normal bacterial growth and therefore bacteria may lose or gain plasmids without causing harm. However, plasmids often contain genes that provide a selective advantage to a bacterium under certain environmental conditions such as the presence of antibiotics, when an antibiotic resistance gene in a plasmid can code for an enzyme capable of denaturing the antibiotic. These types of plasmids provide antibiotic resistance to an increasing number of bacteria, causing serious problems in hospitals and other healthcare environments.
- An **episome** is a unit of genetic material composed of a series of genes, such as a plasmid, that is capable of integrating itself into the chromosomal DNA of the organism and therefore can stay intact and is duplicated with every cell division. It becomes a basic part of the genetic makeup of the organism and therefore is no longer considered a plasmid or separate unit, because it became part of the chromosomal DNA.

Genotype and Phenotype

Genes located on the DNA molecule can be grouped into structural genes that code for proteins, genes that code for RNA, and regulatory genes that control gene expression.

- The **genotype** of an organism represents its exact genetic makeup and, in the case of bacteria, a specific species such as *E. coli* can have various strains, each strain with its specific and often only slightly altered genotype.
- The **phenotype** of an individual organism represents the observable characteristics of that organism. While an organism's genotype has the greatest influence on the phenotype, environmental factors can somewhat alter the appearance. This phenomenon is referred to as phenotypic plasticity, describing the degree to which an organism's phenotype is determined by its genotype. In the case of bacteria, high levels of plasticity indicate that environmental factors such as pH or temperature, or the type of medium they grow on, have a strong influence on the appearance of the bacterial culture.
- The relationship between genotype and phenotype can be simply expressed as: genotype + environment = phenotype.

Mutations

Mutations are changes to the base pair sequence of DNA or RNA, passed on by cell division. Mutations are random events that are unpredictable. The rate of mutation is a measure of the rate of genetic change and is often referred to as *mutant frequency*. The types of mutations can be classified as spontaneous and induced mutations.

- Spontaneous mutations occur naturally with no known cause.
- Induced mutations can occur in nature through exposure to radiation or chemicals affecting the DNA. Genetic changes can also be produced in the laboratory. Physical, chemical, or biological agents that alter the DNA are called *mutagens* or *mutagenic agents*.

A **microlesion** is an injury to the DNA that involves only one base pair. When more than one base pair or several genes are affected the damage is called a **macrolesion.** Mutations can be classified according to the type of change occurring in a gene; these include point mutations, frameshift mutations, inversions, transposons, and reversions.

- **Point mutations** occur when a single nucleotide base is altered. A base substitution involves the replacement of one base pair with another. This type of point mutation represents the most frequent type. When a purine or a pyrimidine replaces another purine or pyrimidine base, the substitution is referred to as a transition. If a purine replaces a pyrimidine or vice versa, the substitution is called a *transversion*. Silent mutations occur when a codon (three-nucleotide sequence; see Chapter 2, Chemistry of Life) is changed by substitution of one base but the codon still contains the code for the same amino acid, and therefore the end product of protein synthesis is the same. However, when a base substitution codes for a different amino acid the end product is different, changing the shape and function of the protein. The consequence can be minor, harmful, or lethal.
- **Frameshift mutations** involve the deletion or insertion of one or more bases. This mutation results in a misreading,

or shift in the reading, of the genetic code, and a different end product. For example, if the original code reads "The dog was bad" and the letter (base) "o" is deleted, the reading would end up as a nonsense message, because the codons are read in three-letter words.

The dog was bad

The dgw asb ad

Small deletions can occur spontaneously. Exposure to radiation or chemical mutagens often results in the loss of several segments of DNA. Ultraviolet radiation promotes the formation of thymine dimers, which is a bonding between two adjacent thymines on the DNA strand. This results in the functional deletion of the thymine from the base sequence on the gene, because the adjacent dimers bond to each other and distort the DNA molecule and therefore prevent transcription at that spot. In ionizing radiation (x-rays and γ rays) large molecules break and leave small, electrically charged (ionized) molecules. Nucleic acids and proteins are particularly susceptible to this type of radiation. In lethal mutation prolonged radiation will cause sufficient cell damage to kill the cell. In deletions nucleotides are removed from the DNA strand, causing a mutation. Mutagens causing deletion include hydrogen peroxide, N-methyl-N-nitrosoguanidine, and manganous chloride.

Additions of one or several bases are insertions and are caused by mutagens called *intercalating agents*.

- **Inversions** are macrolesions in which the order of bases is switched or inverted. The change in the base sequence due to inversions produces nonsense codons with a high probability of gene dysfunction.
- **Transposons** (jumping genes) are genes that move from one segment of DNA to another on chromosomes, on plasmids, or within viruses. They contain inverted repeat segments of bases at the ends and a transposonase gene. Transposonase is an enzyme needed to transpose the sequence. Transposons can contain other genes also, such as drug resistance genes. A transposon can insert itself into chromosomal DNA, interrupting the gene sequence, and therefore is a potential mutagen.
- **Reversions** are mutants that can revert back to the wild-type phenotype. This back mutation restores the original phenotype and can be due to the action of mutagens.

Genetic Transfer in Prokaryotes

Bacteria can obtain new genetic material from another organism that is closely related. This can happen through transformation, transduction, or conjugation. Donors are the cells that transfer DNA and recipients are the cells receiving the DNA .

- **Transformation** is the transfer of free DNA or genetic elements from one cell to another. This process occurs naturally in many bacterial species. Transformation is an important tool in the genetic manipulation of bacteria performed in the laboratory environment. This process is routinely used in genetic engineering.

- **Transduction** is the transfer of DNA from one bacterium to another, via a bacteriophage (virus). Bacteriophages transferring the genetic material are called *transducing particles*. Transfer of a limited number of specific genes is called *specialized transduction* and the transfer of any segment of DNA is *generalized transduction*.
- **Conjugation** is the transfer of genetic material during cell-to-cell contact. This process can take place between mating cells of the same species or between closely related species. In mating types the donor carries a sex pilus (F-pilus) whereas the recipient does not.

Classification of Bacteria and Archaea

Prokaryotes are divided into bacteria and archaea. An abundance of information is available about bacteria, but much less is known about archaea. Archaea tend to live in areas not easily accessible and therefore are not involved in everyday human life. Bacteria, on the other hand, especially pathogenic ones, have been investigated extensively.

Members of the archaea are a group of bacteria that have features differing from the other bacteria. With the exception of thermoacidophiles, which are found in hot acidic springs, the rest of the archaea have cell walls lacking peptidoglycan. Archaea are most often found in unusual or extreme habitats and, based on their habitats, they are classified as

- Methanogens: Methane producers
- Thermophiles: Heat lovers
- Halophiles: Salt lovers

Criteria

Bacteria are unicellular organisms that are structurally diverse and widely distributed. With few exceptions bacteria are capable of living independently under environmental conditions favorable to them. The assignment of a bacterium to a species is not based on the same principles that govern species placement in the plant and animal kingdoms. Because bacteria divide by binary fission, bacterial species are not the result of interbreeding groups and therefore bacteria cannot be classified by means of breeding groups. The offspring may evolve in a different direction through mutation, gene transfer, or selected environmental pressures. Gene transfer from one bacterium to another is difficult to assess because the frequency of occurrence is unknown.

A bacterial **species** is defined as a group of bacteria that exhibit a large number of similar characteristics. The originally described bacterium is referred to as the **prototype.** Any subsequent bacterium isolated that has only a few modifications from the prototype is called a **strain** of the original species prototype. Bacteria are named according to the **binominal system** of nomenclature, which was first proposed by Carolus (Carl) Linnaeus (1707–1778), a Swedish botanist, physician, and zoologist, and who is considered to be the "father of modern

Domain	Bacteria	Archaea	Eukarya

Domain → Bacteria Archaea Eukarya
Kingdom → Monera
Phylum → Proteobacteria
Class → Gammaproteobacteria
Order → Enterobacteriales
Family → Enterobacteriaceae
Genus → *Escherichia*
Species → *E. coli*

FIGURE 6.13 Binominal system of nomenclature developed by Carolus Linnaeus.

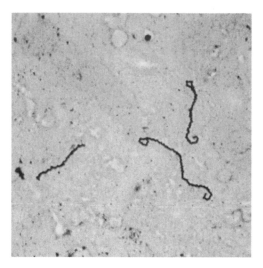

FIGURE 6.14 Leptospira. Silver staining shows the tightly coiled body with hooked ends. From Murray PR, Rosenthal KS, Pfaller MA: *Medical Microbiology*, ed 5, St. Louis, Mosby, 2005.

taxonomy." He classified nature within a hierarchy, starting with kingdoms, which are divided into classes and then into orders, which are divided into genera, followed by division into species (Figure 6.13).

Phenotypic classifications of bacteria involve the microscopic and macroscopic morphologies and were the first used to identify bacteria. For example, bacteria can be classified by Gram-staining properties and by the shape of the individual organism, such as gram-positive cocci. The appearance of bacterial colonies (see Chapter 4, Microbiological Laboratory Techniques) also can be used for identification of the organism. More discriminating methods can then be applied for more specific identification.

Measurements of the presence or absence of specific biochemical markers such as fermentation of specific carbohydrates or the presence of specific enzymes are also used for purposes of identification. Using selected biochemical tests, a high degree of precise identification can be achieved for most isolates. These methods are also useful for subdividing groups of organisms from the same species to identify whether they originate from a common source or not. This method is referred to as biotyping and is of primary use in epidemiology.

Serotyping is a technique by which antigens of a specific cell are identified with marked or labeled antibodies. This method is used primarily to identify microbes that are inert in biochemical settings, difficult to grow, or need to be rapidly identified. As with biotyping, serotyping can also be used to divide the subspecies level for epidemiological purposes. Phage typing and susceptibility of bacteria to various antibiotics are also used for species identification. The latter method, which measures antibiotic susceptibility, is called the *antibiogram pattern method* and has limited discriminatory power.

Analytical characteristics of bacteria can be used to classify genus, species, or subspecies of bacteria also. This method is accurate but labor intensive and the instrumentation used is expensive. Genotypic classification is by far the most precise method for bacterial identification. Genotyping has evolved over the years and has been developed into some simplified methods that can be used in many clinical laboratories.

Classification According to *Bergey's Manual of Systematic Bacteriology*

"Prokaryotes are described in 33 sections of the 4 volumes comprising the first edition of *Bergey's Manual of Systematic Bacteriology* (a second edition is forthcoming)." This section of the chapter provides an overview of some major groups of bacteria important in human health and disease. A more complete outline is illustrated in Appendix A: *Bergey's Manual of Systematic Bacteriology*.

Spirochetes

Spirochetes are a group of helical, motile bacteria with a length from 5 to 500 micrometers (μm). They are flexible and motile with twisting motions of their axial fibrils. These fibrils are a type of endocellular flagella that are wound around their cell body. Free-living spirochetes can be found in various aqueous environments and in association with human or animal hosts. Pathogenic spirochetes include *Treponema pallidum*, *Borrelia burgdorferi*, and *Leptospira interrogans* (Figure 6.14). *Treponema* is the causative agent of syphilis (see Chapter 17, Sexually Transmitted Infections/Diseases), *Borrelia burgdorferi* is the causative agent of Lyme disease, and *Leptospira interrogans* is the causative agent of leptospirosis.

Aerobic/Microaerophilic Helical Vibroid Gram-negative Bacteria

The helical/vibroid gram-negative bacteria are either slightly curved or have multiple helical turns. They are motile with the help of their flagella. These bacteria can live in fresh or coastal waters and some may cause disease in humans or animals. This group of bacteria includes *Campylobacter*, *Helicobacter*, *Bdellovibrio*, and *Vampirovibrio* (Table 6.3). *Bdellovibrio* and *Vampirovibrio* prey on other gram-negative bacteria and on algae.

Gram-negative Aerobic Rods and Cocci

Gram-negative aerobic rods and cocci are a diverse group of bacteria that have been extensively investigated. They are widely

Pathogenic Spirochetes

Disease	Cause	Symptoms	Treatment

Lyme disease	*Borrelia burgdorferi*	Acute: Skin rash, including "bull's-eye" rash; fever, fatigue, headache, muscle and joint aches. Not all symptoms occur in every case of the disease
		Chronic: Fatigue; myalgia; neuropathy, meningitis, and more
			Antibiotics:
			  Early stages: Doxycycline (except in children) and amoxicillin.
			  Refractile or late stages: Prolonged treatment with ceftriaxone

Syphilis	*Treponema pallidum*	Primary, secondary, tertiary, and latent*	Antibiotics in primary and secondary stages: Penicillin, doxycycline, ceftriaxone, or azithromycin
Leptospirosis	*Leptospira interrogans*	Influenza-like symptoms; complications of hepatitis, jaundice, hemorrhage in the liver, uremia bacteriuria, aseptic meningitis; conjunctival hemorrhages	Antibiotics: Doxycycline or penicillin

*See Chapter 17 (Sexually Transmitted Infections/Diseases).

TABLE 6.3 Medically Important Aerobic/Microaerophilic Helical Vibroid Gram-negative Bacteria

Organism	Disease(s)
Campylobacter	Gastrointestinal tract infections: diarrhea, fever, and cramps
Helicobacter pylori	Peptic ulcers, gastritis, duodenitis

TABLE 6.4 Medically Important Gram-negative Aerobic Rods and Cocci

Organism	Disease(s)
Legionella pneumophila	Legionellosis: Pontiac fever, Legionnaires' disease
Neisseria gonorrhoeae	Gonorrhea
Neisseria meningitidis	Meningitis
Bordetella pertussis	Whooping cough
Francisella tularensis	Tularemia
Pseudomonas aeruginosa	Infections in burn victims

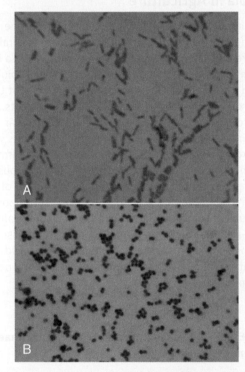

FIGURE 6.15 Gram-negative aerobic rods and cocci. A, Gram stain of *Pseudomonas aeruginosa,* a gram-negative aerobic bacillus. **B,** Gram stain of *Neisseria sicca,* a gram-negative aerobic coccus.

distributed in nature and many are human and animal pathogens. Their metabolism is respiratory in nature and not based on fermentation. Bacteria in this category include *Rhizobium, Legionella, Bordetella,* and *Francisella.* Rhizobia are soil bacteria that fix nitrogen after they are established inside the roots of legumes (Figure 6.15). They cannot fix nitrogen independently, require a plant host, and play a major role in agriculture. Medically important bacteria are shown in Table 6.4.

Facultatively Anaerobic Gram-negative Rods

Facultatively anaerobic gram-negative rods are a large group of bacteria with simple nutritional requirements. With the excep-

tion of the genus *Tatumella,* all motile bacteria in this group have peritrichous flagella. Bacilli are present in soil, water, and in the intestinal tract of animals and humans. Bacteria found in the intestinal tracts of humans and animals are referred to as *enteric bacteria* and include the genera *Escherichia, Salmonella, Shigella, Enterobacter, Proteus,* and *Providencia* (Table 6.5). The best known enteric bacterium is *E. coli* (Figure 6.16), which is an extremely valuable tool used in genetic engineering and recombinant DNA technology. It is often referred to as the *"workhorse"* in molecular biology.

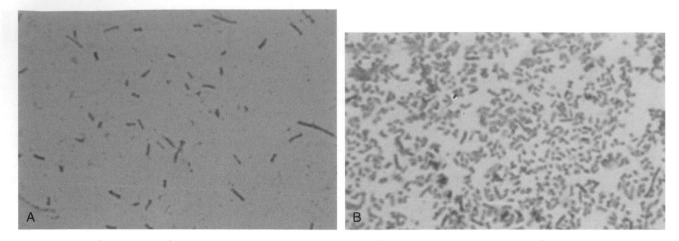

FIGURE 6.16 Facultative anaerobic gram-negative rods. **A,** Gram stain of *Escherichia coli*. **B,** Gram stain of *Proteus vulgaris*.

LIFE APPLICATION]

Rhizobia in Agriculture

Harvesting of protein-rich grain removes much of the nitrogen in the soil, but sufficient amounts are generally left for future crops. Inoculation of legumes with rhizobia is a common practice in agriculture to ensure maximal biological nitrogen fixation to enhance yield potentials without the use of exogenous nitrogen fertilizers. Such inoculants are commercially available in powder, liquid, and granular form.

This inoculation of the roots of leguminous plants with the appropriate species of *Rhizobium* leads to the formation of root nodules that are capable of converting gaseous nitrogen to combined nitrogen through the process of nitrogen fixation. Legumes include economically important plants such as soybeans, clover, alfalfa, peas, and beans. The legume–rhizobia symbiosis is an example of mutualism, in which the bacterium supplies ammonia or amino acids to the plant and receives organic acids as carbon and energy source in return.

TABLE 6.5 Medically Important Facultative Anaerobic Gram-negative Rods

Organism	Disease(s)
Escherichia	Urinary tract infections, peritonitis, meningitis, pneumonia, septicemia
Salmonella	Foodborne illnesses; typhoid fever
Shigella	Bacillary dysentery
Klebsiella	Pneumonia
Enterobacter	Opportunistic infections, most commonly of the urinary and respiratory tracts
Proteus	Urinary tract infections; hospital-acquired wound infection, septicemia, pneumonia in the compromised host
Providenciaz	Urinary tract infections

MEDICAL HIGHLIGHTS]

E. coli O157:H7: The Bad Seed

Escherichia coli is a ubiquitous gram-negative, facultatively anaerobic bacillus that can be found in the intestinal tract of many animals, including humans. Most of the strains of this species are harmless but there are a few that can cause a variety of illnesses, usually associated with infections of the gastrointestinal tract or with nosocomial-type infections. One of the most notorious is *E. coli* O157:H7, also referred to as *enterohemorrhagic E. coli* (EHEC). The vast majority of outbreaks of *E. coli* reported by the media involve this particular strain. Fecal in origin, this strain of bacteria is typically spread through the ingestion of contaminated food or water. Infection can be as subtle as swallowing a mouthful of water while swimming in a lake, or eating food handled by persons who did not wash their hands after using the toilet. Outbreaks have been linked to the consumption of various contaminated food products ranging from ground beef to spinach and tomatoes. Symptoms vary but often include stomach cramps, bloody diarrhea, and vomiting. Most people will recover within 5 to 7 days; however, 5% to 10% of infected people develop a life-threatening complication known as *hemolytic uremic syndrome* (HUS). If not treated quickly, HUS can cause serious damage to the kidneys, which is potentially fatal. With proper treatment most persons with HUS will recover within a few weeks; however, they may suffer some permanent kidney damage. The best ways to prevent an EHEC infection are by washing hands; cooking meats thoroughly; washing raw foods before eating; washing cutting boards between uses, especially when they are used for both meat and raw food preparation; avoiding unpasteurized dairy products and juices; and avoiding water ingestion from a source that may be contaminated, such as a lake or swimming pool.

Coliform Index and Water Testing

Water is essential for life and the ecosystems. The U.S. Environmental Protection Agency (EPA) enforces federal clean water and safe drinking water laws and provides support for municipal wastewater treatment plants. Two bacterial groups, coliforms and fecal streptococci, are commonly used as indicators of possible contamination with sewage because these bacteria are found in human and animal feces. The Coliform Index is used to rate the purity of water on the basis of the count of fecal bacteria. Although coliforms are generally not harmful themselves, they are indicators of the presence of possible pathogenic organisms that also live in human and animal digestive systems.

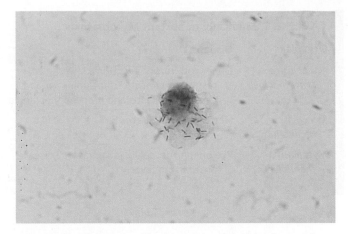

FIGURE 6.17 **Rickettsia.** Gimenez stain of tissue culture cells infected with *Rickettsia*. (From Murray PR, Rosenthal KS, Pfaller MA: *Medical Microbiology*, ed. 5, St. Louis, Mosby, 2005.)

Some of the bacteria found in the gastrointestinal tract of humans are often referred to as coliforms. Coliforms are a group of bacteria, not necessarily enteric, but meeting six criteria to be classified as coliform:

- Gram negative
- Rod shaped
- Facultative anaerobes
- Nonsporulating
- Utilize lactose
- Produce gas

Klebsiella pneumoniae is a coliform found in the normal flora of the mouth and skin, but also in the intestine, and can cause bacterial pneumonia (see Chapter 11, Infections of the Respiratory System). The genus *Citrobacter* can be found in many different environments including soil, water, and wastewater and can also be found in the human intestine. In general, *Citrobacter* does not cause illness but occasionally can be the source of urinary tract infections and infant meningitis.

Anaerobic Gram-negative Rods

Anaerobic gram-negative rods can be straight, curved, helical, motile, or nonmotile. These bacteria are present in the intestinal tract of humans and animals. *Leptotrichia buccalis* and *Fusobacterium* species are frequently found along the gum line and on tooth surfaces. *Bacteroides* are normally commensal, representing a substantial portion of the mammalian gastrointestinal flora, and preventing potential pathogens from colonizing the gut; however, some species are opportunistic pathogens.

Anaerobic Gram-negative Cocci

Anaerobic gram-negative cocci often occur in pairs and are found in the mouth, the intestines, and the vagina. *Veillonella* causes rare opportunistic infections and has a low virulence potential; it is often associated with long-standing gingivitis in dental patients. However, cases of osteomyelitis, bacterial endocarditis, and abscesses in internal organs have been reported in the literature.

TABLE 6.6 Medically Important Rickettsias and Chlamydias

Organism	Disease(s)
Rickettsia rickettsii	Rocky Mountain spotted fever
Rickettsia prowazekii	Epidemic typhus; recrudescent typhus, sporadic typhus
Rickettsia typhi	Endemic or murine typhus
Chlamydia trachomatis	Trachoma, adult inclusion conjunctivitis, neonatal conjunctivitis, infant pneumonia, urogenital infections, lymphogranuloma venereum
Chlamydofilia pneumoniae	Respiratory infections, atherosclerosis
Chlamydophila psittaci	Respiratory infections

Rickettsias and Chlamydias

Rickettsias and chlamydias are very small gram-negative bacteria. The majority of these organisms require a host for replication. In general, rickettsias and chlamydias are rod shaped but also may look coccoidal (Figure 6.17). Host-dependent organisms often cause diseases in humans and animals. Rickettsias need a vertebrate and an arthropod host, whereas chlamydias do not infect invertebrates but have a complex developmental cycle. Medically important organisms include *Rickettsia rickettsii, Rickettsia prowazekii, Rickettsia typhi, Chlamydia trachomatis, Chlamydophila pneumoniae,* and *Chlamydophila psittaci* (Table 6.6). *Orientia tsutsugamushi* is the agent of scrub typhus, a widely endemic disease in Asian Pacific regions that was formerly classified with *Rickettsia*. It is a gram-negative obligate intracellular bacterium belonging to the family Rickettsiaceae.

TABLE 6.7 Medically Important Mycoplasmas

Organism	Disease(s)
Mycoplasma pneumoniae	Upper respiratory infections, lower respiratory infections including tracheobronchitis and bronchopneumonia
Mycoplasma genitalium	Nongonococcal urethritis
Mycoplasma hominis	Pyelonephritis, pelvic inflammatory disease, postpartum fever

TABLE 6.8 Selected Medically Important Gram-positive Cocci

Organism	Disease(s)
Micrococcus	Opportunistic organisms
Staphylococcus aureus	Minor skin infections, pneumonia, meningitis, endocarditis, toxic shock syndrome, septicemia
Streptococcus pyogenes	Pharyngitis ("strep throat"), scarlet fever, pyoderma, erysipelas, cellulitis, necrotizing fasciitis, streptococcal toxic shock syndrome
Streptococcus pneumoniae	Pneumonia, meningitis, bacteremia
Peptococcus and *Peptostreptococcus*	Opportunistic organisms

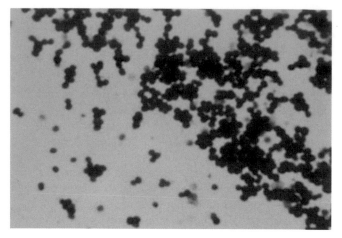

FIGURE 6.18 *Staphylococcus epidermidis*. This is a gram-positive bacterium and a normal resident of the human skin; it can become an opportunistic pathogen.

Mycoplasmas and Ureaplasmas

Mycoplasma and *Ureaplasma* organisms are the smallest free-living bacteria. They are unique among bacteria because they do not have cell walls, resulting in a variable or indistinct shape, and therefore are pleomorphic. They measure 0.3 to 0.8 μm in diameter and are spherical to pear shaped with branched or helical filaments. Because of the absence of the cell wall the mycoplasmas are resistant to penicillins, cephalosporins, vancomycin, and other antibiotics that interfere with cell wall synthesis. Mycoplasmas have special growth requirements and most pathogenic species are host specific. These organisms can cause disease in humans (Table 6.7), animals, and plants.

Gram-positive Cocci

Gram-positive cocci include aerobic and anaerobic spherical cells, ranging from harmless to virulent forms. These cocci include the genera *Micrococcus, Staphylococcus, Streptococcus,* and *Peptococcus*. Some medically important gram-positive cocci are shown in Table 6.8.

- *Micrococci* are aerobic organisms not associated with disease; however; they can be opportunistic pathogens in hosts with a compromised immune system. These

organisms are found in soil, water, dust, and dairy products and are part of the normal flora of the skin.

- *Staphylococci* are gram-positive facultative anaerobes. They can cause a wide variety of diseases in humans and other animals through their production of toxins or tissue invasion. *Staphylococcus* toxins are a common cause of food poisoning because of the heat resistance of the enterotoxin and the ability of staphylococci to grow in foods with relatively low water activity. *Staphylococcus epidermidis* (Figure 6.18) is a commensal organism of the skin, but can cause severe infections in immunosuppressed patients, in those with central venous catheters, and in patients with prosthetic limbs. The pathogenic species *Staphylococcus aureus* produces up to 18 extracellular products that can harm human and animal hosts. Methicillin-resistant *Staphylococcus aureus* (MRSA) is a specific strain that has developed resistance to all penicillins. MRSA infections occur most frequently in hospital and healthcare environments and are commonly termed as a "superbug" infections.

- **Streptococci** are microaerophilic or facultatively anaerobic, organisms that produce lactic acid. The classification of *Streptococcus* spp. is based on the hemolytic patterns of their colonies on blood agar. Alpha hemolysis is due to the reduction of iron in hemoglobin, resulting in partial hemolysins, producing a greenish color on blood agar. Beta hemolysis is a result of complete rupture of red blood cells, resulting in clear areas around bacterial colonies on blood agar. No hemolytic action occurs with the nonhemolytic or gamma-hemolytic strains. Although a number of the *Streptococcus* species are pathogenic (see Table 6.8), many of the species are nonpathogenic and are part of the normal human flora of the mouth, skin, intestine, and upper respiratory tract, but can be opportunistic pathogens. *Streptococcus thermophilus* is not a pathogen and is used in the manufacture of Swiss cheese.

- *Peptococcus* and *Peptostreptococcus* are anaerobic gram-positive cocci and part of the normal flora in the mouth, skin, and gastrointestinal and urinary tracts. They can

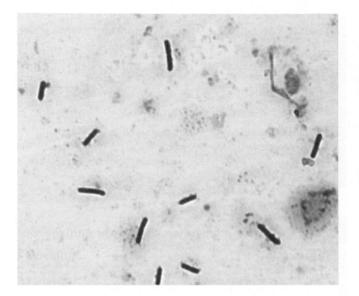

FIGURE 6.19 Bacillus. This micrograph shows the gram-positive, spore-forming *Bacillus cereus*.

TABLE 6.9 Selected Medically Important Endospore-forming Gram-positive Rods and Cocci

Organism	Disease(s)
Bacillus anthracis	Anthrax (cutaneous, gastrointestinal, inhalation)
Bacillus cereus	Gastroenteritis, ocular infections
Clostridium botulinum	Botulism
Clostridium difficile	Antibiotic-associated diarrhea, pseudomembranous colitis
Clostridium perfringens	Gas gangrene, suppurative myositis, myonecrosis, gastroenteritis, food poisoning, necrotizing enteritis
Clostridium tetani	Tetanus

infect normal hosts with a compromised immune system or damaged tissues. Under these conditions the organisms can become pathogenic and can cause brain, liver, breast, and lung abscesses due to septicemia.

Endospore-forming Gram-positive Rods and Cocci

Endospore-forming rods and cocci include the genera *Bacillus* and *Clostridium* (Figure 6.19), both of which play an important role in medicine and the food industry. The spores of these genera are resistant to heat and disinfectants and both genera are widespread in the soil. *Bacillus* species are either obligate aerobes or facultative anaerobes; they include free-living and pathogenic species. Medically important *Bacillus* species include *B. anthracis* and *B. cereus* (Table 6.9). *Bacillus coagulans* is associated with food spoilage, *B. thuringiensis* is an insect pathogen, and *B. subtilis* is an important model organism.

Clostridium perfringens is widely distributed in the environment and can be found as a normal component of decaying matter, in marine sediment, and also in the intestinal tract of humans and other animals. Food poisoning by this organism is a fairly common intestinal intoxication caused by toxins produced by the bacterium. The source of this problem is usually food contaminated by soil or feces or inadequately heated or reheated food (see Chapter 12, Infections of the Gastrointestinal System). *Clostridium tetani* is found in soil as spores or as a parasite in the gastrointestinal tract of animals. The organism produces tetanospasmin, the causative agent of tetanus (see Chapter 13, Infections of the Nervous System and Senses). *Clostridium botulinum* can cause a severe type of food poisoning initiated by the ingestion of foods containing the organism's potent neurotoxin, which is formed during the growth of the bacterium (see Chapter 13).

Regular Nonsporulating Gram-positive Rods

Regular nonsporulating gram-positive rods are obligate or facultative anaerobes with complex nutritional requirements. This group includes *Carnobacterium, Lactobacillus,* and *Listeria.* The organism *Carnobacterium pleistocenium* was discovered in the arctic part of Alaska. It was found in permafrost, and melting ice brought these extremophiles back to a growing vegetative state. The discovery of this organism is of interest to NASA scientists as they investigate the permafrost of Mars for bacterial life. Lactobacilli convert lactose and other sugars to lactic acid and are commonly benign. Some species are used in industry for the production of yogurt, cheese, sauerkraut, pickles, and other fermented foods. *Listeria monocytogenes* is the causative agent of listeriosis. Outbreaks of listeriosis have been attributed to the consumption of hot dogs, deli meats, raw milk, cheeses, raw and cooked poultry, raw meats, ice cream, raw vegetables, and smoked fish, and it has a high mortality rate compared with other food-borne diseases.

Irregular Nonsporulating Gram-positive Rods

Irregular nonsporulating gram-positive rods have unusual shapes (often cubelike), are pleomorphic, and are mostly facultative anaerobes with a few obligate aerobes. Organisms important to humans include but are not limited to the genera *Actinomyces, Corynebacterium,* and *Propionibacterium*. *Propionibacterium shermanii* is used in the production of Swiss cheese. Medically important organisms for this group are shown in Table 6.10.

Mycobacteria

The genus *Mycobacterium* includes gram-positive, aerobic, acid-fast rods that have the tendency to form filaments (Figure 6.20). They are widespread organisms in water, soil, and food sources, whereas some are obligate intracellular parasites (usually infecting mononuclear phagocytes) in animals and humans. Although mycobacteria have a tendency to be difficult to grow in culture, they are classified into two categories, the fast-growing type and the slow-growing type, based on laboratory growth characteristics. In general, mycobacteria can colonize in the host without showing signs and symptoms of host infection. Many people around the world are infected with *M. tuberculosis* and never develop symptoms, yet they are carriers

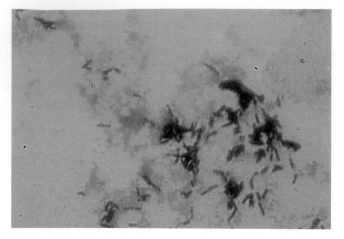

FIGURE 6.20 *Mycobacterium smegmatis*, an acid-fast bacillus.

TABLE 6.11 Selected Medically Important Mycobacteria

Organism	Disease(s)
Mycobacterium tuberculosis	Tuberculosis
Mycobacterium leprae	Leprosy
Nontuberculous mycobacteria (NTM)	Pulmonary disease resembling tuberculosis, lymphadenitis, skin disease, or dispersed disease

TABLE 6.12 Streptomycetes: A Source of Antibiotics

Organism	Antibiotic
Streptomyces griseus	Streptomycin
Amycolatopsis mediterranei	Rifamycin
Saccharopolyspora erythraea	Erythromycin
Streptomyces antibioticus	Oleandomycin

TABLE 6.10 Selected Medically Important Irregular Nonsporulating Gram-positive Rods

Organism	Disease(s)
Actinomyces	Opportunistic pathogens, particularly in the oral cavity, formation of abscesses in mouth, lungs, or gastrointestinal tract
Corynebacterium diphtheriae	Diphtheria
Propionibacterium acnes	Acne
Actinomyces israelii	Periodontal abscesses; lung infections

of the disease. Mycobacterial infections usually are difficult to treat because of their cell wall structure, which is neither truly gram negative nor gram positive. This makes them naturally resistant to many antibiotics whose mechanism of action is the destruction of cell walls (e.g., penicillin). Some medically important mycobacteria are shown in Table 6.11.

Nocardioforms

Nocardioforms are aerobic, gram-positive, catalase-positive rods that form thin branching filaments. They are widespread in the environment, opportunistic, and can cause several diseases, especially in the young, the elderly, and immunocompromised patients. Although *Nocardia* infections are rare it is generally a chronic bacterial infection originating in the lungs and then spreading to other organ systems. The other systems most commonly affected are the brain and skin, but the kidneys, joints, heart, eyes, and bones might be involved. The symptoms of infection vary and depend on the organs involved.

Streptomycetes

Streptomycetes are gram positive, found predominantly in the soil and in decaying vegetation, and most of them are spore forming. In general they are not pathogenic, but many of the

species are important sources of antibiotics (Table 6.12). Very infrequently they cause human disease, most often manifesting itself as a localized, chronic infection of the skin and underlying soft tissue. Invasive *Streptomyces* infections are extremely rare.

Methanogens

Methanogens are archaea that grow in anaerobic environments such as swamps, marshes, marine sediments, sludge, and hydrothermal vents and they produce methane as a metabolic by-product. They are common in wetlands, in the intestinal tracts of ruminants and humans, and are also found in soil with oxygen depletion. They are rapidly killed by the presence of oxygen. There are more than 50 species of methanogens and some of them have been found in extreme environments such as under kilometers of ice in Greenland (see Life Application: Inside a Glacier, in Chapter 1, Scope of Microbiology) or in the hot, dry desert soil. Although methanogens have not been considered to be human pathogens, several research groups are studying methanogens as potential human pathogens, especially in connection with root canal infections. Some methanogens are in endosymbiont relationships with protozoans. Endosymbiosis occurs when one organisms is housed by another, with each of the organisms benefiting from the relationship.

Extreme Thermophiles

Extreme thermophiles are different from bacterial thermophiles because they flourish in extreme heat, with optimal growth temperatures of 50° C or more, and some of them can grow at temperatures up to 150° C under extreme hydrostatic pressure such as in the deep ocean springs. Some of them also can grow in highly acidic environments. These organisms have been of great use in biotechnology because enzymes isolated from thermophiles are able to function under temperatures that would normally denature the enzymes of other organisms. Some of these enzymes are used in the polymerase chain reaction (PCR), a technique of enzymatically replicating small amounts of DNA or DNA fragments (see Chapter 25, Microorganisms in Biotechnology). PCR is commonly used in medical and biological research laboratories for the detection of hereditary diseases, identification of DNA fingerprints, diagnosis of infectious diseases, cloning of genes, paternity testing, and more.

Extreme Halophiles

Archaeal halophiles are aerobic microorganisms that live in environments with high concentrations of sodium chloride, approximately 10 times the salt content of ocean water. Halophiles are coated with a special protein that allows only certain levels of salt to enter the cells. Two of the largest and most studied hypersaline environments are the Great Salt Lake in Utah and the Dead Sea in the Middle East. The extreme halophiles thrive in these environments, sometimes turning the Great Salt Lake a deep red color that is visible from space. Scientists studying these extremophiles on earth hope to find insight in the search for life elsewhere in the universe.

Summary

- Bacteria are prokaryotic unicellular organisms capable of living as an individual cell or attached to others, forming colonies or groupings.
- On the basis of their morphological characteristics they are classified into basic shapes: coccus, spherically shaped; bacillus, rod shaped; spiral, twisted or helical rods; or pleomorphic, variable or indistinct in shape.
- According to their arrangements and grouping after cell division bacteria can be categorized as follows: diplo, in pairs; strep(to), in chains; tetrads, in packets of four; sarcina, in a cube; staph(ylo), in irregular clumps or clusters.
- Bacteria divide primarily by binary fission and their population growth curve can be divided into a lag phase, a logarithmic or exponential growth phase, a stationary phase, and a death phase.
- Bacterial growth can be measured by the increase in cell mass or numbers. Methods include dry weight measurement, turbidity in liquid media, direct cell counts, and viable plate counts.
- Bacterial growth is dependent on nutrient availability as well as the presence of oxygen or absence of oxygen. Depending on the need for oxygen, bacteria are organized as follows: obligate anaerobes, where oxygen is lethal; obligate aerobes, oxygen is required; facultative anaerobes (facultative aerobes), oxygen is not required but its presence benefits the organism's growth; microaerophiles, oxygen is required but in small amounts; or aerotolerant anaerobes, oxygen is not required and its presence neither hinders nor helps the growth of the organism.
- Depending of the source of carbon necessary for bacterial growth, bacteria are classified as photoautotrophs, chemoautotrophs, photoheterotrophs, and chemoheterotrophs.
- Depending on the range of temperature at which bacteria will grow, they are classified as mesophiles, 25° C to 40° C; thermophiles, 45° C and above; psychrophiles, 0° C to 15° C; and psychrotrophs, 25° C to 30° C.
- Bacterial and archaeal chromosomal DNA is a single large circular molecule. These organisms also contain DNA independent of the chromosomal DNA, called *plasmids*, which are generally smaller, circular, self-replicating, and independent of cell division.
- Mutations in bacteria can be classified according to the type of change occurring in the DNA. These changes include point mutations, frameshift mutations, inversions, transposons, and reversions.
- Bacteria can obtain new genetic material from another closely related organism by transformation, transduction, or conjugation.
- Bacteria are named according to the binomial system of nomenclature and are generally classified according to *Bergey's Manual of Systematic Bacteriology*.

Review Questions

1. Straight, rod-shaped bacteria, some of which are endospore forming, are referred to as:
   - **a.** Cocci
   - **b.** Bacilli
   - **c.** Spirals
   - **d.** Vibrios

2. Beadlike chains of cocci formed after cell division along a single axis are called:
   - **a.** Diplococci
   - **b.** Streptococci
   - **c.** Tetrads
   - **d.** Sarcinae

3. Bacteria that use oxygen, but only at low concentration, are classified as:
   - **a.** Obligate aerobes
   - **b.** Microaerophiles
   - **c.** Obligate anaerobes
   - **d.** Aerotolerant anaerobes

4. Bacteria that use organic compounds for both the source of carbon and energy are referred to as:
   - **a.** Photoautotrophs
   - **b.** Chemoautotrophs
   - **c.** Photoheterotrophs
   - **d.** Chemoheterotrophs

5. Microorganisms that show optimal growth at moderate temperatures (between 25° C and 40° C) are called:
   - **a.** Thermophiles
   - **b.** Psychrophiles
   - **c.** Mesophiles
   - **d.** Psychrotrophs

6. A mutation that involves the deletion or insertion of one or more bases is a:
   - **a.** Point mutation
   - **b.** Frameshift mutation
   - **c.** Transduction
   - **d.** Reversion

7. *Treponema pallidum* and *Borrelia burgdorferi* belong to the group of:
   a. Gram-negative aerobic rods and cocci
   b. Anaerobic gram-negative rods
   c. Anaerobic gram-negative cocci
   d. Spirochetes

8. *Legionella* and *Neisseria* are examples of:
   a. Facultative anaerobic gram-negative rods
   b. Gram-negative aerobic rods and cocci
   c. Spirochetes
   d. Anaerobic gram-negative cocci

9. Staphylococci and streptococci are best classified in the group of:
   a. Gram-positive cocci
   b. Gram-negative cocci
   c. Gram-negative aerobic rods and cocci
   d. Anaerobic gram-negative cocci

10. Which of the following is a host-dependent bacterium?
    a. *Mycoplasma*
    b. *Ureaplasma*
    c. *Rickettsia*
    d. *Micrococcus*

11. Bacteria whose overall shape is spherical or nearly spherical are referred to as _____.

12. Microorganisms that acquire energy from light are called _____.

13. Microorganisms that grow only in the presence of oxygen are called _____.

14. Nonchromosomal DNA molecules in bacteria are _____.

15. The transfer of genetic material during cell-to-cell contact is a(n) _____.

16. Describe the different stages of the bacterial population growth curve.

17. Discuss four methods to measure bacterial growth.

18. Describe the nutritional requirement for bacterial growth, with regard to carbon.

19. Discuss the influence of the pH on bacterial growth.

20. Differentiate between genotype and phenotype.

Bibliography

Bauman R: *Microbiology: With Diseases by Taxonomy*, ed 2, 2007, Benjamin Cummings/Pearson Education, San Francisco.

Dunne EF, Burman WJ, Wilson MJ: *Streptomyces pneumonia in a patient with human immunodeficiency virus infection: case report and review of the literature on invasive Streptomyces*, Clin Infect Dis 27:93–96, 1998.

Forbes BA, Sahm, DF, Weissfeld AS: *Bailey & Scott's Diagnostic Microbiology*, ed 12, St. Louis, 2007, Mosby/Elsevier.

Klug WS, Cummings MR, Spencer CA, et al: *Concepts of Genetics*, ed 9, 2009, Benjamin Cummings/Pearson Education, San Francisco.

Madigan MT, Martinko JM, Dunlap PV, et al: *Brock: Biology of Microorganisms*, ed 12, 2009, Benjamin Cummings/Pearson Education, San Francisco.

Mahon CR, Lehman DC, Manuselis G: *Textbook of Diagnostic Microbiology*, ed 3, St. Louis, 2007, Saunders/Elsevier.

Mims C, Dockrell HM, Goering RV, et al: *Medical Microbiology*, ed 3, St. Louis, 2004, Mosby/Elsevier.

Murray PR, Rosenthal KS, Pfaller MA: *Medical Microbiology*, ed 5, St. Louis, 2005, Mosby/Elsevier.

Talaro KP: *Foundations in Microbiology*, ed 6, New York, 2005, McGraw-Hill.

Internet Resources

PubMed, www.pubmed.gov/
Centers for Disease Control and Prevention, http://www.cdc.gov/
emedicine from WebMD, http://www.emedicine.com/
National Institute of Allergy and Infectious Diseases, http://www3.niaid.nih.gov/
National Dairy Council, Cheese, http://www.nationaldairycouncil.org/NationalDairyCouncil/Nutrition/Products/cheesePage4.htm
Vianna ME, Conrads G, Gomes BPFA, et al: Identification and quantification of archaea involved in primary endodontic infections, *J Clin Microbiol* 44:1274–1282, 2006. http://www.asm.org/ASM/files/LeftMarginHeaderList/DOWNLOADFILENAME/000000002036/archaea.pdf
De A, Gogate A: Isolation of *Veillonella* from various clinical specimens and its significance, *Indian Practitioner* 52(7):451–454, 1999. http://www.unboundmedicine.com/medline/ebm/record/12035357.

7

Viruses

OUTLINE

General Structure and Classification
Classification
Morphology
Genome Type
Genome Changes

Viral Multiplication
Multiplication of Bacteriophages
Multiplication of Animal Viruses
Viral Infections

Major Groups of Viruses in Vertebrates
DNA Viruses
RNA Viruses

Subviral Agents
Viroids
Virusoids (Satellites)
Prions

LEARNING OBJECTIVES

After reading this chapter, the student will be able to:
- Describe the two commonly used methods of classifying viruses
- Define and describe capsid, capsomeres, nucleocapsid, virion, and envelope
- Describe and differentiate the types of viral genomes
- Describe and explain the steps in the multiplication of bacteriophages and animal viruses
- Discuss the possible effects of viral infections
- Describe the different kinds of host cell damage caused by viral infections
- Name the DNA viruses infecting and subsequently causing diseases in humans
- Name the RNA viruses infecting and subsequently causing disease in humans
- Compare and contrast viroids and virusoids
- Describe prions and the infections/diseases caused by them

abortive infections
adsorption
bacteriophage
Baltimore classification
    system
capsid
capsomeres
cytocidal infections
cytopathic effects
eclipse period
encapsidation
helical virus
host range
icosahedrons
intracellular
    accumulation phase

International Committee
    on Taxonomy of
    Viruses (ICTV)
lysis
lysis and release phase
lysogenic
lysogeny
lytic
nonpermissive cells
nucleocapsid
oncogenic
permissive cells
persistent infections
prions
prophage
protomeres

provirus
satellites
severe acute respiratory
    syndrome (SARS)
spikes
temperate
uncoating
viral envelope
virion
viroids
virulent
virusoids

WHY YOU NEED TO KNOW

HISTORY

Submicroscopic particles were suspected when mummies with smallpox facial lesions, as well as scattered hieroglyphic accounts of inoculations against these killers, were discovered. Finally, later reports by Edward Jenner—and the milkmaid Sarah Nelmes—of successful vaccinations in the late eighteenth century culminated with the World Health Organization (WHO)-certified eradication of smallpox in 1979. This history suggested an organism smaller than visible bacteria.

Pathogenic microorganisms too small to be seen via light microscopy prompted a Dutch botanist-microbiologist, Martinus Willem Beijerinck (1851–1931), to coin the term *virus* (from the Latin *virus,* meaning toxin, poison). During this same time period (the late nineteenth century) Charles Chamberland made a porcelain filter for isolating these submicroscopic viruses. The tobacco mosaic virus was used in some of the first studies with these filters. The size of the filtered viruses was shown to be several orders of magnitude less than that of bacteria. Dimitri Ivanovski published experiments demonstrating the retained infectious nature of the filterable viral disease-causing agents, after bacteria had been removed by the filtration. Moreover, in the early 1900s, bacteria were even shown to be vulnerable to viral attack by bacteriophages. In 1935, the tobacco mosaic virus was crystallized by Wendell Stanley and identified as a mostly proteinaceous substance, shortly after which time it was further isolated into protein and nucleic acid constituents.

IMPACT

As expected, improved resolution with the advent of electron microscopy afforded the first visible records of viruses. Coupled with advances in biotechnology, the chemical nature of viral composition began to be deciphered, and with it new approaches to viral threats of various magnitudes could be explored. Filterable viruses yielded new functional explanations, and allowed their study for therapy. Diseases such as polio, influenza, AIDS, and rabies are now more accessible to laboratory study, leading to possible treatments to attenuate their effects before human exposure (antibiotics, although effective against bacteria, unfortunately are ineffective against viruses). The invention of the electron microscope made viruses visible and allowed the study of their response to putative chemical therapies or vaccinations.

FUTURE

Once the nature of a virus is visualized, biotechnological approaches via synthetic chemistry, genetic engineering, and computer-assisted screening of designed chemicals can be expeditiously undertaken (see New Drugs in Chapter 21, Pharmacology). These approaches can be applied to improve and test current therapies in use, as well as to develop and test new therapeutic and preventive substances. The complete identification of a virus and its virulence factors will help to design novel approaches to therapy and vaccination against future viral threats.

General Structure and Classification

Viruses are microscopic particles that infect cells of other organisms. They differ from other microorganisms in their structure, biology, and reproduction. Viruses do carry conventional genetic material in the form of DNA or RNA, but they cannot reproduce on their own because they lack the biochemical machinery necessary for replication. Viruses therefore are obligate intracellular parasites capable of infecting both eukaryotic and prokaryotic organisms. A virus that infects bacteria is referred to as a **bacteriophage** or simply phage. For a virus to reproduce, the individual components of the virus must be synthesized by the host cell and then assembled within that cell. In other words, a virus uses the biochemical machinery of its host cell in order to replicate.

Classification

To this date, taxonomic classification of viruses remains difficult because of the lack of fossil records and the ongoing debate about whether they should be considered living or nonliving organisms. At present, virus classification is based mainly on morphology, nucleic acid type, mode of replication, host organisms, and the type of disease they cause.

The **International Committee on Taxonomy of Viruses (ICTV)** is responsible for the development of the current viral classification system. In the early 1990s they devised and implemented rules for the naming and classification of viruses. This system shares several features with the classification system of cellular organisms, such as taxon structure. On the basis of shared properties, the viruses are grouped at the hierarchical levels of order, family, subfamily, genus, and species. The following latinized suffixes are given in italics within the taxon:

Order (-*virales*)

Family (-*viridae*)

Subfamily (-*virinae*)

Genus (-*virus*)

Species (-*virus*)

For the determination of order, the type of nucleic acid DNA or RNA, single or double stranded, and the presence or absence of an envelope are used. In addition, other characteristics such as the type of host, the capsid shape, immunological properties, and the type of disease the virus causes are also considered for further detailed virus classification. An additional classification system is the **Baltimore classification system,** devised by David Baltimore. This system places the virus into one of seven groups distinguishing the viruses on the basis of the relationship between the viral genome and the messenger RNA (Box 7.1). In modern virus classification the ICTV system is used in conjunction with the Baltimore classification system. Although animal and plant virologists both use these systems, the actual application in the process of classification is quite different because of the diversity of viruses.

Morphology

The size of viruses varies from very small, such as the parvovirus at about 20 nm and the poliovirus at 30 nm, to fairly large, such as the vaccinia virus at 400 nm and the poxviruses, which can be up to 450 nm. Most viruses cannot be visualized by light microscopy; therefore electron microscopy is used to examine their structure (see Chapter 1, Scope of Microbiology). However, some viruses are as large as or larger than the smallest bacteria and can be visualized by high optical magnification (Figure 7.1).

An exception to the size of other viruses is a virus discovered in 2003 by a team of French researchers, which named the organism mimivirus. This virus was found in free-living amoebas and has a diameter of 750 nm, which is larger than a *Mycoplasma* bacterium. These organisms also have the largest known viral genome, with about 1000 genes on a double-stranded circular DNA. Mimivirus seems to be an icosahedral particle with a diameter of 400 nm, no envelope, and surrounded by 80-nm fibrils.

Viruses consist of genetic material carried in a "shell" called the *viral coat* or **capsid.** The capsid consists of proteins that are coded by the viral genome. The capsid is a complex and highly organized entity that gives form to the virus and serves as the basis for morphological distinction. Subunits referred to as **protomeres** assemble to form **capsomeres,** which in turn spontaneously aggregate to form the capsid. Proteins associated with nucleic acids are called *nucleoproteins* and the association of viral capsid proteins with viral nucleic acid is referred to as a **nucleocapsid.** At the junction points of the capsomeres, long projections from the nucleocapsids, called **spikes,** are frequently attached (Figure 7.2). These spikes aid in attachment to the host cell membrane receptors. Some viruses have an envelope around the coat and once the virus is fully assembled it is called a **virion.** Depending on the presence or absence of an envelope, viruses are referred to as naked or enveloped viruses (Figure 7.3).

According to the shape and arrangement of capsomeres and the presence of an envelope, viruses can be classified into four distinct morphological types:

- Helical viruses
- Icosahedral viruses
- Enveloped viruses
- Complex viruses

Helical Viruses

Helical capsids have rod-shaped capsomeres, connected along their long axis, resembling a wide ribbon stacked around a central axis forming a helical structure with a central cavity, a hollow tube. As a result, these virions are rod shaped or filamentous and can be short and highly rigid, as in many plant viruses, or long and very flexible, as in many animal viruses. The genetic material can be single-stranded RNA (ssRNA) or single-stranded DNA (ssDNA) and is bound into the protein helix by the interactions between the negative charge on the

BOX 7.1 Baltimore Classification of Viruses

Group I: Double-stranded DNA (dsDNA) viruses
  Order: *Caudovirales* (tailed bacteriophages)
    Family: *Myoviridae*
      Podoviridae
      Siphoviridae
  Unassigned genera
    Family: *Ascoviridae*
      Adenoviridae
      Asfarviridae
      Baculoviridae
      Corticoviridae
      Fuselloviridae
      Guttaviridae
      Herpesviridae
      Iridoviridae
      Lipothrixviridae
      Nimaviridae
      Papillomaviridae
      Phycodnaviridae
      Plasmaviridae
      Polyomaviridae
      Poxviridae
      Rudiviridae
      Tectiviridae
  Unassigned genera
      Mimivirus
Group II: Single-stranded DNA (ssDNA) viruses
  Unassigned bacteriophages
    Family: *Inoviridae*
      Microviridae
  Unassigned viruses
    Family: *Geminiviridae*
      Circoviridae
      Nanoviridae
      Parvoviridae
  Unassigned genera
      Anellovirus
Group III: Double-stranded RNA (dsRNA) viruses
Group IV: Positive-sense single-stranded RNA [(+)ssRNA] viruses
  Order: *Nidovirales*
    Family: *Arteriviridae*
      Coronaviridae
  Unassigned genera
    Family: *Astroviridae*
      Barnaviridae
      Bromoviridae
      Caliciviridae
      Closteroviridae
      Comoviridae
      Dicistroviridae
      Flaviviridae
      Flexiviridae
      Herpesviridae
      Leviviridae
      Luteoviridae
      Marnaviridae
      Nodaviridae
      Picornaviridae
      Potyviridae
      Sequiviridae
      Tetraviridae
      Togaviridae
      Tombusviridae
      Tymoviridae
  Unassigned genera
    Genus: *Benyvirus*
      Cheravirus
      Furovirus
      Hordeivirus
      Idaeovirus
      Machlomovirus
      Ourmiavirus
      Peclavirus
      Pomovirus
      Sadwavirus
      Sobemovirus
      Tobamovirus
      Tobravirus
      Umbravirus
Group V: Negative-sense single-stranded RNA [(−)ssRNA] viruses
  Order: *Mononegavirales*
    Family: *Bornaviridae*
      Filoviridae
      Paramyxoviridae
      Rhabdoviridae
  Segmented negative-stranded viruses
    Family: *Arenoviridae*
      Bunyaviridae
      Orthomyxoviridae
  Unassigned genera
    Genus: *Deltavirus*
      Ophiovirus
      Tenuivirus
      Varicosavirus
Group VI: Reverse-transcribing diploid single-stranded RNA (ssRNA-RT) viruses
    Family: *Metaviridae*
      Pseudoviridae
      Retroviridae
Group VII: Reverse-transcribing circular double-stranded DNA (dsDNA-RT) viruses
    Family: *Hepadnaviridae*
      Caulimoviridae

Medically Important Viruses

Family	Genus (or Subfamily)	Species or Typical Member	Infection/Disease
DNA Viruses			
Parvoviridae	*Erythrovirus*	B19 virus	Erythema infectiosum
Papillomaviridae	*Papillomavirus*	Human papillomavirus (HPV)	More than 60 HPV types: common warts, plantar warts, flat cutaneous warts, etc.
Polyomaviridae	*Polyomavirus*	Polyomavirus	JC virus: Infection of the respiratory system, kidneys, or brain BK virus: Mild respiratory infection
Adenoviridae	*Mastadenovirus*	Human adenovirus 2	Gastrointestinal tract infections, infection of the conjunctiva, central nervous system infections, urinary tract infections
Herpesviridae	*Alphaherpesvirinae*	Herpes simplex virus 1 (HSV-1); human herpesvirus 1 (HHV-1) Herpes simplex virus 2 (HSV-2); human herpesvirus 2 (HHV-2)	HSV-1: Oral and/or genital herpes (predominantly orofacial) HSV-2: Oral and/or genital herpes (predominantly genital)
	Varicellovirus	Varicella-zoster virus (human herpesvirus 3 [HHV-3])	Chickenpox and shingles
	Gammaherpesvirinae	Epstein-Barr virus (EBV) Lymphocryptovirus (HHV-4) Kaposi's sarcoma–associated herpesvirus (HHV-8)	HHV-4: Infectious mononucleosis, Burkitt's lymphoma, CNS lymphoma in AIDS patients, posttransplant lymphoproliferative syndrome, nasopharyngeal carcinoma HHV-8: Kaposi's sarcoma, primary effusion lymphoma, some types of multicentric Castleman's disease
	Betaherpesvirinae	Cytomegalovirus (HHV-5)	Infectious mononucleosis, retinitis, etc.
	Roseolovirus	Roseolovirus (HHV-6, -7)	Sixth disease (roseola infantum or exanthema subitum)
Poxviridae	*Orthopoxvirus*	Smallpox (variola vera) Vaccinia virus	Smallpox—eradicated Vaccinia infections
	Parapoxvirus	Oral virus	Cutaneous lesions
	Molluscipoxvirus	Molluscum contagiosum virus	Wartlike skin lesions
Hepadnaviridae	*Orthohepadnavirus*	Hepatitis B virus	Hepatitis B
RNA Viruses			
Picornaviridae	*Enterovirus*	Poliovirus	Poliomyelitis
	Rhinovirus	Human rhinovirus A	Common cold
	Hepatovirus	Hepatitis A virus	Hepatitis A
	Aphthovirus	Foot-and-mouth disease virus	Foot-and-mouth disease
Caliciviridae	*Calicivirus*	Norovirus	Gastroenteritis
Astroviridae	*Astrovirus*	Human astroviruses (five serotypes)	Gastroenteritis

Medically Important Viruses—cont'd

Family	Genus (or Subfamily)	Species or Typical Member	Infection/Disease
Togaviridae	Alphavirus	Sindbis virus	Sindbis virus disease, polyarthritis and rash
		Ross River virus	Epidemic polyarthritis
		Chikungunya virus	Fever, petechial or maculopapular rash (limbs and trunk), arthralgia or arthritis
	Rubivirus	Rubella virus	Rubella
Flaviviridae	Flavivirus	Yellow fever virus	Yellow fever
		Dengue virus	Dengue hemorrhagic fever
		Tick-borne encephalitis viurs	Encephalitis
	Hepatitis C viruses	Hepatitis C virus	Hepatitis C
Reoviridae	Reovirus	Reoviruses 1–3	Gastrointestinal and respiratory infections
	Rotavirus	Human rotavirus A, B, and C	Gastrointestinal infections
	Orbivirus	Colorado tick fever virus	Colorado tick fever (Mountain tick fever)
Orthomyxoviridae	Influenzavirus A, B	Influenza A and B	Influenza
	Influenza C	Influenza C virus	Influenza
Paramyxoviridae	Paramyxovirus	Newcastle disease virus	Zoonotic: Parainfluenza (influenza-like)
	Morbillivirus	Measles virus (rubeola virus)	Measles
	Rubulavirus	Mumps virus	Mumps
	Pneumovirus	Respiratory syncytial virus	Respiratory tract infections
Rhabdoviridae	Vesiculovirus	Vesicular stomatitis virus	Influenza-like symptoms; malaise, nausea, pain in limbs and back, possible vesicular lesions in mouth, lips and hands, leukopenia
	Lyssavirus	Rabies virus	Rabies
Bunyaviridae	Bunyavirus	Bunyamwera virus La Crosse virus	Various arthropod-transmitted diseases
	Hantavirus	Hantavirus, Puumala virus, Seoul virus	Hemorrhagic fever with renal syndrome
	Nairovirus	Crimean-Congo hemorrhagic fever virus	Crimean-Congo hemorrhagic fever

nucleic acid and the positive charge on the proteins. The nucleocapsid of a naked **helical virus** is rigid and tightly wound into a cylinder-shaped structure. An example is the well-studied tobacco mosaic virus, an ssRNA virus that infects primarily tobacco plants and other members of the *Solanaceae* family (Figure 7.4). Enveloped helical nucleocapsids are more flexible and this type is found in several human viruses such as influenza and measles viruses.

Icosahedral Viruses

Capsids of many virus families are multifaced structures known as **icosahedrons.** These are three-dimensional, geometric figures with 12 corners, 20 triangular faces, and 30 edges (Figure 7.5). This icosahedral capsid symmetry results in a spherical appearance of viruses at low magnification. The arrangement of the capsomeres varies between the viruses and the shape and dimension of the icosahedron depend on the characteristics of its protomeres. Although the basic symmetry of icosahedral viruses is the same there are major variations in the number of capsomeres, and therefore differences in the size of the viruses. The basic triangular face of a small virus is constructed of 3 protomeres, with 60 of these subunits forming the whole capsid. For example, the poliovirus has 32 capsomeres, whereas an adenovirus has 240 capsomeres. During the assembling of an

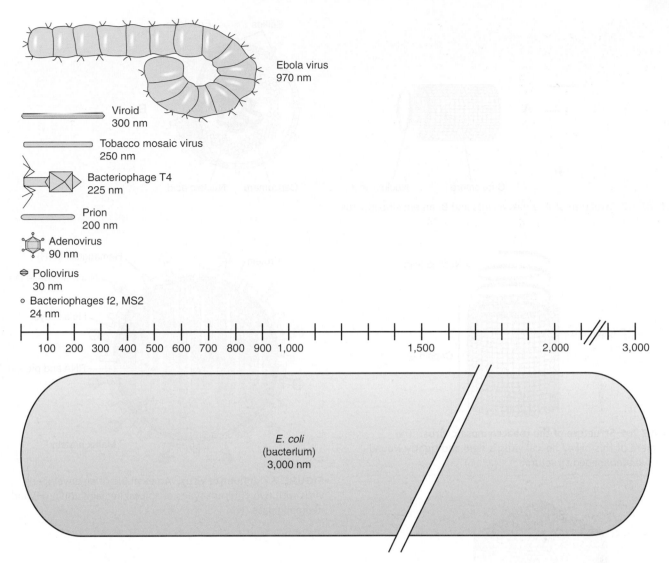

FIGURE 7.1 Size comparison between bacteria, viruses, viroids, and prions.

Labels in figure:
Ebola virus 970 nm
Viroid 300 nm
Tobacco mosaic virus 250 nm
Bacteriophage T4 225 nm
Prion 200 nm
Adenovirus 90 nm
Poliovirus 30 nm
Bacteriophages f2, MS2 24 nm
100 200 300 400 500 600 700 800 900 1,000 1,500 2,000 3,000
E. coli (bacterium) 3,000 nm

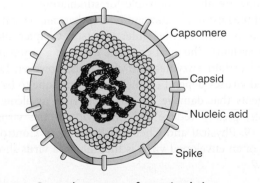

FIGURE 7.2 General structure of an animal virus.

Labels: Capsomere, Capsid, Nucleic acid, Spike

icosahedral virus the nucleic acid is packed into the center, forming a nucleocapsid. Icosahedral viruses can be naked, such as the adenovirus, or enveloped, as the herpes simplex virus (Figure 7.6). Included in this morphological group are the *Iridoviridae* (infect mainly invertebrates), *Herpesviridae, Adenoviridae, Papovaviridae,* and *Parvoviridae.*

Enveloped Viruses

Many viruses have an outer structure, the **viral envelope,** which surrounds the nucleocapsid. Enveloped viruses typically obtain their envelope by budding though a host plasma membrane (see Plasma Membrane in Chapter 3, Cell Structure and Function) but may also include some viral glycoproteins. In some cases the viral envelope is derived from other membranes in the host cell, such as from the membranes of the endoplasmic reticulum or the nuclear membrane. The creation of the viral envelope through the budding process allows the viral particles to leave the host cell without disrupting the plasma membrane and therefore without killing the cell. As a result, some budding viruses can set up persistent infections.

During the formation of the envelope some or all of the host membrane proteins are replaced by viral proteins and some form a layer between the capsid and the envelope. These envelope proteins are glycoproteins; they are exposed to the outside of the envelope as spikes. The lipid bilayer of the envelope is exclusively host specific whereas the majority or all of the glycoproteins are virus specific. The glycoproteins on the surface

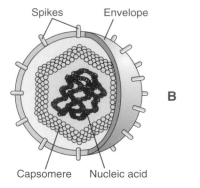
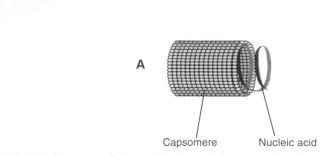

FIGURE 7.3 Structure of **A**, a naked virus and **B**, an enveloped virus.

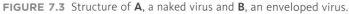

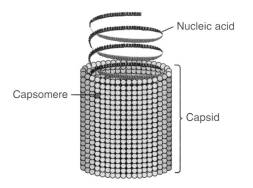

FIGURE 7.4 **Structure of the tobacco mosaic virus.** The capsomere of this naked helical virus is rigid and tightly wound into a cylinder-shaped structure.

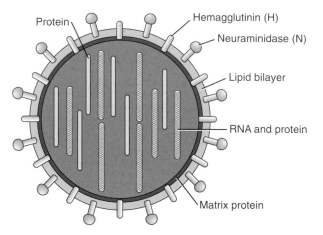

FIGURE 7.7 **Influenza virus.** An example of an enveloped virus with two different types of spikes: hemagglutinin (H) and neuraminidase (N).

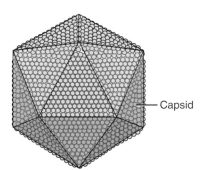

FIGURE 7.5 **Icosahedral virus.** The capsids of these viruses are called *icosahedrons*: three-dimensional, geometric figures with 12 corners, 20 triangular faces, and 30 edges.

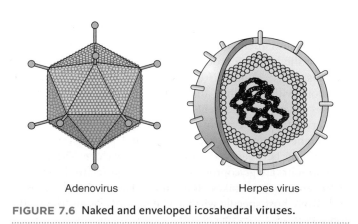

Adenovirus   Herpes virus

FIGURE 7.6 **Naked and enveloped icosahedral viruses.**

of the envelope serve to identify and bind to receptor sites on the plasma membrane of the host. Parts of the viral capsid and/ or envelope are also responsible for stimulating the immune system of the host to produce antibodies that can neutralize the virus and prevent further infection (see Chapter 20, The Immune System). The viral envelope can give a virion protection from certain enzymes and chemicals; however, because enveloped viruses depend on their intact envelope to be infectious, agents that damage the envelope, such as alcohol and detergents, greatly reduce the infectivity of the virus (see Chapter 19, Physical and Chemical Methods of Control). An example of an enveloped virus is the influenza virus shown in Figure 7.7.

Complex Viruses

Complex viruses are a special group of viruses that consist of a capsid that is neither purely helical nor completely icosahedral and that has extra structures such as protein tails or a complex outer wall. The poxviruses are large, complex DNA viruses with an unusual morphology. These viruses lack a regular capsid and the viral genome is associated with proteins within a central disk structure, the nucleoid, which is surrounded by a membrane and two lateral bodies. The nucleoid is surrounded by

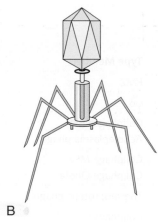

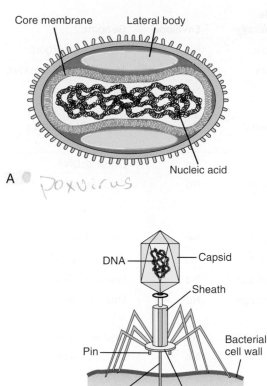

Core membrane   Lateral body

Nucleic acid

A *Poxvirus*

B

DNA — — Capsid

— Sheath

Pin — — Bacterial cell wall

Core   Base plate

FIGURE 7.9 Basic structure of a bacteriophage. Bacteriophages, although different in size and shape, all have a capsid that contains the nucleic acid. Many bacteriophages also have a complex tail that enables the bacteriophage to attach to the host and inject the nucleic acid.

several layers of lipoproteins and a coarse surface of fibrils (Figure 7.8, *A*).

An even more complex group of viruses are bacteriophages, viruses that infect bacteria. In general, bacteriophages have an icosahedral head bound to a polyhedral tail, which is attached to a base plate with many protruding protein tail fibers (Figure 7.8, *B*). Most bacteriophages contain double-stranded DNA (dsDNA); however, ssDNA- and RNA-type phages also exist. There are at least 12 separate groups of bacteriophages (Table 7.1), which are structurally and genetically diverse. Probably the most widely studied bacteriophages are the ones that infect *Escherichia coli,* a bacterium found in the normal flora of the intestinal tract (see Chapter 9, Infection and Disease). These bacteriophages are called *coliphages* and include the lambda phage and the T phages. Bacteriophages exist in different sizes and shapes, but the basic structural features are the same (Figure 7.9):

- **Head** or **Capsid:** All bacteriophages possess a head structure that varies in size and shape. It is made of many copies of one or more different proteins and the nucleic acid is located within this structure. The head or capsid therefore acts as the protective covering for the nucleic acid.

- **Tail:** Many bacteriophages have tails attached to the head, whereas others do not. The tail is a hollow tube that serves as a channel for the nucleic acid to pass through during the process of infecting a bacterium. Its size also varies depending on the phage type. Some of the more complex phages have a tail that is surrounded by a sheath, which contracts during infection of the bacterium. These phages also have a base plate at the end of the tail, with one or more tail fibers attached to it. The base plate and tail fibers play a major role in binding of the bacteriophage to the bacterium. Phages without base plate and tail fibers have other structures involved in binding of the phage to the bacterium.

Genome Type

The genetic information of a virus can be carried in the form of DNA or RNA. It can be dsDNA, ssDNA, dsRNA, or ssRNA. Furthermore, the nucleic acids can be linear or a closed loop. Although both DNA and RNA can be found in viral species, in general the species will contain one or the other. One exception is the human cytomegalovirus, a genus of herpesviruses (in humans known as *human herpesvirus* 5), which contains both a DNA core and several messenger RNA (mRNA) segments. The size of the genome varies substantially between species.

DNA Viruses

Most DNA viruses either belong to Group I or Group II viruses of the Baltimore classification system, with the exception of Group VII viruses, which contain a DNA genome but are classified as reverse-transcribing viruses because they replicate through an RNA intermediate. Their genetic material is DNA and they use DNA-dependent DNA polymerase for replication. The DNA in Group I viruses is dsDNA, whereas Group II viruses have ssDNA. Families of DNA viruses include *Herpesviridae* (genital herpes) and *Poxviridae* (smallpox).

RNA Viruses

RNA viruses use RNA as their genetic material and do not replicate using DNA. They belong to Group II, IV, or V of the Baltimore classification system. Their nucleic acid is usually ssRNA with the exception of reoviruses, which are the only group of dsRNA viruses.

TABLE 7.1 Groups of Bacteriophages

Family or Group	Genus	Type Member	Particle Morphology	Envelope	Genome
Corticoviridae	Corticovirus	PM2	Isometric	No	Supercoiled dsDNA
Cystoviridae	Cystovirus	φ6	Isometric	Yes	Three segments, dsRNA
Inoviridae	Inovirus Plectrovirus	Coliphages fd Acholeplasma phage	Rod	No	Circular ssDNA
Leviviridae	Levivirus Allolevirus	Coliphage MS2 Coliphage Qbeta	Icosahedral	No	1(+)strand (+)ssRNA
Lipothrixiviridae	Lipothrixvirus	Thermoproteus phage 1	Rod	Yes	Linear dsDNA
Microviridae	Microvirus Spirovirus	Coliphages φX174 Spiroplasma phages Mac-1 phage	Icosahedral	No	Circular ssDNA
Myoviridae		Coliphages T4	Tailed phage	No	Linear dsDNA
Plasmaviridae	Plasmavirus	Acholeplasma phage	Pleomorphic	Yes	Circular dsDNA
Podoviridae		Coliphage T7	Tailed phage	No	Linear dsDNA
Siphoviridae	Lambda phage group	Coliphage lambda	Tailed phage	No	Linear dsDNA
Sulfolobus Shibatae virus		SSV-1	Lemon shaped	No	Circular dsDNA
Tectiviridae	Tectivirus	Phage PRD1	Icosahedral	No	Linear dsDNA

dsDNA, Double-stranded DNA; dsRNA, double-stranded RNA; ssDNA, single-stranded DNA.

RNA viruses can further be classified as negative-sense (−s; negative-strand) and positive-sense (+s; positive-strand) RNA viruses depending on whether their nucleic acid is complementary to the viral mRNA or not. In +s RNA the viral RNA is identical to the viral mRNA and therefore translation by the host cell can begin immediately. In contrast, −s viral RNA is complementary to mRNA and must be converted to +s RNA by RNA polymerase before translation can begin. RNA viruses often have high mutation rates due to the absence of DNA polymerase, the enzyme that seeks, finds, and corrects mistakes in genetic material. Families of RNA viruses include *Picornaviridae* (poliomyelitis), *Filoviridae* (Ebola), and *Paramyxoviridae* (measles and the "common cold").

Reverse-transcribing Viruses

All Group VI viruses have an RNA genome, but they replicate via a DNA intermediate. These viruses are dependent on the enzyme reverse transcriptase so that reverse transcription of its genome from RNA into DNA can occur. This DNA can then be integrated into the host's genome by an integrase enzyme. At this point the retroviral DNA is referred to as a provirus. The Group VI viruses include the families *Metaviridae, Pseudoviridae,* and *Retroviridae.*

The Group VII viruses have DNA genomes within the invading viral particles. The DNA genome is transcribed into mRNA to provide a template for protein synthesis, and into pregenomic RNA that is used as the template during genome replication. The virally encoded reverse transcriptase uses the pregenomic RNA as a template for the production of genomic DNA. Group VII includes the families *Hepadnaviridae* and *Caulimoviridae.*

Genome Changes

Viruses have diverse characteristics and the origin of viruses and their genome has been under investigation for decades. Advances in the field of genetics and the availability of genome sequences are beginning to provide some answers to these questions. Gene transfer between host cell genomes and viral genomes has been reported for some DNA viruses including the human herpesviruses. Comparative genomic studies show that more than 30 herpesvirus proteins show significant similarity to human proteins. The genes encoding these proteins may have derived from the human genome. This phenomenon is likely responsible for the high mutation rate in the herpesviruses. Gene transfer and recombination between DNA viruses have also been documented, providing another source for the genetic diversity of viruses.

RNA viruses need RNA-dependent RNA polymerases in order to synthesize new RNA genomes. Unlike DNA polymerases, RNA-dependent RNA polymerases have no proofreading ability and therefore errors often occur. These enzymes are capable of mutations in about 1 of every 10,000 nucleotides, resulting in at least one mutation per genome in each replication cycle. This feature of RNA viruses is one of the reasons for the great variability and rapid evolution of these viruses. Furthermore, RNA viruses can recombine genomes during RNA synthesis if two or more RNA genomes are present in an infected cell. One relevant example of viral genomic exchange is a newly emerged type of coronavirus, the SARS-associated coronavirus, the cause of severe acute respiratory syndrome (SARS). In summary, viruses that attack eukaryotic cells mutate

Avian Influenza in Humans

Although the avian influenza A viruses usually do not infect humans, the World Health Organization (WHO) has recently reported that the virus (H5N1) jumped the species barrier from birds to mammals, including humans. Infections in humans are rare and most occurred after direct contact with infected poultry. In humans, clinical symptoms due to the avian influenza A virus range from conjunctivitis to severe respiratory disease to death. Scientists warn that through mutation or recombination with other influenza viruses, this virus could acquire the ability to spread throughout the human population by person to person contact, resulting in a pandemic disease.

Almost 400 cases of human infection with the H5N1 virus have been reported between November 2003 and June 2008. The WHO maintains situation updates and cumulative reports of human cases of avian influenza A on their website, http://www.who.int/csr/disease/avian_influenza/en/

rapidly and exchange gene segments with other viruses and organisms.

Viral Multiplication

Viruses are acellular organisms and do not replicate through cell division; instead they use host cell machinery and metabolism to produce multiple copies of themselves. Outside the host cell a virus is an inert particle. Host cells for each class of viruses are species specific and often even tissue specific.

Multiplication of Bacteriophages

A bacteriophage (or simply phage) is a virus that infects bacteria and multiplies inside of them. Just like bacteria, bacteriophages are common in all natural environments and their presence is directly related to the numbers of bacteria present. Knowledge of the phage life cycle is necessary to understand one of the mechanisms by which bacterial genes can be transferred from one bacterium to another. Bacteriophages are often used in diagnostic laboratories for the identification of pathogenic bacteria through phage typing, because each phage is highly specific for the bacterium it will invade. Bacteriophages can contain either DNA or RNA as its nucleic acid and the size of the nucleic acid varies depending on the phage. A simple phage might contain only enough nucleic acid to code for 3 to 5 average-sized gene products whereas others may code for more than 100 gene products. Therefore the number of different kinds of proteins and the amount of each will vary depending on the bacteriophage.

The events that occur in the multiplication cycle of bacteriophages include adsorption, penetration, replication, assembly,

maturation, and release. Adsorption represents the recognition process between phage and bacterium, followed by attachment and then penetration of the phage DNA into the bacterium. Replication represents copying of phage nucleic acid, followed by the assembly of phage parts and maturation of the newly formed bacteriophages. The mature phages are then released from the host cell and are ready to infect others. These events are shown in Figure 7.10.

Adsorption

In the first step of successful bacterial infection, a phage must find a susceptible host and attach to the bacterial cell. This **adsorption** is mediated by the tail fibers (or analogous structures on phages without tail fibers), which bind to specific receptors on the bacterial cell surface. Bacterial structures that act as phage receptors include surface molecules of the cell wall, pili, and flagella. The host specificity of the phage is commonly determined by the type of tail fibers of the phage. This first step of attachment of the bacteriophage to the bacterium by the tail fibers is weak and reversible. The second step is irreversible binding of the phage to the bacterium. It is mediated by components of the base plate or by alternative ways in use by bacteriophages that lack these base plates. This firm attachment to the bacterium is irreversible and the phage is positioned for penetration.

Penetration

After the irreversible binding, the bacteriophage is still outside the bacterium and must inject its nucleic acid through the bacterial cell wall and into the cytoplasm of the host. Phages may have a contractile sheath that "constricts" after adsorption, pushing the inner tube through the cell wall of the bacterium and the cell membrane. This allows the phage's nucleic acid to pass through the membrane and enter the bacterial cell. Bacteriophages without a contractile sheath use other mechanisms, such as digestion of portions of the bacterial cell wall, to gain access to the cytoplasm. In general, only the nucleic acid enters the host cell; the rest of the phage remains outside the bacterium. Penetration by some DNA bacteriophages that attach to pili, rather than to the cell wall, results in both the genomic DNA and capsid entering the cytoplasm of the host cell.

Assembly

Once the phage nucleic acid has entered the bacterium the bacterial metabolism shifts to the genetic expression of the viral nucleic acid strand and does not synthesize its own molecules. This change in metabolic activity of the host cell results in the formation of viral molecules such as the following:

- Proteins that seal the damaged bacterial cell wall to prevent premature bacterial cell death
- Enzymes that are necessary to copy the genome of the bacteriophage
- Proteins that are needed for the formation of the capsid head and part of the tail fibers
- Enzymes required for the weakening of the bacterial cell wall in order to lyse the bacterial cell and release the newly assembled bacteriophages

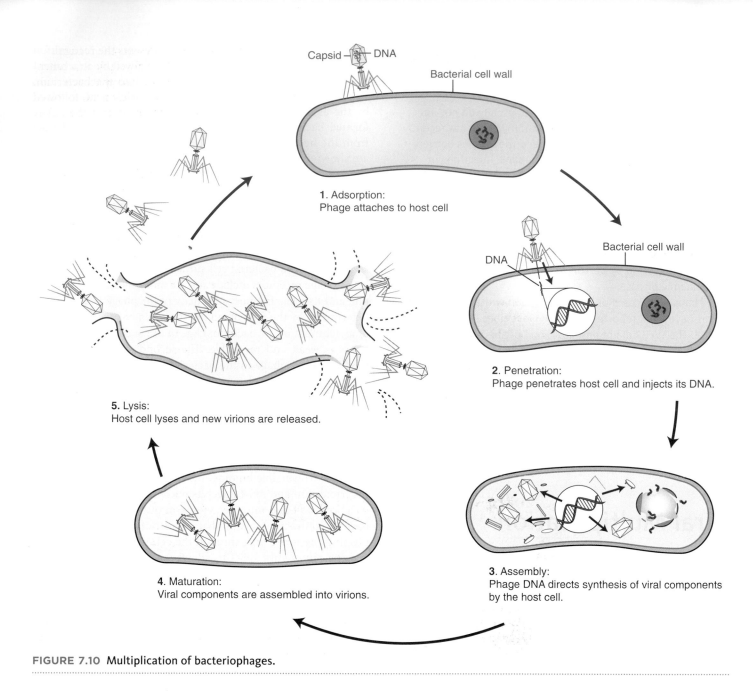

FIGURE 7.10 Multiplication of bacteriophages.

The multiplication of bacteriophages can either result in the **lysis** ("bursting") of the infected bacterium or in a silent viral infection referred to as **lysogeny.**

- **Lytic** or **virulent** phages are phages that after multiplication destroy the bacterium by lysis at the end of the multiplication cycle, releasing the newly formed phages into the environment. This lytic life cycle can be divided into three phases: the eclipse period, the intracellular accumulation phase, and the lysis and release phase.
  - **Eclipse period:** In this phase no infectious phage particles can be found in the host cell. The viral synthesis process utilizes the resources of the host and the phage nucleic acid takes over the biosynthetic machinery to produce phage specific mRNA's to make proteins. In the early phase of this period, early mRNA's code for proteins which are needed for the synthesis of

phage DNA and synthesis of host DNA, RNA and proteins come to an end. After the production of phage DNA late mRNAs and their corresponding proteins are made. These late proteins are structural proteins for the phages and also proteins necessary for the lysis of the host cell.
  - **Intracellular accumulation phase:** The nucleic acids and the structural proteins made in the previous phase are assembled into complete infectious phages that accumulate in the host cell.
  - **Lysis and release phase:** During this phase the bacteria begin to lyse, due to the accumulation of phage lysis proteins, and the phages are released into the environment surrounding the bacterium. Infected bacteria may release up to 1000 bacteriophages.
- **Lysogenic** or **temperate** phages are those that can either multiply by the lytic cycle or undergo adsorption and

Therapeutic Bacteriophages

The term "therapeutic bacteriophages" describes the therapeutic use of lytic bacteriophages for the treatment of pathogenic bacterial infections. In general, the host range of bacteriophages is narrower than that of antibiotics used in the clinical environment. Most bacteriophages are specific for one species of bacteria and may only lyse a specific strain within a species. Many bacteria become resistant to all available antibiotics and cause serious problems in the form of untreatable infections, such as some hospital-acquired infections (see Chapter 9, Infection and Disease), and the basis for possible epidemics.

Phage therapy was first developed in the early 1900s but, because of the emergence of antibiotics in 1941, the Western world shifted interest away from the further use and study of phage therapy. Because of their isolation from Western advances in antibiotic production, Russian scientists continued to develop the already successful phage therapy to treat the wounds of soldiers in field hospitals. As a result, extensive clinical research and implementation of phage therapy continued in Eastern Europe.

In 2006, a biopharmaceutical company (GangaGen, Inc.) began developing phage technology for the treatment of antibiotic-resistant bacterial infections and was awarded a U.S. patent for the invention of "lysin-deficient bacteriophages having reduced immunogenicity" for use in the destruction of pathogenic bacteria, including those resistant to antibiotics. This patent provides an opportunity for phage therapy to be used in both human and veterinary medicine.

penetration into the bacterial host but are not replicated or released at that time. Instead the phage genes are not transcribed, and the phage genome exists in a repressed state. The phage DNA in this stage is referred to as a **prophage,** because it is not a phage but has the potential to produce a phage. In general, the bacteriophage DNA is integrated into the host chromosome and passed on to the daughter cells of the bacterium. The host cell carrying a prophage might not be adversely affected at all and the lysogenic state might persist indefinitely or eventually result in lysis. Lysogeny is a less deadly form of parasitism, allowing the virus to spread without killing the host. On occasion the prophage in a lysogenic cell can be activated, which ultimately results in viral replication and the lytic cycle.

Multiplication of Animal Viruses

The basic stages of multiplication of animal viruses are similar to those seen in bacteriophages. However, several differences are present between the host cells, their viruses, and also in

some steps of the multiplication cycle. The stages of the multiplication cycle for animal viruses include adsorption, penetration, uncoating, replication, assembly, and finally release from the host cell. The duration of the multiplication cycle varies among animal viruses. The basic stages of the cycle in naked and enveloped viruses are shown in Figure 7.11.

Adsorption

The first stage of multiplication is the attachment (adsorption) of the virus to a susceptible host cell. Like bacteriophages, animal viruses are specific to their host cells and they infect only one or a restricted range of host species. This limitation is referred to as the **host range.** For example, hepatitis viruses attack cells in the liver, the mumps virus attacks the salivary glands, and HIV attaches to the CD4 protein of helper T cells (see Chapter 20, The Immune System). They adsorb to specific receptor sites embedded in the plasma membrane of their host, which are generally glycoproteins the host cell requires for its normal cellular functions. The attachment sites on the virus (viral receptors) are distributed over the capsid or envelope of the virus and are generally glycoproteins or proteins. Animal cells that lack receptors for a specific virus are resistant and cannot be infected by that virus. Naked and enveloped viruses differ in their mode of attachment to the host cell. Naked viruses have surface molecules that adhere to the membrane receptor, whereas enveloped viruses possess glycoprotein spikes that bind to the plasma membrane receptors of the host cells (Figure 7.12). The attachment of a virus to its host can be prevented by antibody molecules that are capable of attaching to the viral attachment sites or to the host cell receptors. The presence of these antibodies in the host organism is the most important basis for immunity against viral infections (see Chapter 20).

Penetration

After the adsorption stage is the penetration of the virus into the cytoplasm of the host, either via endocytosis (engulfment) of the whole virus or by fusion of the viral envelope with the plasma membrane, allowing only the nucleocapsid of the virus to enter the cell. Unlike bacteriophages, animal viruses generally do not "inject" their nucleic acid into the host cells; however, on occasion nonenveloped viruses leave their capsid outside the cell while the genome passes into the cell.

Uncoating

When the nucleocapsid is in the host cell cytoplasm the viral nucleic acid is released by a process called **uncoating.** The uncoating process varies between viruses. If penetration occurs by receptor-mediated endocytosis (see Chapter 3, Cell Structure and Function) the entire virus is engulfed by the host cell and becomes enclosed in a vacuole or vesicle. The enzymes in the vacuole or vesicle then dissolve the envelope and the capsid, and the viral genome is released. Another method of entry occurs by direct fusion of the viral envelope with the plasma membrane of the host cell, thereby releasing the nucleocapsid into the cell cytoplasm. Some antiviral drugs (see Chapter 22, Antimicrobial Drugs) exert their effect by preventing the uncoating of the nucleocapsid.

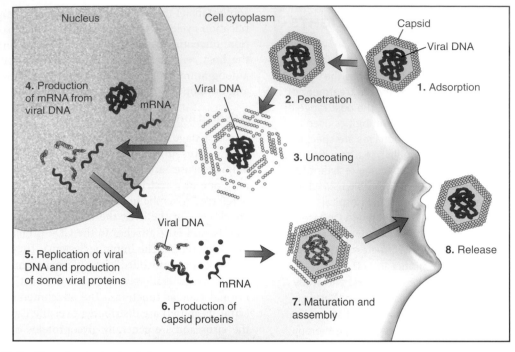

FIGURE 7.11 Multiplication of naked animal viruses.

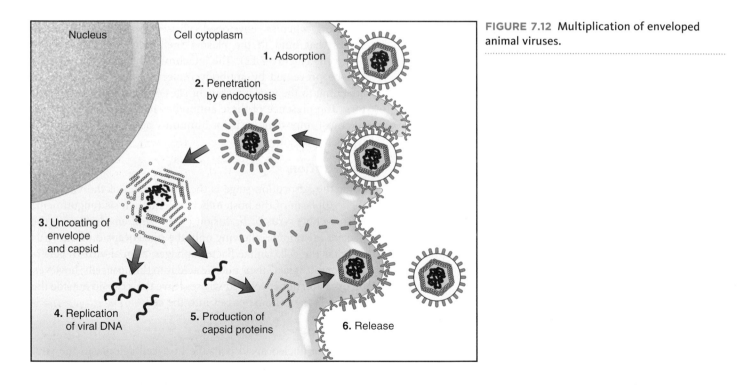

FIGURE 7.12 Multiplication of enveloped animal viruses.

Replication

Synthesis and replication of animal viruses occur immediately after the uncoating process. This phase is highly regulated, complex, and the events proceed depending on whether the nucleic acid of the infecting virus is DNA or RNA.

In the case of DNA viruses, the viral DNA enters the nucleus of the host cell where it is transcribed into early mRNA, which leaves the nucleus and enters the cytoplasm. The early mRNA is then translated into early viral proteins. The early viral pro-

teins deal with the replication of viral DNA and therefore are transported back into the nucleus. Once in the nucleus these proteins become involved in the synthesis of multiple copies of viral DNA, using host DNA polymerase. The copies of the viral genome then act as templates for transcription into late mRNA which leaves the nucleus for translation into late viral proteins in the cytoplasm. The late proteins are structural proteins such as coat and envelope proteins, or core proteins such as enzymes that are transported back into the nucleus for the next stage of the replication phase.

RNA viruses cannot be transcribed in the same manner as DNA viruses, because the host polymerases do not work for RNA. In other words, the RNA virus must provide its own polymerase if transcription is necessary. In the case of dsRNA viruses, one strand is first transcribed by viral polymerase into mRNA. Three separate routes for the formation of mRNA occur in ssRNA viruses:

- An ssRNA with a positive-sense configuration can be used directly as mRNA.
- An ssRNA with a negative-sense configuration must first be transcribed into a positive-sense strand by viral polymerase and can then be used as mRNA.
- Retroviruses use a different route. These viruses have a positive-sense ssRNA that is made into a negative-sense ssDNA, using viral reverse transcriptase present in the nucleocapsid. This process is followed by the formation of dsDNA, which enters the nucleus and becomes integrated into the host DNA. The integrated viral DNA is then transcribed by host polymerase into mRNA.

In all three cases, translation of the viral mRNA occurs at the host ribosomes, producing viral proteins for the final assembly of the virus. In addition to viral protein synthesis the virus must also replicate its nucleic acid. In the early phase the proteins produced are enzymes and regulatory molecules that will allow subsequent replication of viral nucleic acid. The late phase deals with the synthesis of proteins necessary for capsid formation.

Assembly

Once the synthesis of the viral components is complete the assembly phase begins. In this phase, mature viral particles are constructed from a growing quantity of viral components. Commonly, the capsid is produced first as an empty shell that serves as a container for the nucleic acid. This process is called **encapsidation.**

Release

The final phase of viral multiplication is the release stage, which results in the exit of mature virions from the host cell. This process occurs in one of two ways: budding (exocytosis) or cell death (lysis). Nonenveloped viruses mature in the nucleus or cytoplasm and are released when the cell ruptures or lyses. Enveloped viruses, on the other hand, are discharged by budding from:

- The plasma membrane
- The nuclear membrane
- The endoplasmic reticulum
- Or by vesicular formation, without cell death

The nucleocapsid binds to the membrane, which curves around the particle, forming a small pouch (envelope). Whenever a virus uses a host membrane to exit the cell, it always inserts into the envelope specific viral proteins, which represent specific viral antigens. These antigens are used by the virus to gain access into a new host cell. Furthermore, the insertion of viral molecules into the host plasma membrane alters the host

cell, resulting in an antigenically different cell. This expression of viral antigens is a major factor in the development of antiviral immune responses.

Although budding of enveloped viruses causes them to be shed gradually over a period of time without sudden cell death, most active viral infections are ultimately lethal to the cell because of cumulative damage caused by the virus.

Viral Infections

The short- and long-term effects of viral infections in animal cells are well documented and viral infections can have the following outcomes:

- **Abortive infections** are infections of **nonpermissive cells** where no viral production occurs.
- **Lytic** or **cytocidal infections** kill the host cell. This type of infection occurs in **permissive cells,** cells that provide the biosynthetic machinery to support the complete replication cycle of the virus.
- **Persistent infections** are infections that do not cause cell death. They can be:
- Chronic infections that are not lytic but productive. The cellular effects of chronic infections are mostly the same as in acute cytocidal infections with the exception that the production of viruses may be slower, intermittent or limited to only a few cells.
- Latent infections with limited macromolecular synthesis but no virus synthesis. In other words, only restricted expression of the viral genome occurs. The viral gene products are associated with few if any changes in the infected cell.
- Slow infections, characterized by a prolonged incubation period without prominent morphological and physiological changes to the host cell. Although the progression of cellular damage may take years, it is followed by extensive cellular injury and disease.
- Transforming infections, in which the viral nucleic acid may remain in specific host cells indefinitely, and a virus may or may not be produced. The term **oncogenic** transformation refers to the genetic modification of cell proliferation control so that the cell becomes cancerous. DNA or RNA tumor viruses may initiate several changes that convert normal cells into malignant tumor cells (see Genotoxic Effects later in this chapter). Infected cells may also undergo other types of inheritable changes resulting in morphological, physiological, and biochemical alterations that are nononcogenic. In other words, if a virus infects a cell and alters the properties of that cell, the cell is referred to as transformed.

Host Cell Damage

A viral infection is usually associated with changes in the cell morphology, physiology, and biosynthetic events.

Morphological Effects Changes in the morphology of a host cell caused by viral infections are referred to as **cytopathic effects.** Cytopathic effects (CPEs) include the following:

TABLE 7.2 Cytopathic Effects of Selected Viruses

Virus	Cytopathic effect
Adenovirus	Nuclear inclusions; cell clumping
Herpes simplex virus	Cell fusion leading to multinucleated giant cells; nuclear inclusions
HIV	Multinucleated giant cells
Influenza virus	Rounding of cells
Poliovirus	Cell lysis
Rabies virus	Cytoplasmic inclusions: Negri bodies
Reovirus	Cell enlargement; vacuoles and inclusion bodies in cytoplasm
Smallpox virus	Rounding of cells; cytoplasmic inclusions

- Altered shape (i.e., rounding of cells)
- Detachment from tissue surface
- Lysis
- Membrane fusion
- Altered membrane permeability
- Inclusion bodies (either altered host cell structure or accumulation of viral components)
- Apoptosis (programmed cell death)

The specific cytopathic effects caused by different viruses depend on the viruses and the cells they infect. The observations of cytopathic effects can be used in clinical virology to aid in the identification of a viral isolate. Cytopathic changes of selected viruses are listed in Table 7.2.

Physiological Effects. Interaction of a virus with the plasma membrane or intracellular membranes and any subsequent events, such as the addition of viral proteins, can change the physiological characteristics of the host cell. This may include the movement of ions, formation of secondary messengers, and launching of activities that lead to altered cellular activities. Viral proteins incorporated into the plasma membrane of the host cell may also alter its antigenic or immune properties.

Biochemical Effects. A large number of viruses inhibit or alter synthesis of the infected cells' own macromolecules, such as DNA, RNA, and various proteins. Cellular transcription and protein-to-protein interactions may also be altered to promote the production of new viruses. Furthermore, some viruses may stimulate specific cellular biochemical activities in order to increase virus replication.

Genotoxic Effects Genotoxic substances damage DNA either directly, by binding to the DNA, or indirectly leading to DNA damage by affecting enzymes involved in DNA replication. These substances therefore cause mutations, which may or may not lead to cancer. After a viral infection, breakage, fragmentation, rearrangement, or other changes in the host DNA may occur. Double-stranded DNA viruses interact directly with the

host DNA and in some cases the viral DNA becomes integrated at a particular site in the host genome. All parts of the viral genome are expressed in permissive cells, which leads to viral replication, lysis, and cell death. When the viral DNA becomes integrated into the host genome at random sites in nonpermissive cells, only part of the viral genome is expressed. In this case the early control functions of the virus are expressed, while viral structural proteins are not produced. Several DNA viruses such as the hepatitis B virus, the herpesviruses, and the papillomaviruses are potentially initiators of cancer. RNA tumor viruses (retroviruses) usually change cells into malignant cells by integrating their own nucleic acid into the host cell genome and may even produce infectious new viruses. Because RNA is the genome of the mature viral particle it must first be copied to DNA (see Viral Multiplication earlier in this chapter) before integration into the host DNA.

Major Groups of Viruses in Vertebrates

Vertebrate viruses cause disease after they break the natural protective barriers and gain access to underlying tissues and organs. Most viruses are specific to a particular cell or tissue type, but a particular disease may be caused by several viruses that have a common tissue preference. The genome of viruses can consist of either DNA or RNA.

DNA Viruses

Adenoviruses

Adenoviruses belong to the family *Adenoviridae* and most commonly cause respiratory illness. There are 49 immunologically distinct human adenoviruses and, depending on the serotype, they may also cause various other illnesses including gastroenteritis, conjunctivitis, cystitis, and rashes. The symptoms caused by adenovirus-induced respiratory illnesses range from common cold symptoms to pneumonia, croup, and bronchitis. In children adenoviruses typically cause respiratory and gastrointestinal tract infections. Immunocompromised patients are especially vulnerable and susceptible to severe complications of adenoviral infections.

Adenoviruses are linear dsDNA viruses of medium size (90–100 nm), are nonenveloped, and have an icosahedral nucleocapsid. The viruses are unusually stable to chemical or physical agents and also to adverse pH conditions. This allows the virus to survive outside of the human body for prolonged periods of time.

Hepadnaviruses

Hepadnaviruses are part of the family *Hepadnaviridae* and cause hepatitis in humans and animals. These viruses are enveloped virions with a small circular genome of partially double-stranded and partially single-stranded DNA. When the virus enters the host cell, the single-stranded portion is restored to a double strand by a DNA polymer present in the core. One member of the group is the hepatitis B virus (HBV), which

Oncogenic Viruses and Associated Cancers

Virus	Nucleic Acid	Disease	Cancer
Papovaviridae *Papillomavirus* (some)	dsDNA	Warts, genital warts	Cervical cancer
Herpesviridae *Lymphocryptovirus* (Epstein-Barr virus)	dsDNA	Infectious mononucleosis	Burkitt's lymphoma; nasopharygeal carcinoma; may play a role in the development of Hodgkin's disease
Herpesviridae Herpes simplex virus (HSV-2, HSV-8)	dsDNA	Genital herpes	Cervical cancer Kaposi's sarcoma
Hepadnavirus Hepatitis B virus	dsDNA	Hepatitis B	Liver cancer
Adenoviridae	dsDNA	Acute respiratory disease; common cold	Adenocarcinomas
Poxviridae	dsDNA	Smallpox; cowpox	Miscellaneous
Retroviridae	ssRNA	Adult T-cell leukemia; HIV infections	Adult T-cell lymphoma; AIDS

infects hepatocytes where it can persist, causing hepatitis, and can also be a factor in liver cell carcinoma. HBV can cause acute or chronic, symptomatic or asymptomatic disease (see Chapter 12, Infections of the Gastrointestinal System).

Herpesviruses

Herpesviruses *(Herpesviridae)* are a large family of DNA viruses that cause disease in humans and animals. The human herpesviruses are grouped into three subfamilies: *Alphaherpesvirinae,* *Betaherpesvirinae,* and *Gammaherpesvirinae.* This classification is based on differences in viral characteristics such as genome structure, tissue tropism, cytopathology, and site of latent infection, as well as pathogenesis of the disease (Table 7.3). The human herpesviruses are as follows:

- Herpes simplex viruses 1 and 2 (HSV-1 and HSV-2)
- Varicella-zoster virus (VZV)
- Epstein-Barr virus (EBV)
- Cytomegalovirus (CMV)
- Human herpesviruses 6, 7, and 8 (HHV-6, HHV-7, and HHV-8)

The herpesviruses are large enveloped dsDNA (linear) viruses that acquire their envelope by budding from nuclear and plasma membranes of the host cell. They replicate in the nucleus of infected cells and characteristically demonstrate latency, which allows them to exist in a dormant stage for the duration of the host tissue's lifetime. When activated they cause recurrent disease in their hosts (e.g., varicella-zoster virus; see Chapter 10, Infections of the Integumentary System, Soft Tissue, and Muscle). Reactivation of the viruses can occur in response to environmental changes such as ultraviolet light, x-rays, heat, cold, hormonal changes, stress (both physical and emotional), and immune deficiencies.

Papillomaviruses and Polyomaviruses

Papillomaviruses and polyomaviruses were previously grouped in the family *Papovaviridae,* but have been divided into two families, the *Papillomaviridae* and *Polyomaviridae.* Both families can cause host-dependent lytic, chronic, latent, and transforming infections. Papillomaviruses and polyomaviruses are small nonenveloped viruses with circular dsDNA and an icosahedral capsid. Human papillomaviruses cause warts and several types are associated with cancer such as cervical carcinomas.

Parvoviruses

Parvoviridae species are the smallest of the DNA viruses (18 to 26 nm in diameter), and only one member, the B19 agent, is known to infect human cells. All other members are best known for their capacity to cause disease in animals. The parvoviruses have a nonenveloped, icosahedral capsid and the B19 virus genome contains one linear, ssDNA molecule. The B19 virus prefers to replicate in mitotically active cells such as human bone marrow cells, erythroid cells, and erythroid leukemia cells. B19 is the agent of contagious erythema infectiosum, commonly called *fifth disease,* because of the development of a face rash similar to the other four diseases, measles, rubella, scarlet fever, and Dukes' disease.

Poxviruses

Poxviruses are the largest viruses, about 200 nm in diameter and 300 nm in length, with very complex nucleocapsid symmetry. They vary in shape depending on the species, but for the most part they are brick shaped or in oval form, similar to a rounded brick. The viral genome is a large double-stranded linear DNA, fused at both ends. The human poxviruses include variola (genus *Orthopoxirus*), the causative agent for smallpox, and molluscum contagiosum (genus *Molluscipoxvirus*), which can cause benign tumors in humans.

TABLE 7.3 Characteristics of Herpesviridae

Subfamily	Virus	Pathophysiology	Transmission
Herpesdviridae			
Human herpesvirus 1	Herpes simplex virus 1 (HSV-1)	Oral and/or genital herpes (primarily orofacial)	Close contact
Human herpesvirus 2	Herpes simplex virus 2 (HSV-2)	Oral and/or genital herpes (predominantly genital)	Sexually transmitted
Human herpesvirus 3	Varicella-zoster virus (VZV)	Chickenpox and shingles	Respiratory and close contact
Gammaherpesvirinae			
Human herpesvirus 4	Epstein-Barr virus (EBV), lymphocryptovirus	Infectious mononucleosis, Burkitt's lymphoma, CNS lymphoma in AIDS patients, posttransplant lymphoproliferative syndrome, nasopharyngeal carcinoma	EBV: saliva (kissing disease)
Human herpesvirus 8	Kaposi's sarcoma–associated herpesvirus	Kaposi's sarcoma, primary effusion lymphoma, some types of multicentric Castleman's disease	Close contact (sexual), saliva?
Betaherpesvirinae			
Human herpesvirus 4	Cytomegalovirus	Infectious mononucleosis, retinitis, etc.	Close contact, transfusions, tissue transplant, congenital
Human herpesvirus 6 Human herpesvirus 7	Roseolovirus	Sixth disease (roseola infantum or exanthema subitum)	Respiratory and close contact?

The vaccinia virus, another poxvirus related to the smallpox virus, is the "live virus" used in the smallpox vaccine. When given to humans as a vaccine it will help the body to develop immunity to smallpox. The vaccinia virus is best known for the eradication of smallpox, which was announced by the World Health Organization in 1980.

RNA Viruses

Bunyaviridae

Bunyaviridae species are enveloped viruses with a large negative-stranded RNA as their nucleic acid. They are zoonoses and while generally found in animals, certain members in this family can infect humans (Table 7.4). *Bunyaviridae* comprises a group of at least 200 viruses broken down into five genera based on structural and biochemical features: *Bunyavirus, Phlebovirus, Uukuvirus, Nairovirus,* and *Hantavirus.* With the exception of the hantavirus, which is carried by rodents, *Bunyaviridae* species are arthropod-borne.

Coronaviruses

Coronaviruses belong to the family *Coronaviridae* and are cataloged as Group IV of the Baltimore classification system. These viruses are between 80 to 160 nm in diameter, which makes them the largest of the RNA viruses. Coronaviruses are enveloped with a (+) ssRNA genome and helical symmetry. They infect humans and animals, causing respiratory and enteric diseases. The coronaviruses are the second most prevalent cause of the common cold, the rhinovirus being the most common one.

LIFE APPLICATION

Smallpox as Biological Weapon

Smallpox is believed to have originated more than 3000 years ago in India or Egypt, and it is one of the most devastating diseases known to mankind. While effective treatment of the disease has never been developed, Edward Jenner discovered that inoculation with cowpox could protect humans against smallpox. The development of the first live vaccine against small pox in 1796, and its later worldwide distribution, led to the eradication of the smallpox (variola) virus in 1980, resulting in the destruction of reference stocks in the World Health Organization laboratories. However, the virus did not disappear and stocks still exist in the United States and Russia. The natural smallpox virus was successfully eliminated, but the former Soviet Union was stockpiling large amounts of the smallpox virus for use in biowarfare. The U.S. Centers for Disease Control and Prevention (CDC) considers smallpox a category A agent together with anthrax, plague, botulism, tularemia, and viral hemorrhagic fever. These agents have great potential in bioterrorism-biowarfare if acquired by terrorists and/or hostile nations. All these agents could be widely distributed causing serious disease outbreaks. This potential threat has renewed interest in developing new smallpox vaccine programs and programs dealing with the development of potent antiviral drugs.

TABLE 7.4 Examples of *Bunyaviridae* Capable of Infecting Humans

Genus	Insect Vector	Vertebrate Host	Human Pathology
Bunyavirus	Mosquito	Rodents, small mammals, primates, birds, marsupials	Febrile illness, encephalitis
Hantavirus	None	Rodents	Hemorrhagic fever with renal syndrome, adult respiratory distress syndrome, hantavirus pulmonary syndrome, shock, pulmonary edema
Nairovirus	Tick	Hares, cattle, goats, seabirds	Hemorrhagic fever
Phlebovirus	Fly	Sheep, cattle, domestic animals	Rift Valley fever, sandfly fever, hemorrhagic fever, encephalitis, conjunctivitis, myositis

TABLE 7.5 Hepatitis Viruses

Virus	Subfamily	Structure	Transmission
Hepatitis A	Picornavirus	Positive-sense RNA, unenveloped icosahedral capsid	Fecal–oral route, water- or foodborne
Hepatitis B	Hepadnavirus	Enveloped DNA	Paternally by blood or needles, sexual contact, perinatally
Hepatitis C	Flavivirus	Positive-strand RNA, enveloped	Blood-to-blood contact, infected blood, intravenous drug abuse, sexually, transfusion and organ recipients
Hepatitis D	Delta agent (virus)	Negative-sense, single-stranded, closed circular RNA	Needs hepatitis B virus to exist, found in persons infected with the hepatitis B virus
Hepatitis E	Herpesvirus	Nonenveloped, positive-sense, single-stranded RNA	Fecal–oral route, especially contaminated water

The **severe acute respiratory syndrome (SARS)** is caused by the coronavirus SARS-CoV (see Chapter 11, Infections of the Respiratory System, and Chapter 18, Emerging Infectious Diseases).

Hepatitis Viruses

Many of the liver diseases, collectively called *hepatitis*, are caused by viruses, coming from a wide range of viral families (Table 7.5). Each of the hepatitis viruses infects and damages the liver, causing jaundice and the release of liver enzymes. Viral hepatitis is a cause of considerable morbidity and mortality in the human population, both from acute and chronic infection, including chronic active hepatitis, cirrhosis, and hepatocellular carcinoma. Viral hepatitis is a major public health problem throughout the world, affecting several hundreds of millions of people.

Orthomyxoviruses

Orthomyxoviruses belong to the family *Orthomyxoviridae* and include the influenza A, B, and C viruses. The viruses are enveloped with a segmented negative-sense RNA genome. Influenza A and C viruses infect multiple species, whereas influenza B infects mostly humans. Significant human disease is due only to influenza A and B viruses. The type A viruses are the most virulent human pathogens in this group and cause the most severe disease. Influenza viruses are respiratory

TABLE 7.6 Known Flu Pandemics

Name of Pandemic	Date	Estimated Deaths
Asiatic (Russian) flu	1889–1890	1 million
Spanish flu	1918–1920	40 million
Asian flu	1957–1958	1 to 1.5 million
Hong Kong flu	1968–1969	0.75 to 1 million

viruses (see Chapter 11, Infections of the Respiratory System) responsible for the classic flulike symptoms of fever, malaise, headache, and body aches (myalgias). Influenza is one of the most prevalent of the viral infections. The segmented nature of the influenza virus genome makes the development of new strains possible through mutation and rearrangement of gene segments between human and animal strains of the virus. This genetic instability and the resulting emergence of new strains are responsible for the annual flu epidemics and periodic pandemics (see Chapter 18, Emerging Infectious Diseases). The prophylactic vaccines and antiviral drugs that are now available make it possible to prevent serious disease complications in people at risk. Example of known flu pandemics (worldwide) are given in Table 7.6.

Paramyxoviruses

Paramyxoviruses belong to the family *Paramyxoviridae*, which consists of three genera: *Morbillivirus, Paramyxovirus,* and *Pneumovirus.*

- *Morbillivirus* includes the measles viruses.
- *Paramyxovirus* includes the parainfluenza and mumps viruses.
- *Pneumovirus* includes the respiratory syncytial virus.

Paramyxoviruses have a (−) ssRNA genome, are highly pleomorphic and enveloped, with helical nucleocapsid symmetry. The Nipah virus and Hendra virus, zoonosis-causing viruses, are highly pathogenic paramyxoviruses identified in 1998 after outbreaks of severe encephalitis in Malaysia and Singapore. Protection can be provided for the measles and mumps viruses by an effective live vaccine used in the United States and other developed countries. Vaccination programs in these countries make the occurrence of measles and mumps rare.

Picornaviruses

Picornaviruses are viruses belonging to the family *Picornaviridae*. They are one of the largest families of viruses and are the smallest of the RNA viruses. Picornaviruses are nonenveloped viruses with icosahedral nucleocapsids containing a (+) ssRNA as their genome. This RNA is similar to mRNA and can either act as mRNA or can be a template for a replicate form. Picornaviruses are separated into nine distinct genera, with many of them important pathogens of humans and animals. They include *Enterovirus, Rhinovirus, Hepatovirus, Cardiovirus, Aphthovirus, Parechovirus, Erbovirus, Kobuvirus,* and *Teschovirus.*

Two main categories causing a variety of human infections are the enteroviruses and the rhinoviruses. They are distinctly different in the stability of their capsid at low pH as well as in their optimal temperature for growth. The capsid of enteroviruses is stable at the pH 3, which allows them to survive under harsh environmental conditions such as the gastrointestinal tract and sewer systems. They are transmitted by the fecal–oral route. In contrast, the rhinoviruses are acid labile; they infect primarily the nose and throat; and they grow best at 33° C (temperature of the nasal cavity). Enteroviruses replicate at 37° C. The portal of entry (see Chapter 9, Infection and Disease) can be the upper respiratory tract, the oropharynx, and the gastrointestinal tract. Most enteroviruses are cytolytic; they replicate rapidly and cause direct damage to the infected cells. In the case of poliovirus, the virus infects skeletal muscle and gains entry to the nervous system by traveling along the innervating nerve fibers (see Chapter 13, Infections of the Nervous System and Senses). Rhinoviruses are the most common initiators of the common cold and upper respiratory tract infections. There are 115 or more serotypes of rhinovirus; their infections are self-limiting and generally do not cause serious disease.

Rhabdoviruses

Members of the family *Rhabdoviridae* infect plants, insects, fish, birds, and mammals, including humans. Rhabdoviruses are simple viruses that carry their genome in the form of a (−) ssRNA. They encode only five proteins, are enveloped, and have a characteristic bullet-shaped appearance. The most significant pathogen of this group is the rabies virus, causing the almost invariably fatal disease called *rabies*. Until Louis Pasteur developed the rabies vaccine, a bite from a rabid animal always led to certain death. Although rare, it is possible that a person may contract rabies if infectious material from a rabid animal, such as saliva, gains entry directly though their eyes, nose, mouth, or a wound. For protective purposes the rabies vaccine is now given to people at high risk of exposure. People not vaccinated and who have been bitten by an animal or otherwise been exposed to rabies can receive vaccination after the exposure to prevent the disease.

Reoviruses

The name reovirus was given to a group of enteric and respiratory viruses not associated with a particular disease and were considered to be "respiratory, enteric, orphans." Reoviruses are nonenveloped with an icosahedral nucleocapsid and a dsRNA genome. The virion is rather resistant to undesirable environmental and gastrointestinal conditions such as variations in pH and temperature, detergents, and drying. One of the genera of reoviruses is *Rotavirus,* the causative agent of human infantile gastroenteritis (see Chapter 12, Infections of the Gastrointestinal System), a common disease in children. The virus accounts for approximately 50% of all case of diarrhea in children requiring hospitalization because of dehydration. Rotaviral infections are a major problem in underdeveloped countries, where the virus is responsible for more than 1 million deaths per year. Rotaviruses are also one of the causes of "traveler's" diarrhea.

Retroviruses

Retroviruses are classified according to the disease they cause, tissue tropism and host range, virion morphology, and complexity of the genome. The subfamilies of the human retroviruses are *Oncovirinae, Lentivirinae,* and *Spumavirinae* (Table 7.7). The viruses are enveloped, somewhat spherical in shape, and their genome consists of two identical copies of (+) ssRNA. These viruses have a unique replication cycle: they encode an RNA-dependent DNA polymerase (reverse transcriptase), which allows them to replicate through a DNA intermediate. The DNA copy of the viral genome, called a **provirus,** is then integrated into the host cell DNA and thereby becomes a cellular gene.

Togaviruses

Members of the family *Togaviridae* are enveloped (+) ssRNA viruses with icosahedral nucleocapsid symmetry. They include the genera *Alphavirus* and *Rubivirus*. Alphaviruses are found around the world and many of them are pathogenic to humans. The most common results of alphaviral infections include infectious arthritis, encephalitis, rashes, and fever. Alphaviruses are of interest in gene therapy research laboratories for the development of viral vectors for gene delivery.

Rubivirus contains only one recognized species, the rubella virus, and the causative agent of rubella (German measles). In contrast to the other togaviruses, rubella is a respiratory virus (see Chapter 11, Infections of the Respiratory System).

Flaviviruses

Flaviviruses are enveloped viruses with (+) ssRNA and icosahedral nucleocapsid symmetry, making them similar to togaviruses but they differ in their method of replication. Flaviviruses are the causative agents of yellow fever, encephalitis, Dengue fever, and hepatitis C.

Subviral Agents

Subviral agents are substances smaller than a virus but having some viral properties. These are unusual infectious agents with a characteristically small genome, and include **viroids, virusoids (satellites),** and **prions.**

Viroids

Viroids range in size from 15 to 100 nm in diameter, and their RNA genomes are 246 to 375 nucleotides in length. They are all single-stranded circles; replication does not depend on the presence of a helper virus, and no proteins are encoded. They are common plant pathogens causing serious economic problems. Although they do not have a protective protein coat around the nucleic acid, these naked RNA pathogens can cause disease in susceptible plants. These plants include potatoes, tomatoes, cucumbers, palm trees, and certain fruit trees. The current taxonomy of viroids is shown in Table 7.8.

Virusoids (Satellites)

Virusoids or satellites RNAs have genomes from 220 to 388 nucleotides long, their genomes are circular and single stranded, and they have ribozyme activity. Virusoids replicate in the cytoplasm of their host, using an RNA-dependent RNA polymerase. Although the RNA replication is similar to that of viroids, virusoids require that the host cell be infected with a specific helper virus. Virusoids are generally associated with plant infections, but there are similar agents that infect animals. One of these agents infecting humans is the hepatitis delta virus (HDV). For hepatitis D virusoid to function, a cell must be simultaneously infected with the hepatitis B virus. However, there is a significant difference between viroids and HDV: viroids cannot produce proteins whereas HDV produces two proteins named small and large delta antigens.

Prions

Prions (proteinaceous infectious particles) are infectious agents that do not have a nucleic acid genome. Prions are normal proteins in animal tissue, but when these particles become abnormally folded and shaped they become proteinaceous infectious particles that are not cellular organisms or viral particles. In their noninfectious stage they are normal proteins involved in cell-to-cell communication. Once they become infectious prions and come in contact with physiological normally shaped proteins, these particles will transform the normal proteins into abnormally shaped prions. Prions are associated with a variety of neurodegenerative diseases with a slow onset and previously considered to be caused by slow viruses. Prion diseases are transmissible from host to host of a single species, or sometimes from one species to another. They destroy brain tissue, giving it a spongy appearance, and thus also referred to as the transmissible spongiform encephalopathies (TSEs), such as "mad cow disease."

TABLE 7.7 Subfamilies of Retroviruses

Subfamily	Characteristics
Oncovirinae	Associated with cancer and neurological disorders
Type B	Unconventional nucleocapsid in mature virus
Type C	Centrally located nucleocapsid core in mature virion
Type D	Cylindrical nucleocapsid core
Lentivirinae	Slow disease onset: neurologic disorders and immunosuppression; are D-type viruses (cylindrical nucleocapsid core)
Spumavirinae	No clinical disease, but characteristic vacuolated "foamy" cytopathology
Endogenous viruses	Retrovirus sequence that can be integrated into the human genome

TABLE 7.8 Classification of Viroids

Family (Subfamily)	Genus	Species	Hosts
Pospiviroidae	*Pospiviroid*	Potato spindle tuber viroid	Plants
	Hostuviroid	Hop stunt viroid	
	Cocadviroid	Coconut cadang-cadang viroid	
	Apscaviroid	Apple scar skin viroid	
	Coleviroid	Coleus blumei viroid 1	
Avsunviroidae	*Avsunviroid*	Avocado sunblotch viroid	Plants
	Pelamonviroid	Peach latent mosaic viroid	

Examples of Human Prion Diseases

Disease	Transmission	Clinical Signs and Symptoms	Treatment
Creutzfeldt-Jacob disease (CJD)	Spontaneous transformation of normal prion proteins; 10%–15% inherited (autosomal dominant)	Dementia Early neurologic signs: Periodic waves on the electroencephalogram (EEG); presence of "florid plaques" on neuropathology; presence of agent in lymphoid tissue	None known; rapidly progressive and always fatal
Variant Creutzfeldt-Jacob disease (vCJD)	"Mad cow" disease: Contracted when exposed to food contaminated with bovine spongiform encephalopathy (BSE)	Prominent psychiatric/behavioral symptoms; painful dyesthesiasis (distortion of the sense of touch); delayed neurological signs; large amounts of "florid plaques" on neuropathology	Supportive: No specific treatment; fatal
Gerstmann-Sträussler-Scheinker syndrome	Inherited	Various levels of ataxia; dysarthria (slurring of speech), dementia, nystagmus, spasticity, visual disturbances	No cure, no known treatment, only supportive
Kuru	Cannibalism	Unsteady gait, tremors, slurred speech	No cure, no treatment, only supportive

Summary

- Virus classification is primarily based on morphology, nucleic acid type, mode of replication, host organism, and the type of disease caused. The two classification systems used most often are the ICTV system and the Baltimore system.
- Viruses can infect bacteria, plants, and animals.
- In general, viruses are host specific, as well as specific to tissues and cells.
- According to the shape and arrangement of capsomeres and the presence or absence of an envelope, viruses can be classified into four distinct morphological types: helical, icosahedral, enveloped, and complex.
- The viral genome is represented by nucleic acids, either RNA or DNA, which can be in the form of single- or double-stranded molecules.

- Viruses do not replicate through cell division; they use the host cell machinery and metabolism to manufacture multiple copies of themselves. Although similar, the mechanism of replication varies between bacteriophages and animal viruses.
- Viral infections of animal cells can have different outcomes; they can be abortive, lytic, or persistent infections.
- Viral infections are usually associated with changes in the host cells and include morphological, physiological, and biochemical transformations.
- Subviral agents causing infections in plants, human, and animals are classified as viroids, virusoids (satellites), and prions.

Review Questions

1. Viruses can infect:
   a. Plants
   b. Bacteria
   c. Animals
   d. All organisms

2. The correct hierarchical order for virus classification is:
   a. Order, genus, family, subfamily, species
   b. Species, genus, family, subfamily, order
   c. Order, family, subfamily, genus, species
   d. Genus, order, family, subfamily, species

3. Viral capsomeres are composed of subunits called:
   a. Envelopes
   b. Protomeres
   c. Capsids
   d. Nucleoids

4. RNA viruses belong to which of the following groups according to the Baltimore classification system?
   a. I, II, III
   b. II, III, IV
   c. I, IV, V
   d. II, IV, V

5. A phage in a repressed stage is referred to as a(n):
   a. Antiphage
   b. Prophage
   c. Virulent phage
   d. Latent phage

6. The correct sequence of stages in the multiplication of animal viruses is:
   a. Adsorption, penetration, uncoating, replication, assembly, release
   b. Penetration, adsorption, assembly, uncoating, replication, release
   c. Adsorption, uncoating, penetration, replication, assembly, release
   d. Penetration, uncoating, adsorption, replication, assembly, release

7. A persistent infection that is not lytic but productive is called a _____ infection.
   a. Chronic
   b. Latent
   c. Slow
   d. Transforming

8. All of the following are cytopathic effects as a result of a viral infection *except*:
   a. Altered shape
   b. Lysis
   c. Change in antigens
   d. Membrane fusion

9. Which of the following viruses belong to the family *Herpesviridae*?
   a. Epstein-Barr virus
   b. Poxvirus
   c. SARS-CoV
   d. HIV

10. Transmissible spongiform encephalopathies are caused by:
    a. Flaviviruses
    b. Virusoids
    c. Prions
    d. Orthomyxoviruses

11. A virus that infects bacteria is referred to as a(n) _____.

12. Kaposi's sarcoma is caused by human herpesvirus number _____.

13. Members of *Picornaviridae* are _____ viruses.

14. A fully assembled virus is called a(n) _____.

15. Group VI viruses according to the Baltimore classification system include the families *Metaviridae, Pseudoviridae,* and _____.

16. Discuss the two methods of viral classification.

17. Describe host cell damage resulting from viral infections.

18. Name and describe the different morphological types of viruses.

19. Describe and contrast the multiplication of bacteriophages versus animal viruses.

20. Explain and discuss the structure and pathogenicity of subviral agents.

Bibliography

Bauman R: *Microbiology: With Diseases by Taxonomy*, ed 2, 2007, Benjamin Cummings/Pearson, San Francisco.

Forbes BA, Sahm, DF, Weissfeld AS: *Bailey & Scott's Diagnostic Microbiology*, ed 12, St. Louis, 2007, Mosby/Elsevier.

Klug WS, Cummings MR, Spencer CA, et al: *Concepts of Genetics*, ed 9, 2009, Benjamin Cummings/Pearson, San Francisco.

Madigan MT, Martinko JM, Dunlap PV, et al: *Brock: Biology of Microorganisms*, ed 12, 2009, Benjamin Cummings/Pearson, San Francisco.

Mims C, Dockrell HM, Goering RV, et al: *Medical Microbiology*, ed 3, St. Louis, 2004, Mosby/Elsevier.

Murray PR, Rosenthal KS, Pfaller MA: *Medical Microbiology*, ed 5, St. Louis, 2005, Mosby/Elsevier.

Talaro KP: *Foundations in Microbiology*, ed 6, New York, 2005, McGraw-Hill.

Internet Resources

Baron S, editor: *Medical Microbiology*, ed 4, Galveston, 1996, The University of Texas Medical Branch at Galveston. http://www.ncbi.nlm.nih.gov/books/bv.fcgi?rid=mmed

International Committee on Taxonomy of Viruses, ICTVdB Index of Viruses, http://www.ncbi.nlm.nih.gov/ICTVdb/Ictv/index.htm

Centers for Disease Control and Prevention (CDC), http://www.cdc.gov/

MicrobiologyBytes: Virology: Mimivirus, http://www.microbiologybytes.com/virology/Mimivirus.html

CDC, Avian Influenza A Virus Infections of Humans, http://www.cdc.gov/flu/avian/gen-info/avian-flu-humans.htm

World Health Organization, Avian influenza, http://www.who.int/csr/disease/avian_influenza/en/

Microbiology and Immunology On-line, University of South Carolina School of Medicine, Part Two: Bacteriology, http://pathmicro.med.sc.edu/book/bact-sta.htm

indiaPRwire, "GangaGen granted new US patent on therapeutic bacteriophages," http://www.indiaprwire.com/pressrelease/biotechnology/20061004693.htm

EverGreen, Phage Biology and Phage Therapy, http://www.evergreen.edu/phage/phagetherapy/phagetherapy.htm

Phage Therapy Center, http://www.phagetherapycenter.com/pii/PatientServlet?command=static_home

University of Maryland, General Microbiology, List of Lecture Topics, http://www.life.umd.edu/classroom/bsci424/BSCI223WebSiteFiles/LectureList.htm

Microbiology and Immunology On-line, University of South Carolina School of Medicine, Part Three: Virology, http://pathmicro.med.sc.edu/book/virol-sta.htm

MicrobiologyBytes: Virology: Viroids, http://www.microbiologybytes.com/virology/Viroids.html

USDA Agricultural Research Service, VIROIDS!—From Scourge to Boon in the 21st Century? http://www.ars.usda.gov/is/AR/archive/dec99/boon1299.htm

Mayo Clinic, http://www.mayoclinic.com/

World Health Organization, http://www.who.int/en/

CDC, Prion Diseases, http://www.cdc.gov/ncidod/dvrd/prions/

National Institute of Neurological Disorders and Stroke, Disorder Index, http://www.ninds.nih.gov/disorders/disorder_index.htm

Merck Manuals Online Medical Library, Viral Infections, http://www.merck.com/mmhe/sec17/ch198/ch198a.html

8

Eukaryotic Microorganisms

OUTLINE

Introduction

Fungi
Characteristics of Fungi
Life Cycle of Fungi
Classification of Fungi

Algae
Characteristics of Algae
Life Cycle of Algae
Classification of Algae

Protozoans
Characteristics of Protozoans
Life Cycle of Protozoans
Classification of Protozoans

Slime Molds
Cellular Slime Molds
Plasmodial Slime Molds

Helminths
Characteristics of Helminths
Life Cycle of Helminths
Classification of Helminths

LEARNING OBJECTIVES

After reading this chapter, the student will be able to:
- Describe, compare, and differentiate the characteristics of fungi, algae, protozoans, and helminths
- Describe the defining characteristics of fungi and explain the difference between their sexual and asexual reproduction
- Identify the medically important fungi
- Name the defining characteristics of algae, classify them, and describe the difficulties in their classification
- Describe the general characteristics of asexual and sexual reproduction of algae
- Identify the three defining and the common characteristics of protozoans

- Describe the general life cycle of protozoans and explain the importance of the macro- and micronucleus
- Discuss the fundamental differences between cellular and plasmodial slime molds
- Describe the main characteristics of parasitic helminths
- Describe the life cycles of flukes, tapeworms, and roundworms, and classify them into the appropriate categories

KEY TERMS

apical complex
definitive host
dikaryon
coenocytic
cyst
flatworms
harmful algal blooms
   (HABs)
Harmful Algal Bloom-
   related Illness
   Surveillance System
   (HABISS)
heterotrophic

hyphae
intermediate hosts
macronucleus
merozoites
micronucleus
mitosomes
mycelium
mycology
mycorrhizae
National Center for
   Environmental Health
   (NCEH)
plasmodium

roundworms
saprobes
schizogony
scolex
septate hyphae
sporangia
sporangium
sporozoite
tapeworms
thallus
trophozoite

WHY YOU NEED TO KNOW

HISTORY

The bacterial pathogen *Yersinia pestis* has been identified as the causative agent of the "Black Death," or bubonic plague, which killed about a third of the known world's population during several centuries of the Middle Ages. A viral pathogen (influenza virus A subtype H1N1) caused the Great Influenza Pandemic of 1918, which took an estimated 100 million lives over a period of about 9 months in 1918 to 1919! On occasion there are related current outbreaks of bird flu and bubonic plague. The threat of these pandemics is so horrendous that there is a tendency to underplay the significance of other groups of organisms.

However, fungi, algae, protozoans, and helminths have also proven to be significant players in the field of human pathogens. For example, a type of algae containing a neurotoxin is responsible for "red tide" fish kill outbreaks that periodically occur off the shores of the Pacific, New England, and Gulf Coast states. These algae release a cellular product, saxitoxin, which is toxic to fish and other marine life. When shellfish from contaminated waters is consumed by humans it can cause serious neuromuscular problems and/or death, if the condition is untreated. Other protozoans are human pathogens responsible for such diseases as amoebic dysentery, malaria, and toxoplasmosis, to name but a few. Interactions between helminths and humans also result in diseases such as trichinosis, tapeworm infections, elephantiasis, and schistosomiasis. Virtually all the diseases mentioned have been recorded throughout the history of human diseases.

Moreover, in cases such as malaria, once the complex life cycle of the organism (*Plasmodium* spp.) and its vector

(*Anopheles* spp.) was uncovered and understood, great strides were made in eradicating the disease in developed countries, but it is far from eradicated in developing countries. Malaria remains one the most costly and prevalent unconquered human diseases at large in the world. One of the first recorded references to the disease can be found in early Chinese and Hindu writings. It is estimated that malaria—the name comes from the Medieval Italian *mal aria*, or bad air, because it was associated with the foul-smelling odors of the swamps near Rome—has been a pathogen of humans throughout all of recorded history. In the late fifth century BCE, Hippocrates described aspects of the disease in his writings. A series of discoveries were made in the late 1800s by independent researchers and physicians that led to a complete picture of the life cycle of *Plasmodium*, the organism responsible for causing malaria. Sir Ronald Ross, a British army surgeon who, using birds as experimental models, established the major stages of the life cycle, in 1902 received the Nobel Prize for his work. Malaria accounted for much suffering and death among troops participating in the American Civil War, the Spanish–American War, World War II, the Korean War, and the Vietnam War. In an attempt to free the world of malaria, in 1955 the World Health Organization (WHO) began a worldwide program to eradicate the disease. Unfortunately, the program collapsed by 1976 because of the emergence of resistance to DDT (dichlorodiphenyltrichloroethane) by the mosquito vectors that play a critical part in the life cycle and the development of resistance to chloroquine, the drug used to fight *Plasmodium*, the causative protozoan agent.

continued

IMPACT

Malaria is endemic in countries in a belt area roughly about the equator in tropical and subtropical climates. These equatorial countries include South and Central America, Africa, China, the Middle East, India, and Asia. This disease is responsible for about half a billion infections per year; 1 to 3 million deaths per year or, as you read this, about a death every half a minute! If the disease remains uncontrolled, this death rate is estimated to double in 20 years.

Malaria, being a disease associated with poverty, is also a hindrance to economic progress, particularly where it is endemic in developing countries. The disease causes loss of work days, school days, and loss of days/weeks for the caregivers who must be absent from their occupations, not to mention loss of investments from tourism. For example, affected areas such as sub-Saharan Africa, where about 90% of the fatalities occur, cost Africa $12 billion annually, which is about 40% of the total public health expenditure.

With the recognition of extraerythrocytic (latent liver) forms of the disease in the 1980s, new strategies have been viewed to institute better treatment and/or a potential cure or vaccine.

FUTURE

Protection from severe endemic diseases such as malaria is best achieved with vaccines. Some of the ideal characteristics of a vaccine include safety, simple application, life-long protection, low cost, and ease of distribution, to mention a few. Not all these features are obtainable and are generally approached to varying degrees. Prevention and treatment of malaria begin with eradication of the female *Anopheles* mosquito vector followed by the development of a vaccine and treatments that can attack the sporozoite, liver, merozoite, or sexual stages. All of this must be cost-effective as sub-Saharan Africa is also beset by HIV/AIDS and tuberculosis. Given the socioeconomic environment, additional factors of application of successful drug candidates come to play important roles. The Malaria Vaccine Initiative (MVI), sponsored by the Bill & Melinda Gates Foundation; Roll Back Malaria (RBM); and Medicines for Malaria Venture (MMV) of the WHO are examples of complementing programs currently in the works.

Introduction

Eukaryotic organisms differ from bacteria and archaea in many ways including cell size, internal structure, and genetic properties (see Chapter 3, Cell Structure and Function). The classification of eukaryotes has changed over the centuries starting in the late eighteenth century with Linnaeus, who classified all organisms as either plants or animals. At present, instead of the traditional classification schemes, many taxonomists favor classification schemes that are based on distinguishing characteristics at the molecular level. Modern taxonomy attempts to explain the genetic relationships of microbes and place them in groups based on similarities in their biochemical and metabolic characteristics, their nucleotide sequences, as well as their cellular ultrastructure as revealed by electron microscopy. Although universal support for a particular classification scheme has not been reached, many taxonomists favor a scheme similar to the one shown in Figure 8.1.

Many eukaryotic organisms are pathogens, and according to the World Health Organization (WHO, Geneva, Switzerland), parasitic diseases rank among the top 20 microbial causes of death in the world, especially in the developing countries. These pathogens are not only fungi, algae, and protozoans, but also include parasitic helminths. Although helminths are not microorganisms, they play an important role in infectious disease and for that reason are also addressed in this chapter.

Fungi

The study of fungi is called **mycology,** and although more than 100,000 species of fungi are known, only about 200 are pathogenic to humans and animals, and relatively few fungi are virulent enough to be considered primary pathogens (Table 8.1). Moreover, the incidence of fungal infections has been increasing, especially those acquired in hospitals (nosocomial), other institutional settings such as nursing homes, and in people with a compromised immune system.

Fungi have important symbiotic relationships with other organisms and therefore can be beneficial to life in general. For example, they play a major role in the decomposition of dead plant material, and they are the primary decomposers of material such as cellulose, which cannot be digested by animals. The majority of plants are dependent on their symbiotic relationship with **mycorrhizae** (fungi that help the roots of plants to absorb minerals and water from the soil). Fungi provide food for humans in the form of mushrooms and truffles, and they are used in the manufacture of foods and beverages, including breads, alcoholic beverages, citric acid, soy sauce, and some cheeses. Fungi also produce pharmaceuticals such as the antibiotics penicillin and cephalosporin (see Chapter 22, Antimicrobial Drugs, for details). In addition, fungi are of use in the making of the immunosuppressive drug cyclosporine for organ transplant patients, and mevinic acids, which are used in the

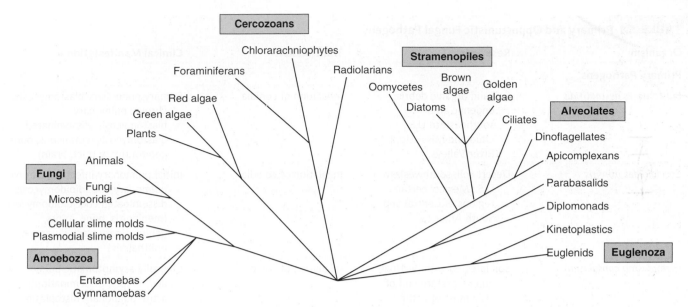

FIGURE 8.1 Phylogenetic tree of eukaryotic organisms. This phylogenetic tree of eukaryotic organisms is based on current knowledge of biochemical, metabolic, and genetic characteristics as well as ultrastructure.

manufacture of cholesterol-reducing drugs. Fungi are also important research tools in genetics and biotechnology (see Chapter 25, Biotechnology).

Characteristics of Fungi

Fungi are eukaryotes but are quite different from plants and animals. Fungal colonies are vegetative structures because they are made up of cells involved in catabolism and growth. Whether microscopic or macroscopic, they generally grow as filamentous, multinucleated organisms that form threadlike filaments called **hyphae,** or as unicellular fungal organisms (Figure 8.2, *A*). Morphologically, fungi are often divided into three groups.

- *Mushrooms:* Mostly macroscopic organisms
- *Yeasts:* Mostly microscopic
- *Molds:* Both microscopic and macroscopic

Most fungi that are identified as human pathogens are microscopic. Hyphae are long, branching filamentous cells of a fungus and they represent its main vegetative growth. A collective mass of the threadlike hyphae is called the **mycelium** (Figure 8.2, *B*). A mycelium can be small, forming colonies too small to see with the naked eye, or they can be extensive, such as *Armillaria gallica,* which was described as extending through 37 acres of forest soil and was estimated to weigh at least 9700 kg.

Depending on environmental conditions such as temperature, fungi can exhibit different morphological characteristics, a condition referred to as dimorphism. They may appear as yeasts, molds, or fleshy fungi. For instance, some fungi can grow as a mold at room temperature (about 25° C) and as yeast at 37° C. Fungi often adapt to an environment that is hostile to bacteria. They are free-living and **heterotrophic** organisms (i.e., they use

organic compounds as their source of carbon). Although fungi, like bacteria, absorb nutrients rather than ingest them, they differ in several nutritional characteristics as well:

- Fungi tend toward maximal growth in a somewhat acidic environment, at about pH 5, which is too acidic for the growth of most bacteria (with such exceptions as *Helicobacter pylori*, which likes to grow at the pH of the human stomach [see Chapter 12, Infections of the Gastrointestinal System]).
- Most fungi are more resistant to osmotic pressure than are bacteria and can grow in relatively high concentrations of sugar or salt.
- Fungi can grow on substances with low moisture content, too low to support bacterial growth.
- Fungi metabolize more complex carbohydrates than bacteria.

Fungi have a cell wall, typically composed of a strong, flexible, nitrogenous polysaccharide called *chitin,* and a plasma membrane that contains ergosterol. Fungi differ from plants because they lack chlorophyll and therefore do not use photosynthesis in their metabolic processes. Moreover, their ribosomal RNA is an 80S rRNA, which is the same as in humans and animals. For medical/treatment purposes, important aspects of fungal metabolism include the following:

- Chitin synthesis and other compounds for use in the cell wall, materials that induce hypersensitivity (see Chapter 20, The Immune System)
- Ergosterol synthesis for the plasma membrane, making the plasma membrane susceptible to antimicrobial agents targeting ergosterol synthesis or ergosterol incorporation into the plasma membrane (see Chapter 22, Antimicrobial Drugs)

TABLE 8.1 Primary and Opportunistic Fungal Pathogens

Organism	Reservoir	Transmission	Clinical Manifestation
Primary Pathogens			
Blastomyces dermatitidis	Soil and organic debris; endemic area southeastern U.S., Ohio and Mississippi River Valleys	Inhalation of conidia	Primary pulmonary blastomycosis; chronic pulmonary blastomycosis; disseminated blastomycosis (cutaneous, bone, genitourinary tract, brain)
Coccidioides immitis	Desert soil; southwestern U.S.; Mexico; certain regions of Central and South America	Inhalation of conidia	Initial pulmonary infection; chronic pulmonary coccidioidomycosis; disseminated coccidioidomycosis (meningitis, bone, joints, genitourinary tract, cutaneous, ophthalmic)
Histoplasma capsulatum	Soil infested with bird/bat guano; eastern half of U.S.; most of Latin America; parts of Asia, Europe, and Middle East	Inhalation of conidia	Clinically asymptomatic pulmonary and "cryptic dissemination"; acute pulmonary histoplasmosis, mediastinitis, pericarditis; chronic pulmonary histoplasmosis
Paracoccidioides brasiliensis	Soil and vegetation; Central and South America	Inhalation of conidia	Diverse clinical manifestations; chronic multifocal involvement (lungs, mouth, nose); juvenile progressive disease (lymph nodes, skin, and viscera)
Opportunistic Pathogens			
Candida spp.	Gastrointestinal mucosa, vaginal mucosa, skin, nails	Gastrointestinal translocation, intravascular catheters	Mucocutaneous candidiasis; oral/vaginal thrush; hematogenous dissemination; hepatosplenic candidiasis; endophthalmitis
Cryptococcus neoformans	Soil infested with bird guano	Inhalation of aerosolized yeast; percutaneous inoculation	Primary cryptoccal pneumonia; meningitis (particularly in HIV-infected patients); hematogenous dissemination; genitourinary cryptococcosis; primary cutaneous cryptococcosis
Aspergillus spp.	Soil, plants, water, pepper, air	Inhalation of conidia; transfer to wounds via contaminated bandages and/or tape	Allergic bronchopulmonary aspergillosis, sinusitis; aspergilloma; invasive aspergillosis (lung, brain, skin, gastrointestinal tract, heart)

- Toxin synthesis
  - Ergot alkaloids
  - Psychotropic agents
  - Aflatoxins
- Ribosomal synthesis

Fungal pathogens can be classified on the basis of their growth forms—filamentous, yeast, or dimorphic—and on the type of infection they can cause. For example, in superficial mycoses, the fungus grows on the surface of the skin or hair. In cutaneous and subcutaneous mycoses, nails and deeper layers of the skin are involved, and in systemic (deep) mycoses, the fungus spreads to internal organs (Box 8.1). Patients with a compromised immune system are especially susceptible to fungal infections. Whereas superficial and cutaneous mycoses are generally mild, systemic mycoses are serious and difficult to treat.

Yeasts

Yeasts exist as single cells that reproduce by budding. However, some species may become multicellular through the formation of connected budding cells referred to as pseudohyphae, or true

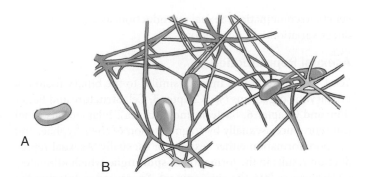

FIGURE 8.2 Fungi. Fungi can exist as **(A)** unicellular organisms, or **(B)** form a mycelium, a mass of hyphae that continues to grow.

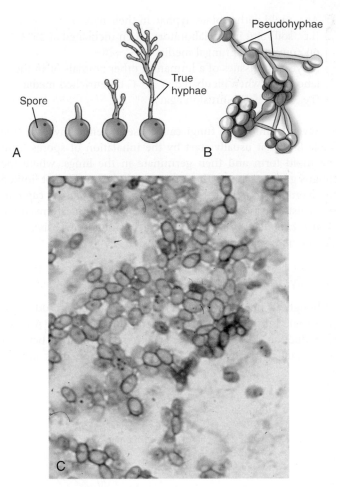

FIGURE 8.3 Yeast. Single yeast cells can reproduce by **(A)** budding or **(B)** become multicellular through the formation of pseudohyphae. **C,** Micrograph of a typical unicellular yeast culture.

BOX 8.1 Disease-causing Fungi
Superficial mycoses
- *Epidermophyton*
- *Microsporum*
- *Trichophyton*
- *Sporothrix*

Deep mycoses
- *Aspergillus*
- *Blastomyces*
- *Candida*
- *Coccidioides*
- *Cryptococcus*
- *Histoplasma*
- *Paracoccidioides*

MEDICAL HIGHLIGHTS

Yeast Infections—Candidiasis: The Fungus Among Us

Candidiasis is an infection that can be caused by more than 20 species of *Candida,* most commonly by *Candida albicans.* These fungi are often part of the normal human flora, but under certain conditions can become opportunistic organisms and cause yeast infections. The most common infections caused by *Candida albicans* are vaginal yeast infections, thrush (oral infection), and diaper rash.

---

hyphae (Figure 8.3). They can be classified according to the presence or absence of capsules, the size and shape of the cells, the mechanism of daughter cell formation, formation of hyphae, presence of sexual spores, and other physiological/genetic data. Yeasts may require oxygen for their metabolic activities as obligate aerobes or may be able to continue their metabolic activities in the absence of oxygen as facultative anaerobes. Yeasts do not require light for their growth.

Molds

Molds are rapidly growing, asexually reproducing fungi that grow on a variety of substances. They are characterized by the development of hyphae (long filaments of cells joined together), which results in colony characteristics that can be used for identification purposes. Hyphae can grow to immense proportions (see *Armillaria gallica,* earlier this chapter). In general, the hyphae in molds contain cross-walls called *septa,* which divide the hyphae into distinct uninuclear, cell-like units called **septate hyphae.** Some classes of fungi have **coenocytic** hyphae, which do not contain septa and appear as long, continuous cells with many nuclei (Figure 8.4). In an appropriate environment, the hyphae grow to form a mycelium that is visible to the naked eye.

Dimorphic Fungi

In general, microscopic fungi can be divided into two basic morphological forms: yeast and molds (hyphae). Some fungi can exhibit both growth forms depending on the conditions in which growth occurs, especially temperature. These fungi are called *dimorphic fungi.* Their patterns of growth are as follows:

- As a mold with septate hyphae in their natural reservoir (i.e., soil) and in the laboratory when incubated at 25° C on conventional fungal media
- As yeast in tissues of a human or other animals or in the laboratory when incubated at 37° C on enriched media (i.e., brain heart infusion agar)

Several dimorphic fungi can cause systemic mycoses (see Table 8.1) that usually start by the inhalation of spores from the mold form and then germinate in the lungs, where the fungus grows as yeast. These fungi include, but are not limited to, *Sporothrix schenckii* (sporotrichosis), *Histoplasma capsulatum* (histoplasmosis), *Blastomyces dermatitidis* (blastomycosis), *Paracoccidioides brasiliensis* (paracoccidioidomycosis), and *Coccidioides* spp. (coccidioidomycosis).

Life Cycle of Fungi

Although all fungi have some means of asexual reproduction (mitosis), most fungi can also reproduce sexually. Asexual reproduction does not involve genetic recombination between two sexual types, whereas sexual reproduction does involve genetic recombination. Sexual reproduction, as expected, introduces variation in a population.

Asexual Reproduction

Yeast typically bud in a manner similar to the binary fission of prokaryotic organisms (see Chapter 3, Cell Structure and Function; and Chapter 6, Bacteria and Archaea). Filamentous fungi can reproduce asexually by fragmentation of their hyphae, and by spore formation either sexually or asexually. Asexual reproduction results in the formation of **sporangia,** which ultimately release spores into the environment. Spores, after entering the respiratory tract, are common causes of infection (see Chapter 11, Infections of the Respiratory System). These asexual spores are often categorized on the basis of the nature and manner of spore development:

- Sporangiospores form inside a sac, the **sporangium,** which is attached to a stalk, the sporangiophore, located on the tips or sides of hyphae. The spores are released when the sporangium ruptures.
- Conidia (conidiospores) are produced at the tips or sides of hyphae but are not enclosed by a saclike structure. Their development involves the pinching off of the tip of a fertile hypha or the segmentation of a preexisting vegetative hypha. They are the most common of the asexual spores and exist in different forms (Figure 8.5):
  - Arthrospore: A rectangular spore, formed when a septate hypha breaks at the cross wall
  - Chlamydospore: A spherical conidium produced by the thickening of a hyphal cell that is released when the surrounding hyphae crack
  - Blastospore: A spore that buds from a parent cell
  - Phialospore: A spore that buds from the mouth of a vase-shaped, spore-bearing cell
  - Microconidium and macroconidium: Spores formed by the same fungus under different conditions, either as

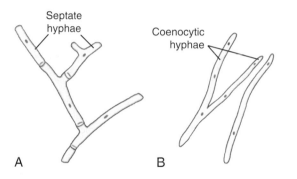

FIGURE 8.4 Hyphae. A, Septate hyphae; **B,** coenocytic hyphae.

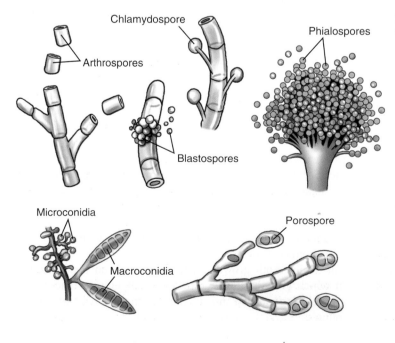

FIGURE 8.5 Types of asexual fungal spores.

one cell (microconidium) or as two or more cells (macroconidium)
- Porospore: A spore that grows out through small pores in a spore-bearing cell

Sexual Reproduction

Sexual reproduction introduces genetic variation into a population. The sexual reproduction phase of fungi, unlike asexual spore formation, introduces variable characteristics into its population. Moreover, sexual reproduction in fungi occurs when nutrients are limited, and/or other conditions are unfavorable for growth. Therefore, by this mechanism, survival of the species through genetic changes is made possible.

Because fungal mycelia are morphologically indistinguishable, rather than using the terms female and male, fungal mating types are designated as "+" and "−." Sexual reproduction of fungi can be summarized into four basic steps, with some differences occurring between groups.

- Haploid (n) cells from a + mycelium and a − mycelium fuse and form a **dikaryon.** This stage is not considered to be diploid or haploid, but is designated as (n + n).
- After a period of time, which ranges from hours to years and maybe even centuries, a pair of nuclei within the dikaryon finally fuses, forming a diploid (2n) nucleus.
- The meiotic cell division that follows restores the haploid state of the organism.
- The haploid nuclei are then divided into + and − spores, reestablishing the + and − mycelia.

Fungal spores are compact and lightweight, and therefore they can be dispersed widely throughout the environment by movement in air, water, and by other living organisms. Spores germinate on arriving at a favorable environment and thus form a new fungal colony within a brief period of time.

Classification of Fungi

Traditionally, fungi are divided into four major subgroups: Zygomycota, Ascomycota, Basidiomycota, and Deuteromycota. Some fungi form partnerships with either green algae or cyanobacteria and are considered a separate group: the lichens.

- *Zygomycota* are coenocytic (multinucleate) molds, most of which are **saprobes** (fungi that derive their nutrition from nonliving organic material); the remaining are obligate parasites of insects or other fungi.
- *Ascomycota* are the primary fungi causing food spoilage. This group also includes plant pathogens, both producing a negative impact on the economy. However, many of the Ascomycota are beneficial and probably the best known fungus in this category is *Penicillium* (Figure 8.6, *A*), the mold responsible for the production of the antibiotic penicillin (see Chapter 22, Antimicrobial Drugs). Another fungus in this group, *Saccharomyces* (Figure 8.6, *B*), ferments sugar to produce alcohol and carbon dioxide, the basic processes necessary in the baking and brewing industries. Furthermore, *Neurospora,* the pink bread mold,

is an important contributor in genetic and biochemical research.
- *Basidiomycota* include mushrooms (fleshy fungi) and other fruiting bodies of fungi (Figure 8.7). Many of the mushrooms are edible and some produce toxins and/or hallucinatory chemicals. In addition, the fungus *Cryptococcus neoformans* grows in the form of yeast in humans and is the leading cause of fungal meningitis. Besides the edible and poisonous forms, Basidiomycota are important decomposers, digesting cellulose and lignin of dead plants, which returns essential nutrients back to the soil.
- *Deuteromycota* are somewhat different than the other subgroups, and sometimes are referred to as "imperfect fungi." Whereas stages of sexual reproduction in the previously described groups have been well established, the sexual stages of Deuteromycota are unknown. Either this group of fungi does not produce sexual spores, or their sexual spores have not been identified at this time (recall that sexual spores may not form diploid nuclei for centuries).
- *Lichens* (Figure 8.8) consist of hyphae (mold) of a fungus and cyanobacteria or green algae. The mold, often an ascomycete, surrounds the photosynthetic cell and provides nutrients, water, and protection from drying out and

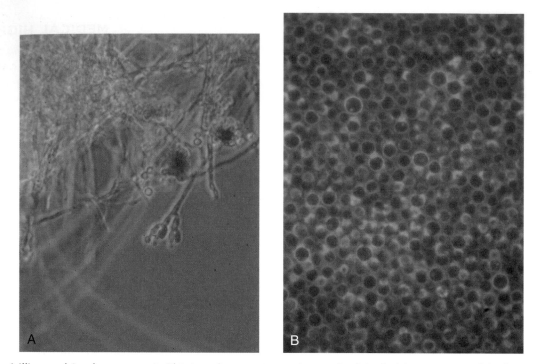

FIGURE 8.6 *Penicillium* and *Saccharomyces*. **A,** This is a phase-contrast micrograph of the fruiting structure of the fungus *Penicillium*, showing spore formation. **B,** This micrograph illustrates a dark-field image of the yeast *Saccharomyces*.

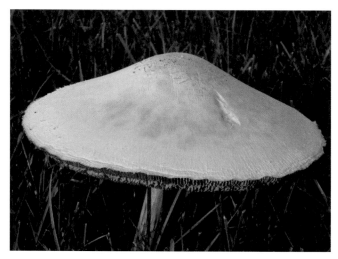

FIGURE 8.7 **Fleshy fungi.** Fungi display a wide variety of structures. This photograph shows a typical mushroom, a fleshy fungus with the cap and stem formed by a thick mat of hyphae that is collectively called a *mycelium*. The overall vegetative structure is called a *thallus*. Courtesy Andrew W. Van Meter.

excessive light. Conversely, the algae or cyanobacterium supplies carbohydrates and oxygen, the by-products of photosynthesis, to the fungus.

Algae

Algae are microscopic, photosynthetic organisms that are widespread in fresh and marine waters. They are a main component in plankton, a community of free-floating microscopic organisms that play an essential role in the aquatic food chain. Other algae are found in the soil, on rocks, plants, and some even exist in hot springs or snow banks. With the exception of *Prototheca,* a genus of unusual nonphotosynthetic algae that are associated with skin and subcutaneous infections in humans and animals, algae are rarely infectious.

Medical concerns involving algae are due primarily to food poisoning caused by toxins of marine algae such as dinoflagellates. Overgrowth of these motile organisms during certain times of the year causes "red tides," so named because they cause the water to turn a deep red color. As marine animals feed, they accumulate the toxin given off by the algae, and this toxin can persist for several months. These events cause severe disruptions in fisheries of the affected waters because filter-feeding shellfish become poisonous to humans because of the algal toxin. This paralytic shellfish poisoning of humans occurs after the consumption of toxin-exposed clams, shellfish, or other invertebrates. The poisoning is marked by severe neurological symptoms that can lead to death. Significantly, cooking does not destroy the toxin and to this date, no antidotes are available.

Another toxic algal form is *Pfiesteria piscicida,* which has been implicated in several episodes of massive fish kills in the United States. Although the disease was first reported in fish it has been observed in humans as well, especially those working around the waters in which an abundance of this organism exists. This newly identified species occurs in at least 20 forms, all of which are capable of releasing the toxin, and both fish and humans develop neurological symptoms and bloody skin lesions. Nutrient-rich agricultural runoff water has been shown to promote a sudden increase in *Pfiesteria.*

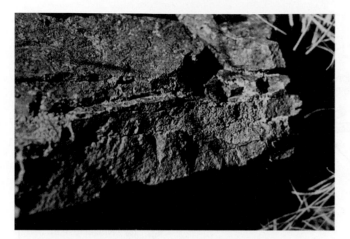

FIGURE 8.8 Lichens. This photo of a lichen shows the yellow fungal hyphae, which are visible to the naked eye. With a microscope one can see that the hyphae of the fungus form a matrix woven around algal cells; together the fungus and algae form a mutualistic association with physiological properties different from those of either of the individual species. From Atlas RM: *Principles of microbiology*, St. Louis, 1995, Mosby-Year Book.

LIFE APPLICATION

Harmful Algal Blooms: Pretty Poisons

Marine and freshwater are full of microscopic organisms, most of which are harmless and provide essential links in the food chain. However, a few species among the phytoplankton (autotrophic component of plankton) can produce potent toxins given opportunistic conditions for growth, causing **harmful algal blooms (HABs).** These algal blooms can occur in both marine and freshwater environments when a particular algal species succeeds in competition with other species and is allowed rapid reproduction. An HAB is a bloom that produces toxins that cause harm to plants and animals; it can kill fish, other aquatic life, and may also be harmful to humans in contact with the contaminated water or fish. Blooms can be caused by several factors, including agricultural runoff, fertilizers, and other environmental changes such as water quality, temperature, nutrients, and change in exposure to sunlight. Algal blooms can appear greenish, brown, reddish-orange, or have no color at all, as is the case with *Pfiesteria piscicida*. The National Center for Environmental Health (NCEH; http://www.cdc.gov/nceh/Information/about.htm) has developed the Harmful Algal Bloom-Related Illness Surveillance System (HABISS; http://www.cdc.gov/hab/surveillance.htm#about) to support public health decision-making in the case of algal blooms in particular areas in the United States.

Characteristics of Algae

All algae have two things in common: all are photosynthetic organisms and all are aquatic. Other than that, they differ in distribution, morphology, reproduction, and biochemical pref-

erences; they are not a unified group. The classification of algae is problematic and has not been completely determined. Historically, the differences in photosynthetic pigments, storage products, and cell wall composition have been used to classify algae into several groups. The groups according to their photosynthetic pigments are as follows: green algae, red algae, brown algae, golden algae, and yellow-green algae.

Life Cycle of Algae

All algae are capable of asexual reproduction. In unicellular algae the nucleus divides by mitosis and when the newly formed nuclei move to the opposite poles of the cell, the cell divides into two new cells by cytokinesis (see Chapter 3, Cell Structure and Function). Multicellular algae also may reproduce asexually by fragmentation, and each fragment is capable of forming a new **thallus** (the entire vegetative structure) or filaments.

Unicellular algae can also reproduce sexually and each algal cell then serves as a gamete, which can fuse with another gamete to form a zygote. This zygote then undergoes meiosis to return to the haploid state. When multicellular algae reproduce sexually, every cell in the reproductive structures of the algae becomes a gamete. The sexual reproduction of many algae can occur by alternation of haploid and diploid generations (Figure 8.9). In these life cycles, the diploid organism undergoes meiosis to produce male and female haploid spores, which then develop into haploid male and female thalli. In some algae, each of these will produce gametes that fuse to form a zygote, which then creates a new diploid thallus.

In some of the algal species, sexual and asexual reproduction can alternate, depending on the available growth conditions. Other species may alternate generations, whereby the offspring resulting from sexual reproduction reproduce asexually, and the next generation then reproduces sexually.

Classification of Algae

As mentioned earlier, the classification of algae is problematic and a summary of the algal groups described in this section and their characteristics is shown in Table 8.2.

- **Chlorophyta** are green algae whose pigments are chlorophylls *a* and *b*. They use sugar and starch as food reserves. Because of these and other similarities with plants, green algae are often considered to be progenitors of plants. Most green algae are unicellular or filamentous, living in freshwater ponds, lakes, and pools (Figure 8.10). They form a characteristic green to yellow scum.
- **Rhodophyta** (red algae) contain a red accessory pigment (thus their name) and use glycogen as their energy-storing molecule. Red algae have cell walls containing agar, a gelatinous substance used as a solidifying substance in microbiological culture media. This polysaccharide has many more applications, including its use as a thickener for soups, jellies, and ice cream, to name a few.
- **Phaeophyta** are commonly referred to as brown algae because of the presence of brown pigments (xanthophylls) in addition to chlorophylls and carotene. Depending on

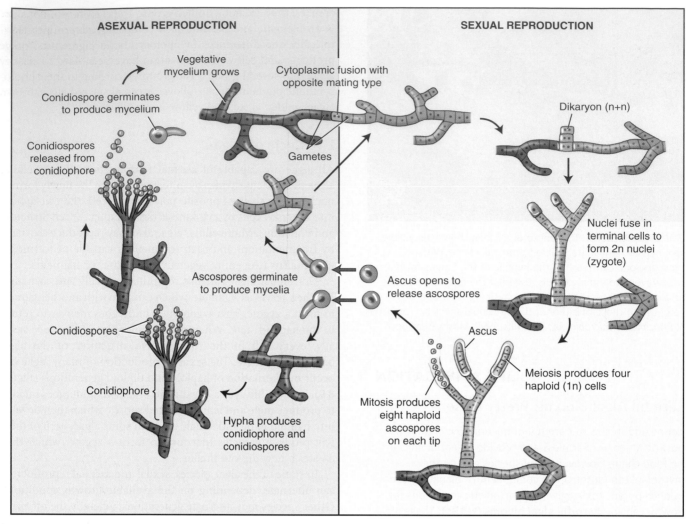

FIGURE 8.9 Asexual and sexual reproduction of algae.

TABLE 8.2 Summary of Algae

Group (Common Name)	Organization	Pigments	Storage Product(s)	Cell Wall	Habitat
Chlorophyta (green algae)	Varies from unicellular, colonial, filamentous, to multicellular	Chlorophylls *a* and *b*, carotene, xanthophylls	Sugar, starch	Cellulose or protein, absent in some	Fresh, brackish, and salt water; terrestrial
Rhodophyta (red algae)	Multicellular	Chlorophyll *a*, phycoerythrin, phycocyanin, xanthophylls	Glycogen (floridean starch)	Agar or carrageenan, some with calcium carbonate	Mostly salt water
Phaeophyta (brown algae)	Multicellular, vascular system, holdfasts	Chlorophylls *a* and *b*, xanthophylls	Laminarin, oils	Cellulose and alginic acid	Brackish and salt water
Chrysophyta (golden algae, yellow-green algae, diatoms)	Mainly unicellular, some filamentous forms, usually some form of motility	Chlorophylls, phycoerythrin, phycocyanin, xanthophylls	Chrysolaminarin	Cellulose, silica, calcium carbonate	Fresh, brackish, and salt water; terrestrial; ice

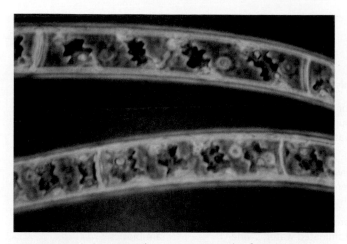

FIGURE 8.10 Spirogyra. This is a micrograph of *Spirogyra*, a filamentous green algae. From Atlas RM: *Principles of microbiology*, St. Louis, 1995, Mosby-Year Book.

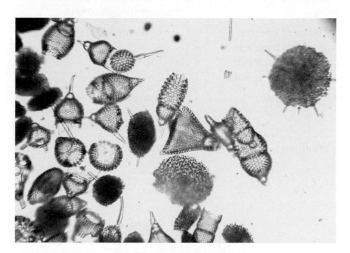

FIGURE 8.11 Diatoms. This is a micrograph of the silica "skeletons" of diatoms, algae in the division Chrysophyta.

the amount of brown pigments, these algae may appear brown, tan, yellow-brown, greenish brown, or green. Most brown algae are marine organisms.

- **Chrysophyta** is a diverse group of algae and some taxonomists lately have grouped them with brown algae because of similarities in the nucleotide sequences and flagellar structure. Diatoms, comprising one taxon in this group (Figure 8.11), have a unique cell wall composed of silica, and are a major component of marine phytoplankton. Phytoplankton include photosynthetic microorganisms that form the basis of food chains in the oceans. Significantly, because of their massive numbers, diatoms are the major source of the world's oxygen.

Protozoans

Protozoans are a group of microorganisms that are defined by three common characteristics: (1) they are eukaryotes; (2) they are unicellular; and (3) they lack a cell wall. Many protozoans are free-living organisms whereas others are potential parasites of humans and other animals. Notably, immunocompromised people are susceptible to all opportunistic organisms, including protozoans. For the most part, infections caused by protozoans are most prevalent in tropical and subtropical nations, but also occur in temperate regions.

Characteristics of Protozoans

Protozoans are unicellular organisms that vary in size and are defined by the three characteristics described in the previous section. Protozoa consist of a diverse group of microbes and with the exception of one subgroup they are motile due to cilia, flagella, and/or pseudopodia (see Chapter 3, Cell Structure and Function). Protozoans may vary in size, but all require a moist environment to survive. Most species live in ponds, streams, lakes, and oceans, whereas others live in moist soil, beach sand, and decaying organic matter. Aquatic protozoans are important components of plankton, the basis of the food chain of aquatic animals.

Most protozoa are chemoheterotrophs and obtain their nutrients from various sources, such as by phagocytizing:

- Bacteria
- Decaying organic matter
- Other protozoans
- Host tissue

However, some protozoans are photoautotrophic, such as the dinoflagellates and euglenoids. These organisms are sometimes classified as algal plants rather than as protozoans, which adds to the problematic nature of their classification.

Protozoans exist in a motile, active, feeding state called the **trophozoite** during times of plentiful food and moisture. If the environment becomes unfavorable for feeding and therefore growth, many species of protozoans are capable of entering a dormant stage in which the organism exists as a **cyst.** In this stage the organisms can be distributed by air, which may play a role in transmitting diseases such as amoebic dysentery. Given appropriate moisture and nutrients the cyst breaks open and becomes an active trophozoite.

A few protozoans are pathogens that infect the human body as intracellular or extracellular parasites. Intracellular parasites infect a wide variety of cells including erythrocytes, macrophages, epithelial cells, muscle cells, and cells of the nervous system. Extracellular parasites reside in the blood, intestine, or urogenital system (Table 8.3).

Life Cycle of Protozoans

The life cycle of protozoans ranges from simple to complex; some exist as trophozoite only, whereas others alternate between the trophozoite stage and the cyst stage. Asexual reproduction by fission, budding, or schizogony is the main method of reproduction in protozoans. **Schizogony** is the term for multiple fission, in which the nucleus undergoes multiple divisions before the cell divides. After the formation of multiple nuclei, small amounts of cytoplasm surround each nucleus, and the

Examples of Protozoal Infections

Organism	Disease	Transmission	Treatment/Drugs of Choice
Entamoeba histolytica	Amebiasis; amoebic dysentery	Ingestion of mature cysts through contaminated food or water	Iodoquinol, paromomycin, metronidazole, tinidazole
Naegleria fowleri	Amoebic meningoencephalitis	Through nose when swimming or diving in warm waters, underchlorinated swimming pools; free-living organism	Various treatments have been used; their effectiveness is unclear because most infections are still fatal
Balantidium coli	Balantidiasis	Fecal–oral route: fecally contaminated water; swine reservoir	Symptomatic treatment; antibiotics
Giardia lamblia (G. *intestinalis*)	Giardiasis	Zoonotic: contaminated water and food	Metrodinazole, tinidazole, nitazoxanide
Leishmania spp.	Leishmaniasis	Sandflea bites	Sodium stibogluconate
Toxoplasma gondii	Toxoplasmosis	Cleaning litterbox of infected cats; eating contaminated raw or partly cooked meat; contaminated drinking water	Pyrimethamine plus sulfadiazine
Plasmodium spp.	Malaria	Bite by infected mosquito	Chloroquine, quinine, primaquine, mefloquine; and some drug combinations
Trichomonas vaginalis	Trichomoniasis	Sexually transmitted	Metronidazole, tinidazole

TABLE 8.3 Protozoans as Parasites in the Human Body

Site of Infection	Organism
Blood	*Plasmodium vivax* (causes malaria) *Trypanosoma brucei* (causes trypanosomiasis)
Central nervous system	Amoebas *Plasmodium vivax* *Toxoplasma* *Trypanosoma*
Intestine	*Cryptosporidium* *Entamoeba* *Giardia* *Cyclospora* *Microsporidia* (can also infect other sites)
Liver	*Entamoeba* *Leishmania*
Skin	*Leishmania*
Urogenital tract	*Trichomonas*

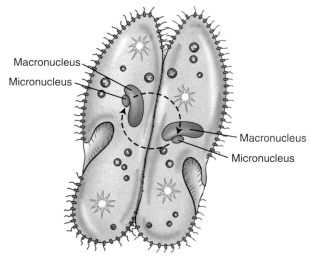

FIGURE 8.12 Conjugation of *Paramecium*. Each cell has a macronucleus, which is responsible for growth, and a haploid micronucleus. During conjugation the two cells fuse and the micronuclei of the two cells fuse. The parent cells, now fertilized, will separate and produce daughter cells with recombined DNA.

initial single cell separates into several daughter cells. Some parasitic species reproduce asexually within host cells by this method.

A few protozoa reproduce sexually by conjugation as seen in the ciliate *Paramecium* (see the next section, Classification of Protozoans). Conjugation is a form of genetic exchange by which members of two different mating types temporarily fuse and exchange nuclei. Each cell has two nuclei (Figure 8.12): a **macronucleus,** responsible for growth, and a haploid **micronucleus,** specialized for carrying out the process of conjugation.

Giardia: The Hiker's Uninvited Companion

Giardia lamblia is a flagellated protozoan, found worldwide in all types of climates, and is the most commonly identified intestinal parasite in the United States. Transmission is usually by the fecal–oral route via contaminated water. It only takes 10 cysts to establish infection and the cysts, which are resistant to the usual levels of chlorine in water treatment plants, can remain viable for more than 2 months in cold water. Giardiasis occurs in cities and other populated areas, but a higher risk for contracting the disease exists for hikers and campers who drink water from streams in remote areas where the water is thought to be pure and safe. The incubation period is usually between 6 and 20 days and the symptoms can range from simple nausea to vomiting, abdominal cramps, fatigue, weight loss, and explosive diarrhea. The symptoms usually persist for 1 to 4 weeks but in some cases can become chronic. To treat giardiasis, the drugs of choice include quinacrine and metronidazole, which have been shown to be effective. Short of filtration, the most effective way to make drinking water safe is to boil it for a minute or to add bleach or tincture of iodine to warm water. Infected individuals must be cautious, as a *Giardia* infection can be contagious. Effective ways to prevent transmission of the disease include proper hand washing and avoidance of swimming in recreational waters for at least 2 weeks after the cessation of disease symptoms.

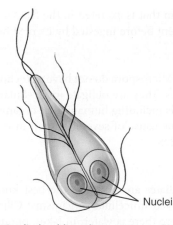

FIGURE 8.13 *Giardia lamblia.* The protozoan *Giardia lamblia* is equipped with flagella to provide whiplike motility for movement through its environment.

When two cells fuse, a micronucleus from each cell migrates to the other cell and fuses with a micronucleus within that cell. After this process is completed the parent cells separate; each is now a fertilized cell, and with later cell division they will produce daughter cells with recombinant DNA. The conjugation of protozoans is completely different from the bacterial process of the same name, discussed in Chapter 6 (Bacteria and Archaea).

The survival of protozoans in unfavorable conditions is due primarily to the variety of methods of reproduction and the ability of some species to form resting stages called *cysts*. A cyst allows the microbe to survive even when temperatures are not ideal, oxygen is unavailable, food is lacking, or toxic chemicals are present. A cyst also permits the parasite to survive outside a host, which is of importance because parasitic protozoa may have to be expelled from one host in order to find a new host.

Classification of Protozoans

Just as with other eukaryotic microorganisms the classification of protozoans has changed and today's taxonomists recognize that previous schemes do not reflect genetic relationships between them. More than two centuries ago Linnaeus classified protozoans as animals. Later, protozoans and algae were grouped into the kingdom Protista, and some taxonomists divided the protozoa into four groups, based on their mode of locomotion: (1) Sarcodina, (2) Mastigophora, (3) Ciliophora, and (4) Sporozoa. For many applications, this grouping according to locomotion is still the most common one. Because taxonomists still revise and refine the classification of protozoa on the basis of electron microscopic findings and even more so on the basis of nucleotide sequencing, this book focuses on medically important protozoans independent of their past, current, or future classification schemes. The groupings in this text are based on both unique morphologies as well as cellular structures and organelles. Protozoans may colonize and infect various areas of the human body, and particular infections have been selected for discussion of infections involving a particular organ system.

Archaezoa

Archaezoa are protists that do not have mitochondria but instead possess **mitosomes**—unique cell organelles that appear to be a remnant of mitochondria, but the function of which has not yet been identified. Mitosomes have been seen only in organisms that do not have mitochondria, including anaerobic or microaerophilic organisms. Because these protozoans do not contain mitochondria they cannot use oxidation for energy transformation. Mitosomes were first described in *Entamoeba histolytica*, an intestinal parasite of humans, and more recently have been identified in some species of *Microsporidia* as well as in *Giardia intestinalis* (also called *Giardia lamblia*). Although there are some similarities between mitochondria and mitosomes, mitosomes do not have genes within them. The genes for the components of these organelles are within the nuclear genome.

Many Archaezoa are spindle shaped and have two or more flagella, located mostly on the anterior (front) end, that are used for whiplike motility and allow the cells to move through their environment (Figure 8.13). Human parasites include *Trichomonas vaginalis* (see Chapter 17, Sexually Transmitted Infections/Diseases) and *Giardia* spp. (see Chapter 12, Infections of the Gastrointestinal System). *Trichomonas vaginalis* lacks a cyst stage and must be transferred from host to host rather quickly before it dries out. *Giardia lamblia,* on the other hand, is a cyst-forming organism that is excreted in the feces and can survive in the environment before ingested by its next host.

Microspora

Like Archaezoa, Microspora do not have mitochondria and also lack microtubules. They are obligate intercellular parasites in a variety of animals including humans. The organisms have been reported to be the cause of several human diseases, mostly in patients with AIDS.

Ciliophora

Ciliophora or ciliates are probably the best known and most frequently observed unicellular organisms. Ciliates are found almost everywhere there is water; in lakes, ponds, oceans, soil, and they can be obligate and opportunistic parasites. As their name indicates, they have cilia by which they either move themselves or move the water around their surface. Some of the ciliates have only one cilium, whereas others are covered with cilia, or have isolated tufts. All ciliates have a macronucleus and a micronucleus and therefore are capable of sexual as well as asexual reproduction. They are predators of bacteria and other single-celled organisms. A commonly studied organism in college teaching laboratories, and a well-known member of this group, is *Paramecium,* found in freshwater environments, especially ponds.

In general, ciliates are harmless, and *Balantidium coli* is the only ciliate pathogenic to humans, causing a disease called *balantidiasis.* It is the largest protozoan parasite of humans and is known to be able to exist as a trophozoite as well as a cyst. It produces proteolytic enzymes that break down and digest the intestinal epithelium (see Chapter 12, Infections of the Gastrointestinal System).

The classification of ciliates has always been difficult and has undergone several changes, especially lately because of the advances in genetic research. Genetic analysis has shown that many ciliates now grouped together on the basis of their morphological similarity are not necessarily genetically closely related. In the future it can be expected that the taxonomy of ciliates, just as for other eukaryotic microbes, will undergo many revisions as genetic technology continues to advance.

Euglenozoa

Euglenozoa are a large group of flagellated protozoa, including a variety of common free-living species and some important parasites, some of which can infect humans. Euglenoids are well-known flagellates, found in freshwater rich in organic materials. Many are photoautotrophs, but others feed by phagocytosis, preying on bacteria and smaller flagellates. The euglenoids have a semirigid plasma membrane and move with the aid of a flagellum located at the anterior end of the cell. The photoautotrophic euglenoids have a red "eyespot," an organelle containing carotene, which senses light and directs the cell in the appropriate direction for photosynthesis. Other euglenoids are facultative chemoheterotrophs and ingest organic matter.

Hemoflagellates are blood parasites, transmitted by the bite of blood-feeding insects. They have long, slender bodies and an undulating membrane, giving them mobility in the circulatory system of the host. The genus *Trypanosoma* (Figure 8.14)

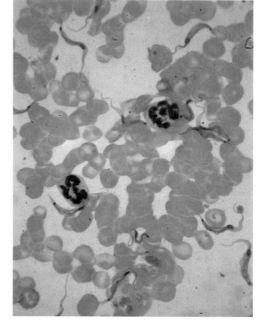

FIGURE 8.14 *Trypanosoma.* This is a micrograph of the *Trypanosoma* protozoa in a blood sample. This protozoan is responsible for causing the diseases African sleeping sickness and Chagas' disease.

includes *T. brucei,* which is transmitted by the tsetse fly and is the causative agent of sleeping sickness (see Chapter 14, Infections of the Circulatory System).

Amoebozoa

Amoebozoa, or amoebas, are a major group of amoeboid protozoans. Most of them are unicellular and common habitants in soil and water. They move by means of cytoplasmic flow, by extending blunt, lobelike projections of the cytoplasm, called *pseudopods* (Figure 8.15). The primary way in which these protozoans obtain nutrition is by phagocytosis, whereby the cell surrounds potential food particles and seals them into vacuoles, where digestion followed by absorption occurs. The only organism pathogenic to humans is *Entamoeba histolytica,* a parasite in the human intestine causing amoebic dysentery (see Chapter 12, Infections of the Gastrointestinal System). *Entamoeba* is transmitted between humans through ingestion of cysts that are present in the feces of infected persons. Another amoeba that can infect humans, typically immunocompromised people, is *Balamuthia,* which has been reported to cause brain abscesses referred to as primary amoebic meningoencephalitis (see Chapter 13, Infections of the Nervous System and Senses). *Balamuthia* is a free-living organism found in water and can enter the body through the lower respiratory tract or through open wounds. The organism cannot be transmitted by person-to-person contact.

Apicomplexa

Apicomplexa are a large group of protozoans characterized by the presence of a unique, complex organelle called the **apical complex** (Figure 8.16). This complex can be visualized only by

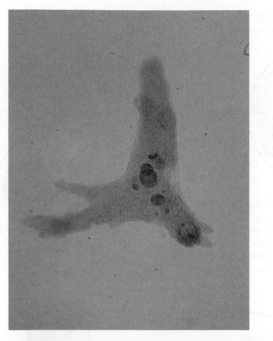

FIGURE 8.15 Amoeba. This is a micrograph of a typical amoeba with its characteristic pseudopods, or "false feet," that allow it to crawl over surfaces.

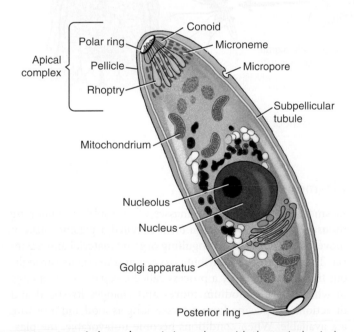

FIGURE 8.16 Apicomplexa. Apicomplexa with the typical apical complex.

electron microscopy and it has been shown to consist of an apical conoid into which the ducts of saclike organelles called *rhoptries* lead. Furthermore, microtubules extend backward from this complex, apparently to support the surface of the organism. These rhoptries are believed to secrete an adhesive substance that facilitates attachment to the host cell, followed by entry of the parasite through the membrane.

Apicomplexans have a complex life cycle requiring transmission between several hosts. An example is *Plasmodium*,

the causative agent of malaria. Malaria is a devastating parasitic disease, endemic to tropical and subtropical areas of Asia, North and South America, the Middle East, North Africa, and the South Pacific. *Plasmodium vivax* is the most common among the four human malaria species: *P. falciparum, malariae, ovale,* and *vivax.* The organism is transmitted through the bite of infected *Anopheles* mosquitoes. The infective stage of *Plasmodium* carried by the mosquito is called the **sporozoite.** Once injected into the human the sporozoites are carried in the bloodstream to the liver, where they undergo schizogony to produce thousands of progeny called **merozoites.** Leaving the liver, the merozoites then invade red blood cells and reproduce. The young trophocytes (cells that provide nourishment to other cells) form ringlike structures referred to as a ring stage, which enlarges and divides repeatedly. Eventually the red blood cells rupture and release more merozoites, which then can infect more red blood cells to perpetuate their asexual reproduction. The waste products of the merozoites are responsible for the resulting fever and chills, characteristics of malaria. Some merozoites develop into male and female sexual forms (gametocytes), which can be picked up by a bite of another *Anopheles* mosquito. The gametocytes then enter the mosquito's intestine and begin their sexual cycle by uniting to form a zygote. The zygote produces an oocyst in which cell division occurs and asexual sporozoites are formed. After rupturing of the oocytes the sporozoites migrate to the salivary glands of the mosquito and the cycle can start again (Figure 8.17).

Other apicomplexans are *Babesia microti, Toxoplasma gondii,* and *Cryptosporidium.*

Babesia microti is a parasite that infects erythrocytes and causes fever and anemia in humans. Before entering the human host, the life cycle of *Babesia* involves a rodent, primarily the white-footed mouse *Peromyscus leucopus,* and a *Babesia*-infected tick that introduces sporozoites into the mouse host. Here the sporozoites undergo asexual reproduction and some parasites differentiate into male and female gametes. Once ingested by an appropriate tick, usually the deer tick *Ixodes dammini,* they undergo a sporogonic cycle resulting in the production of sporozoites (Figure 8.18). Humans enter the cycle when bitten by infected ticks. The sporozoites enter erythrocytes and undergo asexual reproduction, which is responsible for the clinical symptoms of the disease—babesiosis. Humans are dead-end hosts and there is little chance that subsequent transmission occurs from ticks feeding on an infected person. However, human-to-human transmission can occur through blood transfusions.

Toxoplasma gondii is another intracellular parasite in humans and its life cycle includes domestic cats. The organism is the causative agent of toxoplasmosis, which is discussed in Chapter 16 (Infections of the Reproductive System).

Slime Molds

Slime molds have both fungal and amoebal characteristics but are more closely related to amoebas than to fungi. Slime molds

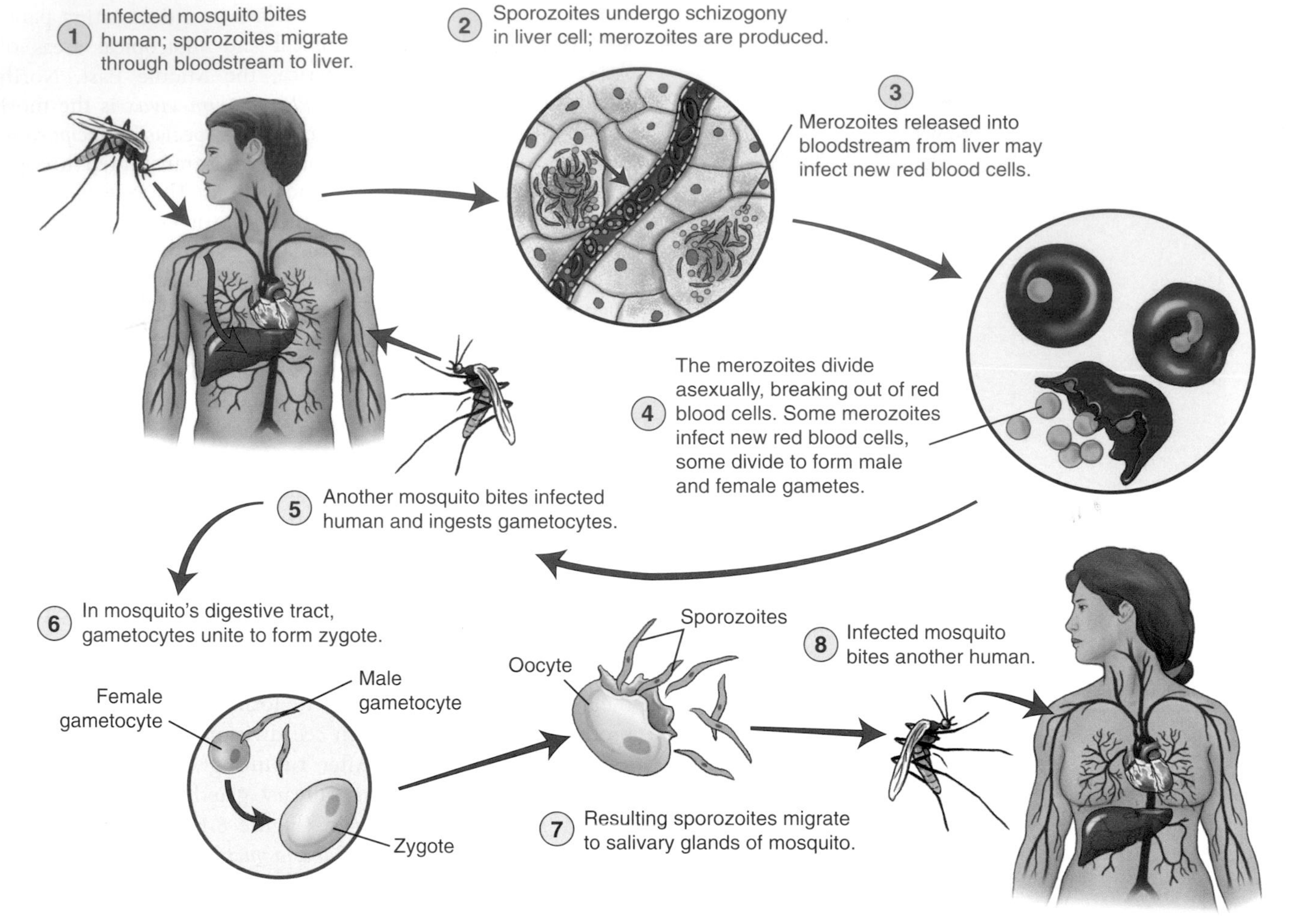

1 Infected mosquito bites human; sporozoites migrate through bloodstream to liver.
2 Sporozoites undergo schizogony in liver cell; merozoites are produced.
3 Merozoites released into bloodstream from liver may infect new red blood cells.
4 The merozoites divide asexually, breaking out of red blood cells. Some merozoites infect new red blood cells, some divide to form male and female gametes.
5 Another mosquito bites infected human and ingests gametocytes.
6 In mosquito's digestive tract, gametocytes unite to form zygote.
Female gametocyte
Male gametocyte
Zygote
Oocyte
Sporozoites
7 Resulting sporozoites migrate to salivary glands of mosquito.
8 Infected mosquito bites another human.

FIGURE 8.17 ***Plasmodium vivax.*** Life cycle of *Plasmodium vivax,* the causative agent of malaria.

appear as cellular slime molds or plasmodial slime molds and are not pathogenic to humans.

Cellular Slime Molds

Cellular slime molds are typical eukaryotic cells that resemble amoebas and spend most of their lives as single amoeboid cells feeding on fungi and bacteria by phagocytosis. Under unfavorable conditions large numbers of these cells aggregate to form a single structure. This aggregation occurs in response to the release of chemicals by some individual amoebas and others respond by migrating toward the released chemical (cyclic adenosine monophosphate, or cAMP). The aggregated amoebas become enclosed in a slimy sheath called a *slug,* which migrates toward light. After migration, the slug begins to form differentiated structures; some form a stalk whereas others go up the stalk and form a spore cap. Most of these differentiate into spores, are released under appropriate conditions, and germinate to become single amoebas (Figure 8.19). Cellular slime molds are of great interest to biologists because they provide a relatively simple and easily manipulated system for understanding cellular migration and aggregation.

Plasmodial Slime Molds

Plasmodial slime molds are masses of protoplasm containing thousands of nuclei. This life form is called a **plasmodium;** it moves as a giant amoeba engulfing organic material and bacteria. These organisms distribute oxygen and nutrients throughout the plasmodium by a process called *cytoplasmic streaming,* in which the plasmodium moves and changes its speed and direction. The plasmodium grows as long as food and moisture are available. When conditions become unfavorable, the plasmodium separates into many protoplasmic groups, each of which forms a stalked sporangium in which spores develop. The spore nuclei undergo meiosis to form haploid cells. On release, in improved conditions, the spores will germinate, fuse, and form diploid cells, which then develop into a multinucleated plasmodium.

Helminths

Helminths are a group of eukaryotic worms that are not microorganisms, yet of interest to microbiologists because parasitic

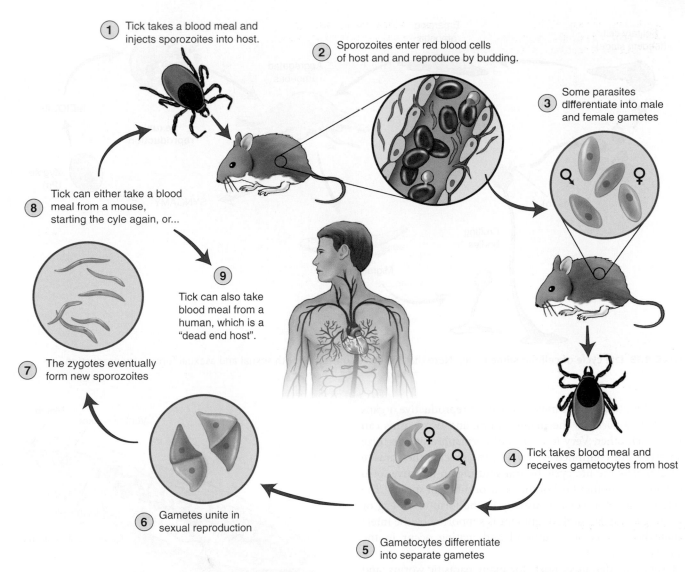

FIGURE 8.18 Life cycle of *Babesia microti*. Note that the cycle consists of both sexual and asexual forms of reproduction.

1. Tick takes a blood meal and injects sporozoites into host.
2. Sporozoites enter red blood cells of host and and reproduce by budding.
3. Some parasites differentiate into male and female gametes
4. Tick takes blood meal and receives gametocytes from host
5. Gametocytes differentiate into separate gametes
6. Gametes unite in sexual reproduction
7. The zygotes eventually form new sporozoites
8. Tick can either take a blood meal from a mouse, starting the cyle again, or...
9. Tick can also take blood meal from a human, which is a "dead end host".

helminths exhibit microscopic infective and diagnostic stages in their life cycle, usually by way of their eggs or larvae. Depending on the life cycle of a specific helminth these microscopic forms are generally found in blood, feces, or urine, and must be distinguished from other microbes.

Characteristics of Helminths

Many parasitic helminths spend much of their life cycle in a mammalian host. Most of the helminths affecting humans are either flatworms (platyhelminths; Platyhelminthes) or roundworms (nematodes; Nematoda). Adult animals are usually large enough to be seen with the naked eye, but the microscope is necessary to identify their eggs and larvae.

All helminths are multicellular eukaryotes that generally contain digestive, circulatory, nervous, excretory, and reproductive systems. Parasitic helminths differ from their free-living counterparts, because parasites must be highly specialized to live inside their hosts. For example, their reproductive system is often dominant over other systems, and the worms may be reduced to a series of flattened sacs filled with ovaries, testes, and eggs to optimize infection. They might lack a digestive system because they can absorb the necessary nutrients from the food of the host and body fluids, or tissues of the host. Motility may be reduced, because the parasites are transferred from host to host. Furthermore, parasitic helminths do not have an extensive nervous system, because they do not have to search for food or adapt to environmental changes.

Life Cycle of Helminths

The life cycle of parasitic helminths includes the fertilized egg (embryo), larva, and adult. It can be extremely complex, involving a succession of **intermediate hosts,** and a **definitive host** for the adult parasite.

Adult helminths may have male reproductive organs in one individual and female reproductive organs in another, in which case the worms are called *dioecious*. Reproduction in these species occurs only when the host contains worms of both sexes.

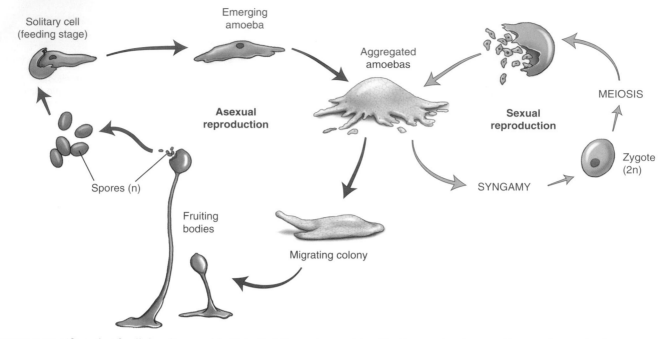

FIGURE 8.19 **Life cycle of cellular slime mold.** Note that the cycle consists of both sexual and asexual forms of reproduction.

If a helminth has both male and female reproductive organs it is called *monoecious* (hermaphroditic), and two worms can fertilize each other. Very few types of hermaphrodites fertilize themselves. For continued survival of the species, the parasite must complete the life cycle by transmitting an infective form to the body of another host of the same or different species. The infective stage of a worm is usually in the form of an egg or larva. In general, larval development is supported by the intermediate host, whereas adulthood and mating occur in the definitive (final) host.

Humans are definitive hosts for many parasitic worms, and the sources of infection include contaminated food, soil, water, or infected animals. The route of infection (see Chapter 9, Infection and Disease) can be by oral intake or skin penetration.

Classification of Helminths

The helminths are classified according to shape, size, and degree of organ development, and by the presence of hooks, suckers, or other special structures. In addition, the mode of reproduction, the type of host, and the morphology of eggs and larvae are also considered in their classification.

Platyhelminths

Members of the phylum Platyhelminthes are dorsoventrally flattened, thus the name **flatworms.** Parasitic flatworms include trematodes and cestodes.

- Trematodes (flukes) are generally flat and leaf shaped, with oral and ventral suckers holding the organism in place (Figure 8.20). They have complex life cycles and their common names are given according to the tissue of the definitive host in which the adults live (e.g., lung fluke, liver fluke, blood fluke).

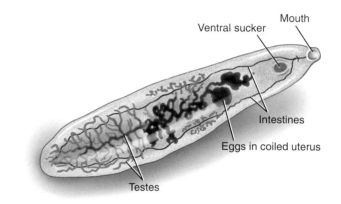
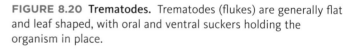

FIGURE 8.20 **Trematodes.** Trematodes (flukes) are generally flat and leaf shaped, with oral and ventral suckers holding the organism in place.

- Cestodes or **tapeworms** are intestinal parasites (see Chapter 12, Infections of the Gastrointestinal System). Adult tapeworms share a basic body structure: a **scolex** (head), a neck, and one or more proglottids (segments; see Figure 8.21). The scolex of the worm attaches to the intestine of the definite host, and the neck is a relatively undifferentiated mass of cells forming new segments—this is where all growth in the adult tapeworm occurs. The body of the worm is composed of successive units of proglottids collectively called *strobila*. It makes the worm look like a strip of tape and this is the source of its common name. Mature proglottids are released from the mature tapeworm and leave the host in its feces. The most mature proglottids are at the tail of the tapeworm and the most immature are closest to the neck.

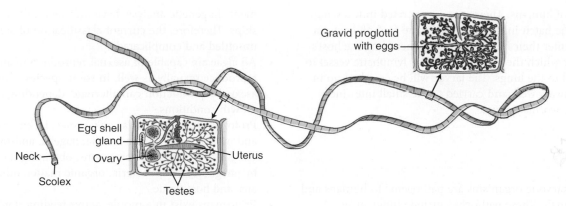

FIGURE 8.21 Cestode (tapeworm) morphology. The scolex attaches the worm to the host tissue. Behind the scolex is the neck region, followed by the proglottids (body segments), which grow from the neck region as long as the worm is attached to the host. The proglottids closest to the neck are immature; those in the middle portion have matured, and the proglottids nearest the end become gravid (full of fertilized eggs). At this point the gravid proglottids break off and leave the host along with the feces.

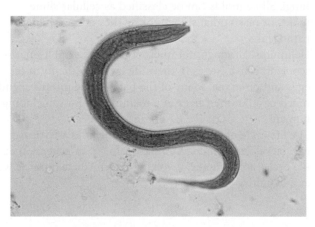

FIGURE 8.22 Hookworms. Hookworms live in the small intestine of humans. Their eggs are excreted in feces, and their larvae hatch in the soil. From Mahon CR, Lehman DC, Manuselis G: *Textbook of diagnostic microbiology,* ed 3, St. Louis, 2007, Saunders.

Nematodes

Nematodes, or **roundworms**, are cylindrical and tapered at each end and are the most numerous multicellular animals on earth. Nematodes possess digestive, nervous, excretory, and reproductive systems, but lack defined circulatory and respiratory systems. They are found everywhere in freshwater, marine, and terrestrial environments. Many are free-living and harmless; others are parasitic and can be pathogenic to plants and animals, including humans. Nematode infections in humans are divided into two categories, depending on whether the eggs or the larvae are the infecting agent.

- *Enterobius vermicularis,* the pinworm or seatworm, spends its life in a human host. The adult worms reside in the large intestine, from where it migrates to the anal area to deposit its eggs (hence the name, seatworm). The eggs can then be transmitted to another host by ingestion or via a fomite (contaminated clothing or bedding). *Ascaris lumbricoides* (a large roundworm that infects humans) is a

parasite without an intermediate host. It spends its adult life in the human small intestine and feeds primarily on predigested food. Eggs can be excreted with feces and are able to survive in soil for long periods of time until accidentally ingested by another host. The eggs hatch in the small intestine and the larvae dig out of the intestine into the bloodstream. They are transported to the lungs, where they grow and eventually are coughed up, swallowed, and returned to the intestine for maturation into adults.

- *Necator americanus* and *Ancylostoma duodenale* are also called *hookworms* (Figure 8.22), and live in the small

MEDICAL HIGHLIGHTS

Ascariasis: Nematode Freeloaders

The most prevalent intestinal worm infections are caused by nematodes and are generally transmitted by contact with soil contaminated with human feces containing nematode eggs. The most common human worm infection is due to *Ascaris lumbricoides,* a large roundworm that ranges in length from 6 to 13 inches. The infections are common throughout the world in both temperate and tropical areas, but are more prevalent in areas of poor sanitation, and are usually a result of human carelessness. Often, symptoms may not occur in infected individuals; however, they are active carriers of the infection.

Eggs are swallowed and pass to the intestine, where they develop into larvae. The larvae can penetrate the intestinal wall, enter the circulatory system, and reach the lungs. A large number of larvae within the lungs at any point in time may cause pneumonia. Once in the lungs the larvae will travel via the bronchial tree to the pharynx, where they are swallowed. On entering the small intestine again the larvae will grow, mature, and mate, and their progeny will be released into the environment to find a new host.

intestine of humans. Their eggs are excreted in feces, and their larvae hatch in the soil. The larvae feed on bacteria and can enter their human host by penetrating the host's skin, after which they enter a blood or lymphatic vessel to be carried to the lungs. The larvae will be coughed up in sputum, swallowed, and carried to the small intestine, where the worms mature.

Summary

- Many eukaryotic organisms are pathogenic to humans and other animals. These pathogens include fungi, algae, protozoans, and helminths.
- Fungi are vegetative structures that generally grow as filamentous, multinucleate organisms (a mass of hyphae forms a mycelium), or they grow as unicellular fungi. Fungi are free-living, heterotrophic organisms that can appear as yeasts, molds, or fleshy fungi.
- Fungal reproduction can be asexual (mitosis) or sexual. Asexual reproduction results in the formation of sporangia and can occur at any time, whereas sexual reproduction generally occurs under conditions that are unfavorable for growth. Sexual reproduction provides variability of characteristics, making survival of the species more likely.
- Algae are aquatic, photosynthetic organisms, but they differ in distribution, morphology, reproduction, and biochemical preferences. Historically, algae were classified according to their photosynthetic pigments, but advance-

ments in genetic analysis have indicated different relationships. Therefore, the current classification of algae is unsettled and complicated.

- All algae are capable of asexual reproduction and most can reproduce sexually as well. In some species sexual and asexual reproduction can alternate, depending on the given growth conditions.
- Protozoans are unicellular eukaryotes, lacking cell walls, and most are motile due to cilia, flagella, and/or pseudopodia. Most are chemoheterotrophs, obtaining their nutrients by phagocytosis of bacteria, organic matter, other protozoans, and host tissue.
- Protozoans exist in a motile, active feeding state called the *trophozoite,* or in a dormant state called a *cyst.* Many are human parasites and their life cycle ranges from simple to complex.
- Slime molds have both fungal and amoebal characteristics, but they are more closely related to amoeba than to fungi. Slime molds can be classified as cellular slime molds or plasmodial slime molds. They are not human pathogens.
- Helminths, although not microorganisms, exhibit microscopic infective stages in their life cycles in the form of eggs and/or larvae. Many of the parasitic helminths spend much or all of their lives in a mammalian host, including humans.
- The life cycle of parasitic helminths includes a fertilized egg, larval stage, and the adult organism. In general, their life cycles are complex, involving intermediate hosts as well as a definitive (final) host.

Review Questions

1. The antibiotics penicillin and cephalosporin are produced by:
   a. Algae
   b. Slime molds
   c. Fungi
   d. Protozoans

2. Fungi are free-living _____ organisms.
   a. Autotrophic
   b. Chemotrophic
   c. Heterotrophic
   d. Phototrophic

3. Algae that contain agar in their cell walls belong to the:
   a. Chrysophyta
   b. Rhodophyta
   c. Chlorophyta
   d. Phaeophyta

4. Diatoms, major components of marine phytoplankton, belong to:
   a. Chrysophyta
   b. Rhodophyta
   c. Chlorophyta
   d. Phaeophyta

5. The process by which the nucleus of protozoans undergoes multiple divisions before the cell divides is called:
   a. Budding
   b. Mitosis
   c. Schizogony
   d. Fragmentation

6. The eukaryotes known for the presence of a macronucleus and a micronucleus are:
   a. Algae
   b. Fungi
   c. Protozoans
   d. Slime molds

7. *Plasmodium* is:
   a. A type of algae
   b. A protozoan
   c. A slime mold
   d. A helminth

8. *Toxoplasma gondii* belongs to which group of eukaryotic organisms?
   a. Algae
   b. Fungi
   c. Protozoans
   d. Helminths

9. A scolex is a structure found in:
   a. Algae
   b. Fungi
   c. Protozoans
   d. Helminths

10. Which of the following is commonly referred to as a pinworm?
   a. *Enterobius vermicularis*
   b. *Necator americanus*
   c. *Ascaris lumbricoides*
   d. *Ancylostoma duodenale*

11. The study of fungi is called _____.

12. The vegetative structure of algae is referred to as a(n) _____.

13. The unique cell organelle found among the Archaezoa, which appears to be a remnant of mitochondria, is called a(n) _____.

14. Masses of protoplasm containing thousands of nuclei are a characteristic of _____.

15. The common name for nematodes is _____.

16. Describe the classification of fungi with emphasis on the medically important species.

17. Describe the general characteristics of algae and their possible life cycles.

18. Name and describe three protozoans that are human parasites.

19. Describe the fundamental difference between cellular and plasmodial slime molds.

20. Describe the basic structure of cestodes (tapeworms) and their life cycle.

Bibliography

Adl SM, Simpson AG, Farmer MA, et al: *The new higher level classification of eukaryotes with emphasis on the taxonomy of protests.* J. Eukaryot. Microbiol. 52(5) 2005, pp 399–451.

Bauman R: *Microbiology: with diseases by taxonomy*, ed 2, 2007, Benjamin Cummings/Pearson Education, San Francisco.

Lehne RA: *Pharmacology for nursing care*, ed 6, St. Louis, 2007, Saunders/Elsevier.

Leon-Avila G, Tovar J: *Mitosomes of Entamoeba histolytica* are abundant mitochondrion-related remnant organelles that lack a detectable organellar genome, Microbiology 150:1245–1250, 2004.

Smith M, Bruh J, Anderson J: *The fungus Armillaria bulbosa is among the largest and oldest living organisms*, Nature 356:428–431, 1992.

Talaro KP: *Foundations in Microbiology*, ed 6, 2008, McGraw-Hill, New York.

Totora GJ, Funke BR, Case CL: *Microbiology: An introduction*, ed 9, 2007, Benjamin Cummings/Pearson Education, San Francisco.

Tovar J, Fischer A, Clark CG: *The mitosome, a novel organelle related to mitochondria in the amitochondrial parasite Entamoeba histolytica*, Mol Microbiol 32:1013–1021, 1999.

Internet Resources

"The Influenza Pandemic of 1918" (by Molly Billings, 1997, 2005), http://virus.stanford.edu/uda/

Blackwell Publishing, "New classification of eukaryotes has implications for AIDS treatment, agriculture and beyond," http://www.wiley.com/bw/press/pressitem.asp?ref=533

University of Sydney, Introduction to Fungal Reproduction & Dispersal, http://bugs.bio.usyd.edu.au/Mycology/Reprodn_Dispersal/introduction.shtml

New York State Department of Health, Babesiosis Fact Sheet, http://www.health.state.ny.us/diseases/communicable/babesiosis/fact_sheet.htm

emedicine from *Web*MD, Balantidiasis, http://www.emedicine.com/MED/topic203.htm

Woods Hole Oceanographic Institution, Harmful Algae, http://www.whoi.edu/redtide/

Centers for Disease Control and Prevention (CDC), Environmental Hazards & Health Effects, Harmful Algal Blooms (HABs), http://www.cdc.gov/hab/

Texas Parks and Wildlife, Harmful Algal Blooms (HABs), http://www.tpwd.state.tx.us/landwater/water/environconcerns/hab/

CDC, CDC'S Harmful Algal Bloom-related Illness Surveillance System, http://www.cdc.gov/hab/surveillance.htm#about

CDC, National Center for Environmental Health (NCEH), About NCEH, http://www.cdc.gov/nceh/Information/about.htm

CDC, Division of Parasitic Diseases, Parasitic Disease Information, Fact Sheet, Ascaris Infection, http://www.cdc.gov/ncidod/dpd/parasites/ascaris/factsht_ascaris.htm

Infection and Disease

[OUTLINE

Host–Microbe Relationship
    Symbiosis
    Normal Flora (Microbiota)
    Opportunistic Pathogens

Stages of Infection
    Portal of Entry
    Virulence and Pathogenicity
    Portal of Exit
    Etiology of Infectious Diseases

Epidemiology and Public Health
    Diseases in the Population
    Reservoirs
    Modes of Transmission

Healthcare-associated (Nosocomial) Infections
    Types of Nosocomial Infections
    Transmission
    Antimicrobial Resistance in Healthcare Settings
    Control and Prevention

[LEARNING OBJECTIVES

After reading this chapter, the student will be able to:
- Name and differentiate between the different types of symbiotic relationships, and explain how microbes of the normal flora can become opportunistic pathogens
- Identify and describe the portals by which pathogens gain excess to the body and how pathogens exit the body
- Explain the difference between contamination and infection, as well as the stages and nature of infections, and discuss virulence, virulence factors, and pathogenicity
- Define etiology; and explain Koch's postulates including its limitations
- Name and explain the terms used to describe the different patterns of infection in a population
- Explain the different approaches used in epidemiology to study the diseases in a population
- Describe the different reservoirs of infectious agents

- Explain the different ways of disease transmission and describe the classification of infectious diseases
- Describe the nature and types of healthcare-associated (nosocomial) infections, and discuss the monitoring and information systems initiated and administered by the Centers for Disease Control and Prevention (CDC) to help in the control of these infections
- Discuss the transmission and prevention of healthcare-associated infectious diseases

KEY TERMS

acute infections	evasion of host defenses	pathogen
adhesion	exogenous	pathogenicity
airborne transmission	experimental	primary infection
amensalism	epidemiology	resident flora
analytical epidemiology	focal infections	secondary infection
autoinoculation	fomite	sepsis
bacteremia	foodborne transmission	septicemia
bodily fluid transmission	iatrogenic	sporadic
chronic infections	index case	subclinical infection
colonization	indirect contact	symbiosis
commensalism	infection	systemic infection
contamination	invasins	toxemia
descriptive epidemiology	invasion	toxigenic
direct contact	local infections	toxins
transmission	microbiota	transient flora
droplet	mixed infections	vectors
endemic	mutualism	viremia
endogenous	normal flora	virulence
epidemic	opportunistic pathogen	virulence factors
epidemiology	pandemic	waterborne transmission
etiology	parasitism	

WHY YOU NEED TO KNOW

HISTORY

Combating infection and disease has been throughout history, and continues to be now, as essential as the need for food and shelter. The causes of infection and disease have been and continue to be equally problematic. As pointed out in Chapter 1 (Scope of Microbiology), it wasn't until the seventeenth century that the application of van Leeuwenhoek's light microscope revealed "animalcules," suggesting theories that microorganisms could be a cause of disease.

With improved technology and refinement of scientific logic, Robert Koch, Louis Pasteur, and others in the late 1800s developed what has come to be known as *"Koch's postulates."* These four postulates are the foundation of the germ theory of disease, and they have been used to identify numerous disease-causing organisms. In a laboratory setting with agar culture plates, Koch demonstrated the cause of anthrax to be *Bacillus anthracis.*

IMPACT

Advances in technology have shown some shortcomings in Koch's postulates, but these same technological advances have also offered solutions to them. By uncovering causes of disease in the laboratory setting, new drugs and therapies, including vaccines, for prevention are and continue to be developed.

The concept that it is possible to eradicate a disease of pandemic proportions, such as smallpox, became a reality when the World Health Organization (WHO) announced the eradication of smallpox in December 1979. The marshalling of worldwide knowledge via computer and other technologies provide the resources to develop a plan of action under which humankind can operate if they so choose.

FUTURE

With today's global connectivity, both through the movement of populations and the import/export of products along with increased mobility within national or local populations, the threat of the rapid spread of disease will remain a significant challenge for all levels of healthcare professionals. Whether combating the increasing threat of nosocomial infections, which is exacerbated by the emergence of antibiotic-resistant strains of organisms, or conducting research to determine host–pathogen relationships and the vector of transmission, all those in the healthcare and related fields will be instrumental in preventing the next outbreaks of infectious diseases. A local or institutional problem has the potential to expand into an epidemic if healthcare workers do not possess a working knowledge of infection and disease.

Host–Microbe Relationship

Microbes are found everywhere on earth and the interaction of humans with microorganisms is inevitable, complex, and not always completely understood. Under normal circumstances, humans and other animals are free of microbes in utero, but during birth the newborn is exposed to microbes, which will start to colonize the infant's intestine. From this time on humans and microbes establish a symbiotic relationship that lasts a lifetime.

Symbiosis

Symbiosis is the term that describes a close relationship between two different types of organisms in a community. Depending on the outcome of this relationship, symbiosis can be classified as mutualism, commensalism, parasitism, or amensalism (Table 9.1):

- **Mutualism:** Mutualism is a relationship between two organisms in which both members benefit from the interaction. For example, in the large intestine of humans, *Escherichia coli* releases vitamins during the breakdown of nutrients that are not digestible by the human gastrointestinal (GI) tract, but necessary for the survival of the bacteria. The vitamins released by *E. coli* can easily be absorbed by the intestinal epithelium of the human large intestine. As shown in the Life Application, probiotics are also examples of mutualism between specific bacterial species and the human gastrointestinal tract.
- **Commensalism:** Commensalism is a term used for a symbiotic relationship in which one of the organisms benefits and the other is neither harmed nor helped. Many microorganisms in the **normal flora** of the human skin and mucous membranes are commensals. Examples include certain saprophytic mycobacteria that inhabit the ear and external genitals, living on secretions and removed cells. These organisms do not appear to bring benefit or harm to the host.
- **Parasitism:** In parasitism one organism benefits, while the other is harmed, either slightly or to such an extreme that the host will be killed. A parasite that is capable of causing disease is called a **pathogen.** Species of bacteria, protozoans, algae, and fungi all can be microscopic human

pathogens. Larger pathogens include the parasitic worms and biting arthropods.
- **Amensalism:** Amensalism is an interaction between two species in which one organism can hamper or prevent the growth and/or survival of another, without being positively or negatively affected by the other organism. A familiar example is *Penicillium,* a mold that secretes penicillin, a chemical capable of killing a wide range of bacteria (see Chapter 22, Antimicrobial Drugs).

Normal Flora (Microbiota)

A newborn's first contact with microorganisms occurs while traveling through the birth canal, where lactobacilli residing in the mother's vagina will become the predominant organisms in the newborn's intestine. The next exposure of the newborn to microorganisms occurs with the beginning of breathing, and this is soon followed by feeding. From then on, other orally acquired bacteria such as *E. coli* will begin to colonize the large intestine and will remain there throughout life. In other words, starting at birth the human body enters a state of dynamic equilibrium with microorganisms. In addition, throughout a person's life, other microorganisms will establish residency in mucous membranes that are open to the external environment, on the skin and its derivatives (Figure 9.1). Mucous membranes open to the external environment include those of the respiratory tract (Figure 9.2), gastrointestinal tract (Figure 9.3), and urogenital tract (Figure 9.4). The microbes that establish themselves on the skin and mucous membranes usually do not cause disease and constitute the normal flora (**microbiota**) of the human body. This normal flora consists of resident or transient microbes:

- A **resident flora** remains part of the normal flora throughout the life of a person. An example would be *Staphylococcus epidermidis,* a resident of the skin, or *E. coli,* which is part of the intestinal flora. A detailed listing of the various organisms that reside in/on the human body is provided in Table 9.2.
- A **transient flora** can be found in the same locations as the resident flora, but remains in the body for only a few hours, days, or months before it vanishes. These organisms cannot survive for reasons such as competition with other microorganisms for nutrients, elimination by the host's immune system, or chemical and physical changes in the

TABLE 9.1 Symbiotic Relationships

Symbiosis Type	Organism 1	Organism 2	Example
Mutualism	Benefits	Benefits	*Escherichia coli* in human large intestine
Commensalism	Benefits	Neither harmed, nor helped	Many microbes that make up the normal flora of the human skin and mucous membranes
Parasitism	Benefits	Harmed	Tuberculosis bacterium in the human lung; certain protozoans, fungi, and helminths
Amensalism	Not affected	Impedes or restricts	*Penicillium* (mold) secretes penicillin, which kills certain bacteria

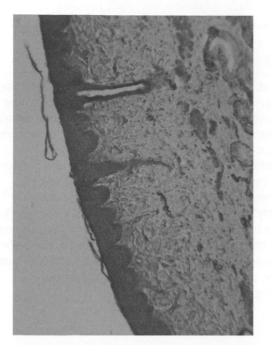

FIGURE 9.1 **Skin.** Micrograph of the skin, showing the protective layer of epidermis with the underlying connective tissue of the dermis.

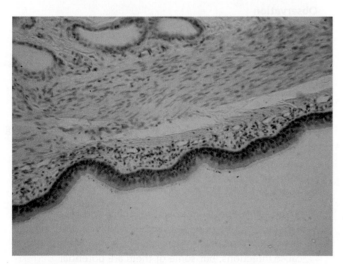

FIGURE 9.2 Ciliated epithelium (mucous membrane) of the respiratory tract.

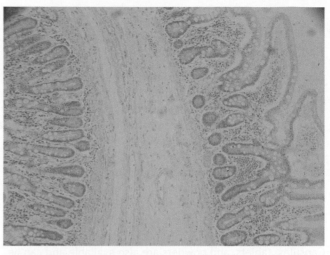

FIGURE 9.3 Typical epithelial lining (mucous membrane) of the gastrointestinal tract.

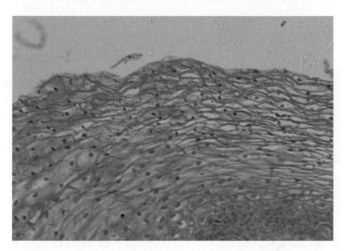

FIGURE 9.4 Mucous membrane of the urogenital tract.

body of the host. An example would be *Bacillus laterosporus,* sometimes found in the intestines; when present the organism helps to keep fungal populations such as *Candida* in check.

Opportunistic Pathogens

In general, this balance between the normal flora and the human host can be maintained, but when the balance is interrupted for whatever reason, the microorganisms can cause infection and disease. They become opportunistic pathogens. An **opportunistic pathogen** does not cause disease in its normal habitat in a healthy person, but can cause infection under con-

ditions of immune suppression, changes in the normal flora, or when a member of the normal flora gains access into an area of the body it normally does not inhabit.

- *Compromised immune system immune suppression (see Chapter 20, The Immune System):* Any factors that suppress or weaken the immune system can enable opportunistic pathogens to cause infections and disease. These factors include acute and chronic diseases, especially those involving the immune system directly (e.g., AIDS); malnutrition, stress (emotional and physical), age (very young or very old), the use of radiation and chemotherapy in the treatment of cancer, or the use of immunosuppressive drugs in transplant patients.
- *Changes in the normal flora:* The normal flora plays a somewhat protective role regarding pathogens, because it takes up space, uses available nutrients, and releases toxic waste products, all of which present a problem for arriving pathogens, which must compete well enough to become established to infect and cause disease in the desired host. This condition is acknowledged as microbial competition

Probiotics: Yogurt as Medicine?

One often-used definition of probiotics, developed by the World Health Organization (WHO), is that they are live microorganisms, mostly bacteria, which when taken in proper amounts result in a health benefit for the host. These bacteria are called "friendly" or "good" bacteria and are the same or similar to the normal flora found in healthy individuals. For centuries, home remedies and medicinal folklore have suggested that some fermented milk products conferred a certain health benefit to the user. Modern probiotic products have taken forms other than just milk products, such as by the addition of probiotics to juices and soy beverages. Capsules, tablets, and powders are also available and can be added to food products or directly ingested. The list of potential health benefits of probiotics is growing, some of which have specific potential in the control of infectious

diseases. These include competition of "friendly" bacteria with pathogens, replenishment of normal intestinal flora after depletion caused by antibiotics, and stimulation of certain immune system components. Thus far research has uncovered some rather minor side effects such as mild digestive discomfort, but there is also a potential infection problem when introducing bacteria into a host with an already depressed immune system. In these cases the normally "friendly" bacteria may become opportunistic pathogens and require treatment with antibiotics. Concerns have also been raised about overstimulation of the immune system, effects of metabolic activities as a result of increased bacterial numbers, or gene transfers between pathogens and probiotic microorganisms.

TABLE 9.2 Normal Flora in Selected Regions of the Human Body

Region	Genera	Observation
Skin	*Staphylococcus, Propionibacterium, Corynebacterium, Micrococcus, Acinetobacter, Candida* (fungus), *Malassezia* (fungus)	The varied environment of the skin results in locally dense or sparse populations, depending on moisture, temperature, and exposure to the environment. In general, the microbes live on the outer layer of the skin, in hair follicles, and in pores of glands
Eyes (conjunctiva)	*Staphylococcus, Propionibacterium, Micrococcus, Corynebacterium*	Although the microbiota is similar to that of the skin, tears reduce the normal flora and prevent others from colonizing
Upper respiratory tract	*Fusobacterium, Haemophilus, Lactobacillus, Moraxella, Staphylococcus, Streptococcus*	Microbes that are part of the normal flora are potential pathogens, but are generally kept at bay by an intact immune system, by nasal secretions, and by the ciliary escalator of the trachea
Mouth (upper digestive tract)	*Fusobacterium, Haemophilus, Lactobacillus, Staphylococcus, Streptococcus, Actinomyces, Treponema, Corynebacterium, Candida* (fungus)	Although saliva does contain antimicrobial substances, the moisture, warmth, and continuous supply of food support many microorganisms. Normally these microbes do not cause infections, but some of them are potential pathogens
Lower digestive tract	*Escherichia coli, Bacteroides, Fusobacterium, Lactobacillus, Enterococcus, Enterobacter, Bifidobacterium, Citrobacter, Proteus, Klebsiella, Candida* (fungus)	The large intestine contains the largest amount of resident microbes. Bacteria are mostly anaerobes but some facultative anaerobes also present
Female urogenital tract	*Lactobacillus, Bacteroides, Clostridium, Staphylococcus, Streptococcus, Candida* (fungus), *Trichomonas* (protozoan)	As the pH of the vagina changes so does the microbial flora. Flow of urine prevents extensive colonization of the urethra and urinary bladder
Male urogenital tract	*Lactobacillus, Bacteroides, Fusobacterium, Mycobacterium, Peptostreptococcus, Staphylococcus, Streptococcus*	Flow of urine prevents excessive colonization of microbes in the urethra or urinary bladder

or antagonism. When the normal flora changes for any reason it may allow one of the members to become an opportunistic pathogen and thrive. Examples include vaginal yeast infections by *Candida albicans* in women after prolonged antibiotic therapy, or oral thrush also caused by *Candida* spp. in cancer patients after chemotherapy. Other conditions that change the normal flora include hormonal changes, stress, changes in the diet, or exposure to an excessive number of pathogenic organisms.

- *Entrance of a member of the normal flora into areas of the body where it is not present under normal conditions:* This can occur after injury, in burn victims, or even when an intestinal organism such as *E. coli* enters the urethra, where it then becomes opportunistic.

Stages of Infection

In terms of infection in the human body, **contamination** refers to the presence of microbes in or on the body, or on objects. Contaminants can reach the body in food, drink, by air, or they can be introduced by wounds, insect bites, and sexual intercourse. The outcome of a contamination varies. Some microbes remain at the site at which they first came in contact with the body, such as on the skin and mucous membranes; they do not cause harm and become part of the resident (normal) flora, or a transient flora. To initiate an infection the microorganism must gain entry into the host and its tissues. The term **infection** refers to the presence and growth of a microorganism in the body, with the exception of organisms in/on the normal flora. Notably, an infection may or may not cause disease.

Portal of Entry

The site where a pathogen enters the body is referred to as the *portal of entry,* which can be the skin, mucous membranes, the placenta, or the so-called *parenteral route* (other then the digestive tract route). The source of the infectious agent can be exogenous, from outside the body, or endogenous, in which case the organism is already in the body, such as in the normal flora.

Portals of entry are generally the same areas that support normal flora: the skin and the mucous membranes of the gastrointestinal, respiratory, and urogenital tracts (Figure 9.5). The majority of pathogens have their preferred portal of entry, which provides the necessary habitat for further growth and eventual spreading. Most often, if a pathogen enters the wrong portal, infection will not occur. For example, influenza virus uses the respiratory mucosa as its portal of entry, where it may successfully infect its host, but when limited to contact with the skin only, influenza virus will not cause an infection. Some infectious agents can enter via more than one portal of entry, such as the skin and mucous membranes, where the infection then can lead to various diseases. For example, *Streptococcus* and *Staphylococcus* have adapted to several portals of entry such as the skin and the urogenital and respiratory tracts.

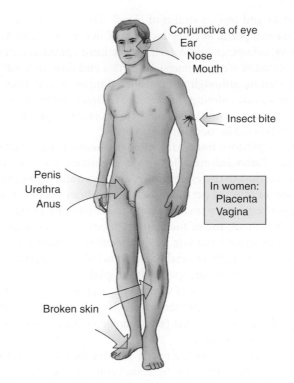

FIGURE 9.5 Portals of entry. The portals of entry for microbes include the skin (broken skin, insect bites); the mucous membranes of the gastrointestinal, respiratory, and urogenital tracts; as well as the conjunctiva and the placenta.

Skin

The top layer of the skin, the epidermis, consists of a thick layer of keratinized dead cells that is the first line of defense against microbial invasion; however, some pathogens can enter the body through natural openings in the skin, such as hair follicles and sweat glands. Damage to the skin in the form of abrasions, cuts, punctures, and scrapes opens the skin to contaminants, which ultimately can cause infection. Moreover, larvae of some parasitic worms burrow through the skin to get to the underlying tissues, and some fungi use digestive enzymes to gain entry to the soft tissues.

Mucous Membranes

Mucous membranes line all the body cavities and the canals that come in contact with the outside, such as the canals of the gastrointestinal, respiratory, and urogenital tracts, as well as the conjunctiva, the thin membrane covering the eye and the underside of the eyelids. The skin and the outer layer of the mucous membranes are composed of tightly packed epithelial cells. However, in contrast to the epidermis, the mucosal lining is thin, moist, and warm, and composed of living cells.

- The gastrointestinal (GI) tract serves as the portal of entry for pathogens present in food, liquid, and other ingested substances. Microorganisms that can survive in the GI tract are adapted to survive the action of digestive enzymes and environments that undergo drastic changes in the pH. Enteric bacterial pathogens include *Salmonella, Shigella,*

Vibrio, and certain strains of *E. coli.* Viruses using the GI tract as a portal of entry include poliovirus, hepatitis A virus, echovirus, and rotavirus. The most common enteric protozoans are *Entamoeba histolytica* and *Giardia lamblia.* Helminths, although not considered microbes, are infectious agents entering through the GI tract and include trematodes, cestodes, and nematodes (see Chapter 8, Eukaryotic Microorganisms).

- The respiratory tract is the most frequently used portal of entry. Pathogens are able to enter the mouth and nose by air, via dust particles, moisture, and respiratory droplets from an infected person. Mucous membranes that line the upper respiratory tract are continuous with the membranes of the sinuses and of the auditory tubes, and pathogens can be transferred from one site to the other. Examples of bacteria using this portal of entry include the causative agents of sore throat, meningitis, diphtheria, and whooping cough. Examples of viral agents include those causing the common cold, influenza, measles, meningitis, mumps, rubella, and chickenpox (see Chapter 11, Infections of the Respiratory System).
- The urogenital tract is a portal of entry for pathogens that are generally contracted by sexual contact (see Chapter 17, Sexually Transmitted Infections/Diseases). However, girls and women who are not sexually active are also susceptible to lower urinary tract infections because of the close proximity of the anus to the female urethra. Therefore urinary tract infections caused by *E. coli,* as opportunistic organisms, are more common in women than men. Vaginal yeast infections are common in women who are under stress; taking birth control pills, antibiotics, and/or steroids; who are pregnant; or because of other factors. Vaginal yeast infections are usually due to an overgrowth of *Candida albicans.*
- The conjunctiva is generally a good barrier against infectious agents, but some bacteria such as *Haemophilus aegyptius* (pinkeye), *Chlamydia trachomatis,* and *Neisseria gonorrhoeae* can easily attach to this membrane.

Placenta

The placenta, an organ formed by maternal and fetal tissues, is usually an effective barrier against microorganisms that may be present in the maternal circulation. However, some microbes can cross the placenta and infect the embryo or fetus, sometimes causing spontaneous abortions, birth defects, or premature births.

Parenteral Route

Technically the parenteral route is not a portal of entry, but a means of bypassing other portals of entry. In this manner, pathogens are introduced directly into the subcutaneous tissue, as happens with punctures by a nail, thorn, or contaminated needles. This way of pathogen entry can also be achieved by cuts, bites, stab wounds, deep abrasions, or surgery.

Virulence and Pathogenicity

After pathogens have gained entry into the body they must undergo adhesion and several other steps to be able to multiply, thereby causing an infection and possible disease.

Virulence refers to the degree of **pathogenicity** or disease-evoking power of a specific microbe. Virulence therefore is the degree of pathogenicity of a microbe and is based on **virulence factors.** A pathogen is a microorganism that is capable of causing disease. The ability of a microorganism to cause disease is directly related to the number of infecting organisms, the portal of entry, the host defense mechanisms (see Chapter 20, The Immune System), and the intrinsic characteristics of the bacteria and their virulence factors. These include the following:

- **Adhesion:** Adhesion is the first and probably the most crucial step in infection, because without adhesion to the host cells or tissue, the microbes will be removed by ciliary motion (see Chapter 3, Cell Structure and Function), sneezing, coughing, swallowing, urine flow, flow of tears,

---

Pathogens That Cross the Placenta

Microbe	Pathogen	Condition	Effect on Unborn
RNA viruses	Lentivirus (HIV)	AIDS	Immunosuppression (AIDS)
	Rubivirus	German measles	Severe birth defects or death
DNA viruses	Cytomegalovirus	Usually asymptomatic	Deafness, microcephaly, mental retardation
	Parvovirus B-19	Erythema infectiosum	Abortion
Bacteria	*Treponema pallidum*	Syphilis	Abortion, multiorgan birth defects, syphilis
	Listeria monocytogenes	Listeriosis	Granulomatosis infantiseptica, death
Protozoans	*Toxoplasma gondii*	Toxoplasmosis	Abortion, epilepsy, encephalitis, microcephaly, mental retardation, blindness, anemia, jaundice, rash, pneumonia, diarrhea, hypothermia, deafness

or intestinal peristalsis. Bacteria must first bind to the host cell, via pili, fimbriae, or specific membrane receptor sites. Viral adhesion occurs by capsid or envelope proteins. The mechanism of the adhesion process can be nonspecific or specific:

- Nonspecific adhesion involves nonspecific attractive forces or interactions the microorganism uses to move toward the eukaryotic host. These interactions and forces can include the following:
  - Hydrophobic interactions
  - Electrostatic attraction
  - Atomic and molecular vibrations
  - Brownian movement
  - Recruitment and trapping by biofilms (see Chapter 6, Bacteria and Archaea)
- Specific adhesion involves a permanent lock-and-key interaction between complementary molecules on each cell surface and under normal physiological conditions this attachment becomes irreversible. Examples of such specific attachments/adhesions are illustrated in Table 9.3.

- **Colonization:** Another essential step in the development of an infection is the establishment of the pathogen at the portal of entry once adhesion of the pathogen has occurred. Human pathogens usually colonize tissues that are in contact with the external environment, such as the urogenital tract, the digestive tract, the respiratory tract, and the conjunctiva of the eye. Some virulent bacteria may produce special proteins that allow them to colonize these parts to cause disease.

- **Invasion:** The invasive qualities of a pathogen may be aided by the production of extracellular substances, allowing it to disrupt host cell membranes, breaking down the primary and secondary defensive barriers of the host. These substances are referred to as **invasins** (Table 9.4) and their activity then facilitates the growth and spread of the pathogen.

- **Evasion of host defenses:** The ability to avoid the host response can be due to the presence of a capsule, the production of proteins that bind to the host cell antibodies, or mutation of the organism to alter its antigenicity. Various strategies are used by microbes to avoid being eliminated by the host phagocytes, but usually they involve blocking one or more steps of phagocytosis (see Chapter 20, The Immune System). Some of these strategies include but are not limited to the following:
  - Avoidance of contact with phagocytes by invading or remaining in regions that are inaccessible to phagocytes or are not patrolled by them. Some pathogens induce minimal or no inflammation to avoid provoking an

TABLE 9.3 Examples of Specific Adhesions of Bacteria to the Host

Species	Adhesion Factor	Host Receptor	Site	Disease
Chlamydia	Unknown	Sialic acid	Conjunctival or urethral epithelium	Conjunctivitis or urethritis
Bordetella pertussis	Fimbriae	Galactose on sulfated glycolipids	Respiratory epithelium	Whooping cough
Escherichia coli, enteropathogenic	Type 1 fimbriae	Species-specific carbohydrate(s)	Intestinal epithelium	Diarrhea
E. coli, uropathogenic	Type 1 fimbriae	Complex carbohydrate	Urethral epithelium	Urethritis
E. coli, uropathogenic	P pili	Globobiose linked to ceramide lipid	Upper urinary tract	Pyelonephritis
Mycoplasma	Membrane proteins	Sialic acid	Respiratory epithelium	Pneumonia
Neisseria gonorrhoeae	N-Methylphenyl-alanine pili	Glucosamine–galactose carbohydrate	Urethral/cervical epithelium	Gonorrhea
Staphylococcus aureus	Cell-bound protein	Amino terminus of fibronectin	Mucosal epithelium	Various
Streptococcus mutans	Glycosyltransferase	Salivary glycoprotein	Pellicle of tooth	Dental caries
Streptococcus pneumoniae	Cell-bound protein	N-Acetylhexosamine–galactose disaccharide	Mucosal epithelium	Pneumonia
Streptococcus pyogenes	Protein F	Amino terminus of fibronectin	Pharyngeal epithelium	Sore throat
Streptococcus salivarius	Lipoteichoic acid	Unknown	Buccal epithelium of tongue	None
Treponema pallidum	Peptide in outer membrane	Surface protein	Mucosal epithelium	Syphilis
Vibrio cholerae	N-Methylphenylalanine pili	Fucose and mannose carbohydrate	Intestinal epithelium	Cholera

TABLE 9.4 Survey of Bacterial Invasins

Invasin	Organism(s) Producing Invasin	Mechanism
Hyaluronidase	Streptococci, staphylococci, clostridia	Assaults the matrix of connective tissue by depolymerizing hyaluronic acid
Collagenase	*Clostridium histolyticum, Clostridium perfringens*	Breaks down collagen
Neuraminidase	*Vibrio cholerae, Shigella dysenteriae*	Degrades neuraminic acid of the intestinal mucosa
Kinases	Streptococci and staphylococci	Converts plasminogen to plasmin, which digests fibrin
Leukocidin	*Staphylococcus aureus*	Disrupts neutrophil membranes and causes discharge of lysosomal granules
Streptolysin	*Streptococcus pyogenes*	Repels phagocytes and disrupts phagocyte membrane, causing discharge of lysosomal granules
Hemolysins	Streptococci, staphylococci, clostridia	Phospholipases or lecithinases that destroy erythrocytes and other cells by lysis
Phospholipases	*Clostridium perfringens*	Destroys phospholipids of the plasma membrane
Lecithinases	*Clostridium perfringens*	Destroys lecithin in cell membranes
Anthrax EF	*Bacillus anthracis*	An adenylate cyclase that causes increased levels of intracellular cAMP
Pertussis AC	*Bordetella pertussis*	An adenylate cyclase that causes increased levels of intracellular cAMP and subsequent increase in respiratory secretions

cAMP, Cyclic adenosine monophosphate.

intense immune response. Other organisms inhibit phagocyte chemotaxis; for example, *Clostridium* produces a toxin that inhibits neutrophil chemotaxis. In addition, some bacteria hide their antigenic surface so that phagocytes do not recognize the organism as non-self.

- Inhibition of phagocytic engulfment is used by some bacteria that have substances on their surfaces that inhibit phagocytic activity or engulfment.
- Survival inside phagocytes, either neutrophils or macrophages, is another way by which some microbes can resist killing. These organisms are considered intracellular parasites.
- Yet another, aggressive strategy used by some organisms is to produce products that kill or damage phagocytes either before ingestion or after ingestion.
- **Toxins:** Another virulence factor is determined by the ability of the organism to produce enzymes, exotoxins, and endotoxins that will damage the host cells or interfere with a vital host cell function. Toxins constitute a major virulence factor.

Toxins

An organism that produces toxins is called **toxigenic**. This is an underlying mechanism by which many microorganisms, especially bacteria, produce disease.

Chemically, bacterial toxins are either lipopolysaccharides associated with the cell wall of gram-negative bacteria, or proteins released from the bacterial cell. Toxins associated with the cell wall are called *endotoxins*, and proteins released from a

bacterium are referred to as *exotoxins* (Figure 9.6). Bacterial toxins are among the most powerful toxins known to humankind.

Exotoxins

Exotoxins are typically soluble proteins secreted by bacterial cells during their exponential growth phase. They can act at sites other than the location of the infection and bacterial growth. Often the toxins produced are species specific and associated with a particular disease (Table 9.5). For example, *Clostridium tetani* is the only organism to produce the tetanus toxin, and *Corynebacterium diphtheriae* makes diphtheria toxin. As with other proteins, these enzymes can be denatured by heat, acid, and proteolytic enzymes (enzymes that break down proteins).

Like enzymes, many bacterial exotoxins are substrate specific and generally the site of damage caused by the toxin indicates the location of the substrate for that particular toxin. This has led to naming these toxins according to their target, such as enterotoxin, neurotoxin, leukocidin, or hemolysin to name a few.

Endotoxins

Endotoxins are lipopolysaccharides and structural components of gram-negative bacterial cell walls (e.g., Shiga toxin). Endotoxins are released from the cell walls during lysis initiated by an effective host defense or by the action of antibiotics. After release, these toxins can also act on sites remote from the original site of infection and growth. In contrast to exotoxins, endotoxins are less potent and less specific in their actions. Because

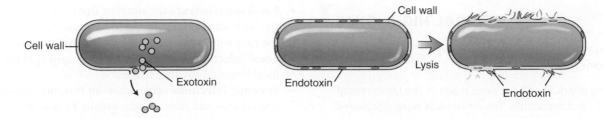

FIGURE 9.6 Actions of exotoxins and endotoxins. Exotoxins *(left)* are produced within the bacterial cells and released into the environment. Endotoxins *(right)* are components of the bacterial cell wall and are released when the bacterial cell lyses due to the immune response or antibiotic treatment.

TABLE 9.5 Examples of Bacterial Exotoxins

Organism	Toxin	Activity	Pathology
Bacillus anthracis	Anthrax toxin (EF)	Edema factor (EF) causes increased levels of intracellular cAMP in phagocytes and the formation of ion-permeable pores in membranes	Hemolysis
Bordetella pertussis	Adenylate cyclase (AC) toxin	Causes increased levels of cAMP in phagocytes and the formation of ion-permeable pores in membranes	Hemolysis; whooping cough
Escherichia coli	Heat-labile (LT) toxin	Increases the level of cAMP in cells of the GI tract, causing secretion of water and electrolytes	Severe abdominal cramps; bloody diarrhea; high fever
	Heat-stable (ST) toxin	Stimulates guanylate cyclase, promotes secretion of water and electrolytes from intestinal epithelium	Severe abdominal cramps; bloody diarrhea; high fever
Pseudomonas aeruginosa	Exotoxin A	Inhibits protein synthesis	Various
Vibrio cholerae	Cholera enterotoxin	Increases the level of cAMP in cells of the GI tract, causing secretion of water and electrolytes	Cholera
Clostridium botulinum	Botulinum toxin	Disrupts secretion of acetylcholine at neuromuscular synapse, preventing muscular contraction	Botulism
Clostridium tetani	Tetanus toxin	Prevents the breakdown of acetylcholine by enzymes at the neuro-muscular synapse, causing constant muscle contraction	Tetanus

cAMP, Cyclic adenosine monophosphate; *GI,* gastrointestinal.

these toxins are lipopolysaccharides and not proteins, they are heat stable and even boiling for 30 minutes does not destabilize them. However, certain oxidizing agents such as superoxide, peroxide, and hypochlorite have been reported to be effective in neutralizing them. A general comparison between bacterial exotoxins and endotoxins is presented in Table 9.6.

Portal of Exit

To infect others, pathogens must leave the infected patient by a portal of exit. Oftentimes this is the same as the portal of entry, such as the entrance and exit of infectious particles in and out of the respiratory system. However, pathogens can also leave the

host by excretion/secretion in various parts of the body, by defecation, or via blood. Secretory substances such as nasal secretions, saliva, sputum, respiratory droplets, tears, and earwax, are also ways by which pathogens can exit a host and infect another, usually by casual contact.

Etiology of Infectious Diseases

As mentioned earlier, not all infections cause disease and it is essential to differentiate between an infection and a disease. An infection is the colonization of a host by an infectious agent. When an infectious agent causes pathological changes and interferes with the normal functioning of the body it is termed

Microbial Enzymes versus Blood Clots and Bronchitis

Interesting discoveries have been made in the treatment of blood clots and bronchitis. The treatments were discovered in an unusual place: in the proteolytic enzymes produced by a bacterium and a fungus. For centuries the Japanese have used a fermented food product called *natto,* which was known to contribute to healthy skin and cardiovascular health, and to help prevent osteoporosis. Studies have shown that the enzyme produced by the fermenting bacterium *Bacillus natto* is effective at dissolving blood clots, potentially preventing heart attacks and strokes. This enzyme, called *nattokinase,* can dissolve clots even faster than plasmin, the main clot-dissolving enzyme produced by the body. Furthermore, nattokinase is longer acting and also has been shown to stimulate the body to produce more of its own clot-dissolving enzymes such as plasmin and urokinase.

In the case of bronchitis, an enzyme from the fungus *Aspergillus melleus* has been shown to reduce the painful inflammation and mucus associated with bronchitis. According to studies, the enzyme breaks down proteins in the mucus, making it less viscous and "sticky" and thus reducing mucus buildup and inflammation of the affected tissue.

TABLE 9.6 Comparison of Bacterial Exotoxins and Endotoxins

Feature	Exotoxin	Endotoxin
Chemical nature	Protein	Lipopolysaccharides
Location	Extracellular	Part of cell wall
Specificity	High degree	Low degree
Potency	Relatively high	Relatively low
Denatured by heat	Yes	No
Antigenic	Yes	Yes
Toxoid*	Yes	No

*A toxoid is an endotoxin modified so that it is no longer toxic, but still causes the host to generate antitoxin.

infectious disease. The study of the cause of disease is called **etiology.**

Patterns of Infection

Infections have varied patterns and are named accordingly as local infections, focal infections, systemic infections, mixed infections, acute and chronic infections, and primary and secondary infections.

- **Local infections** are the simplest ones; the organism enters the body and remains confined to a specific tissue. This is the case with boils, fungal skin infections, and warts.
- **Focal infections** occur when the pathogen spreads from a local infection to other tissues.
- **Systemic infections** occur when an infection spreads to several sites and tissue fluids, usually by way of the circulatory system.
  - **Septicemia** is a systemic infection caused by the multiplication of pathogens in the blood. This condition is a common example of **sepsis,** a toxic inflammatory condition arising from the spread of microbes.
  - **Bacteremia** represents the presence of bacteria in the blood.
  - **Toxemia** refers to the presence of toxins in the blood.
  - **Viremia** is the term used to describe viruses in the blood.
- **Mixed infections** occur when several infectious agents concurrently establish themselves at the same site. Some mixed infections are synergistic infections in which microbes cooperate in breaking down the tissue.
- **Acute infections** are infections that appear rapidly, with pronounced (severe) symptoms, but then rapidly vanish.
- **Chronic infections** have usually less severe symptoms than acute infections, but they persist for long periods of time.
- A **primary infection** is an initial infection, which is followed by complications due to another microbe.
- A **secondary infection** follows a primary infection. In general, secondary infections are caused by a different microbe, which gains access to the body through a lesion of either the skin or the mucous membrane damaged by the first pathogen, or they can be microbes of the normal flora that become opportunistic because of a compromised immune system.
- A **subclinical infection** is one that does not cause any apparent symptoms, and can be carried over long periods of time without causing symptoms of illness in the individual.

Koch's Postulates

The germ theory of disease was proposed by Louis Pasteur and Robert Koch (see Chapter 1, Scope of Microbiology). Although Louis Pasteur was convinced that microbes caused disease in humans he was not able to link a specific microbe with a particular disease. After many years of experimentation, Koch was able to establish that specific microorganisms cause specific diseases. Koch developed a series of conditions—postulates—that must be met to identify a particular microbe as pathogenic and the cause of a particular disease. Using his postulates he proved that *Bacillus anthracis* is the causative agent for anthrax and that *Mycobacterium tuberculosis* causes tuberculosis. This concept is now known as *Koch's postulates* (Figure 9.7), and can be summarized as follows:

- The suspected pathogen must be present in every case of the disease, and absent in healthy individuals.
- The pathogen must be isolated from the diseased host and grown in pure culture outside the host.

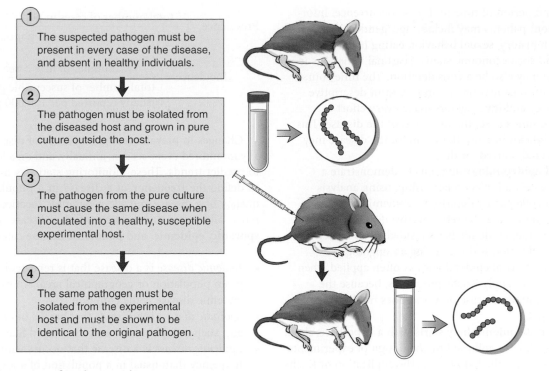

FIGURE 9.7 Illustration of Koch's postulates.

- The pathogen from the pure culture must cause the same disease when inoculated into a healthy, susceptible experimental host.
- The same pathogen must be isolated from the experimental host and be shown to be identical to the original pathogen.

Exceptions to Koch's Postulates

Although Koch's postulates provide the basics of the etiology of infectious disease, they are not always appropriate to use, for the following reasons:

- Some pathogens cannot be cultured in the laboratory.
- Many infectious diseases can be caused by several different pathogens.
- A particular pathogen can cause different diseases, depending on the portal of entry.
- Some diseases are caused by a combination of pathogens, such as liver infections caused by both the hepatitis B virus and the hepatitis D virusoid. The latter cannot cause infection without the hepatitis B virus. Other exceptions are polymicrobial diseases caused by biofilms.
- Some pathogens are exclusively human pathogens and ethical considerations prevent human inoculation to prove Koch's postulates. These exceptions include diseases caused by viruses or animal parasites. Also, *Rickettsia* and *Chlamydia* are obligate intracellular parasites without an animal model.

Although Koch's postulates do not always seem to apply, scientists have found other means to reach the desired outcome of the postulates by following other routes. Furthermore, Koch's postulates are at work in the food industry, where microbes need to be carefully monitored, and the desired microbe must be isolated in the desired end product. Despite the challenges Koch's postulates remain useful for confirming microbial roles in infection, disease, and other processes. The concepts used to prove cause have been employed as modules of proof in other scientific disciplines. For example, Eccles used a similar pattern to show that acetylcholine (ACh) was a chemical transmitter in the central nervous system, which established mammalian neurotransmission as being chemical, when it had previously been promoted as electrical.

Epidemiology and Public Health

Epidemiology is the study of the distribution and causes of disease in populations, and serves as the foundation of interventions needed in the interest of public health and preventive medicine. Epidemiologists study how many people or animals are affected, where they are distributed, and the outcome of the disease, such as recovery, death, and disability. In addition, they study the factors that influence the distribution and outcome of the disease. Epidemiologists use three basic approaches to study the dynamics of diseases in populations: descriptive, analytical, and experimental.

- **Descriptive epidemiology** is the collecting and tabulating of data concerning the disease. These data generally include information about the affected individuals and the location and period of time of disease occurrence. Information about patients may include age, gender, occupation, health history, sexual behavior, eating habits, travel history, and socioeconomic status. Seasonal variations in the climate may also be a consideration. The time course and chain of transmission are important in descriptive epidemiology and investigators make every effort to identify the **index case,** the first case, of the disease. This might be difficult because the victim of the disease may have recovered, moved, or died.

- **Analytical epidemiology** attempts to demonstrate a probable cause-and-effect relationship, using analysis of the data collected by descriptive epidemiology. Analytical studies may be retrospective if the data are analyzed after an epidemic has subsided, or prospective if the data collection is done during an ongoing epidemic. Analytical epidemiology is often applied when it is unethical to apply Koch's postulates, because the disease is a human disease only and does not have an animal model.
- **Experimental epidemiology** starts with a hypothesis about a particular disease, followed by the design of experiments and studies to test the hypothesis. The application of Koch's postulates is a perfect example of experimental epidemiology.

Epidemiology is a subject of major importance to state and federal public health departments. The Centers for Disease Control and Prevention (CDC) is the central source of epidemiological information in the United States. The CDC publishes the *Morbidity and Mortality Weekly Report (MMWR),* which can be viewed at the CDC website (www.cdc.gov). This publication contains data on morbidity (the incidence of specific notifiable diseases), and mortality (the number of deaths associated with a particular disease). The morbidity rate reflects the number of people affected by a particular disease during a given time in relation to the total population. The mortality rate shows the number of deaths resulting from a disease in a population during a given period of time in relation to the total population. The *Morbidity and Mortality Weekly Report* is of interest to microbiologists, physicians, and other healthcare and public health professionals. Nationally notifiable infectious diseases are diseases that must be reported by physicians to the U.S. Public Health Service and are shown in Box 9.1. A well-developed network of individuals and agencies keeps track of infectious diseases at the local, district, state, national, and international levels. The CDC shares its information and statistics with the World Health Organization (WHO) for the purpose of worldwide tabulation and control.

Diseases in the Population

Diseases in a population can be reported as the prevalence of the disease, which is the total number of existing cases in the entire population, or the disease can be measured by incidence, which is the number of new cases over a certain period of time compared with the general healthy population. The equations used to determine these rates are as follows:

$$Prevalence = \left(\frac{total\ number\ of\ cases\ in\ population}{total\ number\ of\ persons\ in\ population} \right) \times 100 = \%$$

$$Incidence = \left(\frac{number\ of\ new\ cases}{total\ number\ of\ susceptible\ persons} \right)$$
(usually reported per 100,000 persons)

Changes in prevalence and incidence of diseases are generally monitored every season, annually, and on a long-term basis to predict trends. These monitoring statistics make it possible to define the frequency of a disease in a population. The frequency of a disease and the geographic location of the occurrence allow for classification of the disease into **endemic, sporadic, epidemic,** and **pandemic** disease categories.

- *Endemic disease* is a disease that is repeatedly present in a given population or geographical area. An example of an endemic disease is the common cold.
- *Sporadic disease* is a disease that breaks out only occasionally, such as typhoid fever in the United States.
- *Epidemic disease* is a disease that occurs with greater frequency than usual in a population of a given area. Influenza is an example of a disease that can occasionally reach epidemic proportions.
- *Pandemic disease* is a worldwide epidemic such as AIDS and the influenza of 1918.

Reservoirs

For an infectious disease to continue to exist, its causative agent(s) must have a permanent place to reside. Sites where pathogens are maintained as a source of infection are called *reservoirs of infection.* These can be in the form of animal, human, or nonliving reservoirs.

Animal Reservoirs

Many of the pathogens that normally infect animals, either domesticated or wild, also can affect humans. Diseases that occur primarily in animals and can be transmitted to humans are referred to as *zoonoses* (Table 9.7). Humans can be infected by zoonoses by several routes: direct contact with the infected animal; contact with animal waste, or with waste-contaminated food or water; contact with dust from contaminated hides, fur, or feathers; consumption of infected animal products; or through the medium of insect vectors. Humans often are the definitive (final) host for zoonotic pathogens and usually are not a significant reservoir for reinfection of animal hosts. However, zoonotic diseases transmitted by blood-sucking arthropods are likely to be transmitted back to the species of the animal host.

Human Carriers

The main reservoir for human infectious agents is the human body. People with an obvious infectious disease are easily identified and precautions can be put in place to avoid transmission of the disease. However, many individuals may be infected and remain asymptomatic for years and never become sick. People who are infected and do not show any symptoms are referred

BOX 9.1 Nationally Notifiable Infectious Diseases

- Acquired immunodeficiency syndrome (AIDS)
- Anthrax
- Arboviral neuroinvasive and nonneuroinvasive diseases
  - California serogroup virus disease
  - Eastern equine encephalitis virus disease
  - Powassan virus disease
  - St. Louis encephalitis virus disease
  - West Nile virus disease
  - Western equine virus disease
- Botulism
  - Botulism, foodborne
  - Botulism, infant
  - Botulism, other (wound and unspecified)
- Brucellosis
- Chancroid
- *Chlamydia trachomatis,* genital infections
- Cholera
- Coccidioidomycosis
- Cryptosporidiosis
- Cyclosporiasis
- Diphtheria
- Ehrlichiosis
  - *Ehrlichia chaffeensis*
  - *Ehrlichia ewingii*
  - *Anaplasma phagocytophilum*
  - Undetermined
- Giardiasis
- Gonorrhea
- *Haemophilus influenzae,* invasive disease
- Hansen's disease (leprosy)
- Hantavirus pulmonary syndrome
- Hemolytic uremic syndrome, postdiarrheal
- Hepatitis, viral, acute
  - Hepatitis A, acute
  - Hepatitis B, acute
  - Hepatitis B, perinatal infection
  - Hepatitis C, acute
- Hepatitis, viral, chronic
  - Chronic hepatitis B
  - Hepatitis C infection (past or present)
- HIV infection
  - HIV infection, adult/adolescent (age ≥ 13 yr)
  - HIV infection, child (age ≥ 18 mo and < 13 yr)
  - HIV infection, pediatric (age < 18 mo)
- Influenza-associated pediatric mortality
- Legionellosis
- Listeriosis
- Lyme disease
- Malaria
- Measles
- Meningococcal disease

- Mumps
- Novel influenza A virus infections
- Pertussis
- Plague
- Poliomyelitis, paralytic
- Poliovirus infection, nonparalytic
- Psittacosis
- Q fever
  - Acute
  - Chronic
- Rabies
  - Rabies, animal
  - Rabies, human
- Rocky Mountain spotted fever
- Rubella
- Rubella, congenital syndrome
- Salmonellosis
- Severe acute respiratory syndrome–associated coronavirus (SARS-CoV) disease
- Shiga toxin–producing *Escherichia coli* (STEC)
- Shigellosis
- Smallpox
- Streptococcal disease, invasive, Group A
- Streptococcal toxic shock syndrome
- *Streptococcus pneumoniae,* drug resistant, invasive disease
- *Streptococcus pneumoniae,* invasive disease, nondrug resistant, in children less than 5 years of age
- Syphilis
  - Syphilis, primary
  - Syphilis, secondary
  - Syphilis, latent
  - Syphilis, early latent
  - Syphilis, late latent
  - Syphilis, late, unknown duration
  - Neurosyphilis
  - Syphilis, late, nonneurological
  - Syphilitic stillbirth
- Syphilis, congenital
- Tetanus
- Toxic shock syndrome (other than streptococcal)
- Trichinellosis (trichinosis)
- Tuberculosis
- Tularemia
- Typhoid fever
- Vancomycin-intermediate *Staphylococcus aureus* (VISA)
- Vancomycin-resistant *Staphylococcus aureus* (VRSA)
- Varicella (morbidity)
- Varicella (deaths only)
- Vibriosis
- Yellow fever

Data from http://www.cdc.gov/ncphi/disss/nndss/PHS/infdis.htm (accessed April 29, 2009).

TABLE 9.7 Examples of Zoonoses

Disease	Infectious Agent	Animal Reservoir	Mode of Transmission
Viral			
Rabies	Lyssavirus spp.	Bats, skunks, raccoons, foxes, dogs	Direct contact via bite or scratch of infected animal
Hantavirus pulmonary syndrome	Hantavirus spp.	Rodents, primarily deer mice	Inhalation of viruses from dried feces and urine or direct contact with rodent saliva, feces, or urine
Yellow fever	Flavivirus spp.	Monkeys	Bite of *Aedes* mosquito
Influenza (some)	Influenza virus	Swine, birds	Direct contact
Bacterial			
Anthrax	*Bacillus anthracis*	Domestic livestock	Direct contact with infected animals, inhalation
Brucellosis	*Brucella* spp.	Domestic livestock	Direct contact with contaminated meat, milk, or animal
Lyme disease	*Borrelia burgdorferi*	Deer	Tick bites
Rocky Mountain spotted fever	*Rickettsia rickettsii*	Rodents	Tick bites
Typhus	*Rickettsia prowazeki* *Rickettsia typhi*	Rodents	Louse bites
Bubonic plague	*Yersinia pestis*	Rodents	Flea bites
Leptospirosis	*Leptospira* spp.	Wild animals, domestic dogs and cats	Direct contact with urine, soil, water
Psittacosis (parrot fever)	*Chlamydia psittaci*	Birds, especially parrots	Direct contact, bird droppings
Salmonellosis	*Salmonella* spp.	Poultry, rats, reptiles	Ingestion of contaminated food and water
Fungal			
Ringworm	*Trichophyton* spp. *Microsporum* spp. *Epidermophyton* spp.	Domestic animals	Direct contact
Protozoan			
Malaria	*Plasmodium* spp.	Monkeys	Bite of *Anopheles* mosquito
Toxoplasmosis	*Toxoplasma gondii*	Cats and other animals	Ingestion of contaminated meat, inhalation of pathogen, direct contact
Helminthic			
Tapeworm infestation	*Dipylidium caninum*	Dogs	Ingestion of larvae transmitted in dog saliva
Fasciola infestation	*Fasciola hepatica*	Sheep, cattle	Ingestion of contaminated meat
Trichinellosis	*Trichinella spiralis*	Pigs, bears	Ingestion of undercooked contaminated meat

to as *carriers.* They are able to infect others without necessarily knowing that they are carriers. It is believed that these healthy carriers have an immune system response that prevents them from getting the disease.

Nonliving Reservoirs

Nonliving reservoirs of infection include soil, water, and food. Soil is a great environment for pathogens such as fungi, helminths, and bacteria. If the soil is contaminated with fecal material it can contain organisms normally present in the intestinal tract of humans and other animals, and ultimately is responsible for gastrointestinal disease. In addition, the soil can harbor pathogens such as *Clostridium botulinum,* the causative agent of botulism, and *C. tetani,* which causes tetanus. Water can potentially be contaminated with feces and urine containing parasitic worm eggs, pathogenic protozoans, bacteria, and viruses. Contamination with infectious agents can also include foods improperly prepared or stored.

Modes of Transmission

Infectious diseases are transmitted either by a reservoir or via a portal of exit to a portal of entry of another host, or by **autoinoculation** (self-inoculation). Infectious agents can be transmitted to a host in many ways, including contact, vehicle, or vector transmission.

Contact Transmission

In contact transmission the pathogen is spread from one host to another either by direct contact, indirect contact, or respiratory droplets.

- **Direct contact** transmission involves direct physical contact of the infectious agent between hosts, such as by person-to-person contact; no intermediate object is involved. Common forms of direct contact transmission are touching, kissing, and sexual intercourse. Examples of pathogens transmitted this way include agents causing respiratory tract infections, staphylococcal infections, measles, scarlet fever, and sexually transmitted diseases. Zoonoses can also be transmitted from an animal reservoir to a human by direct contact through touching, biting, or scratching. Furthermore, direct transmission is possible within a single individual with poor personal hygiene when putting fingers in the mouth that are contaminated with fecal material.
- **Indirect contact** transmission occurs when the pathogen is transmitted from the reservoir to the susceptible host by a **fomite**—a nonliving object. Fomites can be tissues, handkerchiefs, towels, bedding, toys, clothes, diapers, money, eating utensils, drinking cups/glasses, medical equipment and devices, contaminated needles, and any other items that can harbor or transmit pathogens. Contaminated needles are a common fomite for the transmission of HIV and hepatitis B and C.
- **Droplet** transmission occurs when infectious agents are transmitted through respiratory droplets that travel a distance less than 1 meter. These droplets are released into the environment by normal exhaling, laughing, coughing, or sneezing. Sneezing is the most effective form of droplet transmission. Examples include the transmission of the common cold, influenza, pneumonia, and pertussis.

Vehicle Transmission

Any transmission of pathogens that require some sort of medium is considered a vehicle transmission. Modes of transmission in this category include airborne, waterborne, and foodborne transmissions, as well as transmission through bodily fluids and intravenous fluids. Foodborne, waterborne, and airborne diseases are also shown in the Healthcare Applications tables of Chapter 1 (Scope of Microbiology).

- **Airborne transmission** refers to the spread of pathogens by droplet nuclei (droplets of mucus), other aerosols, and dust that travel more than 1 meter from the reservoir to the host. Aerosols may originate from coughing or sneezing and from air conditioning and other cooling systems. Pathogens can attach themselves to dust particles and be transmitted by air via sweeping, mopping, changing of bed linens, changing of clothes, or simple dusting.
- **Waterborne transmission** generally occurs through untreated or poorly treated sewage. Many gastrointestinal diseases including giardiasis, amebic dysentery, and cholera are transmitted by water. Waterborne shigellosis and leptospirosis can also be transmitted via this route. Fecal–oral infections are the major source of diseases in the world as pathogens such as *Schistosoma* worms and enteroviruses are shed in feces, get into the water supply, subsequently enter the gastrointestinal mucosa or skin, and then cause disease elsewhere in the body.
- **Foodborne transmission** generally involves pathogens in or on foods that are incompletely cooked, poorly processed under unsanitary conditions, not refrigerated, or poorly refrigerated. This type of contamination can be by normal microbial flora, with zoonotic pathogens, and with parasitic worms that alternate between human and animal hosts. Viruses such as the hepatitis A virus can also be transmitted this way.
- **Bodily fluid transmission** needs to be considered, especially in healthcare workers, who must take precautions when handling these fluids, which can potentially be contaminated with pathogens. Blood, urine, saliva, and other bodily fluids can be reservoirs for different pathogens. Examples of diseases that can be transmitted via this route include AIDS, hepatitis, and herpes.

Vector Transmission

Vectors are animals, usually arthropods, that carry pathogens from one host to another. Vectors can transmit the pathogens either biologically or mechanically (Box 9.2).

- *Biological vectors* transmit pathogens, but also serve as host for a part of the pathogen's life cycle. Biological vectors important to human diseases are biting insects, including mosquitoes, ticks, lice, fleas, blood-sucking flies or bugs, and mites.
- *Mechanical vectors,* on the other hand, do not have to be a host for the pathogen, but passively carry the agents to a new host by their feet or other body parts, such as happens with flies.

BOX 9.2 Arthropod Vectors

Biological Vectors
- *Mosquitoes:* Malaria, yellow fever, elephantiasis, dengue, viral encephalitis, West Nile virus
- *Ticks:* Lyme disease, Rocky Mountain spotted fever, babesiosis, ehrlichiosis
- *Fleas:* Bubonic plague, endemic typhus
- *Lice:* Epidemic typhus
- *Blood-sucking flies:* African sleeping sickness, river blindness
- *Blood-sucking bugs:* Chagas' disease
- *Mites:* Scrub typhus

Mechanical Vectors
- *Houseflies:* Foodborne illness
- *Cockroaches:* Foodborne illness

Healthcare-associated (Nosocomial) Infections

Nosocomial infections are infections acquired in the course of treatment in a hospital or hospital-like setting, but secondary to the patient's original conditions. Infections obtained by patients or healthcare providers while they are treated or working in a healthcare setting such as a hospital, clinic, nursing home, dental office, and other healthcare facility are referred to as *healthcare-associated infections* (HAIs). HAIs are among the top 10 leading causes of death in the United States. In the latest update (2009) by the CDC, it is estimated that in American hospitals alone HAIs account for an estimated 1.7 million infections and 99,000 associated deaths each year (Box 9.3).

The CDC developed the National Nosocomial Infections Surveillance (NNIS) system in the early 1970s to monitor the incidence of HAIs and their associated risk factors and pathogens. The purpose of the system is to help infection control professionals and hospitals stay up to date on the rapidly expanding science and practice of infection prevention and control, and to be able to better manage endemic and epidemic episodes of HAI. This voluntary system included approximately 300 hospitals in 2005, at which time it started to undergo a major redesign into a web-based knowledge management and adverse events reporting system. This system is now called the *National Healthcare Safety Network* (NHSN), and is a secure Internet-based surveillance system that integrates patient and healthcare personnel safety surveillance systems managed by the Division of Healthcare Quality Promotion (DHQP) at the CDC. Initially enrollment into the system was given to a limited number of facilities in 2005, followed by a national open enrollment for hospitals and outpatient hemodialysis centers in 2007.

Types of Nosocomial Infections

Healthcare facilities, by their very nature, are filled with sick people capable of shedding a variety of pathogens from different portals of exit. Furthermore, people with infections and/or diseases have a stressed, weakened, and often a compromised/suppressed immune system, making them even more susceptible to any infectious or opportunistic agents. Healthcare-associated infections can be categorized as exogenous, endogenous, and iatrogenic infections.

> **BOX 9.3 Types of Healthcare-associated Infections in the United States**
>
> - 32% of all healthcare-associated infections (HAIs) are urinary tract infections
> - 22% surgical site infections
> - 15% pneumonia
> - 14% bloodstream infections
> - 9% other (meningitis, gastroenteritis)
> - 8% skin infection

- **Exogenous** HAIs are caused by pathogens in the healthcare environment, shed from sick people.
- **Endogenous** infections are caused by microbes in the normal flora of a patient, which become pathogenic because of a variety of factors associated with the healthcare setting. These factors include the state of the patient's immune system, immovability (bedridden), diet, and many others. Another factor is the use of antimicrobial drugs that may inhibit some of the normal flora, allowing the overgrowth of others, causing superinfections in the absence of the usual competition. Superinfections, however, are not limited to healthcare settings.
- **Iatrogenic** infections are a set of infections that may result from the use of medical procedures such as the use of catheters, invasive diagnostic procedures, and surgery.

Nosocomial infections can be caused by a variety of organisms (Table 9.8), some of which cause specific infections and disease; others have the capacity to cause a variety of infections, depending on their portal of entry. Bacteria that gain entrance to the bloodstream have the chance to settle at a site different from the site of entry if not treated promptly. Septicemia is less common, but can occur when surgery is performed on an infected area or an area where bacteria normally grow (i.e., intestine).

Transmission

Because of the large number and variety of pathogens in the healthcare environment and the compromised state of the patients, the routes and chain of transmission constitute an ongoing concern for healthcare providers and their patients. The principal routes of concern are as follows:

- Direct contact transmission from hospital staff to the patient
- Visitor to patient
- Patient to patient via activities of staff members
- Indirect contact transmission through fomites
- Airborne transmission through the healthcare facility's ventilation system

Therefore certain hospital areas are reserved for specialized care, including burn, hemodialysis, recovery, intensive care, and oncology units. Unfortunately, these environments also provide a risk for an epidemic spread of nosocomial infections from patient to patient.

Diagnostic and certain therapeutic procedures provide a possible route of transmission through fomites. For example, the urinary catheter, commonly used to drain the urinary bladder, is a fomite in many nosocomial infections. Intravenous catheters, used for the delivery of fluids, nutrients, or medication, need to penetrate the skin and can be a potential fomite for infection. Other potential fomites are the various components of respiratory equipment, needles, and surgical dressings. All these potential ways of transmission are the reason for the use of many control measures aimed at the prevention of nosocomial infections in the healthcare environment.

TABLE 9.8 Infectious Diseases That May Be Acquired in Healthcare Facilities

Pathogen	Disease
Acinetobacter	Variety, ranging from pneumonia to serious blood or wound infections
Blood-borne pathogens	
Hepatitis B	Hepatitis
Hepatitis C	Hepatitis
HIV/AIDS	HIV/AIDS
Burkholderia cepacia	Respiratory infections, pneumonia, especially in patients with cystic fibrosis
Clostridium difficile	Diarrhea, colitis
Clostridium sordellii	Pneumonia, endocarditis, arthritis, peritonitis, myonecrosis, toxic shock syndrome (gynecologic infections)
Creutzfeldt-Jakob prion	Creutzfeldt-Jakob disease
Ebola	Viral hemorrhagic fever
Enteric bacteria	Gastrointestinal infections
Hepatitis A	Hepatitis
Influenza viruses	Influenza
Methicillin-resistant *Staphylococcus aureus* (MRSA)	Potentially life-threatening infections such as pneumonia, surgical site infection, bloodstream infections
Mumps virus	Mumps
Norovirus	Gastroenteritis
Parvovirus	Erythema infectiosum (fifth disease)
Poliovirus	Poliomyelitis (rare)
Rubella virus	Rubella
Coronavirus	SARS
Pseudomonas aeruginosa	Infections in burn patients
Streptococcus pneumoniae (drug resistant)	Meningitis, bacteremia, pneumonia, otitis media
Mycobacterium tuberculosis	Tuberculosis
Varicella	Chicken pox
Vancomycin-intermediate *Staphylococcus aureus* (VISA)	Potentially life-threatening infections such as pneumonia, surgical site infection, bloodstream infections
Vancomycin-resistant enterococci (VRE)	Various infections

SARS, Severe acute respiratory syndrome.

Antimicrobial Resistance in Healthcare Settings

Drug-resistant pathogens are becoming an increasing threat to the population (see Chapter 18, Emerging Infectious Diseases), particularly in healthcare settings. Of all patients with nosocomial infections in the United States, 99,000 annually die as a result of their infection. More than 70% of the bacteria causing these infections are resistant to at least one of the drugs commonly used to treat them. Persons infected with drug-resistant organisms generally have longer hospital stays and require second- or third-choice drugs that may be less effective and more toxic.

Control and Prevention

Each healthcare facility has a safety program, policies, and procedures (see Chapter 5, Safety Issues) that will include procedures and precautions designed to reduce the incidence of HAIs. These procedures are aimed at preventing the transmission of pathogens to patients and healthcare personnel. In general, these measures include disinfection, medical asepsis (good housekeeping, hand washing, bathing, sanitary food handling, proper hygiene, measures to prevent the spread of pathogens between patients), surgical asepsis, and isolation of contagious and particularly susceptible patients.

Any source of agents that can cause nosocomial infections must be kept clean and disinfected, including items such as humidifiers, which provide both a suitable environment for bacteria to grow and a method of airborne transmission. Furthermore, according to the CDC hand washing is the single most important means of preventing the spread of infection. It has been shown in several studies that effective hand washing by all medical and support staff significantly reduced (by 50%) deaths from nosocomial infections when the hospital personnel followed strict guidelines about washing their hands frequently. Unfortunately, it has been reported by the CDC that on average healthcare workers wash their hands only 40% of the time before interacting with patients.

All accredited hospitals have an infection control committee and most hospitals have at least one infection control nurse, epidemiologist, or specialized microbiologist. The role of these individuals is to identify problem sources such as improper adherence to hospital guidelines for disease prevention and control, and the occurrence of antibiotic-resistant strains of bacteria.

The CDC has published guidelines and recommendations for the prevention of healthcare-associated infections, including guidelines for the protection of patients, guidelines for the protection of healthcare workers, and other guidelines and recommendations for other topics dealing with infection control. All these guidelines are available at the CDC website.

Summary

- Under normal circumstances the newborn is initially exposed to microbes during birth, followed by many more exposures. This is the start of the development of a relationship between humans and microbes. The relationship between two different types of organisms is referred to as *symbiosis,* and, depending on the outcome of the relationship, symbiosis is classified as mutualism, commensalism, parasitism, or amensalism.

- Microorganisms that establish residency on the skin and in the mucous membranes that open to the external environment, and do not cause disease, represent the normal flora.
- Whenever the balance between the normal flora and the human host is interrupted, the microorganisms of the normal flora can cause infection and disease—they become opportunistic pathogens.
- Contamination is the presence of microbes in or on the body; it can result in infection and disease, and the microorganisms can enter the host via several possible portals of entry.
- After gaining entry into the host, the pathogen must undergo adhesion and several other steps to be able to cause an infection, but not all infections cause disease.
- Infections have varied patterns, and when an infectious agent causes pathological changes and interferes with the normal functioning of the body it is termed infectious disease; the study of the cause of the disease is called *etiology.*

- Robert Koch established a series of conditions—postulates—that must be met to identify a particular microbe as pathogenic and the cause of a particular disease. Although these postulates provide the basics of the etiology of an infectious disease, they are not always applicable.
- Epidemiology is the study of the distribution and causes of diseases in a population, and is the foundation for necessary interventions in the interest of public health. It is a subject of major importance for state and federal public health departments. Diseases in a population are reported as the prevalence of the disease, measured by incidence, which is the number of new cases over a certain period of time compared with the healthy population.
- For an infectious disease to continue to exist, its causative agent must have a permanent place to reside, a reservoir of infection. Infectious agents can be transmitted to a host by contact, vehicle, or vector transmission.
- Healthcare-associated (nosocomial) infections (HAIs) are infections acquired as a result of treatment or working in healthcare facilities. Healthcare facilities serve sick people, capable of shedding pathogens. Transmission of pathogens and the development of resistant strains in this setting are becoming an increasing problem to public health.

Review Questions

1. Which type of symbiosis benefits both members?
   a. Mutualism
   b. Parasitism
   c. Commensalism
   d. Pathogenesis

2. The mold that produces penicillin is an example of:
   a. Parasitism
   b. Mutualism
   c. Commensalism
   d. Amensalism

3. The presence of microbes in or on the body is a(n):
   a. Infection
   b. Disease
   c. Contamination
   d. Adhesion

4. All of the following areas of the human body contain normal flora *except* the:
   a. Peritoneum
   b. Urethra
   c. Vagina
   d. Mouth

5. Bacterial endotoxins are:
   a. Proteins in the cell wall
   b. Secreted into the environment
   c. Components of the gram-positive cell wall
   d. Components of the gram-negative cell wall

6. When a pathogen spreads from the original site to other tissues or organs it is called a(n) _____ infection.
   a. Local
   b. Focal
   c. Natural
   d. Acute

7. A disease that is generally present in a given population is:
   a. Pandemic
   b. Epidemic
   c. Sporadic
   d. Endemic

8. Which of the following is *not* considered to be a vehicle transmission?
   a. Airborne
   b. Droplet
   c. Foodborne
   d. Bodily fluid

9. Which of the following is likely to be the most frequently used portal of entry?
   a. Skin
   b. Gastrointestinal tract
   c. Respiratory tract
   d. Conjunctiva

10. Infections that may result from the use of catheters are classified as:
    a. Iatrogenic infections
    b. Local infections
    c. Exogenous infections
    d. Endogenous infections

11. The symbiotic relationship in which one of the organisms benefits and the other is not harmed or helped is referred to as _____.

12. A flora found in the same location as the resident flora, but which remains only for a given amount of time, is called a(n) _____ flora.

13. A microorganism capable of causing disease is called a(n) _____.

14. A vector that transmits pathogens and also serves as host for a part of the pathogen's life cycle is a(n) _____ vector.

15. A worldwide epidemic is considered a(n) _____ disease.

16. Describe how microbes of a normal flora in the human body can become opportunistic pathogens.

17. Describe the three basic approaches used by epidemiologists to study the dynamics of a disease in a population.

18. Discuss Koch's postulates and its limitations.

19. Describe the necessary steps a microbe must take before it can cause infection and disease.

20. Discuss healthcare-associated (nosocomial) infections (HAIs).

Bibliography

Bauman R: *Microbiology: with diseases by taxonomy*, ed 2, San Francisco, 2007, Benjamin Cummings/Pearson Education.

Forbes BA, Sahm DF, Weissfeld AS: *Bailey & Scott's diagnostic microbiology*, ed 12, St. Louis, 2007, Mosby/Elsevier.

Grimes JD: *Koch's postulates—then and now*, Microbe 1(5):223–228, 2006.

Klevens M, Edwards JR, Richards CL Jr, et al: *Estimating healthcare-associated infections and deaths in U.S. hospitals, 2002*, Public Health Reports 122:160–166, 2007.

Mims C, Dockrell HM, Goering RV, et al: *Medical microbiology*, ed 3, St. Louis, 2004, Mosby/Elsevier.

Murray PR, Rosenthal KS, Pfaller MA: *Medical microbiology*, ed 5, St. Louis, 2005, Mosby/Elsevier.

Talaro KP: *Foundations in microbiology*, ed 6, New York, 2008, McGraw-Hill.

Totora GJ, Funke BR, Case CL: *Microbiology: an introduction*, ed 9, San Francisco, 2007, Benjamin Cummings/Pearson Education.

Internet Resources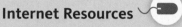

Todar's Online Textbook of Bacteriology, http://www.textbookofbacteriology.net/

CDC, Smallpox: 30th Anniversary of Global Eradication, http://www.cdc.gov/Features/SmallpoxEradication/

CDC, Nationally Notifiable Infectious Diseases, United States, 2007, http://www.cdc.gov/ncphi/disss/nndss/phs/infdis2009.htm

Thacker SB: Epidemiology and public health at CDC, *MMWR Morb Mortal Wkly Rep 55*(Suppl. 2):3–4, 2006, http://www.cdc.gov/mmwr/preview/mmwrhtml/su5502a2.htm

CDC, National Nosocomial Infections Surveillance System (NNIS), http://www.cdc.gov/ncidod/dhqp/nnis.html

CDC, Healthcare-associated Infections (HAIs), http://www.cdc.gov/ncidod/dhqp/healthDis.html

10

Infections of the Integumentary System, Soft Tissue, and Muscle

OUTLINE

Introduction

Bacterial Infections
Staphylococcal Infections
Streptococcal Infections
Acne
Leprosy

Viral Infections
Warts
Herpes Simplex Infections
Varicella-Zoster Infections
Molluscum Contagiosum
Roseola Infantum
Smallpox

Fungal Infections (Mycoses)
Tineas
Cutaneous Candidiasis
Subcutaneous Mycoses

LEARNING OBJECTIVES

After reading this chapter, the student will be able to:
- Classify bacterial skin infection based on the layers of skin and soft tissue involved
- Identify and describe the different kinds of staphylococcal skin infections
- Identify and describe the different kinds of streptococcal skin infections
- Explain the causes of acne and leprosy
- Describe the different kinds of warts and their causative agent
- Discuss skin infections caused by herpesviruses
- Discuss the importance of smallpox
- Describe the different kinds of tineas
- Describe cutaneous candidiasis
- Discuss subcutaneous mycoses

abscess
boils
candidiasis
carbuncles
chromoblastomycosis
dermatophytes
dermis

epidermis
folliculitis
furuncles
hypodermis
Langerhans cells
mycetoma

mycoses
necrotizing infections
pyogenic exudate
spreading infections
subcutaneous layer
tincas

WHY YOU NEED TO KNOW

HISTORY

Hands are one of the most efficient and direct instruments for transferring microbes and/or pathogens to the main port of entry in the body—the mouth. They are also one of the most efficient and direct methods for pathogens to be collected and subsequently transferred to other ports of entry, such as breaks in the skin. The average person carries between 10,000 and 10 million bacteria per hand. Ignaz Semmelweis (July 1, 1818 to August 13, 1865), a Hungarian physician, is one of the first practitioners to understand and connect the relationship between hands and the transfer of bacteria to portals of entry. His assessment of the cause and the use of the information helped to cure the ravages of puerperal (childbed) fever. The current medical practice of that time (mid-1800s at about the same time the germ theory of disease was being formulated) was for physicians to proceed directly from an autopsy to the live patient without washing anything, least of all hands. In fact, the crusts of blood, pus, and some necrotic tissue residues were wiped on and left on the lapels of their coats to show they had "experience." In addition, the medical bureaucracies were highly resistant to any changes in their established practices that did not include anything resembling hygiene, but did include belief in miasmas ("bad air") and balance of the "four humours" (see Why You Need to Know: History in Chapter 2, Chemistry of Life). Actually, the miasmas were generated from the stench of rotting flesh from dead tissues and cadavers. The germ theory of disease had not yet been developed. Then a fellow physician and close friend of Semmelweis died from a scalpel wound with symptoms not unlike those of patients with puerperal fever.

IMPACT

Ignaz Semmelweis postulated that the odor came from some residue on the patients or cadavers and that if this was removed then the puerperal fever might be altered. He extended his washing to remove the stench and included instruments used to examine patients and cadavers, medical students' hands, midwife personnel, and all who came in contact with puerperal fever. The results were dramatic. Death rates in the wards and elsewhere plummeted from more than 30% to 1%! Yet, the "establishment" was unwilling (see Semmelweis reflex, below) to accept the cause of death and dying from puerperal fever as a result of their time-honored practices. Finally, the wisdom and evidence of Semmelweis, Koch, Pasteur, Lister, and others prevailed during the mid- to late 1800s as the germ theory gradually became accepted.

Joseph Lister (April 5, 1827 to February 10, 1912), "the father of modern antisepsis," was aware of the work of Semmelweis and that of other germ theory advocates; however, he used carbolic acid (phenol) instead of chlorinated soaps to disinfect hands, surgical instruments, and operating fields. Carbolic acid was used to deodorize sewage and his reasoning, like that of Semmelweis, was to get rid of the source of the odor. In addition, one of Lister's nurses developed contact dermatitis to the carbolic acid and he had Charles Goodyear make rubber surgical gloves for protection. He further acknowledged Semmelweis's earlier work by stating, "Without Semmelweis, my achievements would be nothing."

FUTURE

Bureaucratic rejection without examination of experimental evidence has given rise to the "Semmelweis reflex" or dismissal out of hand, as an automatic reflex to new, challenging ideas without the benefit of thought or experimentation.

Soaps and detergents are definitely effective tools to slow down or prevent transmission of microbes. The development of antimicrobacterial soaps has led to the use of these products in most households, public places, and in the healthcare environment. While the use of these antibiotic products is essential in healthcare facilities, concern is growing over the overuse of antibacterial household cleaning and hygiene products for fear of the possible development of antimicrobial drug resistance. Appropriate hand washing with regular soap and water has proven effective under most circumstances. The Centers for Disease Control and Prevention, in conjunction with many scientific groups, is currently studying the possible consequences of overuse of certain antibacterial products.

Introduction

The skin provides an efficient, significant barrier against invading microbes and thus represents the first line of defense against infection (see Chapter 20, The Immune System). The human skin and mucous membranes host many bacterial species as part of their normal flora (see Chapter 9, Infection and Disease). Although these organisms normally do not cause infections in intact skin, any break in the skin can lead to a range of infections, from treatable to life-threatening skin conditions. There are many types of skin infections caused by different organisms such as bacteria, viruses, fungi, and parasites. Microbial disease of the skin may result from the following:

- A break in the skin, allowing microorganisms to enter the body
- Systemic infections, which also manifest themselves in the skin (see the Healthcare Application table)
- Toxin-mediated skin damage due to the production of microbial toxins at a site in the body distant from the point of original infection

Persons with certain conditions or diseases can be at greater risk for such infections; such people include but are not limited to those with:

- Diabetes, because of poor blood flow to the skin
- AIDS, because of a compromised immune system
- Burns, because of a large area of exposed and open skin and underlying tissue areas
- Medical treatments such as chemotherapy, which depress the immune system

To understand the different types of skin infections and infections of the underlying tissue it is important to understand tissue structure. The skin is composed of three layers: the epidermis, dermis, and subcutaneous tissue or hypodermis (Figure 10.1).

- The **epidermis** is composed of five layers of epithelial tissue, where the cells are constantly formed by the innermost layers through mitosis. Within the epidermis are **Langerhans cells,** which are dendritic cells that play a role in defense against invading microbes (see Chapter 20, The Immune System).
- The **dermis** consists of two layers: the superficial papillary layer (closest to the epidermis) and a deeper reticular layer. The papillary layer is composed of loose connective tissue and contains blood capillaries that service the epidermis and cutaneous receptors. The reticular layer consists of irregular dense connective tissue surrounding blood vessels, hair follicles, nerves, sweat glands, and sebaceous glands. The epidermis is anchored to the dermis by a basement membrane.
- The **hypodermis** or **subcutaneous layer** is made of loose connective tissue with abundant adipose (fat) cells.

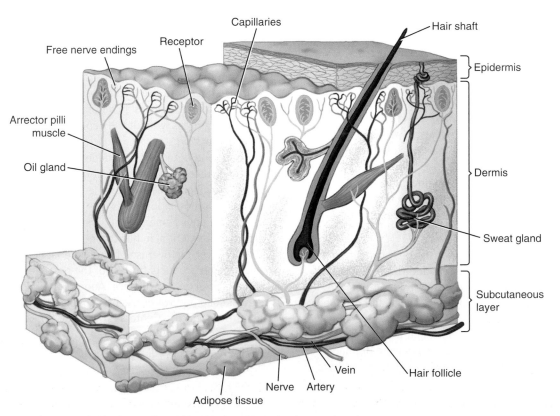

FIGURE 10.1 Basic structure of the skin with epidermis, dermis, and subcutaneous layer.

Skin Manifestations of Systemic Bacterial and Fungal Infections

Disease	Cause	Skin Manifestation
Toxic shock syndrome	*Staphylococcus aureus* and some streptococci	Rash and desquamation due to bacterial toxin
Scarlet fever	*Streptococcus pyogenes*	Erythematous rash caused by bacterial erythrogenic toxins
Syphilis	*Treponema pallidum*	Disseminated infectious rash in the secondary stage of the disease
Enteric fever	*Salmonella typhi*	"Rose spots" containing bacteria
Meningitis, septicemia	*Neisseria meningitidis*	Petechial or maculopapular lesions containing bacteria
Septicemia	*Pseudomonas aeruginosa*	Ecthyma gangrenosum
Typhus	*Rickettsia prowazeki* *Rickettsia typhi*	Macular or hemorrhagic rash
Blastomycosis	*Blastomyces dermatitidis*	Papule or pustule development into granuloma lesions containing fungus
Cryptococcosis	*Cryptococcus neoformans*	Papule or pustule most commonly on the face or neck

Bacterial Infections

Bacterial infections of skin, soft tissue, and muscle can be classified on an anatomical basis, depending on the layers of skin and soft tissue involved:

- **Abscesses:** An abscess is a localized collection of pus in an area of tissue that is infected. It is a defensive mechanism of the body to prevent the spread of infectious material to other areas of the body. Abscesses can occur in any kind of solid tissue but most frequently on the skin surface, where they are easily visible. They may be superficial pustules or pimples, furuncles or **boils,** carbuncles or pyogenic groups of hair follicles, and deep skin abscesses.
- **Spreading infections:** Can be limited to the epidermis, such as is the case for impetigo, or can involve the subcutaneous fat, as in cellulitis.
- **Necrotizing infections:** These infections result in the death of the infected tissue (necrosis). Some of these infections spread with alarming rapidity (i.e., "flesh-eating bacteria") along the surface of the muscles, causing an interruption of blood flow. Because the immune system uses the bloodstream for the purposes of defense, the cells of the immune system and their antibodies cannot reach the infected area; hence the infection can spread rapidly and may be difficult to control. In the case of a necrotic infection, death is not uncommon, even with the appropriate treatment.

Staphylococcal Infections

Staphylococcal infections are among the most common bacterial skin infections. Staphylococci are part of the normal flora on the skin and in the nose of healthy adults. In general, these bacteria do not cause harm, except when there is a break in the skin, burns, or other injuries allowing the organism to enter through the mechanical skin barrier and cause infection. Staphylococcal infections range from mild to life-threatening. People susceptible to staphylococcal infections include newborns, breastfeeding women, people with skin disorders, and people with a weakened immune system, such as those with diabetes and cancer.

Furuncles (Boils)

Staphylococcus aureus is the most common cause of boils and persons who are carriers of the virulent strain of *Staphylococcus aureus* often go through recurrent boils. Exposure to *Pseudomonas aeruginosa* and/or *Pseudomonas folliculitis* in hot tubs or swimming pools may also lead to **furuncles.** The infection begins in a hair follicle (**folliculitis**) and subsequently spreads into the surrounding dermis (Figure 10.2). Furuncles can occur in the hair follicles anywhere on the body but are most commonly found on the face, neck, armpit, buttocks, and thighs. At first the lesion presents itself as a firm, red, painful nodule and then develops into a large, painful mass that often drains large amounts of **pyogenic exudate** (pus). Collections of furuncles can fuse to form **carbuncles,** a large infected mass, which may drain through several sinuses or develop into an abscess. Drainage to the inside can result in access of the bacteria to

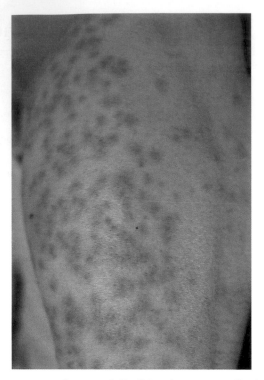

FIGURE 10.2 *Pseudomonas folliculitis.* This is a superficial infection that begins in a hair follicle and subsequently spreads into the underlying dermis. (From Cohen J, Powderly WB: *Infectious diseases,* ed 2, St. Louis, 2004, Mosby.)

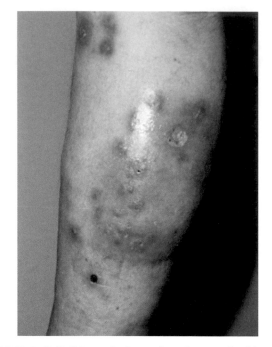

FIGURE 10.3 Cellulitis on the lower leg, characterized by redness, nodules, and swelling. (From Mahon CR, Lehman DC, Manuselis G: *Textbook of diagnostic microbiology,* ed 3, St. Louis, 2007, Saunders.)

underlying sites, which can then be the cause of serious infections such as peritonitis, empyema, meningitis, or systemic poisoning (septicemia). Furuncles may heal on their own if they drain properly. Warm moist compresses encourage furuncles to drain and therefore speed up the healing processes. Deep or large lesions most often need to be lanced or drained surgically.

Cellulitis

Cellulitis is an acute infection of the dermis and subcutaneous tissue usually caused by *Staphylococcus aureus,* streptococci, or other bacteria. The origin of the infection is either a superficial skin lesion such as a boil or ulcers resulting from trauma. Cellulitis is characterized by redness, swelling, warmth, and pain or tenderness and develops within a few hours or days of the trauma. It occurs most commonly on the lower legs (Figure 10.3) and the arms or hands, but other areas of the body may be involved. Regional lymph nodes become enlarged and the patient suffers malaise, chills, and fever. Systemic antibiotics as well as local compresses and analgesics are usually necessary.

Impetigo (Pyoderma)

Impetigo is a superficial skin infection limited to the epidermis, common in infants and children. People who play contact sports (e.g., football, wrestling) are also susceptible, regardless of age. *Staphylococcus aureus* is an organism that can cause highly contagious infections such as impetigo in neonates, causing a threat in neonatal care units. In older children impe-

tigo may also be caused by group A β-hemolytic streptococci. Scratching, direct contact with hands, eating utensils, or towels can easily be vectors to spread the infection. Lesions start with red or pimple-like sores most commonly on the face, arms, and legs. The small vesicles rapidly enlarge, fill with pus, and subsequently rupture to form yellowish-brown crusty masses (Figure 10.4). Because of autoinoculation with hands, towels, and clothes, additional vesicles develop around the primary site of infection. The treatment of impetigo depends on the age of the child and the severity of the infections and may include hygienic measures, topical treatment, and oral antibiotics in more severe cases.

Streptococcal Infections

Most often streptococcal skin infections are secondary to a primary lesion caused by another organism. Streptococci can cause cellulitis and impetigo as described previously. Although uncommon because of antibiotic treatment, glomerulonephritis may occur after streptococcal infections.

Erysipelas

Erysipelas is a type of acute infection generally caused by group A *Streptococcus.* Historically, the face was the most commonly involved site of infection, but now it accounts for approximately 20% of cases and the legs are most often affected (Figure 10.5). Erysipelas can be distinguished from cellulitis by the raised advancing edges and sharp borders. In general, oral antibiotics such as penicillin (see Chapter 21, Pharmacology, and Chapter 22, Antimicrobial Drugs) are used to treat the infection;

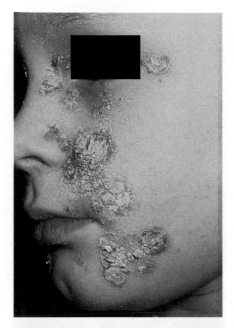

FIGURE 10.4 **Impetigo.** A superficial skin infection, limited to the epidermis with the typical yellowish-brown crusty masses. (Courtesy of MJ Wood. From Mims C, Dockrell HM, Goering RV, et al: *Medical microbiology,* ed 3, St. Louis, 2004, Mosby.)

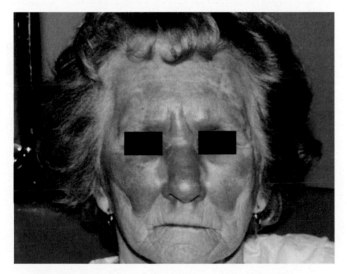

FIGURE 10.5 **Erysipelas of the face caused by group A** *Streptococcus.* (From Mahon CR, Lehman DC, Manuselis G: *Textbook of diagnostic microbiology,* ed 3, St. Louis, 2007, Saunders.)

however, severe cases, with complications such as bacteremia (bacteria in the blood), might require the use of intravenous antibiotics.

Acute Necrotizing Fasciitis

Necrotizing fasciitis ("flesh-eating bacteria"; see Medical Highlights) is an uncommon infection of the deep layers of the skin and subcutaneous tissue. Although a mixture of aerobic and anaerobic bacteria is often present at the original site of infection, the severe inflammation and tissue necrosis seem to be due primarily to the actions of a highly virulent strain of *Streptococcus pyogenes* (gram-positive, group A β-hemolytic *Streptococ-*

cus), the organism responsible for "strep throat." These infections typically originate in the mucous membranes (e.g., the throat) or skin. Necrotizing fasciitis is a progressive, rapidly spreading, inflammatory infection causing secondary necrosis of subcutaneous tissue and adjacent fascia. Proteases, which are tissue-destroying enzymes released by the pathogen, are the cause of the necrosis. The infected area becomes noticeably inflamed, painful, and enlarged, and symptoms of dermal gangrene are apparent. Systemic toxicity accompanied by fever, tachycardia, hypotension, mental confusion, disorientation, and possibly organ failure occur. Immediate and aggressive treatment is essential, including surgical removal of all infected tissue, accompanied by aggressive antimicrobial therapy, fluid replacement, and possible amputation to prevent further spread of the infection. The mortality rate is estimated to be 40% to 60%.

MEDICAL HIGHLIGHTS

Flesh-eating Bacteria

The expression "flesh-eating bacteria" is somewhat sensational, but the fact remains that bacteria causing the condition of necrotizing fasciitis do attack and destroy the subcutaneous (soft) tissue, which then becomes gangrenous. Although this condition is not new, it is rare, and has recently captured the attention and imagination of the public mostly because of coverage generated by the various news media.

The infection takes place in soft tissues below the skin, affecting fat and the fascia covering the tendons and muscles, and spreads extremely rapidly to kill these tissues because of lack of blood, after which the gangrenous, necrotized systems must be removed or necrotizing fasciitis may become systemic, resulting in death. Treatments are available but they must be instituted rapidly, before the disease becomes systemic. Patients with chronic illnesses such as cancer, diabetes, and advanced kidney disease requiring dialysis are at greater risk of developing gangrenous invasive group A streptococci (GAS) from the same bacterial group A streptococci that are responsible for "strep throat." Yet, there is no evidence that the risk of getting flesh-eating disease is increased when group A *Streptococcus* is detected in patients with strep throat. In fact, fewer than one child in a million will get the flesh-eating disease; statistically, there is a better chance (100 times better) of dying in an automobile accident than of necrotizing fasciitis.

Keeping the skin intact and clean are the two most important preventive actions to be taken. Proper washing of hands and the judicious (not excessive) use of antibiotic ointments on even small breaks in the integument is essential. Alertness to flulike symptoms during the flu season should be followed up with appropriate common sense behaviors such as regular visits for medical checkups and staying away from crowds of people after initiating treatment with antibiotics.

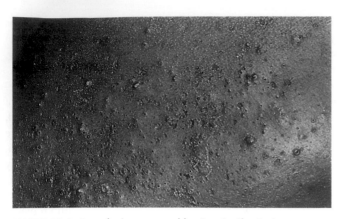

FIGURE 10.6 Acne lesions caused by *Propionibacterium acnes.* (Courtesy of A du Vivier. From Mims C, Dockrell HM, Goering RV, et al: *Medical microbiology,* ed 3, St. Louis, 2004, Mosby.)

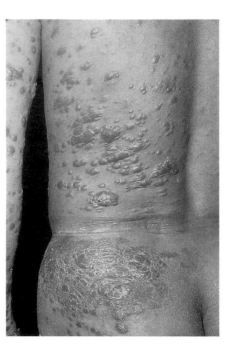

FIGURE 10.7 Multibacillary leprosy. This case shows lepromatous leprosy with multiple nodules, each containing many bacteria. (From Cohen J, Powderly WB: *Infectious diseases,* ed 2, St. Louis, 2004, Mosby.)

Acne

Acne is caused by *Propionibacterium acnes,* a bacterium present on the skin of most people. It lives on fatty acids secreted by sebaceous glands, which in adolescence have increased activity due to hormonal changes (Figure 10.6). This excessive amount of sebum released results in the formation of whiteheads and blackheads, and the breakdown of sebum by *P. acnes* causes local inflammation and the eruption of pimples, sometimes causing skin lesions (folliculitis) that can result in permanent scar formation. *P. acnes* can be treated with antibiotics and antibacterial preparations; however, tetracycline-resistant *P. acnes* is becoming common.

Leprosy

Leprosy (Hansen's disease) is caused by *Mycobacterium leprae* and previously affected millions of people worldwide. Although leprosy still represents a health problem in parts of Africa, Asia, the South Pacific, and some South American countries, according to the World Health Organization (WHO) the global number of new cases detected annually has decreased dramatically, and continues to do so. Leprosy is not highly contagious and prolonged exposure to a source is necessary for infection. Transmission of the infection is related to overcrowding and poor hygiene; it generally occurs by direct contact and aerosol inhalation. The clinical manifestations vary but generally affect the skin, mucous membranes, and nerves (see Chapter 13, Infections of the Nervous System and Senses). The chronic disease is classified as borderline, paucibacillary, or multibacillary leprosy.

- *Borderline leprosy* is the most common form; the skin lesions, or macules, resemble those of tuberculoid leprosy (i.e., hypopigmented areas without feeling, due to destruction of nerve tissue by the immune response) but are more numerous and irregular."
- *Paucibacillary leprosy* is characterized by one or more hypopigmented skin macules and damaged peripheral

nerves, resulting from attack by inflammatory cells of the immune response.
- *Multibacillary leprosy* is associated with symmetric skin lesions, nodules, thickened dermis, and damage to the nasal mucosa (Figure 10.7). Typically there is no loss of feeling because patients with this form of leprosy do not mount an effective immune response.

The mechanism of pathogenicity is relatively unknown because the organism cannot be grown on artificial culture medium, making it difficult to study in the laboratory environment. Laboratory diagnosis of *M. leprae* therefore depends on microscopic examination of skin biopsies. Treatment of leprosy includes antibiotics, rehabilitation, and education. In the case

TABLE 10.1 Bacterial Infections of the Skin

Infection	Common Cause	Treatment
Folliculitis, furuncles, carbuncles	*Staphylococcus aureus*	Moist heat to drain boil; topical antibiotics (e.g., 2% erythromycin), oral antibiotics
Cellulitis	*Staphylococcus aureus* *Streptococcus pyogenes*	Cool, wet dressing on infection site; oral antibiotics
Impetigo	*Staphylococcus aureus* *Streptococcus pyogenes*	Topical and oral antibiotics
Erysipelas	Group A *Streptococcus*	Oral antibiotics; intravenous antibiotic in severe cases (bacteremia)
Acute necrotizing fasciitis	Group A *Streptococcus*	Surgical removal of infected tissues, aggressive antimicrobial treatment, fluid replacement
Acne	*Propionibacterium acnes*	Topical antibacterial preparations, oral antibiotics
Leprosy	*Mycobacterium leprae*	Antibiotics, rehabilitation, education

of immunocompromised patients drug treatment might be required over the entire lifetime. An overview of bacterial skin infections is given in Table 10.1.

Viral Infections

Viruses are the most common causes of acute infections that do not necessarily require hospitalizations. This section deals with viral infections that involve the integument, but also can engage other systems as well. Some viruses can enter through a break in the skin; some can be introduced through an insect bite. Only a few viruses gain access to the human body via an animal bite, hypodermic needles, blood transfusion, or acupuncture. A summary of viral skin infections is provided in Table 10.2. Some viruses enter through the respiratory system and cause skin lesions. These include the viruses causing measles, rubella, and chickenpox (see Chapter 11, Infections of the Respiratory System).

- *Measles:* Measles is caused by a paramyxovirus of the genus *Morbillivirus*. Measles is an acute, highly communicable respiratory disease that also manifests itself as a characteristic skin rash. It is a generalized, maculopapular, erythematous rash that begins after the fever starts (see Chapter 11). In general, the area where the rash starts is the head, followed by spreading to cover most of the body and often causing extreme itching.
- *Rubella:* Also called *German measles,* rubella is caused by the rubella virus of the family Togaviridae. This is also a respiratory infection (see Chapter 11) with additional manifestation in the skin, in the form of a rash that appears on the face and then spreads to the trunk and limbs. The rash appears as pink dots under the skin on the first or third day of the illness and then disappears after a few days without peeling of the skin. The condition is generally fairly benign but is a major concern in pregnant

women because the disease can cause congenital rubella, a serious condition for the fetus (see Congenital Rubella in Chapter 23, Human Age and Microorganisms).
- *Chickenpox* and *shingles:* These are discussed in the section Varicella-Zoster Infections, later in this chapter.

Warts

Warts are the result of a common viral infection caused by the human papillomavirus (HPV). They are generally small, rough tumors, most often located on the hands and feet.

The virus is transmitted by direct contact with an individual or by fomites such as a towel. Autoinoculation is sometimes responsible for the spreading of warts in an individual. Different types have been identified according to shape (Figure 10.8), site affected, and type of HPV:

- *Common wart:* Raised with roughened surface; grayish-yellow or brown in color, mostly on hands, around nails, and knees
- *Flat wart:* Small, smooth, flattened, tan or flesh colored; may occur in large numbers, commonly on the face, neck, hands, wrists, and knees
- *Filiform* or *digitate wart:* Fingerlike (threadlike) wart; common on the face, near eyelids and lips
- *Plantar wart:* Hard lump, occasionally painful; often shows multiple black specks in the center; found at pressure points on soles of the feet
- *Mosaic wart:* A group of tightly clustered plantar-type warts, found on hands or soles of the feet
- *Genital wart:* Often occur in clusters, can be tiny or can spread into large masses in the genital area; warts on the genitals are contagious and the virus is transmitted to another person during oral, vaginal, or anal sex (see Chapter 17, Sexually Transmitted Infections/Diseases)

Warts in children and adolescents often disappear on their own. The treatment of warts depends on their length of time on

TABLE 10.2 Common Viral Infections of the Skin

Infection	Common Cause	Treatment
Warts	Human papillomavirus	Application of salicylic and lactic acid; freezing with liquid nitrogen; electrodesiccation; immunotherapy; laser surgery
Cold sores	HSV-1 or HSV-2 (less common)	Antiviral topical ointments, antiviral oral medications
Chickenpox	Varicella-zoster virus	No medical treatment (generally); antihistamine to relieve itching; antiviral in high-risk cases
Shingles	Varicella-zoster virus	Bed rest; topical agents; cool compresses to affected skin areas; antiviral medications; steroids; antidepressants and anticonvulsants if needed
Roseola infantum	HHV-6 and HHV-7	Treatment for fever
Molluscum contagiosum	*Molluscum contagiosum*	No treatment necessary in people with a functioning immune system
Smallpox	Variola virus	Vaccination

HHV, Human herpesvirus; *HSV*, herpes simplex virus.

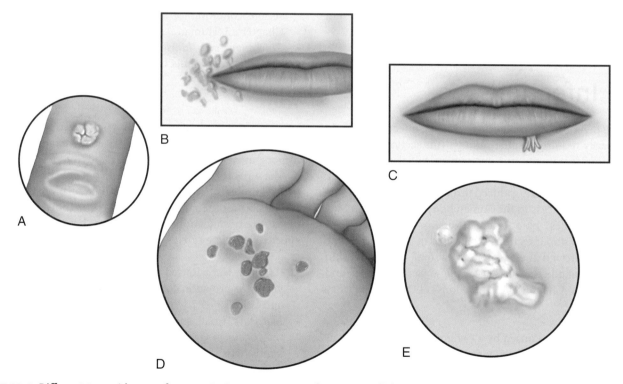

FIGURE 10.8 **Different types/shapes of warts. A,** Common wart; **B,** flat wart; **C,** filiform wart; **D,** plantar wart; **E,** mosaic wart.

the skin, location, type, and also their severity. Treatment may include the application of salicylic and lactic acid to soften the infected area, freezing the wart with liquid nitrogen, electrodesiccation, or laser surgery.

Herpes Simplex Infections

Herpes infections generally manifest themselves as painful, watery blisters in the skin or mucous membranes of the lips, mouth, or the genitals (Figure 10.9). The herpes simplex virus has two strains: herpes simplex virus 1 and 2 (HSV-1 and HSV-2). HSV-1 usually causes infections on the lips and in the mouth (fever blisters), whereas HSV-2 is primarily responsible for genital herpes. It should be noted that both strains can potentially infect both general regions. All herpesviruses have the capacity to remain latent in the ganglia of the sensory fibers innervating a particular area of the skin. Subsequent infections therefore have the tendency to appear in the same areas. HSV is transmitted by direct contact of lips or genitals during the time when the sores are present or just before they appear. The

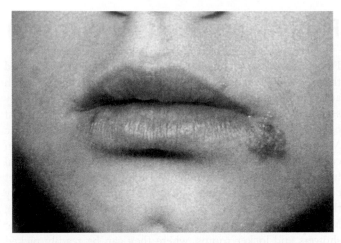

FIGURE 10.9 Recurrent herpes simplex infection: cold sore. (From Hart CA, Broadhead RL: *Color atlas of pediatric infectious diseases*, London, 1992, Wolfe.)

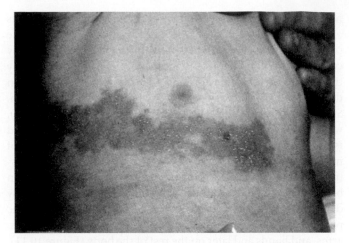

FIGURE 10.10 Shingles along a thoracic dermatome. (From Murray PR, Rosenthal KS, Pfaller MA: *Medical microbiology*, ed 5, St. Louis, 2005, Mosby.)

mechanism(s) of reactivation of the virus are poorly understood but several factors have been identified to cause reoccurrence: ultraviolet light, x-rays, heat, cold, hormonal imbalance, and emotional or other stress factors. Herpes can also be transmitted during childbirth and the disease can be fatal to the infant. Both viruses can also cause morbidity and mortality in an immunosuppressed person.

Treatment is available in the form of antiviral medications, which reduce the duration of the symptoms and accelerate healing, but do not cure the condition or limit the ability of the virus to establish latency or recurrent infections.

Varicella-Zoster Infections

The varicella-zoster virus (VZV), a herpesvirus, is the causative agent for chickenpox, and when recurring later in life it causes herpes zoster, also called *shingles*. This virus is transmitted by respiratory droplets or by any contact with secretions of the respiratory tract of an infected individual. Therefore the primary infection begins in the mucosa of the respiratory tract, and then progresses by the bloodstream throughout the body and to the skin. VZV has some characteristics in common with HSV, such as the ability to create latent infections of neurons, and therefore having the ability to cause recurrent disease and the formation of blister-like lesions.

The primary disease caused by VZV is chickenpox, which is usually relatively mild in children but more severe if it affects adults. Because the virus is latent, it can be reactivated in older adults or in people with impaired immunity. Once reactivated, the virus replicates along the neural pathways and infects the skin, causing a characteristic rash along the entire dermatome (Figure 10.10).

Molluscum Contagiosum

Molluscum contagiosum is caused by a poxvirus, the molluscum contagiosum virus or MCV. This viral skin infection causes raised, pearl-like papules or nodules in the skin and is common in children. Lesions in children are frequently apparent on the face, neck, armpit, arms, and hands, but may occur anywhere on the body except the palms and the soles. The virus is contagious and in children is transmitted through direct contact, saliva, or shared articles of clothing, including towels. In adults, molluscum infections are most often spread by sexual contact and usually affect the genitals, lower abdomen, buttocks, and inner thighs. The skin lesions are flesh-colored, dome-shaped, pearly in appearance, and generally not painful, but can itch or become irritated. Molluscum lesions in people with normal immune systems may disappear in 6 to 9 months but can also persist through autoinoculation. The lesions may be extensive in people with AIDS or other conditions that affect the normal functioning of the immune system. Treatment, if necessary, depends on the patient's age, overall heath, and medical history; on the location and number of lesions; and involves a variety of topically applied substances as well as cryosurgery and laser therapy.

Roseola Infantum

Roseola infantum or sixth disease is caused by human herpesvirus type 6 (HHV-6) and HHV-7 (roseolovirus). It is a self-limiting disease affecting children between 6 months and 3 years of age and is characterized by a high fever of 102° F to 104° F (39° C to 40° C) and a generalized body rash. In some cases, the high fever can cause febrile convulsions due to a sudden rise in body temperature. Once the fever subsides, after 3 to 5 days the rash appears, usually starting on the trunk and spreading to the limbs. The rash disappears within hours to a day.

Smallpox

Smallpox is an acute contagious disease caused by the variola virus, a member of the orthopoxvirus family. It is one of the most devastating diseases known to humans and for centuries epidemics swept across continents, drastically reducing the population. The virus can be spread from person to person by contact with skin lesions or via secretions of the respiratory tract. The disease, for which no effective treatment has been developed, kills approximately 30% of the infected population. Survivors show characteristic deep pitted scars (pockmarks), which are most prominent on the face. The incubation period is usually 12 to 14 days and is followed by the sudden onset of influenza-like symptoms such as fever, malaise, headache, prostration, and severe back pain; when the digestive system becomes involved, abdominal pain and vomiting occur. A few days later, when the body temperature falls, the characteristic pimples associated with the disease start to erupt in the mouth, arms, and hands and later on the rest of the body (Figure 10.11). These pimples, now called *macules*, are still small but the patient is at the most contagious stage.

In 1967 the WHO started a campaign to eradicate smallpox by vaccination (originally developed by Edward Jenner) with a live attenuated strain of the vaccinia virus. After successful vaccination campaigns throughout the world, the WHO certified the eradication of smallpox in 1979. Cultures of the virus are kept by the Centers for Disease Control and Prevention (CDC) in the United States and at the Russian Vector Institute for Virology in Novosibirsk, Siberia. Concern about the use of smallpox by bioterrorists resulted in the preparation of contingency plans by many countries to deal with potential threats (see Chapter 24, Microorganisms in the Environment and Environmental Safety). These plans include the stockpiling of the smallpox vaccine. In December 1999, the WHO Advisory Committee on Variola Virus Research concluded that the then current vaccine supplies to prevent and control a smallpox outbreak were limited. As a result, a number of governments have chosen to examine their stocks, test their potency, and consider whether more vaccine is required. At present, the United States has a big enough stockpile of the smallpox vaccine to vaccinate everyone in the United States in the event of a smallpox emergency (CDC information).

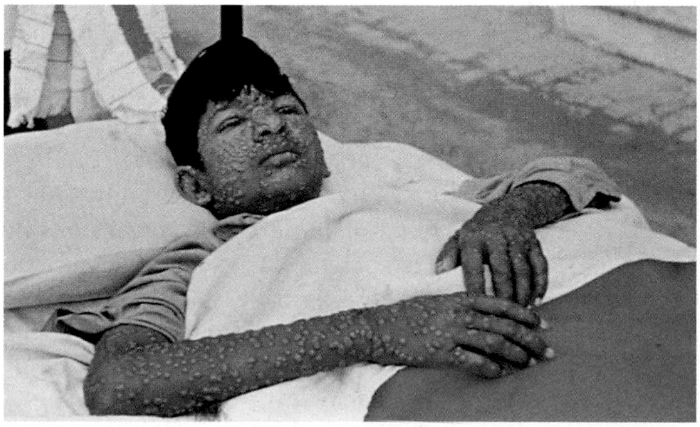

FIGURE 10.11 **Characteristic pimples associated with smallpox.** (From Murray PR, Rosenthal KS, Pfaller MA: *Medical microbiology,* ed 5, St. Louis, 2005, Mosby.)

Fungal Infections (Mycoses)

Fungal infections of the skin are referred to as **mycoses,** and they are common and usually mild. However, in people with a compromised immune system, fungi can cause potentially serious diseases. Fungi are parasites or saprophytes; they exist off living or dead organic matter (see Chapter 8, Eukaryotic Microorganisms). Some fungi infect humans only; others can cause disease in other animals as well. Although the natural fungal habitat is the soil, they are often transmitted by direct contact with an infected person, an animal, or indirectly through contact with a fomite (e.g., a towel, or the floor). Many fungi live on damp surfaces such as the floors in public showers and locker rooms, where they can be readily picked up by direct contact. Fungi also prefer moist areas of the human body such as skin folds, between the toes, and genital areas. A summary of common fungal infections is illustrated in Table 10.3.

Tineas

Tineas refer to fungal infections superficially affecting the outer layers of the skin, the nails, and the hair. The causative agents live off the dead, keratinized cells of the epidermis. The most important fungi that cause disease of skin, hair, and nails are called **dermatophytes.** Tinea is a common skin inhabitant and may cause several types of superficial skin infections, named depending on the area of the body infected. As the fungus grows it spreads out in a circle, leaving normal-looking skin in the middle. This ringlike formation is why this type of infection is called *"ringworm"* (Figure 10.12), but contrary to its name it is not caused by a worm, but by fungi causing tinea.

Tinea Capitis

Tinea capitis is an infection of the scalp causing itchy, red areas, destroying the hair and leaving bald patches. This infection is common in school-aged children and may result from infection with *Microsporum canis,* transmitted by cats and dogs, or by *Trichophyton tonsurans,* which is transmitted by humans. The infection can also be transmitted by infected items (fomites) such as hats, combs, clothing, or other such objects. Oral antifungal medications are recommended for treatment.

Tinea Corporis

Tinea corporis affects the body almost anywhere; on the arms, legs, or chest, in particular on nonhairy parts. The lesion is characterized by a round, erythematous ring of vesicles or papules with a clear center, customary for "ringworm" infections. Symptomatic pruritus or a burning sensation is not unusual. Tinea corporis is contagious and can be acquired from infected individuals; through contaminated items, shower floors and walls, as well as pool surfaces. The infection can also be spread by pets, in particular by cats. Topical, over-the-counter antifungal medications are often effective. Severe or chronic infections may require oral antifungal medications, and

TABLE 10.3 Examples of Fungal Skin Infections

Infection	Common Cause	Treatment
Tinea capitis	*Trichophyton tonsurans* *Microsporum audouinii* *Microsporum canis*	Oral antifungal medications
Tinea corporis	*Trichophyton rubrum* *Microsporum canis* *Trichophyton tonsurans* *Trichophyton verrucosum*	Topical over-the-counter medications; severe or chronic infections, oral antifungals and antibiotics
Tinea cruris	*Trichophyton rubrum* *Epidermophyton floccosum*	Self-care; over-the-counter topical medications
Tinea unguium	*Trichophyton rubrum* *Trichophyton mentagrophytes* var. *mentagrophytes*	Oral antifungal medications and local fungicides (might take months for treatment)
Tinea versicolor	*Malassezia furfur*	Over-the-counter topical medications; severe cases, prescription-strength topical and/or oral medication
Tinea pedis	*Trichophyton rubrum* *Trichophyton mentagrophytes* var. *interdigitale* *Epidermophyton floccosum*	Over-the-counter antifungal powders, sprays, or creams
Cutaneous candidiasis	*Candida albicans*	Topical antifungal medications
Chromoblastomycosis	*Cladophialophora carrionii* *Fonsecaea pedrosoi* *Fonsecaea compacta* *Phialophora verrucosa*	Oral antifungal drugs, cryosurgery; antibiotics to prevent secondary infection
Mycetoma	*Acremonium falciforme* *Acremonium recifei* *Acremonium nidulans* *Exophiala jeanselmei* *Leptosphaeria senegalensis* *Madurella grisea* *Madurella mycetomatis* *Neotestudina rosatii* *Pseudallescheria boydii* *Pyrenochaeta romeroi*	Depends on etiological agent and extent of disease; drug combinations over extended period of time
Sporotrichosis	*Sporothrix schenckii*	Oral potassium iodide; itraconazole

antibiotics may be given to prevent secondary bacterial infections. Furthermore, if transmitted by a pet, the pet should also be treated.

Tinea Versicolor

Tinea versicolor is caused by the yeast *Malassezia furfur* (formerly *Pityrosporum ovale*) and is commonly found on the human skin; it is therefore not contagious to others. The pathogenicity of this particular fungus seems to be associated with a change from its yeast form to the hyphal form, which occurs under special conditions such as in warm and humid environments. This fungal infection often affects the skin of young people, and spots are commonly present on the back, underarms, upper arms, chest, lower legs, and neck. The spots produced are either reddish-brown or lighter than the surrounding area. In people with dark skin tones, hypopigmentation is common, and in people with lighter skin color hyperpigmentation is more common. Treatment includes over-the-counter topical applications, but in severe cases prescription-strength topical and/or oral medication might be required. Although tinea versicolor does not leave permanent skin discoloration, the skin may remain uneven in color for several weeks, even after successful treatment.

Tinea Cruris

Tinea cruris is a fungal infection of the groin area and is commonly referred to as *"jock itch."* The infection occurs most commonly in adult men and can be triggered by friction from clothes and prolonged wetness in the groin area as occurs during sweating. The condition causes itching and a burning sensation and the affected area may appear red, tan, or brown, with flaking, peeling, or cracking skin. Tinea cruris can be

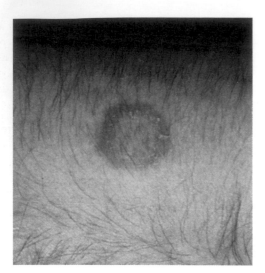

FIGURE 10.12 Typical tinea lesion with its round appearance, thus often referred to *"roundworm."* (Courtesy of AE Prevost. From Mims C, Dockrell HM, Goering RV, et al: *Medical microbiology*, ed 3, St. Louis, 2004, Mosby.)

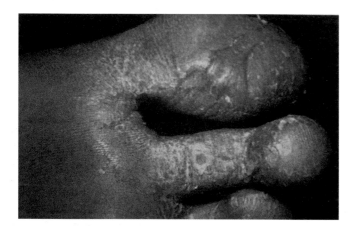

FIGURE 10.13 **Athlete's foot.** Lesions between the toes are symptoms of tinea pedis. (From Bergquist L, Pogosian B: *Microbiology*, St. Louis, 2000, Saunders.)

passed from one person to the next by direct skin-to-skin contact or by contact with unwashed clothing such as athletic supporters; hence the term "jock itch." The condition usually responds to self-care within 2 weeks if the skin is kept clean and dry, topical over-the-counter antifungal or drying powders are applied, and tight damp clothing is avoided.

Tinea Unguium

Tinea unguium, also called *onychomycosis,* infects the nails, particularly the toenails. The infection can occur directly in the nail itself or can result from an untreated fungal infection of the foot. Tinea unguium produces nails that look white and opaque, and are thick and brittle. People at risk for this infection are those with diabetes and/or peripheral vascular disease, older women, and people of any age who wear artificial nails. In addition, people who are required to wear close-fitting rubber foot-

wear at work and people living in a warm humid climate are also more likely to acquire this infection.

Treatment might require several months and usually includes oral antifungal medication as well as local fungicides. Onychomycosis is difficult to cure and may return even after treatment.

Tinea Pedis

Tinea pedis, commonly called *"athlete's foot,"* thrives in warm and humid conditions. The infection is most frequently due to *Trichophyton rubrum, T. interdigitale,* and *Epidermophyton floccosum.* Of all the tinea infections, athlete's foot is the most common. It generally causes cracked, flaking, peeling skin between the toes and the affected areas are commonly red. Itchiness, burning, or stinging and blisters, oozing, or crusting may occur as well (Figure 10.13). The infection may also spread to the heels, palms, and between the fingers. Athlete's foot is contagious and can be obtained through direct contact or fomites such as shoes, stockings, showers, or pool surfaces (see Life Application: Athlete's Foot). The afflicted feet may have a foul odor and secondary bacterial infections are not uncommon, which adds to the inflammation and possible necrosis. Over-the-counter antifungal powders, sprays, or creams can help to control the infection.

Cutaneous Candidiasis

Cutaneous **candidiasis** is a skin infection caused by the fungus *Candida. Candida albicans* is a widespread yeast and occurs as part of the normal flora in the oral cavity, genitalia, large intestine, and also the skin of about 20% of people. Healthy people usually keep infections due to *Candida* spp. in check. In immunocompromised patients, the use of certain antimicrobial drugs, inadequate nutrition, and certain diseases may

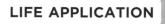

LIFE APPLICATION

Athlete's Foot

Tinea pedis—athlete's foot—affects people of all ages but is more common in adults than children. The fungus is typically picked up from the floors of showers, locker rooms, bathrooms, changing rooms, swimming pools, steam rooms, and exercise facilities in general. Unless the floors in these warm and moist environments are disinfected frequently, the fungal spores can persist for months or years in these environments. Walking barefoot on a communal floor or sharing a towel can result in infection. Certain common sense precautions can help prevent troublesome athlete's foot infections. They include the following: the wearing of cotton socks during exercise, and of thongs or sandals when walking on a communal floor; frequent airing of shoes; avoidance of occlusive footwear; thorough drying of feet after bathing or swimming; use of antifungal powders; and keeping feet clean and dry.

cause infections with this organism in a variety of systems. Cutaneous candidiasis may involve almost any skin surface but usually prefers warm, moist, and creased areas such as armpits and groins. *Candida albicans* is a common cause of diaper rash in infants, where the organism finds warm and moist conditions ideal for growth. The organisms can also cause infections of the nails and around the corners of the mouth. Other areas include the hands of people who routinely wear rubber gloves, the area around the groin, the crease of the buttocks, and the skin folds under large breasts. Diabetes, obesity, and the use of antibiotics and/or oral contraceptives increase the risk for cutaneous candidiasis. Treatment of the condition involves general hygiene; keeping the skin dry and exposed to air is also helpful, and topical antifungal medications can be used.

Subcutaneous Mycoses

The term *subcutaneous mycosis* indicates a fungal disease in which the pathogen penetrates the dermis or even deeper layers during or after a skin trauma. Three general types of subcutaneous mycoses exist, but the pathogens have only a few characteristics in common and belong to different taxonomic groups. These types are as follows: chromoblastomycoses, mycetomas, and sporotrichosis. Subcutaneous mycoses occur predominantly in the tropics, because of the geographical distribution of the pathogens, ecological factors, and also can be a result of scarcity of adequate medical facilities/treatment in these regions.

Chromoblastomycoses

Chromoblastomycosis is a chronic localized infection of the subcutaneous tissue characterized by verrucoid lesions of the skin, usually located in the lower extremities. It is limited mostly to the subcutaneous tissue without involvement of bone, tendon, or muscle. The original site of infection may be very small, often caused by vegetative material such as thorns or splinters, and the infection builds at the site over a period of months or years. Small red papules will appear but the lesions are usually not painful and patients often do not seek medical care. Satellite lesions may occur as the disease develops; the rashlike areas may enlarge, become raised irregular plaques, and sometimes become tumors with a cauliflower-like appearance. Although the prognosis for small lesions is good, severe cases of the infection are difficult to cure. Some antifungal drugs given orally and cryosurgery have been shown to have some effectiveness. Antibiotics may be given to prevent and/or treat bacterial superinfections, which may occur as a result of these mycoses.

Mycetomas

Mycetoma is a chronic infection that begins as a subcutaneous nodule after injury and may penetrate deeper into the tissue, sometimes even to the bone. Mycetoma may be caused by several fungi and/or actinomycetes, which are bacteria that, like fungi, form filaments. Both types of organisms are found in the soil and on plant material of tropical regions, and are often associated with injuries of the feet. As the infection progresses from the original site it characteristically swells and the middle of the lesion caves in, ulcerates, and discharges pus and grains. Eventually sinus tracts (holes) form, which also are pyogenic with grains that are filled with the microorganism. Considerable deformity occurs, which makes walking difficult. Furthermore, mycetoma may cause itching or burning sensations along with secondary bacterial infections, which are common. Because of the wide range of causative microorganisms, the treatment of mycetoma depends mainly on its etiological agent and the extent of the disease. Treatment with combinations of drugs over extended periods of time has met with some degree of success; however, severe infections may require more heroic interventions such as amputation of the infected foot or hand.

Sporotrichosis

Sporotrichosis, the third general class of subcutaneous mycoses, is caused by *Sporothrix schenckii*, a fungus found in the soil, in sphagnum moss, hay, and other plant material in all parts of the world. The fungus enters the skin through small cuts or punctures from thorns, barbs, pine needles, or wires. At risk are people working with thorny plants, sphagnum moss, and hay. The fungus is not spread by person-to-person contact. Initial symptoms are small painless bumps resembling insect bites and can be red, pink, or purple. The bump occurs at the site of fungal entry, usually on a finger, hand, or arm. Additional bumps follow that resemble boils, and heal very slowly. The occurrence of the initial bump may be any time from 1 to 12 weeks after exposure; however, in most instances they appear within 3 weeks. The infection usually spreads along cutaneous lymphatic channels of the involved extremity. Sporotrichosis formerly was treated with oral potassium iodide and now most often with itraconazole, a new drug with fewer side effects. Sporotrichosis can usually be prevented by wearing gloves and long sleeves when working with plant or wire material that can prick the skin. Skin contact with sphagnum moss should be avoided because it has been implicated as a source of the fungus in a number of outbreaks, especially in plant nurseries.

Summary

- The skin is the first line of defense against infection and any break in the skin may result in invasion by pathogens or opportunistic organisms. A wide range of organisms is associated with skin infections and disease.
- Microbial disease of the skin may occur as a result of a break in the intact skin, systemic infections manifesting themselves in the skin, or toxin-mediated skin damage due to microbial toxins at different areas of the body.
- Bacterial skin infections are classified on an anatomical basis, depending on the layers of skin and soft tissues involved, as abscesses, spreading infections, or necrotizing infections.
- Bacterial skin infections include staphylococcal infections such as furuncles, carbuncles, cellulitis, and impetigo;

streptococcal infections; acute necrotizing fasciitis; acne; and leprosy.

- Some viruses can enter through a break in the skin or via an insect bite and some viruses have a different port of entry and manifest themselves in skin lesions. Skin infections include warts, herpes simplex infections, varicella-zoster infections, molluscum contagiosum, roseola infantum, and smallpox.

- Measles, rubella, and chickenpox are respiratory diseases, but also show skin lesions.
- Most fungal infections are superficial, involving the outer layers of the skin, the nails, and hair. These infections include tineas and cutaneous candidiasis.
- Subcutaneous mycoses occur when pathogens penetrate the dermis and deeper layers. The three general types are chromoblastomycoses, mycetomas, and sporotrichosis.

Review Questions

1. Langerhans cells, which play a role in defense against microbes, are located in the:
   a. Epidermis
   b. Dermis
   c. Hypodermis
   d. Subcutaneous layer

2. The papillary layer of the skin is part of the:
   a. Epidermis
   b. Dermis
   c. Hypodermis
   d. Subcutaneous layer

3. Which of the following organisms is the causative agent for skin infections and toxic shock syndrome?
   a. *Escherichia coli*
   b. *Staphylococcus aureus*
   c. *Treponema pallidum*
   d. *Propionibacterium acnes*

4. Which of the following is a type of acute infection generally caused by group A *Streptococcus*?
   a. Necrotizing fasciitis
   b. Impetigo
   c. Erysipelas
   d. Acne

5. The organism often called *"flesh-eating bacteria"* is:
   a. *Staphylococcus aureus*
   b. *Staphylococcus epidermidis*
   c. *Streptococcus pyogenes*
   d. *Propionibacterium acnes*

6. Acne is caused by:
   a. *Staphylococcus aureus*
   b. *Staphylococcus epidermidis*
   c. *Streptococcus pyogenes*
   d. *Propionibacterium acnes*

7. Warts are commonly caused by:
   a. Human papillomavirus
   b. Herpesvirus
   c. HIV
   d. Varicella-zoster virus

8. Herpes simplex infections on lips and in the mouth are most commonly caused by:
   a. HSV-1
   b. HSV-2
   c. HSV-6
   d. HSV-7

9. "Athlete's foot" is caused by:
   a. Tinea capitis
   b. Tinea corporis
   c. Tinea versicolor
   d. Tinea pedis

10. Diaper rash in infants is commonly caused by:
    a. *Sporothrix schenckii*
    b. Actinomycetes
    c. *Candida albicans*
    d. *Malassezia furfur*

11. Leprosy is caused by _____.

12. Infections that result in the death of infected tissue are called _____ infections.

13. Chickenpox and shingles are caused by the _____ virus.

14. Fungal infections of the skin are referred to as _____.

15. A tinea infection in the groin area is commonly called "_____."

16. Describe the different types of warts according to shape and site affected.

17. Describe the most common staphylococcal skin infections.

18. Describe the most common streptococcal skin infections.

19. Discuss the occurrence of smallpox and smallpox vaccination.

20. Describe the different types of subcutaneous mycoses.

Bibliography

Bauman R: *Microbiology: with diseases by taxonomy*, ed 2, San Francisco, 2007, Benjamin Cummings/Pearson.

Forbes BA, Sahm, DF, Weissfled AS: *Bailey & Scott's diagnostic microbiology*, ed 12, St. Louis, 2007, Mosby/Elsevier.

Mims C, Dockrell HM, Goering RV, et al: *Medical microbiology*, ed 3, St. Louis, 2004, Mosby/Elsevier.

Murray PR, Rosenthal KS, Pfaller MA: *Medical microbiology*, ed 5, St. Louis, 2005, Mosby/Elsevier.

Thibodeau GA, Patton KT: *Anatomy and physiology*, ed 6, St. Louis, 2007, Mosby/Elsevier.

Internet Resources

Aiello AE, Marshall B, Levy SB, Della-Latta P, Lin SX, Larson E. Antibacterial cleaning products and drug resistance. *Emerg Infect Dis* [serial on the Internet]. 2005 Oct [accessed November 14, 2008]. http://www.cdc.gov/ncidod/EID/vol11no10/04-1276.htm

The Merck Manuals Online Medical Library, http://www.merck.com/mmhe/index.html

CDC, Division of Foodborne, Bacterial and Mycotic Diseases (DFBMD), Leprosy (Hansen's Disease), http://www.cdc.gov/nczved/dfbmd/disease_listing/leprosy_ti.html

World Health Organization, Leprosy Elimination, http://www.who.int/lep/en/

CDC, Emergency Preparedness and Response, Smallpox Vaccine, Smallpox Fact Sheet, http://www.bt.cdc.gov/agent/smallpox/vaccination/facts.asp

Noble SL, Forbes RC, Stamm PL: Diagnosis and management of common tinea infections, *American Family Physician*, July 1998 (accessed May 6, 2009). Copyright © 1998 by the American Academy of Family Physicians. http://www.aafp.org/afp/980700ap/noble.html

The University of Adelaide, Australia, Mycology Online, Chromoblastomycosis, http://www.mycology.adelaide.edu.au/Mycoses/Subcutaneous/Chromoblastomycosis/

11

Infections of the Respiratory System

OUTLINE

Introduction

Bacterial Infections
    Streptococcal Infections
    Other Common Infections
    Rare and Opportunistic Infections

Viral Infections
    Common Cold
    Influenza
    Viral Pneumonia
    Hantavirus Pulmonary Syndrome
    Severe Acute Respiratory Syndrome (SARS)

Fungal Infections
    Histoplasmosis
    Coccidioidomycosis
    Blastomycosis
    Pulmonary Aspergillosis

LEARNING OBJECTIVES

After reading this chapter, the student will be able to:

- Name the criteria necessary for microbes to cause an infection of the respiratory system
- Identify the microbes typically present in the normal flora of the respiratory tract
- Name the different streptococcal respiratory infections; describe the transmission, symptoms, and treatment for each
- Discuss drug-resistant *Streptococcus pneumoniae* disease
- Describe the transmission and treatment of mycoplasmal and chlamydial pneumonias
- Discuss pertussis, tuberculosis, and their treatments
- Describe rare and opportunistic respiratory infections caused by bacteria
- Compare and contrast the common cold and influenza, and their prevention and treatment
- Describe infections of the respiratory system caused by fungi and the treatment of their infections
- Describe the common symptoms of upper and lower respiratory system infections, the possible treatments, and prevention

KEY TERMS

bronchi
bronchial tree
ciliary escalator
flu
influenza

larynx
lungs
normal flora
pertussis
pharyngitis

pharynx
pneumonia
scarlet fever
tuberculosis (TB)

WHY YOU NEED TO KNOW

HISTORY

Exposure to about 8 microbes per minute, or approximately 10,000 per day, makes the respiratory tract one of the most common sites for pathogenic infection in the body, as it is in direct contact with the physical environment and the microorganisms contained therein. Couple this with its warm, moist, barrier-layered surfaces and you have excellent conditions for trapping particles to allow for infections. From the common cold to pneumonia, the respiratory tract has been an avenue for the introduction of viruses and bacteria that have persisted with us through the ages, producing disease ranging in severity from merely irritable to lethal. The name "cold" is perhaps a misnomer that was used to describe the season in which the symptoms became more prevalent or the action of the organisms on thermogenesis, which is the process by which the body generates heat or energy by increasing the metabolic rate. The process of thermogenesis can be triggered by conditions such as wet hair, body parts exposed to drafts, or extended periods of time waiting in low temperatures.

Common cold symptoms were recorded in ancient Egypt and Hippocrates referred to the disease in the 400s BC. Early American Indian, Mayan, and Aztec cultures recorded descriptions of the cold; Aztec treatments consisted of chili pepper, honey, and tobacco mixtures.

Wet feet and wet clothes as possible causes for the common cold were stated early in the 1700s and 1800s by John Wesley and William Buchan, respectively. After the discovery of viruses in the late 1800s and their association with the common cold, acute viral nasopharyngitis became the descriptive name of this malady. While the role of bacteria in the germ theory of disease held sway early on, antibiotics failed to cure colds because of their viral cause although they did alleviate accompanying bacterial irritations and secondary infections.

Pneumonia, a respiratory tract disease, occurs as a result of inflamed alveoli filling with fluid, which prevents them from transporting gases needed to support life on a minute-by-minute basis. There are multiple causes of pneumonia, such as bacterial, viral, fungal, or parasitic infections as well as chemical or physical injury; or it may be a secondary condition to another illness such as alcohol abuse or cancer. Severe acute respiratory syndrome (SARS) is caused by the highly contagious SARS coronavirus, which first occurred in 2003 after initial outbreaks in China. According to the World Health Organization (WHO) more than 8000 people worldwide became sick in the 2003 outbreak and of these 774 died.

IMPACT

While the common cold negatively impacts school and work attendance, it positively contributes to visits to physicians and drugstores. This most common of afflictions suffered by humans conservatively costs just under $8 million dollars in visits to physicians and just under $3.5 billion dollars in over-the-counter and prescription drug costs per year. In addition to medically related costs, just under 200 million school days are missed by students each year and just under 130 million workdays by their parents to stay at home with them. Add this to the workdays missed by employees and cold-related work loss is in excess of $20 billion per year.

Pneumonia is common in all age groups but is the leading cause of death among the elderly and those who are chronically or terminally ill. Vaccines are effective for some pneumonia-causing agents, unlike the common cold, which has no cure, only supportive care.

FUTURE

At present, there are no vaccines for the common cold and no cure. Efforts to develop effective vaccines for viral pneumonia should be continued. Other than a well-functioning immune system, the most promising protection from viral infections in general seems to be via a vaccine. Otherwise, treatment to give symptomatic relief is the only approach.

Introduction

The respiratory tract consists of the nasal cavity, the **pharynx, larynx, bronchial tree,** and **lungs.** Structurally and functionally the system can be divided into upper and lower respiratory systems (Figure 11.1).

- The upper respiratory system includes the nose, pharynx, and associated structures.
- The lower respiratory system consists of the larynx, trachea, **bronchi,** and lungs.

The lining of the respiratory tract is a mucosal epithelium that serves as a barrier against microbial invasion; however,

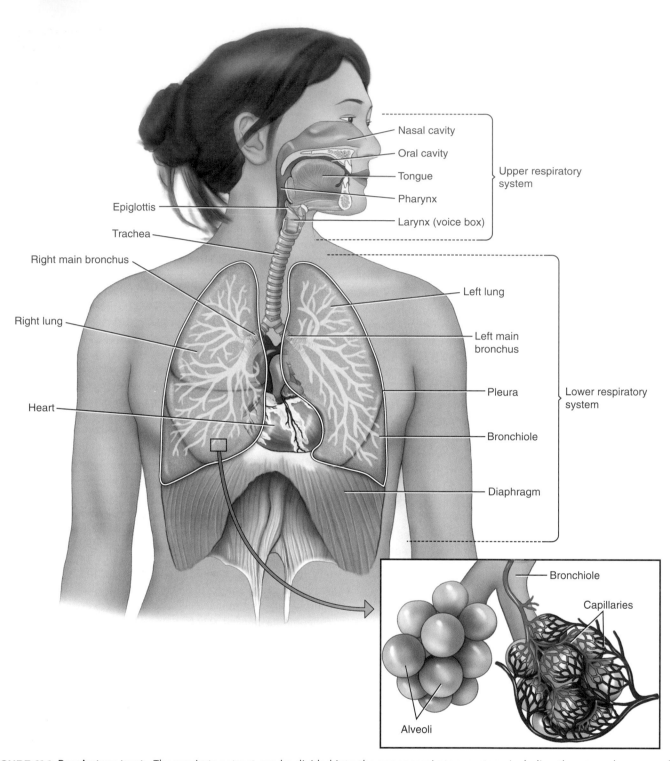

FIGURE 11.1 Respiratory tract. The respiratory tract can be divided into the upper respiratory system, including the nose, pharynx, and associated structures; and the lower respiratory system, consisting of the larynx, trachea, bronchi, and lungs.

it is not as effective as an intact skin barrier. The mucosal lining of the respiratory tract has a moist and relatively warm environment suitable for microbes. Moreover, microbes may be trapped in the mucous layer and by way of the **ciliary escalator** transported to the pharynx and then swallowed. The **normal flora** (see Chapter 9, Infection and Disease) of the respiratory system contains a large number of bacteria

that help to maintain a healthy state of the host by competing with potential pathogenic organisms. The microorganisms of the normal flora are usually harmless but they can become opportunistic pathogens when the host immune system is depressed, or when damage occurs to the mucosal membrane. Infections of the respiratory system can be caused by bacteria, viruses, and fungi. For an infection of the respiratory system to occur due to an exogenous agent the following criteria must be met:

- A sufficient number (dose) of infectious agent must be inhaled.
- The infectious agents must be airborne or contained in droplet nuclei.
- The infectious organism must remain alive and viable while in the air.
- The organism must find susceptible tissue in the host, suitable for attachment and growth.
- Once in the respiratory tract the organism must colonize the surfaces before it can cause disease.

Bacterial Infections

Most of the upper respiratory tract mucosa is colonized by normal flora. The most common bacteria found in the normal flora of the upper respiratory tract are *Staphylococcus aureus* and *S. epidermidis*. In addition, aerobic corynebacteria can be cultured from nasal surfaces. Moreover, small numbers of *Strep-* *tococcus pneumoniae, Neisseria meningitidis,* and *Haemophilus influenzae* can be found in the nasopharynx of some individuals. α-Hemolytic streptococci including *S. mitis, S. mutans, S. milleri,* and *S. salivarius* are considered important organisms in this area because it is believed that these bacteria protect against invasion by pathogenic streptococci; however, these same organisms can also cause tooth decay and periodontal disease if unchecked.

Bacterial infections of the respiratory tract can be caused by *Staphylococcus, Streptococcus, Klebsiella, Haemophilus, Bordetella, Corynebacterium, Mycobacterium, Legionella, Mycoplasma, Chlamydia,* and *Coxiella.* Infections caused by inhabitants of the normal flora can occur and appear as secondary infections after damage to the mucosal lining, usually caused by a viral infection such as the common cold. A summary of bacterial infections acquired through the respiratory system is given in Table 11.1.

Streptococcal Infections

The genus *Streptococcus* is composed of spherical gram-positive bacteria well known for being responsible for "strep throat," but is also capable of causing meningitis, pneumonia, endocarditis,

TABLE 11.1 Bacterial Infections Acquired Through the Respiratory Tract

Illness/Disease	Organism(s)	Target of Infection	Transmission
Streptococcal pharyngitis (strep throat)	Group A *Streptococcus*	Pharynx	Nasal or salivary secretions; person-to-person contact
Scarlet fever	*Streptococcus pyogenes*	Pharynx, tongue	Direct contact with infected person; nasal droplets; fomites such as shared drinking glasses
Drug-resistant *Streptococcus pneumoniae* disease (DRSP)	*Streptococcus pneumoniae*	Pharynx, lungs, alveoli	Person-to-person contact
Mycoplasmal pneumonia	*Mycoplasma pneumoniae*	Lungs; mucous membranes	Nasal secretions among people in crowded environments
Chlamydial pneumonia	*Chlamydia pneumoniae*	Lungs	Inhalation of respiratory droplets
Pertussis (whooping cough)	*Bordetella pertussis*	Trachea—ciliated epithelial cells	Inhalation of respiratory droplets
Tuberculosis	*Mycobacterium tuberculosis*	Lungs	Inhalation of respiratory droplets
Staphylococcal pneumonia	*Staphylococcus aureus; S. pneumoniae*	Lungs	Nosocomial; complication after influenza
Haemophilus infections	*Haemophilus influenzae*	Pharynx, bronchi, lungs	Inhalation of respiratory droplets
Klebsiella pneumonia	*Klebsiella pneumoniae*	Lungs	Nosocomial
Diphtheria	*Corynebacterium diphtheriae*	Respiratory membranes	Inhalation of respiratory droplets
Legionellosis	*Legionella pneumophila*	Lungs	Inhalation of contaminated water mist
Psittacosis ("parrot fever")	*Chlamydia psittaci*	Lungs	Inhalation of dried bird excrements or secretions
Inhalation anthrax	*Bacillus anthracis*	Lungs	Inhalation of spores
Q fever	*Coxiella burnetii*	Lungs	Inhalation of contaminated droplets excreted by infected animals

erysipelas, necrotizing fasciitis (see Chapter 10, Infections of the Integumentary System, Soft Tissue, and Muscle), and toxic shock syndrome. The virulence of group A *Streptococcus* seems to be increasing worldwide.

Strep Throat (Streptococcal Pharyngitis)

Strep throat or streptococcal **pharyngitis** is caused by group A *Streptococcus* bacteria and is the most common bacterial infection of the throat. Although this infection can occur at any age, it is most common in children between the ages of 5 and 15 years. Strep throat is transmitted by person-to-person contact via nasal secretions or saliva (sneezing and/or coughing) by an infected individual or a carrier. On occasion, contaminated food, especially milk and milk products, may be the cause of the infection.

The infection occurs with higher frequency in the late fall, winter, and early spring. Most sore throats are caused by viruses, not by bacteria, and therefore the Centers for Disease Control and Prevention (CDC, Atlanta, GA) recommends that antibiotics not be used unless the test for streptococcal infection proves to be positive, because bacterial resistance to certain antibiotics has been reported. However, if results are positive for *Streptococcus,* patients should receive antibiotics to minimize transmission and to reduce the risk of further complications, such as rheumatic fever.

Scarlet Fever

Scarlet fever is an upper respiratory disease also caused by an infection with a group A β-hemolytic streptococcus *(Strepto-*

coccus pyogenes) (Figure 11.2) and once was a serious childhood disease but now is generally treatable. The incubation period is 1 to 2 days and typically begins with a fever and sore throat, but might also exhibit chills, vomiting, abdominal pain, and malaise. The exotoxin produced by the bacteria is responsible for the "strawberry" tongue (Figure 11.3) as well as the characteristic fine rash on the chest, neck, groin, and thighs. The treatment of scarlet fever is the same antibiotic treatment as for strep throat, and complications with appropriate treatment are rare.

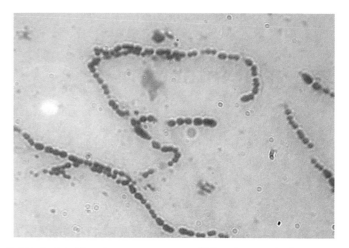

FIGURE 11.2 *Streptococcus pyogenes.* This micrograph shows a Gram stain of *S. pyogenes,* a gram-positive coccus that is usually arranged in chains. This bacterium is typically found in the oral cavity and throat. The organism is responsible for a variety of infections including strep throat, tonsillitis, and necrotizing fasciitis.

MEDICAL HIGHLIGHTS

Complications of Strep Throat (Rheumatic Fever)

Rheumatic fever is an inflammatory disease that can develop as a rare complication to untreated or undertreated strep throat caused by group A *Streptococcus.* Although not as common in the United States as it was before the ready availability and use of antibiotics, it is still prevalent in developing countries. Rheumatic fever presents itself 18 to 20 days after an attack of strep throat, causing joint pain and possible heart valve disease. The exact pathogenesis or mechanism of the disease remains unclear, but is thought to result from an autoimmune response. The disease affects primarily children between the ages of 6 and 15 years. Also, individuals who have suffered rheumatic fever are more likely to develop repeated infections from future exposure to group A *Streptococcus.* On occasion, patients develop carditis that leads to congestive heart failure. Treatment of rheumatic fever includes relief of the symptoms, destruction of group A *Streptococcus,* and prevention of future infections. In addition, untreated group A streptococcal infections can result in poststreptococcal glomerulonephritis (PSGN), a condition that may result in destruction of the glomeruli in the kidneys and ultimately can cause renal failure.

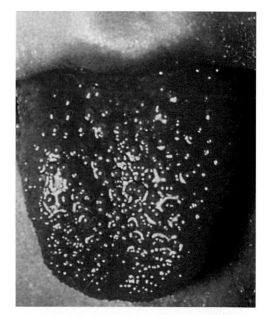

FIGURE 11.3 Scarlet fever. "Strawberry" tongue with its prominent papillae. (Courtesy of WE Farrar. From Mims C, Dockrell HM, Goering RV, et al: *Medical microbiology,* ed 3, St. Louis, 2004, Mosby.)

Streptococcus pneumoniae

Streptococcus pneumoniae is a gram-positive, encapsulated α-hemolytic diplococcus (Figure 11.4), also known as *pneumococcus,* and is a common cause of mild respiratory illness, but also a major source of pneumonia. Other than pneumonia the organism is also capable of causing pharyngitis, sinusitis, otitis media, meningitis, osteomyelitis, septic arthritis, endocarditis, peritonitis, pericarditis, cellulitis, and brain abscess. *S. pneumoniae* is a common inhabitant of the nasopharynx of healthy people, but can be the cause of disease when the organism reaches other areas such as the eustachian tubes, nasal sinuses,

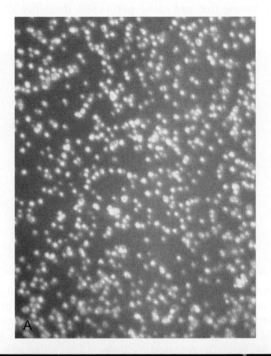

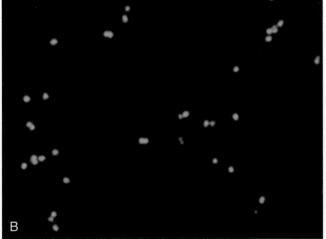

FIGURE 11.4 *Streptococcus pneumoniae. Streptococcus pneumoniae* is a gram-positive coccus; the cocci are usually arranged in pairs (diplococci). In a large percentage of the population this organism is part of the normal flora of the mouth and throat; however, it can cause pneumonia. **A,** Dark-field image showing the diplo, or paired, arrangement of many of the cells. **B,** Capsule stain illustrating the arrangements of the cells and the thick capsule surrounding them.

and lungs. Furthermore the organism can be found in larger numbers in environments where people spend a lot of time in close proximity and it can be transmitted by person-to-person contact or by inhalation. If the organism is inhaled and not removed by the ciliary escalator (such as in smokers, in whom the cilia have been damaged or degenerated), or the mucous membranes are damaged by a viral infection, the bacteria can attach or even penetrate the mucosa. Once the organism succeeds in getting to a site where it normally is not found it will stimulate the immune system of the host, resulting in the attraction of leukocytes (see Chapter 20, The Immune System). The capsule of *S. pneumoniae* is resistant to phagocytosis and if immunity is not present the alveolar macrophages are incapable of destroying pneumococci. In this case the bacterium spreads into the bloodstream, where it most likely causes bacteremia. The organism then can get to other areas of the body, causing the conditions mentioned earlier. The virulence of *S. pneumoniae* is a direct result of its capsule and the encapsulated (smooth) strains are the ones causing disease, whereas the nonencapsulated (rough) strains are avirulent.

The onset of bacterial pneumonia can vary from gradual to sudden. In severe cases patients may have fever, shaking chills, shortness of breath, cough with rust-colored or greenish mucus, and pleuritic chest pain. Fever and sputum production may be absent in elderly persons with pneumococcal pneumonia. Pneumonia can sometimes appear in a mild form, often referred to as *"walking pneumonia,"* in which symptoms are slight or absent. The risk for bacterial pneumonia is highest for young children, the elderly, people with chronic medical conditions (e.g., heart disease, lung disease, and diabetes), and persons who have a suppressed immune system. Because bacterial pneumonia can easily be passed from one member of the community to another, it can manifest itself in a condition referred to as *"community-acquired pneumonia."* This form of the disease occurs worldwide and is a major cause of death among all age groups.

MEDICAL HIGHLIGHTS

Drug-resistant *Streptococcus pneumoniae*

Streptococcus pneumoniae was isolated by Louis Pasteur more than 100 years ago and the organism has been in the research arena ever since then. In the past, isolates of *S. pneumoniae* were consistently susceptible to penicillin, but now penicillin-resistant and multidrug-resistant strains have emerged and are widespread in some communities, especially in the health care settings. According to the CDC, *S. pneumoniae* is a leading cause of morbidity and mortality in the United States, with an estimated 3000 cases of meningitis, 50,000 cases of pneumonia, and more than 7,000,000 cases of otitis media annually. The full extent of the problem with drug-resistant *S. pneumoniae* (DRSP) is, however, unknown because it is not a reportable condition in most of the United States.

Vaccination is available for the prevention of pneumococcal pneumonia. Two vaccines are currently available: the pneumococcal conjugate vaccine, which is part of the routine infant immunization schedule, and the pneumococcal polysaccharide vaccine used for adult immunization. Vaccination with the pneumococcal polysaccharide vaccine is recommended for all adults age 65 years and older and for persons 2 to 64 years of age with certain chronic illnesses or immunocompromising conditions. Without vaccination the treatment of choice used to be penicillin; however, because of overuse of antibiotics nearly all strains of *S. pneumoniae* previously susceptible to penicillin show resistance to penicillin as well as to other antibiotics.

Drug-resistant *Streptococcus pneumoniae* Disease

Drug-resistant *Streptococcus pneumoniae* disease (DRSP) manifests itself as pneumonia, bacteremia, otitis media, meningitis, peritonitis, and sinusitis. These conditions can be caused by an organism that is resistant to one or more commonly used antibiotics. Overuse of antimicrobial agents is a contributing factor to the emerging resistance and spread of resistant strains. Transmission occurs by person-to-person contact and the risk groups are mostly the elderly, children 2 years of age or older, persons who attend or work at child care centers, immunocompromised patients (e.g., those with AIDS), and also persons who recently used antimicrobial agents. Outbreaks of DRSP have been reported in nursing homes, child care centers, and in institutions for HIV-infected people. A pneumococcal conjugate vaccine is available and its use is preventing many infections due to drug-resistant pneumococci. Future increased use of the vaccine, systematic surveillance, and routine testing for the drug-resistant strains might slow down the emerging drug resistance of this bacterium.

Other Common Infections

Mycoplasmal Pneumonia

Mycoplasma pneumoniae, a small bacterium that lacks a cell wall (Figure 11.5), is the cause of primary atypical pneumonia, a relatively mild pneumonia, which usually affects people younger than 40 years of age. Transmission occurs by respiratory droplets through inhalation or person-to-person contact. The incubation period lasts 10 to 14 days and epidemics can occur, especially in crowded areas such as in schools, among military personnel, in homeless shelters, and within a family. Symptoms may last 1 to 3 weeks, starting with fatigue, a sore throat, and a dry cough. It resembles influenza at the beginning, followed by worsening of the cough, which eventually produces sputum. Although it is usually a mild condition and most people recover without treatment, severe cases require antibiotic treatment. It should be noted that because of the lack of a cell wall these organisms are resistant to penicillin and other β-lactam antibiotics (see Chapter 22, Antimicrobial Drugs), which act by interrupting the formation of peptidoglycan crosslinks of bacterial cell walls.

Chlamydial Pneumonia

Chlamydia pneumoniae, now called *Chlamydophila pneumoniae*, is one of the major causes of pneumonia or bronchitis and is

characterized by a gradual onset of cough, with little or no fever. The spectrum of the illness can range from asymptomatic infections to severe disease. Transmissions occur through respiratory secretions of an infected individual and all ages are at risk; however, according to the CDC, it is most common in school-age children. Because the disease is easily passed from one member of the community to another it can give rise to "community-acquired pneumonia." The infection can be treated with antibiotics and generally the drug of choice is erythromycin.

Pertussis (Whooping Cough)

Pertussis, also known as *whooping cough,* is a highly contagious disease caused by *Bordetella pertussis,* an extremely small, aerobic, gram-negative coccobacillus (Figure 11.6). It is a serious disease that can cause permanent disability and even

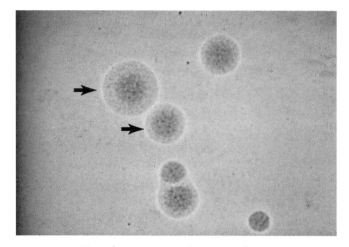

FIGURE 11.5 *Mycoplasma pneumoniae. Mycoplasma pneumoniae* is a small bacterium that lacks a cell wall and is responsible for an estimated 2 million cases of pneumonia in the United States annually, including approximately 100,000 hospitalizations. (From Forbes BA, Sahm DF, Weissfeld AS: *Bailey & Scott's diagnostic microbiology,* ed 12, St. Louis, 2007, Mosby.)

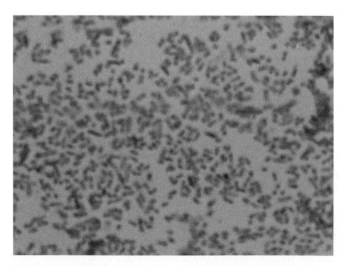

FIGURE 11.6 *Bordetella pertussis. Bordetella pertussis* is a gram-negative coccobacillus (pleomorphic) and the causative agent of whooping cough.

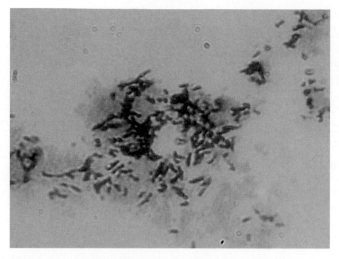

FIGURE 11.7 *Mycobacterium.* This micrograph illustrates an acid-fast stain of *Mycobacterium smegmatis*, an organism with a similar morphology to *M. tuberculosis*, the causative agent of tuberculosis.

death. Pertussis is easily spread from person to person by airborne droplets discharged from the mucous membranes of infected people. Initial symptoms occur about a week after exposure and resemble those of the common cold. The severe coughing spells start approximately 10 to 12 days later and these spells may lead to vomiting. The coughing often ends with a "whoop" noise caused when the patient is trying to take a breath. Despite the availability of, and high coverage with vaccines, pertussis is one of the leading causes of vaccine-preventable deaths worldwide. Ninety percent of all cases occur in the underdeveloped countries and most deaths involve infants who are either not vaccinated or incompletely vaccinated. Treatment with effective antibiotics, if started early, shortens the infectious period but usually does not alter the outcome of the disease.

Tuberculosis

Tuberculosis (TB) is a deadly infectious disease caused by *Mycobacterium tuberculosis* (Figure 11.7). TB is transmitted through the air when an infected person coughs, sneezes, or even talks. Moreover, TB is no longer a disease of the past; it is still a leading killer of young adults worldwide. TB is a chronic condition that usually infects the lungs, but other parts of the body might be involved as well. Most people infected with the organism do not show symptoms, but have latent tuberculosis. According to the World Health Organization (WHO, Geneva, Switzerland) estimate, annually 8 million people worldwide will develop active TB with nearly 2 million deaths. The risk for development of the disease is higher in the first year after infection, but the disease still can occur much later.

After the first effective antibiotic treatments were introduced (1940s and 1950s), the incidence of tuberculosis in the United States declined. The decline in new cases ended in 1985 and the incidence of TB started to rise again. According to the National Institute of Allergy and Infectious Diseases (NIAID, Bethesda, MD), several factors are responsible for this resurgence, such as the following:

- The HIV/AIDS epidemics: People with HIV have an immunocompromised immune system and are more likely to develop active TB, even shortly after first infection.
- Increased numbers of foreign-born nationals who enter the United States from places that have a high incidence of TB cases: These places include Africa, Asia, and Latin America. More than half of the TB cases in the United States are among foreign-born nationals now living here.
- Failure of patients to complete the prescribed antibiotic treatment: These patients stay infectious longer and transmit the disease to more people. Furthermore, incomplete antibiotic treatment can contribute to antibiotic-resistant strains of *M. tuberculosis*.
- Increasing number of elderly in the United States: The increase in the aging population in the United States results in greater numbers residing in long-term facilities. Many of these elderly have declining health and may develop active TB from an infection they obtained much earlier in life.

Initial symptoms of active TB include weight loss (hence in the past, the disease was referred to as *consumption*), fever, night sweats, and loss of appetite. In the case of vague symptoms the infection might go unnoticed and can go into remission or become more chronic and debilitating. These symptoms include cough with chest pain and bloody sputum. Treatment is possible with appropriate antibiotics, which are generally effective, and most people can be cured. Successful treatment can last up to 12 months or longer, using different types of antibiotics. The success of the treatment also depends on the strain of the organism with which the patient is infected. Antibiotic-resistant strains are more difficult to treat, require different drugs, and an increased time of treatment might be necessary. If a person is infected with a strain that is resistant to two or more drugs the condition is called *multidrug-resistant TB* (MDR-TB), which is much more difficult to cure.

Tuberculosis can largely be prevented. In the United States health care providers attempt to identify people infected with *M. tuberculosis* as early as possible to prevent the development of active TB and the spread of the disease. Infected persons will receive isoniazid (INH) every day for 6 to 12 months to prevent active TB. Hospitals isolate people with active TB in controlled environments until spreading is no longer a threat.

TB vaccines are available and the WHO suggests that they be used in countries of the world where the disease is endemic. The vaccine is produced from a live weakened bacterium related to *M. tuberculosis* and is recommended for administration to infants.

Several new and better vaccines for the prevention of TB infection are being developed and have entered clinical trials in the United States. At present, health experts in the United States do not recommend the use of the vaccine for general use in this country because it makes the screening procedures for infected individuals more difficult. The TB skin test, also known as the *tuberculin PPD test*, is used for screening purposes and will show positive results in persons who currently has TB or were exposed or vaccinated in the past. The test is based on the fact that an encounter with *M. tuberculosis* produces a delayed

Tuberculosis and Air Travel

In the early 1990s reports of tuberculosis (TB) transmission during long flights raised serious concerns among public health officials and airlines. These reports included the most dangerous form of TB—the multidrug-resistant TB (MDR-TB). The World Health Organization (WHO) published the first guidelines in 1998, defining the extent of the problem, the potential risks, and recommendations for travelers, physicians, health authorities, and airlines. In addition to raised awareness of the risk for TB transmission on board an aircraft, other airborne diseases caused major international public health emergencies, involving the actual or potential transmission of infection during international flights. Furthermore, the increased incidence of MDR-TB in the following years has raised special concerns in relation to the international spread of particularly dangerous strains of *Mycobacterium tuberculosis.* A revised third edition of "Tuberculosis and Air Travel: Guidelines for Prevention and Control" was prepared by the WHO in collaboration with the International Civil Aviation Organization, the International Air Transport Association, international experts in tuberculosis and other infectious diseases, as well as leading authorities in public health and travel medicine. This new edition was published in 2008 and is available online (see references).

In 2007, these guidelines did not prevent extensive air travel by Andrew Speaker, a resident of Atlanta, Georgia. Although diagnosed with an antibiotic-resistant strain of TB just before his travel, he claims that he was not adequately warned of the risk of spreading the disease on a long trip in a confined area such as an airplane. On his return to the United States, after traveling to France, Greece, Italy, the Czech Republic, and Canada, he was served with an isolation order by the Centers for Disease Control and Prevention (CDC). The legal problems in dealing with a situation such as this are complex and still under review by several organizations, including the CDC.

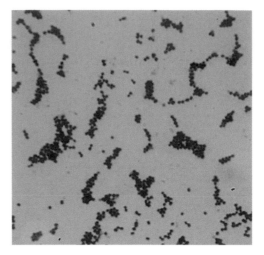

FIGURE 11.8 *Staphylococcus aureus. Staphylococcus aureus* is a gram-positive coccus arranged in grapelike clusters. This is a ubiquitous bacterium that can cause a variety of infections and diseases.

people with another debilitating illness. Although the illness is rare, it is serious and causes death in about 15% to 40% of the cases. Treatment is usually a type of penicillin; however, more strains of *Staphylococcus* are becoming resistant to these and the use of other antibiotics such as vancomycin may be required. Staphylococcal pneumonia also has been reported to be the cause of severe complications after the 2003–2004 influenza seasons.

Haemophilus Infections

Many *Haemophilus* species are part of the normal flora in the upper airways of children and adults and most of them rarely cause disease. However, *Haemophilus influenzae,* a gram-negative coccobacillus (Figure 11.9), is a common cause of infection (bronchiolitis) in children and chronic bronchitis in adults, and occasionally meningitis.

H. influenzae and *S. pneumoniae* are sometimes isolated from the same individual. The transmission occurs by aerosols from an infected individual. Children are routinely and successfully vaccinated against *Haemophilus influenzae* type b, especially for the prevention of meningitis.

Klebsiella pneumoniae

Klebsiella pneumoniae is a gram-negative, encapsulated bacillus found in the normal flora of the mouth, skin, and intestines. It is an opportunistic pathogen that can cause bacterial pneumonia that is most often hospital-acquired (nosocomial) or occurs in nursing homes. Other people at risk are infants, older people, alcoholics, and people with chronic diseases, such as immune disorders. The infection is serious and persons are treated with antibiotics, supplemental oxygen, and intravenous fluids. Despite treatment the death toll ranges from 25% to 50% of infected patients.

Diphtheria

Diphtheria is caused by *Corynebacterium diphtheriae,* a facultative anaerobic, gram-positive bacillus (Figure 11.10), which attacks the throat and nose. It is an upper respiratory illness

hypersensitivity skin reaction (see Chapter 20, The Immune System) to certain components of the bacterium.

Rare and Opportunistic Infections

Staphylococcal Pneumonia

Respiratory infections due to staphylococci are relatively rare in the healthy adult but are common opportunistic organisms in compromised hosts in hospitals and other institutions, causing hospital-acquired and institution-acquired pneumonia. *Staphylococcus aureus,* a gram-positive coccus (Figure 11.8), causes only 2% of community-acquired pneumonias, but 10% to 15% of hospital-acquired pneumonias are due to this organism. These infections most likely occur in people who are hospitalized with another disease and often involves the very young, the old, and

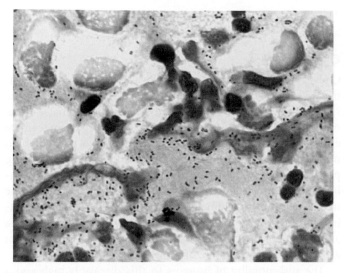

FIGURE 11.9 *Haemophilus influenzae.* *Haemophilus influenzae* is a gram-negative coccobacillus (pleomorphic) commonly found in the upper respiratory tract. The bacterium can cause pneumonia, epiglottitis, and meningitis. (From Murray PR, Rosenthal KS, Pfaller MA: *Medical microbiology,* ed 5, St. Louis, 2005, Mosby.)

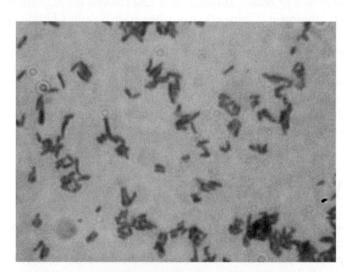

FIGURE 11.10 *Corynebacterium diphtheriae.* *Corynebacterium diphtheriae* is a gram-positive, nonsporing, rod-shaped to pleomorphic bacterium that causes diphtheria. Note the unique arrangement of the bacilli, which are often parallel along the long axis of the rods or in V- or W-shaped clumps, sometimes referred to as a *"Chinese character"* arrangement. This is due to a process called *"snapping division,"* by which reproducing cells divide along the long axis of the cells instead of the ends of the cells.

characterized by a sore throat, low-grade fever, and the formation of a pseudomembrane on the tonsils and pharynx. The formation of the pseudomembrane can cause life-threatening respiratory obstruction. It is a highly contagious disease easily spread by direct physical contact or aerosol secretions from an infected individual. Once the infection takes place the bacterium produces an exotoxin that can potentially spread via the bloodstream to other organs such as the heart and cause significant damage.

A vaccine is available and because of widespread routine childhood immunization, diphtheria is rare in the United States and in many other countries. It is reemerging in some parts of the world where immunization practices are not strictly followed. Other risk factors include crowded environments and poor hygiene.

Diphtheria is a medical emergency and delay in treatment can result in long-term heart disease. Treatment includes antitoxin to eliminate the toxin and antibiotics to eliminate the toxin-producing bacteria themselves. Recovery from the illness is slow and the death rate from diphtheria is 10% in infected patients.

Legionellosis

Legionellosis is an illness caused by *Legionella pneumophila,* a gram-negative bacillus found in water sources in the environment. The disease has two distinct forms:

1. Pontiac fever, a relatively mild respiratory infection
2. Legionnaire's disease, a serious and potentially fatal form of pneumonia. Legionnaire's disease received its name in 1976 when an outbreak of pneumonia occurred in people attending a convention of the American Legion in Philadelphia.

Legionellosis is contracted when people inhale water mist containing the bacteria. Mist-producing devices that potentially can contain *Legionella* include air-conditioning systems in homes, workplaces, hospitals, or other public gathering places. Legionellosis is not spread from person to person, but only through contaminated water sources.

The symptoms of Pontiac fever include fever and muscle aches but do not include pneumonia, and infected persons usually recover within 2 to 5 days without requiring treatment. Persons with Legionnaire's disease show more severe symptoms, including high fever, chills, and a cough that might or might not produce sputum. Other symptoms may include muscle aches, headache, tiredness, loss of appetite, and occasionally diarrhea. Chest x-rays often indicate signs of pneumonia. Distinguishing Legionnaire's disease from other pneumonias is difficult on the basis of symptoms alone; specific tests are needed for a safe diagnosis. These tests include detecting *Legionella* in sputum and body fluids, or finding specific antibodies in the blood of the patient. Legionnaire's disease can be treated with antibiotics.

Psittacosis

Psittacosis is an infection caused by *Chlamydia psittaci,* an obligate intracellular bacterium found in bird droppings. The illness is also known as *parrot disease, parrot fever,* and *ornithosis.* In birds the infection is referred to as *avian chlamydiosis* and *Chlamydia* is shed by infected birds through feces and nasal discharges, which can remain infectious for months. Psittacosis is a rare zoonotic infection and is spread from birds to humans. People at risk include bird owners, pet shop employees, workers in poultry-processing plants, and veterinarians. The symptoms of the disease include fever, chills, headache, muscle aches, dry cough, and often pneumonia. The incubation period after inha-

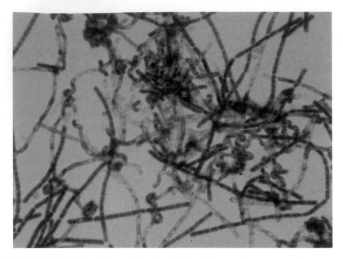

FIGURE 11.11 *Bacillus anthracis.* This micrograph represents a simple stain of *B. anthracis*, a gram-positive, spore-forming bacillus that can cause anthrax. The bacterium is part of the typical soil flora.

lation of dry bird secretions is 5 to 19 days. The infection is treated with antibiotics.

Inhalation Anthrax

Anthrax is an acute infectious disease caused by *Bacillus anthracis,* a gram-positive, spore-forming, facultative anacrobe (Figure 11.11), commonly found in wild and domestic vertebrates. The disease is zoonotic and can occur in humans if a person is exposed to an infected animal, tissue from an infected animal, or spores of the bacterium. The infection can be attained through the skin, by inhalation, or ingestion. There is no known transmission of anthrax from person to person. Symptoms of the disease vary depending on how it was acquired. Symptoms commonly occur within 7 days, but can take up to 60 days. Inhaling the spores only means that a person has been exposed to the disease; it does not mean that symptoms automatically appear, because the bacterial spores must germinate before the actual disease occurs. Once the spores germinate, they release several toxins that cause internal bleeding, swelling, and tissue necrosis. Anthrax spores can remain viable in the environment for 50 years.

The initial symptoms of anthrax when the bacterial spores are acquired through inhalation are similar to those of a common cold, including fever, chills, sweating, fatigue, malaise, headache, cough, shortness of breath, and some chest pain. After several days the symptoms usually progress to the second stage with fever, severe breathing problems, and shock. Cutaneous anthrax appears as a large, deep lesion on the skin, and gastrointestinal anthrax causes lesions in the intestinal tract, often with intestinal bleeding. Antibiotic therapy administered after known or suspected exposure can help prevent the disease. Several antibiotics are effective against anthrax; however, if the second stage has been reached, inhalation anthrax is usually fatal. Vaccination has been developed and is available to select U.S. military personnel, but not to the general public. Anthrax spores and their use in bioterrorism are discussed in Chapter 24 (Microorganisms in the Environment and Environmental Safety).

Q Fever

Q fever is a zoonotic disease caused by *Coxiella burnetii,* a gram-negative, coccobacillus that can form sporelike structures. The species is distributed globally and affects sheep, goats, cattle, dogs, cats, birds, rodents, and ticks. The organism can be excreted in milk, urine, and feces and is also shed in high numbers in the amniotic fluid and placenta during the birthing process. *Coxiella* is resistant to heat, drying, and common disinfectants, and therefore it can survive for long periods of time in the environment. Humans can acquire the infection by inhaling the organism from contaminated barnyard dust, birth fluids, and excreta of infected herd animals. Bites from infected ticks are another possible mode of transmission.

The susceptibility of humans to this disease is high and a small number of organisms appear to be causing the disease. The incubation time depends on the number of organisms that infect the patient, but symptoms usually occur within 2 to 3 weeks of exposure. Symptoms of acute Q fever include fever, headache, muscle pains, cough, chest pain during breathing, shortness of breath, jaundice, and clay-colored stools. Antibiotic treatment is most effective when started early. Chronic Q fever develops in persons who have not been treated effectively within 6 months of the initial exposure and management may require a combination of drugs and prolonged duration of treatment. Because of the nature of the agent (resistant to heat and drying) and human susceptibility to the organism it could be developed for use in biological warfare and, like anthrax, is considered a potential terrorist weapon.

Viral Infections

Although many bacteria are part of the resident normal flora of the upper respiratory system, a large number of viruses are probably part of the transient flora of the nasopharyngeal cells as well. Not all infections of cells cause disease, and such infections might not be apparent because of the lack of symptoms. Moreover, most virions that are able to reach the lungs are destroyed by alveolar macrophages. Nevertheless, an estimated 90% of acute upper respiratory and approximately 50% of lower respiratory infections are caused by viruses (Table 11.2).

Common Cold

A great many varieties of viruses are frequent invaders of the nasopharynx and are responsible for the common cold. The common cold is normally mild and self-limiting. The common cold is the most frequent of all human diseases and typically lasts 3 to 5 days. Symptoms of the common cold usually involve rhinitis, a runny nose, nasal congestion, and sneezing. A sore throat, cough, headache, or other symptoms may be present as well. The nasal secretions usually become thicker within 1 to 3 days and may be yellow or green in appearance. In children with asthma the common cold is the most prevalent trigger of asth-

Pneumonias

Organism	Features	Transmission	Treatment/Prevention
Streptococcus pneumoniae	Shaking chills, fever, pleuritic chest pain, cough, rust-colored or greenish mucus	Inhalation of droplets	Pneumococcal conjugate vaccine; pneumococcal polysaccharide vaccine; antibiotics (amoxicillin, cephalosporins, erythromycin, azithromycin, clarithromycin, fluoroquinolones)
Haemophilus influenzae	More common in patients with COPD, alcoholics, and the elderly	Inhalation of respiratory droplets	*Haemophilus influenzae* type b vaccine; antibiotics (cephalosporins, amoxicillin-clavulanate, azithromycin, fluoroquinolones, trimethoprim-sulfamethoxazole)
Legionella pneumophila	High fever, chills, cough with or without sputum, muscle aches, headache, tiredness, loss of appetite, occasionally diarrhea	Inhalation of water mist; not spread between people	Antibiotics (erythromycin, azithromycin, fluoroquinolones)
Mycoplasma pneumoniae	Fatigue, sore throat, dry cough; eventually sputum production	Close contact; inhalation of respiratory secretions	Mild cases may not require treatment; home care includes rest, high-protein diet, and adequate fluid intake; severe cases treated with antibiotics (erythromycin, doxycycline, azithromycin, clarithromycin fluoroquinolones)
Chlamydia pneumoniae	Gradual onset of cough, little or no fever	Inhalation of respiratory secretions	Antibiotics (erythromycin, doxycycline, azithromycin, clarithromycin, fluoroquinolones)
Staphylococcus aureus	Multiple bilateral nodular infiltrates with central cavitations; common in patients with cystic fibrosis	IV drug use, inhalation of droplets, postinfluenza	Antibiotics—usually penicillin, but many strains are becoming resistant and other antibiotics may have to be used (cephalosporins, nafcillin, oxacillin, vancomycin)
Klebsiella pneumoniae	Opportunistic in infants, older people, alcoholics, people with chronic disease	Mostly nosocomial; also community-acquired	Antibiotics, supplemental oxygen, intravenous fluids
Bacillus anthracis	Fever, chills, sweating, fatigue, malaise, headache, cough, shortness of breath, chest pain, shock; formation of skin eschars, gastrointestinal hemorrhaging	Inhalation of spores, ingestion or penetration through a break in the skin	Vaccination for U.S. military personnel, not for general population; antibiotics for about 60 days (ciprofloxacin, penicillin, doxycyline)
Viral pneumonia; can be caused by several viruses including influenza viruses, parainfluenza, adenovirus, rhinovirus, herpes simplex virus, respiratory syncytial virus, hantavirus, and cytomegalovirus	Fever, dry cough, headache, muscle pain, and weakness; followed by increasing breathlessness, high fever, and worsened cough that may produce a small amount of mucus	Person-to-person contact; respiratory droplets	Supportive care including humidified air, increased fluids, and oxygen; serious forms can be treated with antiviral medications

Pneumonias—cont'd

Organism	Features	Transmission	Treatment/Prevention
Histoplasma capsulatum	Fever, headache, nonproductive cough	Inhalation of fungal spores	Mild cases resolve without treatment; antifungal drugs (itraconazole, ketoconazole)
Coccidioides immitis	Cough, chest pain, fever, chills, night sweats, headache, muscle stiffness, rash, blood-tinged sputum, weight loss, wheezing, and more	Inhalation of airborne arthroconidia	Acute form usually fades without treatment—symptomatic treatment may be recommended; severe disease should be treated with antifungal medications (amphotericin B, ketoconazole, fluconazole, itraconazole)
Blastomyces dermatitidis	Cough with possible brown or bloody mucus, shortness of breath, sweating, fever, fatigue, malaise, weight loss, joint stiffness, muscle stiffness, rash, chest pain	Inhalation of fungus from soil	Mild infections of the lungs do not require treatment; severe infections need antifungal medication
Aspergillus	Chest pain, cough (dry, or producing blood or phlegm), shortness of breath, fever, joint pain, weight loss	Inhalation of spores	Antifungal medication (amphotericin B, itraconazole, voriconazole, caspofungin)

COPD, Chronic obstructive pulmonary disease; *IV,* intravenous.

TABLE 11.2 Viral Infections Acquired Through the Respiratory Tract

Illness/Disease	Organism(s)	Target of Infection	Transmission
Common cold	Adenovirus	Respiratory tract	Respiratory droplets
	Rhinovirus	Upper respiratory tract	Respiratory droplets; fomites; person-to-person contact
Influenza	Influenza virus	Lungs, respiratory tract	Inhalation of airborne viruses; via fomites
Mumps	Mumps virus (paramyxovirus)	Upper respiratory cells	Respiratory secretions
SARS	SARS coronavirus	Lungs	Inhalation of airborne viruses

SARS, Severe acute respiratory syndrome.

matic symptoms. Colds also are a common precursor of ear infections, but congested ears during the common cold are not necessarily a sign of a bacterial infection, but just fluid buildup as a side effect of the cold.

More than 1 billion colds caused by over 200 viruses occur in the United States each year. Children average three to eight colds a year while adults average two to four infections annually. Children usually get colds from other children and when a new strain shows up in a school or day care center it is highly contagious and rapidly spreads throughout the class. Parents usually obtain the infection from their school-aged children. Transmission can occur through aerosols, but most commonly the disease spreads by contaminated hands or fomites. People are most contagious for the first 2 to 3 days, less contagious in the following days, and generally contagion free by day 7 to 10.

There is no specific treatment for a cold except plenty of rest and lots of fluids to relieve symptoms. Over-the-counter medication may help to relieve these symptoms, but will not shorten the duration of the disease. Antibiotics should not be used to treat the common cold because of its viral origin, and they should be given only if signs of a secondary bacterial infection occur.

Influenza

Influenza viruses are primary causes for epidemics and endemic diseases of the respiratory system. **Influenza (flu)** is caused by orthomyxoviruses. They are RNA viruses designated as types A, B, and C. The viruses spread from person to person mainly through coughing or sneezing by infected people, or by fomites and then by hand from touching the mouth, nose, or eyes.

Influenza viruses A and C are capable of infecting a variety of species, whereas influenza B infects primarily humans. Type A viruses are the most virulent human pathogens among these three types of flu viruses and cause the most severe disease state. Because influenza viruses kill epithelial cells, the first line of defense of the lung against infection is broached and flu patients become more susceptible to bacterial infections than do healthy individuals. This susceptibility is likely to be further increased due to a virus-induced immune suppression, common in influenza patients.

The influenza genome is not a single piece of nucleic acid, but instead consists of 8 pieces of segmented negative-sense RNA, encoding 11 proteins. Two of these proteins, hemagglutinin and neuraminidase, large glycoproteins, are well characterized and found on the outside of the viral particles (Figure 11.12, A and B). Neuraminidase is an enzyme involved in the release of the progeny viruses from infected cells. Hemagglutinin is a lectin that mediates the binding of the virus to target cells and the subsequent entry of the viral genome into the host. After the release of the newly produced influenza viruses the host cell dies.

Influenza viruses can be subdivided into different strains based on their antigenic characteristics (Box 11.1). New influ-

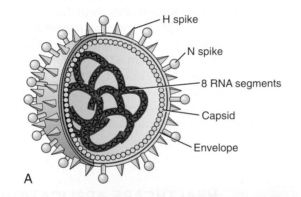

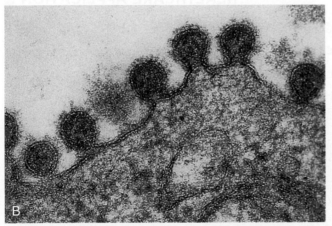

FIGURE 11.12 A, This illustration shows a typical influenza virus with the surface hemagglutinin and neuraminidase glycoproteins on the surface of the virus. **B,** An electron micrograph of the budding process of new viral particles from an infected cell. (Courtesy D. Hockley. From Mims C, Dockrell HM, Goering RV, et al: *Medical microbiology*, ed 3, St. Louis, 2004, Mosby.)

enza virus variants are the result of frequent antigenic changes (i.e., antigenic drift) resulting from point mutations during viral replication. These rapid mutations are partially due to the absence of RNA-proofreading enzymes. As a result, RNA-dependent RNA transcriptase makes a single-nucleotide insertion error about once every 10,000 nucleotides, making almost every newly formed influenza virus a potential mutant. The influenza B viruses undergo antigenic drift less frequently than the influenza A viruses.

Manifestation of flu signs and symptoms during an outbreak of the flu is usually sufficient for the diagnosis of influenza. These symptoms include the following:

- Fever
- Headache
- Fatigue
- Dry cough
- Sore throat
- Runny or stuffy nose
- Muscle aches
- Gastrointestinal symptoms: Nausea, vomiting, and diarrhea can occur and are more common in children than in adults

Laboratory tests such as immunofluorescence or enzyme-linked immunosorbent assay (ELISA) can be used to distinguish between viral strains if necessary. Complications that occur with influenza include bacterial pneumonia, ear infections, sinus infections, dehydration, and worsening of chronic existent medical conditions, such as congestive heart failure, asthma, or diabetes.

Epidemics of influenza in the United States typically appear during the winter months, causing disease among all age groups. Every year millions of Americans are infected and an estimated 36,000 Americans die of influenza-related illness. Especially vulnerable are people with a weak immune system such as the very young, the elderly, and those with a compromised immune system as a result of cancer therapy or disease. Influenza vaccination, that is, the annual "flu shot," is the primary method for preventing the flu and its possible complications. Vaccination can prevent hospitalization and death among people at risk, but also will reduce flu-associated respiratory illnesses among people of all age groups. According to the Advisory Committee on Immunization Practices (ACIP), a part of the CDC, annual influenza vaccinations are recommended for people at high risk

---

BOX 11.1 Serotypes of the Influenza A virus

- H1N1: Spanish flu
- H2N2: Asian flu
- H3N2: Hong Kong flu
- H5N1: Pandemic threat in 2006–2007 flu seasons (avian influenza)
- H7N7: Unusual zoonotic potential
- H1N2: Endemic in humans and pigs
- H9N2, H7N2, H7N3, H10N7

for influenza-related complications, and persons who live with or care for persons at high risk (Box 11.2).

Viral Pneumonia

Half of all pneumonias are believed to be caused by viruses such as the influenza virus, adenovirus, coxsackievirus, varicella-zoster virus, measles virus, cytomegalovirus, and respiratory syncytial virus. Symptoms of viral pneumonia include fever, nonproductive cough, rhinitis, myalgia, and headache; however, different viruses cause different symptoms.

Most cases of viral pneumonia are mild and fade away without treatment within 1 to 3 weeks. More serious cases may require hospitalization and people typically at risk are those with an impaired immune system. Antibiotics are ineffective in treating viral pneumonia, but the more serious forms of viral pneumonia can be treated with antiviral medications. Furthermore, other supportive care includes the use of humidified air, increased fluid intake, and oxygen. Hospitalization may be required to prevent dehydration and to help with breathing. Complications can result in respiratory failure, liver failure, heart failure, and sometimes bacterial infections can follow a viral infection, resulting in a more serious form of pneumonia.

Hantavirus Pulmonary Syndrome

Hantavirus pulmonary syndrome (HPS) is a deadly disease caused by a group of viruses called *hantaviruses*. It is carried by rodents and humans can contract the disease when they come into contact with infected rodents, their urine, and/or droppings. Person-to-person transmission has not been reported. HPS first appeared in the United States in 1993, but it has been found and recognized by authorities since 1978 in South America and Asia.

A hantavirus infection at first appears similar to a severe cold or influenza and is accompanied by fever and muscle aches. The infection then quickly progresses to severe respiratory difficulties and to acute respiratory distress syndrome (ARDS), with fatalities occurring in 30% to 40% of cases. In ARDS, gas exchange and therefore oxygen uptake in the lungs is severely impaired, compromising the functionality of all the organs of the body. Although some experimental use of antiviral drugs has been done, at present the main treatment for ARDS is mechanical ventilation.

Rodent control in and around homes is essential and the CDC has issued guidelines for rodent extermination and avoidance for residents, workers, campers, and hikers in affected areas. HPS has been publicized as an emerging infectious disease as well as an agent considered to be a possible bioterrorist threat.

Severe Acute Respiratory Syndrome (SARS)

SARS is a respiratory illness caused by the SARS coronavirus. The original outbreak (November 2002) seems to have originated in mainland China. The disease spread worldwide over several months before the outbreak was curtailed with help from and coordination by the WHO. This first global outbreak of SARS was reported to have a mortality rate of 9.6% between 2002 and 2003 (see Health Care Application: Global SARS Outbreak).

SARS seems to be transmitted by close person-to-person contact, most readily by respiratory droplets depositing on the mucous membranes of a nearby individual. SARS can be life-threatening and the symptoms include high fever, headache, body aches, and a dry cough, followed by pneumonia. Some patients may develop diarrhea as well. Symptoms usually appear 2 to 10 days after exposure, but in most cases symptoms appear within 2 or 3 days and about 10% to 20% of cases require assisted mechanical ventilation. Support with antipyretics, supplemental oxygen, and additional ventilatory support as needed, constitute the only treatment available to date.

BOX 11.2 Groups of People Recommended for Annual Influenza Vaccination

Persons at high risk for influenza-related complications and severe disease
- Children aged 6-59 months
- Pregnant women
- Persons aged 50 years and older
- Persons of any age with certain chronic medical conditions

Persons who live with or care for people at high risk
- Household contacts who have frequent contact with persons at high risk and who can transmit influenza to those persons at high risk
- Health care workers

HEALTHCARE APPLICATION

Global SARS Outbreak (November 2002–July 2003)*

Country	Cases	Deaths
China	5327	348
Hong Kong	1755	298
Taiwan	671	84
Canada	250	38
Singapore	206	32
United States	75	0
Vietnam	63	5
Philippines	14	2
Other	76	6
Total	8436	812

*Source: Centers for Disease Control and Prevention (http://www.who.int/csr/sars/country/2003_07_09/en/)

Fungal Infections

Fungi can cause infections of the skin, hair, nails and also of the respiratory system. Respiratory diseases caused by fungi most commonly involve the lungs and are referred to as *deep mycoses*. These diseases include histoplasmosis, coccidioidomycosis, blastomycosis, and aspergillosis (Table 11.3). Dimorphism in some fungi (see Fungi in Chapter 8, Eukaryotic Microorganisms) can aid in infection as the single-celled yeast can more easily spread throughout the body via the bloodstream.

Histoplasmosis

Histoplasma capsulatum (Figure 11.13) infections are generally acute respiratory infections that occur in all age groups and in both sexes. The disease affects primarily the lungs and occasionally other organs. The infections are more frequent in adult males, probably because of more frequent occupational exposure. Transmission occurs by inhalation of airborne conidia of the fungus (see Chapter 8). Reservoirs of the organism can be found in soil around old chicken houses, starling bird roosts, and bat caves.

Most infected persons do not have apparent symptoms, but the acute infection shows symptoms that resemble those of

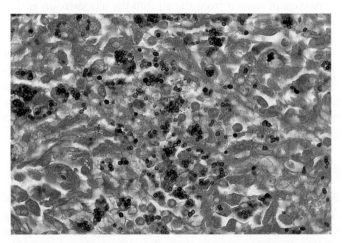

FIGURE 11.13 *Histoplasma capsulatum.* This is a micrograph of *H. capsulatum*, a fungus whose yeast cell stage causes the disease histoplasmosis. (From Forbes BA, Sahm DF, Weissfeld AS: *Bailey & Scott's diagnostic microbiology,* ed 12, St. Louis, 2007, Mosby.)

tuberculosis, usually occurring 10 days after exposure. Symptoms after extensive exposure to the fungus include fever, headache, and nonproductive cough. A progressive form of the disease generally occurs in the young and elderly, and including anyone with immune deficiency. *H. capsulatum* is an intracellular parasite that first attacks the alveolar macrophages in the lungs. The macrophages then disperse the fungus via the blood and lymph, and the disease can become disseminated. Mild cases may not require treatment; others can be treated with antifungal drugs. If untreated this form is fatal. To reduce the risk of infection the following precautions can be taken:

- Avoid areas that may be reservoirs of the fungus, such as areas of accumulating bird guano.
- Persons having to work in areas where there is a risk of exposure to *H. capsulatum* should consult the National Institute for Occupational Safety and Health (NIOSH, Washington, DC) document "Histoplasmosis: Protecting Workers at Risk" (available at http://www.cdc.gov/niosh/docs/2005-109/). This particular document contains information about work practices and personal protective equipment designed to reduce the risk of infection.

Coccidioidomycosis

The causative agent of coccidioidomycosis is *Coccidioides immitis* (Figure 11.14), which resides in the soil of certain parts of the southwestern United States (Arizona, California, Nevada, New Mexico, and Texas), parts of Mexico, and areas in South America. Reservoirs include desert soil, rodent burrows, archaeological remains, and mines. Transmission occurs by inhalation of airborne arthroconidia. Exposure often occurs after natural disasters such as dust storms and earthquakes, potentially exposing thousands of people. This type of exposure is also possible after disturbance of soil by humans. Dust that covers material from endemic areas can also serve as the vehicle of infection; these materials include but are not limited to Native American pots, blankets, and other items sold to tourists, especially in recreational areas.

Although about 60% of the infections fail to cause symptoms, the other 40% result in symptoms ranging in degree from mild to severe. The disease manifests itself as acute, chronic, or disseminated. Symptomatic infections present as cough, chest pain, fever, chills, night sweats, headache, muscle stiffness, muscle aches, joint stiffness, neck and shoulder stiffness, rash,

---

TABLE 11.3 Fungal Infections Acquired Through the Respiratory Tract

Illness/Disease	Organism(s)	Target of Infection	Transmission
Pulmonary blastomycosis	*Blastomyces dermatitidis*	Lungs	Inhalation of spores from dust
Histoplasmosis	*Histoplasma capsulatum*	Alveolar macrophages in lungs	Inhalation of spores near bird droppings
Coccidioidomycosis	*Coccidioides immitis*	Alveolar spaces of lungs	Inhalation of spores
Pneumocystis pneumonia	*Pneumocystis carinii*	Lungs	Inhalation of spores
Aspergillosis	*Aspergillus* spp.	Lungs	Inhalation of spores

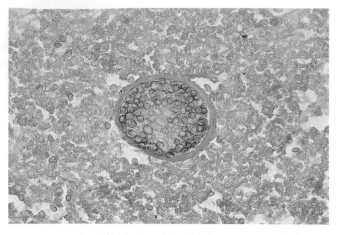

FIGURE 11.14 *Coccidioides immitis.* This is a micrograph of *C. immitis*, a dimorphic fungus that causes coccidioidomycosis. (From Forbes BA, Sahm DF, Weissfeld AS: *Bailey & Scott's diagnostic microbiology*, ed 12, St. Louis, 2007, Mosby.)

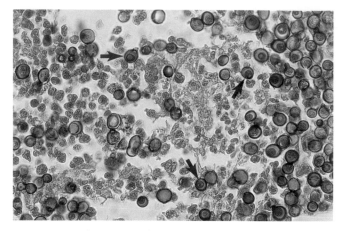

FIGURE 11.15 *Blastomyces dermatitidis.* This is a micrograph of *B. dermatitidis*, a dimorphic fungus whose yeast cell stage can cause blastomycosis, a systemic fungal infection. (From Forbes BA, Sahm DF, Weissfeld AS: *Bailey & Scott's diagnostic microbiology*, ed 12, St. Louis, 2007, Mosby.)

blood-tinged sputum, loss of appetite, weight loss, wheezing, excessive sweating, change in mental status, and sensitivity to light. The acute form of the disease usually fades away without treatment; bed rest and treatment of the flulike symptoms may be recommended. The acute form may become chronic or result in a widespread infection throughout the body. The outcome of chronic infections, if treated, is usually good, but relapses may occur. These relapses usually occur in people with a compromised immune system. If the disease becomes disseminated to other organ systems it can result in a high mortality rate. Disseminated or severe disease should be treated with antifungal medications.

Blastomycosis

Blastomycosis is an acute or chronic infection caused by the pathogen *Blastomyces dermatitidis* (Figure 11.15). Spores of the fungus generally enter the body by inhalation to affect primarily the lungs, but occasionally spread via the bloodstream to other areas of the body, including the skin. The reservoirs for *Blastomyces dermatitidis* are primarily wood and soil. Blastomycosis is considered a rare infection and occurs primarily in the south–central and Midwestern United States and Canada. In addition, infections have also been observed in widely scattered areas of Africa. The disease often affects people with a compromised immune system, such as patients receiving transplants and patients undergoing chemotherapy.

Blastomycosis of the lung may be asymptomatic but generally presents itself in one of the following ways:

- A flulike condition with fever, chills, myalgias, headache, and a nonproductive cough that resolves itself within days
- An acute illness with symptoms similar to those of bacterial pneumonia, including high fever, chills, a productive cough (brown or bloody mucus), and pleuritic chest pain
- A chronic illness resembling tuberculosis or lung cancer. The symptoms include low-grade fever, a productive cough, night sweats, and weight loss

- A speedy, progressive, and severe disease that causes acute respiratory distress syndrome (ARDS), a life-threatening condition that causes lung swelling and fluid buildup in the air sacs. This condition is a medical emergency, because the fluid inhibits gas exchange and therefore the passage of oxygen from the air into the bloodstream is compromised.

If the blastomycosis infection stays in the lungs it may not require medication unless it becomes severe. When blastomycosis spreads and affects other areas of the body, antifungal treatment will be required that may have to be continued for months. Untreated systemic infections slowly worsen and can become lethal.

Pulmonary Aspergillosis

Pulmonary aspergillosis is caused by one or more species of *Aspergillus* (Figure 11.16), a mold commonly found in decaying plants, stored hay, compost piles, bird droppings, and any site where excess dust accumulates. Given the appropriate conditions, the organism forms large amounts of spores that are ultimately released into the environment, where they may remain suspended for long periods of time. *Aspergillus* spp. can also be found in the hospital environment, including showerheads, hospital water storage tanks, and potted plants. *Aspergillus* conidia (spores) are small, can easily be transmitted by inhalation, and subsequently may colonize in the upper or lower respiratory tracts. The respiratory tract is the most frequent and most important portal of entry for this fungus. At present there is no evidence of person-to-person transmission. Pulmonary aspergillosis has been subdivided into four major forms:

- Primary acute pneumonia
- Formation of a "fungus ball" (aspergilloma) within preexisting cavities that have developed in areas of previous lung disease such as tuberculosis or lung abscess

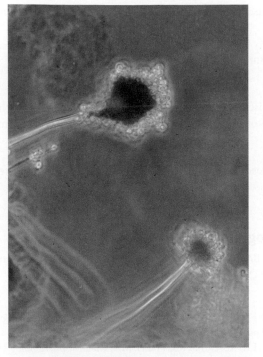

FIGURE 11.16 *Aspergillus* spp. This is a micrograph of *Aspergillus*, an opportunistic fungal pathogen that can cause a variety of diseases collectively called *aspergillosis*.

- Allergic bronchopulmonary aspergillosis (ABPA), characterized by inflammation of the bronchi and/or alveoli. This condition may be similar to asthma or pneumonia, and many patients with ABPA also have asthma. Asthmatic patients and people with cystic fibrosis represent the highest at-risk group for allergic aspergillosis
- Secondary pulmonary (invasive) aspergillosis as an opportunistic systemic infection in immunocompromised patients. This is a serious infection with pneumonia and can spread to other parts of the body

The main treatment for aspergillosis is provided by antifungal drugs, which are sometimes administered intravenously. Antifungal medication does not work for allergic reactions and the use of steroids and relief medications such as bronchodilators may be necessary under these circumstances. A fungus ball generally does not require treatment unless bleeding into the lung occurs, in which case surgical removal of the fungal mass may be required.

Summary

- Structurally and functionally the respiratory system can be divided into the upper respiratory tract including the nose, pharynx and associated structures, and the lower respiratory system consisting of the larynx, trachea, bronchi, and lungs.
- The upper respiratory tract is colonized by normal flora commonly represented by *Staphylococcus aureus* and *S. epidermidis*, but other organisms also might be part of the normal flora, typically in much lower numbers.
- Bacterial infections of the respiratory tract can be caused by *Staphylococcus, Streptococcus, Klebsiella, Haemophilus, Bordetella, Corynebacterium, Mycobacterium, Legionella, Mycoplasma, Chlamydia,* and *Coxiella*.
- Bacterial infections caused by the normal flora are generally secondary infections commonly occurring after damage to the mucosal lining due to viral infections such as the common cold.
- Other opportunistic infections involve bacteria that normally do not cause infection in the healthy adult, but are common in people with a compromised immune system.
- Rare and opportunistic bacterial infections include staphylococcal pneumonia, *Haemophilus* infections, *Klebsiella* pneumonia, diphtheria, legionellosis, psittacosis, inhalation anthrax, and Q fever.
- Many different viruses are frequent intruders of the nasopharynx and are responsible for the common cold, a normally self-limiting infection, and the most frequent of all human diseases.
- Primary causes for epidemics and endemic diseases of the respiratory system are the influenza viruses, which are capable of rapid mutations. Epidemics in the United States usually occur during the winter months, causing disease among all age groups, and can be potentially dangerous for the very young, the old, people with chronic diseases, and immunocompromised persons.
- In addition to the common cold and influenza, viral pneumonia, hantavirus pulmonary syndrome, and SARS are viral infections transmitted via the respiratory system.
- Respiratory diseases caused by fungi most commonly involve the lungs. They are referred to as *deep mycoses,* and include histoplasmosis, coccidioidomycosis, blastomycosis, and aspergillosis.

Review Questions

1. All of the following are structures of the lower respiratory system *except:*
   a. Lungs
   b. Pharynx
   c. Bronchi
   d. Trachea

2. Scarlet fever is caused by:
   a. *Staphylococcus aureus*
   b. *Staphylococcus epidermidis*
   c. *Streptococcus pyogenes*
   d. *Streptococcus pneumoniae*

3. Which of the following organisms is commonly found in the normal flora of the upper respiratory system?
   a. *Staphylococcus aureus*
   b. *Mycoplasma pneumoniae*
   c. *Bordetella pertussis*
   d. *Klebsiella pneumoniae*

4. Whooping cough is caused by:
   a. *Streptococcus pneumoniae*
   b. *Bordetella pertussis*
   c. *Haemophilus influenzae*
   d. *Corynebacterium diphtheriae*

5. Which of the following cannot be and should not be treated with antibiotics?
   a. Strep throat
   b. Tuberculosis
   c. Common cold
   d. Diphtheria

6. Tuberculosis *cannot* be transmitted by:
   a. Fomites
   b. Coughing
   c. Talking
   d. Sneezing

7. The most virulent pathogen of the human flu virus is type:
   a. A
   b. B
   c. C
   d. D

8. SARS is a respiratory illness caused by:
   a. *Streptococcus*
   b. Coronavirus
   c. *Histoplasma*
   d. Type A virus

9. Which of the following geographic areas contains reservoirs for *Coccidioides immitis*?
   a. France
   b. South Africa
   c. Arizona
   d. Iowa

10. The formation of a "fungus ball" within preexisting cavities is a common development in:
    a. Blastomycosis
    b. Pulmonary aspergillosis
    c. Coccidioidomycosis
    d. Histoplasmosis

11. *Streptococcus pneumoniae* is a gram-_____ bacterium.

12. Rheumatic fever is a rare complication of _____.

13. Parrot fever is caused by _____.

14. Legionellosis affects mainly the _____.

15. Hantaviruses, which can cause disease in humans, are carried by _____.

16. Describe the different types of respiratory infections caused by streptococcal species.

17. Discuss the reemergence of tuberculosis and MDR-TB.

18. Name the two distinct forms of legionellosis.

19. Discuss organisms that enter the human body via the respiratory tract and that can be a potential bioterrorism threat.

20. Describe the most common fungal respiratory infections.

Bibliography

Forbes BA, Sahm DF, Weissfeld AS: *Bailey & Scott's diagnostic microbiology*, ed 12, St. Louis, 2007, Mosby/Elsevier.

Mahon CR, Lehman DC, Manuselis G: *Textbook of diagnostic microbiology*, ed 3, St. Louis, 2007, Saunders/Elsevier.

Mims C, Dockrell HM, Goering RV, et al: *Medical microbiology*, ed 3, St. Louis, 2004, Mosby/Elsevier.

Murray PR, Rosenthal KS, Pfaller MA: *Medical microbiology*, ed 5, St. Louis, 2005, Mosby/Elsevier.

Thibodeau GA, Patton KT: *Anatomy and physiology*, ed 6, 2007, Mosby/Elsevier.

Internet Resources

Todar's Online Textbook of Bacteriology, http://www.textbookofbacteriology.net/

CDC, Diseases and Conditions, Seasonal Flu, http://www.cdc.gov/flu/

CDC, National Center for Infectious Diseases, Infectious Disease Information, Pneumonia, http://www.cdc.gov/Ncidod/diseases/submenus/sub_pneumonia.htm

Hageman JC, Uyeki TM, Francis JS, et al: Severe community-acquired pneumonia due to *Staphylococcus aureus*, 2003–04 influenza season, *Emerg Infect Dis* [serial on the Internet]. 2006 Jun [accessed November 15, 2008]. Available from http://www.cdc.gov/ncidod/EID/vol12no06/05-1141.htm

Merck Manuals Online Medical Library, Hospital-Acquired and Institution-Acquired Pneumonia, http://www.merck.com/mmhe/sec04/ch042/ch042c.html

National Institute of Allergy and Infectious Diseases, Tuberculosis (TB), http://www.niaid.nih.gov/factsheets/tb.htm

World Health Organization, Tuberculosis and Air Travel: Guidelines for Prevention and Control, http://www.who.int/tb/publications/2008/WHO_HTM_TB_2008.399_eng.pdf

12

Infections of the Gastrointestinal System

OUTLINE

Introduction
Resident Microbial Flora
Dental Caries
Periodontal Disease
Gastroenteritis

Bacterial Infections/Illnesses
Bacterial Infections
Bacterial Intoxications

Viral Infections
Rotaviruses
Astroviruses and Caliciviruses
Noroviruses
Adenoviruses
Hepatitis

Fungal Infections
Candidiasis
Aspergillosis
Ergotism

Parasitic Infections
Protozoans
Helminths

LEARNING OBJECTIVES

After reading this chapter, the student will be able to:
- Identify the normal flora for each part of the gastrointestinal tract
- Describe the common infections that can occur in the oral cavity
- Describe gastroenteritis: its symptoms and possible causes
- Explain the difference between bacterial infections and bacterial intoxication
- Describe the causes, symptoms, transmission, prevention, and possible treatments of peptic ulcer, salmonellosis, typhoid fever, shigellosis, campylobacteriosis, and yersiniosis
- Identify and differentiate between the different types of *Escherichia coli* gastroenteritis

- Describe the causes, transmission, prevention, and possible treatments of botulism, staphylococcal intoxication, bacillus intoxication, and cholera
- Name the organisms responsible for most common outbreaks of viral gastroenteritis, and discuss prevention and treatments
- Discuss the mycoses that can affect the gastrointestinal system in both healthy and immunocompromised persons
- Describe the parasitic infections that are common in the United States, and describe those that are limited primarily to underdeveloped countries

KEY TERMS

amebiasis
ascariasis
aspergillosis
bacterial infection
bacterial intoxication
botulism
candidiasis
campylobacteriosis
caries
cryptosporidiosis

dental plaque
gastroenteritis
gastrointestinal (GI)
   tract
giardiasis
gingivitis
hepatitis
listeriosis
mucosa
necatoriasis

necrotizing ulcerative
   gingivitis
peptic ulcers
periodontitis
salmonellosis
shigellosis
taeniasis
typhoid fever

WHY YOU NEED TO KNOW

HISTORY

Throughout recorded history diseases such as cholera, dysentery, and typhoid fever have firmly established their place in the annals of human suffering. These fall into a large grouping of diseases known collectively as *gastrointestinal/ digestive system diseases* or *diseases of the upper and/or lower alimentary systems*. These diseases are caused by a wide range of organisms including bacteria, viruses, fungi, protozoans, and helminths. They can be as mild as an upset stomach or, in extreme cases, cause the victim's death.

The history of this group of diseases also includes the interesting story of Mary Mallon, a cook living in New York in the early 1900s (see Medical Highlights: Asymptomatic Disease Carriers: Typhoid Mary). Also, during the American Civil War, Willie Lincoln, the beloved son of Abraham and Mary Lincoln, died from typhoid fever, probably contracted from the water supply of the White House, which came untreated from the Potomac River.

The actual mechanisms of pathogenicity are also varied and can be as subtle as a simple case of a parasite robbing the host of nutrients or as complex as the infection pathway of the bacteria *Listeria monocytogenes*. The diversity of these organisms and their effects on the human digestive system makes them a significant concern in the area of public health.

IMPACT

Whether studying the cholera epidemics that occurred throughout the 1800s here in the United States, which claimed more than 200,000 lives, or a severe diarrhea epidemic that left more than 1500 dead in the Congo in only a 3-week period in 1997, the significant impact of gastrointestinal diseases can easily be demonstrated.

Today, with threats of terrorism in the United States and abroad, the potential of microorganisms as bioweapons is taken seriously. In addition to the widely publicized "anthrax letters" sent to the U.S. Senate starting on September 18 of 2001, in 1984 a cult in Oregon sprayed *Salmonella* on food at a restaurant salad bar in an attempt to sway a local election by sending the voting residents to hospital beds instead of voting booths. Recent recalls of food products ranging from peanut butter to spinach to beef, which contained pathogens affecting primarily the gastrointestinal system, are further examples of how these microorganisms can impact society. Contaminated products adversely affect public health and also cause serious economic problems in the form of massive recalls and legal actions generated by victims of the pathogen-tainted products.

FUTURE

As long as human beings consume water and naturally grown food, there will be an interaction between microbes and the human digestive system. Most of these will be harmless. Improvements in food processing and handling as well as advances in waste management and attention to personal and public hygiene have gone a long way toward preventing and controlling diseases of the digestive system. Advances such as food irradiation show promise in improving the quality of marketed food products. Recently, products that can improve the body's defenses against microorganisms that target the gastrointestinal system have appeared on the market. For example, a yogurt product containing a culture of bacteria that is normally present in the intestine has shown some promise in assisting the body's immune response to potential pathogens.

Introduction

The **gastrointestinal (GI) tract** is a common and easily accessible portal of entry for microbes or their toxins, with the ability to cause infection, inflammation, and/or disease. Foodborne diseases are a major concern worldwide. Contaminated food, water, and fomites, if they gain access through the fecal–oral route, all are capable of infecting the gastrointestinal system. Moreover, microbial infections and diseases of the gastrointestinal tract are the second most common cause of illnesses in the United States, with respiratory illnesses being the most common. A summary of organisms causing disease of the digestive system is provided in Table 12.1.

The GI tract, also referred to as the *digestive tract,* is a tube-like structure starting at the oral cavity (mouth); proceeding to the pharynx, esophagus, stomach, small intestine, and large intestine; and terminating at the anus (Box 12.1). Together with its accessory organs, the biological function of the digestive system (Figure 12.1) is to digest and absorb nutrients for all cells of the body, to enable them to function.

The lining of the GI tract is a mucosal lining, and like the skin it acts as the first line of defense against microbes (see Chapter 20, The Immune System). However, it does not have a dead layer of cells as the skin does and therefore it is not as efficient a defense mechanism. On the other hand, it does provide a moist and warm environment, perfect for microbial growth. As with other portals of entry, the GI tract has a

TABLE 12.1 Summary of Disease-causing Organisms in the Digestive System

Organism	Source	Symptoms	Treatment
Oral Cavity: Bacteria			
Actinomyces	Normal flora	Periodontal disease, dental caries	Brushing, flossing, fluoride; limit sugars
Fusobacterium nucleatum	Normal flora	Pulmonary infections/abscesses; trench mouth	Brushing, flossing, fluoride; limit sugars; penicillin for infections
Lactobacillus	Normal flora	Dental caries	Brushing, flossing, fluoride; limit sugars
Streptococcus mitis *S. mutans* *S. sanguis*	Normal flora	Dental caries	Brushing, flossing, fluoride; limit sugars
Treponema sp.	Contaminated food or water; poor oral/dental hygiene	Fever, bleeding and painful gums, foul odor (trench mouth)	Metronidazole, penicillin, azithromycin
Veillonella	Normal flora	Dental caries	Penicillins
Oral Cavity: Viruses			
Paramyxovirus family: Mumps virus	Salivary and respiratory secretions	Swelling of parotid glands, fever, loss of appetite, headache, damage to reproductive organs in patients past puberty	Mumps vaccine for prevention; no antiviral therapy available
Herpes simplex virus	Direct contact, fomites, contaminated food or water	Blisters/lesions of mouth or throat, fever	Acyclovir
Oral Cavity: Fungi			
Candida albicans	Normal flora of lower GI tract	Nausea, vomiting, pustules on tongue or in throat, skin rash, heart valve damage	Amphotericin B and fluconazole
Gastrointestinal Tract: Bacteria			
Bacillus cereus	Contaminated food	Nausea, diarrhea, vomiting	No recommended antibiotic treatment; fluid replacement
Bacteroides	Normal flora	Diarrhea, fever	Clindamycin
Campylobacter jejuni	Contaminated food	Fever, abdominal pain	No recommended antibiotic treatment, erythromycin used in severe cases; fluid replacement

Continued

TABLE 12.1 Summary of Disease-causing Organisms in the Digestive System—cont'd

Organism	Source	Symptoms	Treatment
Campylobacter fetus	Contaminated food	Bloody diarrhea	No recommended antibiotic treatment; erythromycin used in severe cases; fluid replacement
Clostridium perfringens	Contaminated food	Abdominal pain, diarrhea	Electrolyte/fluid replacement
Clostridium botulinum	Contaminated food	Loss of muscle control, slurring of speech, difficulty in swallowing and/or breathing, eventual muscle paralysis	Botulism antitoxin, artificial respirator
Clostridium difficile	Contaminated food	Colitis, nausea, vomiting	Clindamycin
Escherichia coli	Contaminated food	Nausea, diarrhea; certain strains will cause intestinal bleeding	Fluid replacement; gentamicin, polymyxin; fluoroquinolone and bismuth preparations help prevent *E. coli* gastroenteritis
Helicobacter pylori	Contaminated food or water	Abdominal pain, vomiting, belching, bleeding if ulcers form	Combination of two antibiotics (metronidazole, tetracycline, amoxicillin, or clarithromycin) plus medication to reduce or suppress stomach acid
Salmonella enteritidis	Contaminated food	Fever, nausea, cramps, diarrhea	No recommended antibiotic treatment unless it invades other tissue or blood; fluid replacement
Salmonella typhi	Contaminated food	Fever, continual headache, nausea, cramps, diarrhea	Vaccine available
Shigella dysenteriae *S. flexneri* *S. sonnei*	Contaminated food	Nausea, cramps, intestinal bleeding (*S. dysenteriae* only), diarrhea	Ampicillin, co-trimoxazole; fluid replacement
Staphylococcus aureus	Contaminated food, direct contact	Nausea, cramps, diarrhea	
Vibrio cholerae	Contaminated food or water	Vomiting, muscle cramps, severe watery diarrhea	Preventive vaccine; rapid fluid and electrolyte replacement
Gastrointestinal Tract: Viruses			
Rotaviruses	Contaminated food or water	Vomiting, slight fever, watery diarrhea	No antiviral treatment; fluid replacement
Hepatitis A, E	Contaminated food or water	Nausea, abdominal pain, dark urine, jaundice	Vaccine for type A
Norwalk virus	Contaminated food or water	Nausea, vomiting	No vaccine, no antiviral treatment
Gastrointestinal Tract: Fungi			
Aspergillus flavus	Contaminated food, usually peanuts	Liver damage (cirrhosis)	Amphotericin B, voriconazole
Claviceps purpurea	Contaminated food, usually cereal grains or mushrooms	Reduced blood flow to extremities, causing gangrene; hallucinations, muscle spasms, and seizures	Nifedipine for spasms, seizures—drug detoxification protocol

TABLE 12.1 Summary of Disease-causing Organisms in the Digestive System—cont'd

Organism	Source	Symptoms	Treatment
Gastrointestinal Tract: Protozoa			
Balantidium coli	Contaminated food or water	Nausea, weakness, weight loss, abdominal pain, diarrhea, vomiting	Tetracycline, iodoquinol, metronidazole
Cryptosporidium parvum	Contaminated food or water, oral–fecal contamination	Nausea, weakness, weight loss, abdominal pain, persistent diarrhea, vomiting	Spiramycin, nitazoxanide for children from 1 to 11 yr old
Entamoeba histolytica	Contaminated food or water	Nausea, weakness, weight loss, abdominal pain, diarrhea, vomiting, bloody stool	Metronidazole plus iodoquinol, paromomycin
Giardia lamblia	Contaminated water	Malaise, nausea, weakness, weight loss, cramps, diarrhea	Metronidazole, furazolidone, tinidazole, quinacrine
Gastrointestinal Tract: Helminths			
Taenia saginata (tapeworm)	Ingestion of contaminated meat	Vague abdominal discomfort, few symptoms if any, anemia	Niclosamide (praziquantel, paromomycin, or quinacrine)
Echinococcus granulosus	Ingestion of eggs of organism found in soil, dust, food, water, clothing, etc.	Formation of hydatid cysts	Surgical removal of cysts; mebendazole, albendazole
Enterobius vermicularis (pinworm)	Ingestion of eggs of organism found in soil, dust, food, water, clothing, air, etc.	Itching of anal region, restlessness, irritability, poor sleep, nervousness	Pyrantel pamoate, mebendazole
Necator americanus (hookworm)	Contact with contaminated soil	Usually no symptoms, sometimes a cough, shortness of breath, diarrhea, nausea, vomiting; anemia can result in mental retardation in children	Mebendazole, pyrantel pamoate
Ascaris lumbricoides	Ingestion of eggs of organism found in soil, dust, food, water, clothing, etc.	Usually no symptoms, occasional bouts with fever, trouble breathing, coughing, and wheezing	Mebendazole, piperazine
Trichinella spiralis	Ingestion of contaminated meat	Abdominal pain, diarrhea, fever, muscle pain, swelling around the eyes, rash	Mebendazole, steroids with thiabendazole
Trichuris trichiura (whipworm)	Fecal–oral route	Small numbers—asymptomatic; large numbers—abdominal pain, weakness, bloody diarrhea, weight loss	Mebendazole

normal flora that also helps to protect against pathogens via competition.

Resident Microbial Flora

The GI tract resident (normal) microbial flora is a complex and diverse ecosystem containing a large collection of micro-organisms that flourish in the nutrient-rich environment provided by the digestive system. The type and amount of flora vary within the different areas of the GI tract, with increasing numbers as one moves from the upper GI tract areas to the large intestine. The normal flora of the intestine may prevent infection by competing or interfering with pathogens or potentially pathogenic organisms. Treatment with antibiotics that

Oral cavity

Oropharynx

Esophagus

Stomach
- Fundus
- Body
- Pylorus

Small Intestine
- Duodenum
- Jejunum
- Ileum

Large Intestine
- Cecum
- Colon
  - Ascending colon
  - Transverse colon
  - Descending colon
  - Sigmoid colon
- Rectum
- Anal Canal

upset the balance of the normal flora may favor infections by exogenous pathogens and also the overgrowth of endogenous pathogens.

Oral Cavity

The normal microbial flora of the oral cavity is complex, with bacteria representing the largest population. More than 700 bacterial species have been detected in the adult oral cavity, but more than 50% of these have not been cultured in the laboratory at this time. At birth the oral cavity is sterile but rapidly becomes colonized by organisms from the environment, especially from the mother during the first breastfeedings. At this time *Streptococcus salivarius* is dominant, but the complexity of the flora continues to increase with time. Oral bacteria include streptococci, lactobacilli, staphylococci, corynebacteria, aerobes, *Bacteroides*, various types of spirochetes, and anaerobes.

Stomach

The stomach contains few bacteria because of its high acidity, which makes it a relatively hostile environment for bacteria. Bacteria swallowed with food and those dislodged from the mouth will be drastically lowered in number because of this acidity. However, some bacteria do survive this extreme environment and are moved on into the small intestine. It is all about numbers: the more bacteria are ingested with food, the more will survive and be transported into the next part of the GI tract.

One organism that has been discovered to live in the human stomach is *Helicobacter pylori*, a gram-negative, microaerophilic, spiral-shaped bacterium (Figure 12.2). The organism is highly motile due to its flagella and moves through the stomach lumen until it burrows into the stomach's **mucosa** to a depth where the pH is essentially neutral. It is estimated that about 30% to 50% of the earth's population is colonized by *H. pylori*. Although colonization of the bacterium in the stomach is not necessarily a problem, *H. pylori* is the cause of most cases of gastritis and peptic ulcers (see Bacterial Infections later in this chapter).

Small Intestine

The small intestine provides a friendlier environment for microbial survival than does the stomach. However, because of rapid peristalsis and emptying of pancreatic juice and bile into the first portion of the duodenum, it is difficult for bacteria to colonize the small intestine because they get washed out. As a result the bacterial population, especially in the first portions of the small intestine, remains relatively low. Gram-positive bacteria, mainly lactobacilli and *Enterococcus faecalis,* are inhabitants of this part of the GI tract. The bacterial population increases at the end of the small intestine, and enteric rods and *Bacteroides* can also colonize this part of the GI tract. Intestinal bacteria are capable of metabolizing some compounds that the human digestive tract cannot, which leads to more efficient utilization of food.

Large Intestine

The flow rate in the large intestine is much slower than in the small intestine and bacteria have time to colonize and reproduce, reaching a high concentration. About 1000 species are present including enteric rods, streptococci, clostridia, and lactobacilli. The predominant species are anaerobic *Bacteroides* and bifidobacteria, which greatly outnumber *Escherichia coli.* The colon serves as a holding tank for bacteria that participate in the last stages of food digestion. Intestinal bacteria can metabolize polysaccharides that cannot be broken down by human enzymes (e.g., cellulose) and they also synthesize vitamins K and B, which then can be absorbed by the GI tract. Approximately 20% of the feces of a healthy person consists of bacteria, most of which come from the colon.

Dental Caries

The oral cavity provides a good environment for a variety of microorganisms to flourish. Teeth, the tongue, and the salivary glands are accessory organs of digestion in this area. Microbial life on teeth was first observed by van Leeuwenhoek (see Chapter 1, Scope of Microbiology), who noticed that even after washing his teeth with vinegar, only microbes on the outer layer were killed, not those in the deeper layers.

The enameled surface of the teeth (Figure 12.3) is hard and does not shed cells, which allows microorganism to attach and form a biofilm known as **dental plaque.** If not removed on a regular basis it can lead to cavities (**caries**) or other periodontal problems such as **gingivitis** (inflammation of the gums). The microorganisms responsible for the formation of dental plaque (Figure 12.4) are almost entirely bacteria, normally present in the oral cavity. Under usual circumstances, these bacteria (e.g., fusobacteria and actinomycetes) do not cause damage; however,

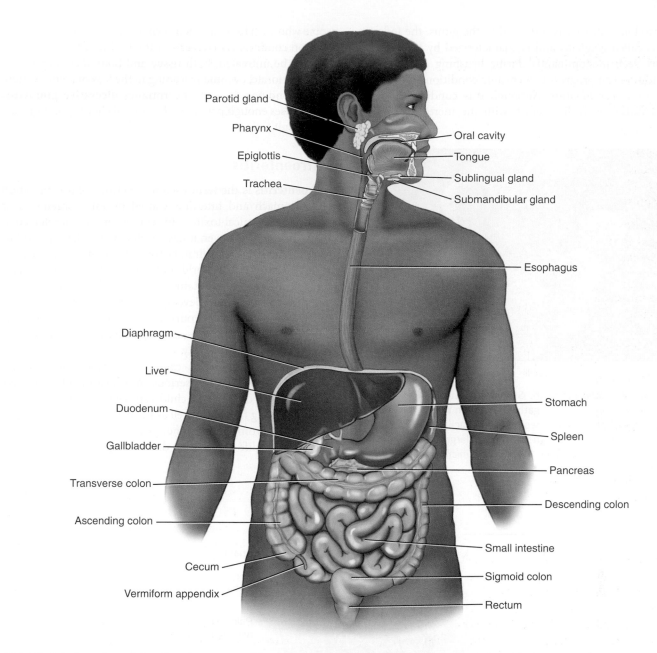

FIGURE 12.1 Overview of the digestive system. The digestive system consists of the gastrointestinal (GI) tract and its accessory organs. The GI tract includes the mouth, pharynx, esophagus, stomach, small intestine, large intestine, anal canal, and anus. The accessory organs are the teeth, tongue, salivary glands, liver, gallbladder, and pancreas.

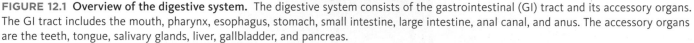

failure to remove these biofilms by regular brushing of the teeth will cause the organisms closest to the tooth surface to change to anaerobic respiration. Anaerobic respiration of bacteria converts sucrose and other carbohydrates into lactic acid, which consequently leads to the demineralization of the adjacent tooth surface, resulting in dental caries.

Periodontal Disease

Periodontal diseases include gingivitis and **periodontitis,** serious infections that if not treated can lead to decay, subsequent tooth loss, and systemic infection. Although the main cause of periodontal disease is dental plaque and an overpopulation of established oral bacteria, other factors also affect the health of the oral cavity. These factors include the following:

- Smoking/tobacco use has been shown to be one of the most significant risk factors in the development and progression of periodontal disease.
- Genetic predisposition to periodontal disease has been suggested by several studies and reported by the American Academy of Periodontology.
- Pregnancy, puberty, stress, medications, diabetes, grinding one's teeth, poor nutrition, and other systemic diseases also have been implicated in the development of periodontal diseases.

If periodontal disease is restricted to the gums, the inflammation is called *gingivitis* and is characterized by bleeding of the gums, seen predominantly during brushing of the teeth. This condition can progress to a chronic condition and is then referred to as *periodontitis*. Although this condition usually does not cause much discomfort, with the increase in older people who wish to retain their own teeth, it has become a more common condition of concern. If the health of the gums continues to be untreated, both tissue and bone that support the teeth deteriorate, eventually leading to the loss of teeth. A more serious condition is acute **necrotizing ulcerative gingivitis,** which causes enough pain to make normal chewing an unpleasant, difficult task.

Gastroenteritis

Gastroenteritis is the term used to describe the inflammation of the stomach and intestine, caused by microorganisms or ingestion of chemical toxins. This condition is often referred to as *"stomach flu"*; however, it has absolutely no relation to influenza (flu), which is a respiratory tract infection. Gastroenteritis transpires all over the world and affects people of every age, race, and socioeconomic status, and is a leading cause of death among children of underdeveloped countries. Intestinal infections have a tendency to flourish wherever people congregate, such as schools, dormitories, and other living or working areas with high population density.

Although gastroenteritis causes discomfort and inconvenience, it is generally not serious in a healthy adult. At-risk groups include children in child care centers and the elderly living in nursing homes, as well as people with chronic diseases and/or a compromised immune system. In theses cases gastroenteritis can be life-threatening due to dehydration and electrolyte imbalance.

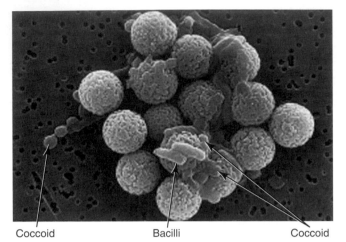

Coccoid   Bacilli   Coccoid

FIGURE 12.2 *Helicobacter pylori.* Scanning electron micrograph of *Helicobacter pylori,* a gram-negative bacterium that is the most common cause of gastritis and peptic ulcers. Bacillus and coccoid forms of the organism are shown attached to large beads. (From Murray PR, Rosenthal KS, Pfaller MA: *Medical microbiology,* ed 5, St. Louis, 2005, Mosby.)

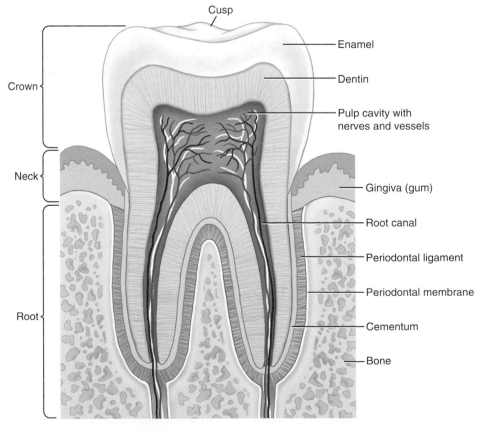

FIGURE 12.3 Cross-section through a typical molar tooth.

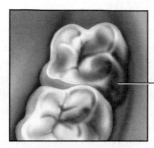

Plaque/biofilm

FIGURE 12.4 Dental plaque. Biofilm (dental plaque) covering the tooth provides an attachment environment for oral bacteria. When bacteria metabolize carbohydrates they often produce acid, which results in decay of the tooth.

LIFE APPLICATION

The Folly of Fashion

The human oral cavity contains a wide variety of microorganisms, a number of which are pathogens or opportunistic pathogens. The bacterial genera *Actinomyces, Bacteroides, Fusobacterium, Streptococcus, Lactobacillus, Veillonella,* and *Prevotella,* and the fungus *Candida albicans,* are typically present in the oral cavity and each has the potential to cause local or even systemic infections. Fortunately, the oral mucosa along with saliva and its antimicrobial properties provide an effective barrier. Any time the protective barrier is damaged by a cut or other injury, the organisms are able to penetrate into deeper tissue and potentially enter the circulatory system. The risk of infection from dental surgery is high and dentists often precede the surgery with an antibiotic regimen to prepare the body for the onslaught of bacteria that will gain access to the bloodstream through the gums.

One particular fashion, oral piercing, has been linked to an increase in infections in and originating from the oral cavity. Statistics from major universities such as Ohio State and organizations such as the Academy of General Dentistry show a direct link between oral piercing and an increase in damage to the oral cavity along with subsequent infections. One dental group noted that their research indicated that one in every five oral piercings resulted in infection. Conditions such as prolonged bleeding, swelling of tissue, damage to the teeth and gums, cheek infections, nerve damage, bacteremia, and in some extreme cases endocarditis have been traced back to oral piercing.

The main symptom of gastroenteritis is mild to severe diarrhea, but it also may include loss of appetite, nausea, vomiting, cramps, and other abdominal discomfort. On occasion muscle aches, headache, and a low-grade fever may also occur. Causes of gastroenteritis include, but are not limited to:

- Contaminated food (with organisms or its toxins)
- Contaminated water
- Contact with an infected person
- Unwashed hands
- Dirty food utensils
- Contaminated work spaces

The infectious form of gastroenteritis can be transmitted from person to person, especially if someone with diarrhea does not thoroughly wash their hands after a bowel movement. Transmission also can occur through sharing of eating utensils, towels, or through contaminated food or water. Gastroenteritis can also be obtained through the ingestion of bacterial toxins, which results in toxemia and does not involve an active infection.

Bacterial Infections/ Illnesses

Bacteria are the most common cause of foodborne illness, which can be caused by the bacteria themselves, their toxins, or both. A **bacterial infection** occurs when a pathogen enters the

MEDICAL HIGHLIGHTS

A New Weapon in Food Safety: Food Irradiation

Many cases of gastrointestinal problems have been found to originate from contaminated food products. One can readily find recent news headlines with numerous reported cases of food-related gastroenteritis outbreaks. From *Salmonella enteritidis* in peanut butter to *E. coli* in ground beef, bacterial contamination in food has become a problem both as a health and as an economic issue. Improvements in sanitation and development of rigorous inspection requirements such as the Hazard Analysis and Critical Control Points program have contributed significantly toward reducing contamination of food products during processing and packaging.

In addition to these measures, the process of food irradiation is gaining acceptance with the public and corporate world alike and has the potential to make a significant impact in decreasing bacterial contamination of food. Irradiation uses high-energy electrons, gamma rays, or x-rays to destroy the chemical bonds of DNA, thus killing the microorganism. The level of radiation used is low and does not leave a radioactive residue, yet is effective enough to either pasteurize or sterilize the food product without negatively affecting its nutritional value or producing undesirable chemical by-products.

The process of food irradiation was first developed for commercial purposes in the 1960s, with much of the research being generated by NASA and the space program.

In 1984, the U.S. Secretary of Health and Human Services endorsed the use of irradiation for food. The number of irradiated food products on the market is increasing rapidly with only a small increase in cost.

GI tract, adheres, and multiplies (see Chapter 9, Infection and Disease). A **bacterial intoxication** occurs when toxins produced by bacteria contaminate food or water and then are introduced to the human body.

Bacterial Infections

The term infection implies the invasion and colonization of cells or tissues by a microorganism. Therefore, discussions of the following conditions involve illnesses due to infection of the gastrointestinal system with specific bacteria.

Helicobacter Peptic Ulcer

Peptic ulcers are a common illness in the United States, and 1 in 10 Americans will experience an ulcer at some time during their lifetime. Ulcers are a form of damage to the gastrointestinal mucosa caused by long-term use of antiinflammatory agents; conditions such as cancer of the esophagus, stomach, pancreas; or by a bacterium, *Helicobacter pylori*. This bacterium is helical, microaerophilic, motile, and gram negative. Many scientists believe that the majority of peptic ulcers are caused by this organism. Although most infected people do not develop an ulcer, others do. The transmission of *H. pylori* is not fully understood, but food and water, as well as kissing, are likely to be responsible. Unlike other organisms, *H. pylori* can survive in the acidic environment of the stomach because it produces an enzyme that can neutralize acids, and allows the bacterium to attach to the intestinal mucosa, damage it, and cause an ulcer by allowing the stomach acids access to the underlying tissue. The symptoms of a peptic ulcer include weight loss, poor appetite, bloating, burping, nausea, and vomiting. Ulcers caused by *H. pylori* can be treated with antibiotics, H_2 blockers, proton pump inhibitors, and stomach-lining protector drugs.

Salmonellosis

Salmonellosis is a gastroenteritis caused by *Salmonella* species, which belong to the family Enterobacteriaceae. They are rod-shaped, gram-negative, facultative anaerobic, nonsporing microorganisms, and their normal habitat is the intestinal tracts of many animals, including humans. *Salmonella* species cause typhoid fever, paratyphoid fever, and foodborne illnesses in humans. Because of the complicated taxonomy of *Salmonella*, the disease-causing species have been reclassified into a single species, *Salmonella enterica*, which has numerous serovars (serotypes). Therefore, instead of the conventional name of *Salmonella typhi* the serotype is now often referred to as *Salmonella enterica* serotype Typhi. From the pathological standpoint *Salmonella* can be divided into serotypes that are typhoidal and nontyphoidal.

Most people infected with *Salmonella* develop diarrhea, fever, and abdominal cramps 12 to 72 hours after infection. The incubation time and severity of resulting illness are proportional to the number of organisms ingested. The illness usually subsides within 5 to 7 days and most people do not require treatment. However, if dehydration occurs because of severe diarrhea, the patient may need to be hospitalized, and if the infection spreads to the bloodstream prompt antibiotic treat-

ment is necessary to prevent septicemia and death. Infants, the elderly, people with chronic disease, and immunocompromised patients are more likely to develop a severe illness. Although the infection is usually treatable, the World Health Organization (WHO, Geneva, Switzerland) has pointed out an increase in the incidence of antibiotic-resistant strains of *Salmonella*, potentially caused by the long-term use of antibiotics in both the poultry and beef industries.

Salmonellosis is usually caused by consumption of foods of animal origin that have been contaminated with *Salmonella*, such as raw or undercooked eggs, poultry, untreated milk products, and meat or other items contaminated with feces. People with salmonellosis should avoid food preparation until they no longer carry the bacterium. Preventive measures include, but are not limited to:

- Avoiding raw or undercooked eggs, poultry, or meat
- Careful monitoring of homemade foods that include raw eggs (e.g., hollandaise sauce, salad dressings, ice cream, mayonnaise, cookie dough, and frostings)
- No consumption of nonpasteurized dairy products
- Avoidance of any chance of cross-contamination between raw and cooked foods
- Separation of uncooked meats from produce, cooked foods, and ready-to-eat foods
- Appropriate washing of hands, cutting boards, countertops, knives, and other utensils after handling uncooked foods
- Washing of hands before and after handling food
- Hand washing after handling reptiles or birds, or after contact with pet feces

According to the Centers for Disease Control and Prevention (CDC, Atlanta, GA), approximately 40,000 cases of salmonellosis are reported annually in the United States alone. But because the milder cases are usually not reported or diagnosed, the actual number of infections may be 30 or more times greater than 40,000. Seasonally, salmonellosis is more common in the summer months than in winter. Also, children are at greater risk of contracting the illness.

Typhoid Fever

Typhoid fever is an acute, life-threatening illness caused by the most virulent serotype of *Salmonella enterica*, serotype Typhi, a rod-shaped, flagellated, gram-negative bacterium. Typhoid fever is transmitted through contaminated food or water, or through close contact with an infected person; it is not found in animals, and is transmitted only via human feces. *Salmonella enterica* serotype Typhi lives only in humans and persons with typhoid fever carry the bacteria in their bloodstream and intestinal tract. Some people exposed to and infected by the organism do not develop the disease, or might have a minor illness and subsequently recover and thus only be carriers of the disease (see Medical Highlights: Asymptomatic Disease Carriers: Typhoid Mary). Typhoid fever is more common in areas of the world where hand washing is not common, and where water is contaminated with human waste.

Symptoms of typhoid fever include a sudden onset of sustained fever as high as 39° C to 40° C (103° F to 104° F), severe

Salmonella: More than 2000 "Flavors"

The genus *Salmonella* includes a number of pathogenic organisms that have become a serious problem for the food industry. In 2004, almost 40,000 cases of nontyphoid *Salmonella* infections were reported in the United States alone, along with an estimated 600 deaths. Some health experts estimate that the number exceeds 2 million cases of salmonellosis, as many cases go unreported. The most common sources for these types of infections are poultry products, eggs, dairy products, and other food types that are prepared on work surfaces where uncooked poultry has also been prepared. Although there are four different forms of *Salmonella* infections, the most common form of salmonellosis is gastroenteritis.

According to most taxonomic classification schemes there are only two or three species of *Salmonella;* however, there are a large number of serotypes within each subspecies. Moreover, within the species containing most of the human pathogens, there are presently more than 2000 unique serotypes! When not causing gastroenteritis, the pathogenic serovars also can cause bacteremia, particularly in the very young, the very old, or in otherwise immunocompromised individuals.

headache, nausea, abdominal pain, either constipation or diarrhea, and occasionally is accompanied by hoarse cough. Antimicrobial therapy shortens the clinical course of typhoid fever and also reduces the risk of death, but antibiotic resistance is a frequent problem as with so many other microbes.

Although typhoid fever is rare in industrialized countries, it remains a serious health threat in the underdeveloped world. According to the CDC, worldwide an estimated 22 million cases of typhoid fever and 200,000 deaths occur each year. Reported cases in the United States are mostly from recent international travelers. At greatest risk are travelers to South Asia and developing countries in Asia, Africa, the Caribbean, and Central and South America. Visitors to South Asia are at the highest risk for infections that are multidrug resistant. Although typhoid vaccination is available it is not required for international travel, but recommended by the CDC for travelers to areas where there is a recognized risk of exposure to the organism.

Paratyphoid fever, also known as *enteric fever*, is similar to typhoid fever, but generally milder. It is caused by *Salmonella enterica* serovars Paratyphi. Three species of *Salmonella* are responsible for this illness: serovars A, B, and C, all of which are transmitted by means of contaminated water or food. Although the agent of typhoid fever is carried only by humans, paratyphoid fever can be transmitted from animals or animal products to humans, or from person to person. Enteric fever is rare in the United States and of the reported cases approximately 60% are acquired during travel to Mexico, India, or South America.

Asymptomatic Disease Carriers: Typhoid Mary

Mary Mallon (September 23, 1869—November 11, 1938), a hard-working Irish immigrant, was born in County Tyrone, Ireland in poverty and worked her way up the ladder in the United States to a top-salaried position as chief household cook in the New York City area between the years 1900 and 1907. Because of prevalent prejudicial attitudes against the Irish at that time, working class immigrants in other household labor positions were paid barely a living wage. Although she was successful in her job, she was an unwitting asymptomatic carrier of typhoid fever, infecting 22 people, 1 of whom died during this period of time. During her lifetime as a cook and a healthy carrier of typhoid fever, it is estimated that she infected 53 people, 3 of whom died. She simply could not accept that she—a healthy, hard-working Irish girl who had no known history of illness could possibly be an asymptomatic carrier of a disease and refused to be tested when confronted by health authorities. Her stubborn, steadfast denials led to forced quarantines. Even her attempt to change her name to Mary Brown, so that she could continue to work in the higher salaried position of domestic cook, was unsuccessful. Eventually she was seized by the public health authorities and quarantined for life on North Brother Island outside New York City. Mallon died at the age of 69 years from pneumonia some 6 years after a paralytic stroke. Typhoid bacteria were identified in her gallbladder at autopsy.

Today, any asymptomatic carrier is referred to as a *"Typhoid Mary"*; a more recent example is the American Andrew Speaker, suspected as being a carrier of the drug-resistant XDR-TB tuberculosis strain. Mr Speaker flew on a commercial aircraft to Europe and back and was placed in quarantine upon his return. This was later found to be a less dangerous, less drug-resistant MDR-TB strain.

Shigellosis

Shigellosis, also called *bacillary dysentery*, is an infectious disease caused by four species of *Shigella: boydii, dysenteriae, flexneri,* and *sonnei.* These bacteria are gram-negative, non–spore-forming, rod-shaped bacteria present only in the gastrointestinal tracts of humans, apes, and monkeys.

The infective dose is small, as the organism is somewhat resistant to the pH of the stomach. Once in the pH environment of the small intestine the organisms proliferate rapidly and continue down the GI tract to adhere to epithelial cells of the large intestine, the primary site of action for the illness. *Shigella* then multiplies in the cells, spreads to neighboring cells, and produces Shiga toxin that destroys tissues, resulting in dysentery.

The infection causes diarrhea that is often bloody, fever, and stomach cramps starting within a day or two of exposure. Five to 7 days after onset, the infection usually subsides. As with other infectious diseases, the very young, the very old, and immunocompromised people are at highest risk. With children less than 2 years of age, the infection may also be associated with febrile seizures (seizures due to high fever). Many different organisms cause diarrhea and bloody diarrhea; therefore it is essential to perform laboratory tests for a definite diagnosis, before selecting the appropriate antibiotic for treatment.

The CDC monitors the frequency of occurrence of *Shigella* infections in the country, and assists local and state health departments investigating outbreaks, to determine means of transmission and to implement control measures. An estimated 18,000 cases of shigellosis occur annually in the United States and are responsible for less than 10% of reported outbreaks of foodborne illness. Many of the mild cases of shigellosis remain undiagnosed and are not reported. The actual number of infections is likely to be much greater. The most common species reported in the United States is *S. sonnei,* which causes relatively mild dysentery. In underdeveloped countries this infection is far more common and is present in the communities most of the time.

Shigella is passed from one infected person to the next, by stool or soiled fingers of one person to the mouth of another. This type of transmission occurs when basic hygiene and hand-washing habits are inadequate, and is particularly common among toddlers who are not fully toilet-trained. *Shigella* can also be transmitted through food as a result of unsanitary handling by people preparing food.

If many cases of *Shigella* occur at the same time it may be due to problems in a restaurant or in the food or water supply in that given area. Any type of community-wide outbreak needs to be addressed by the city, county, and state public health departments, to ensure the safety of the water and food supplies.

Campylobacteriosis

Campylobacteriosis in humans is usually caused by *Campylobacter jejuni, C. fetus,* and *C. coli.* These bacteria are vibrioid or helical, gram-negative, motile microaerophiles. According to the CDC, *C. jejuni* is the leading cause of bacterial diarrhea in the United States, affecting primarily children below the age of 5 years and also young adults between the ages of 15 to 29 years. Worldwide the bacterium is blamed for causing between 5% and 14% of all diarrheal illness. The illness usually lasts for 2 to 5 days but has been reported to last as long as 10 days.

Transmission can occur by handling raw poultry, eating undercooked poultry, drinking nonchlorinated water or raw milk, or handling human or animal feces without following with appropriate hand-washing procedures. In addition to poultry and cattle waste as sources of the bacteria, feces from puppies, kittens, and birds can also contain this microorganism.

As with so many gastrointestinal illnesses caused by microorganisms, the infection is self-limiting and does not require special treatment. However, in the more serious cases antibiotic treatment can be provided. Only a few people will develop complications to the infection.

Escherichia spp. Gastroenteritis

Escherichia coli is a member of the normal intestinal flora and is normally harmless or useful by suppressing the growth of pathogenic organisms. *E. coli* also synthesizes vitamins that are absorbed by the human large intestine. However, *E. coli* does have pathogenic strains. These strains have specialized fimbriae that enable the organism to adhere to the intestinal epithelial cells and disrupt the microvilli. Once the strain colonizes the small intestine, it produces enterotoxins responsible for the illness. Intestinal disease caused by *E. coli* include enterotoxigenic *E. coli* (ETEC), enteroinvasive *E. coli* (EIEC), enteropathogenic *E. coli* (EPEC), enteroaggregative *E. coli* (EAggEC), and enterohemorrhagic *E. coli* (EHEC).

- Enterotoxigenic *E. coli* (ETEC) is the cause of diarrhea in infants and travelers in underdeveloped countries or areas where sanitation is poor. It is generally acquired by ingestion of contaminated food and water and the organism colonizes the small intestine. The illness can vary from minor discomfort to severe, cholera-like symptoms. The enterotoxins produced are heat-labile (LT) and/or heat-stable (ST) toxins.
- Enteroinvasive *E. coli* (EIEC) penetrates and multiplies in the epithelial cells of the colon, resulting in destruction of these cells. The clinical symptoms are similar to those of *Shigella* dysentery (dysentery-like diarrhea) with fever. EIEC is an invasive organism but does not produce LT or ST toxins.
- Enteropathogenic *E. coli* (EPEC) is similar to EIEC and also does not produce LT or ST toxins, although it has been reported that the organism produces an enterotoxin similar to that of *Shigella*.
- Enteroaggregative *E. coli* (EAggEC) is accompanied by persistent diarrhea in young children. In addition to its toxin (enteroaggregative ST-like toxin) it also produces a hemolysin related to one made by strains of *E. coli* that commonly cause urinary tract infections.
- Enterohemorrhagic *E. coli* (EHEC) is currently represented by a single strain, the serotype O157:H7. This serotype produces large quantities of one or more related potent toxins, capable of producing severe damage to the intestinal lining. These toxins are closely related to the toxin produced by *Shigella dysenteriae* and cause diarrhea with abundant bloody discharge. It is frequently life-threatening because of its toxic effects on the kidneys (hemolytic uremia).

Yersiniosis

Yersinia enterocolitica, the causative agent of yersiniosis, can cause a variety of symptoms depending on the age of the infected patient; those infected are most commonly the young. This organism is a gram-negative, facultatively anaerobic rod. Symptoms, typically starting 4 to 5 days after exposure, include fever, abdominal pain, and diarrhea that can last 3 weeks or longer. Although relatively infrequent, symptoms of the infection in adults and older children are sometimes confused with appendicitis, because of the right-sided abdominal pain and fever. Most infections resolve on their own, and only severe cases require antibiotic treatment. The infection is most often acquired by consuming contaminated food, unpasteurized milk, or untreated water. The preparation of raw pork intestines is particularly risky.

Listeriosis

Listeriosis is an illness caused by the microorganism *Listeria monocytogenes*. This gram-positive, nonsporing rod is a facultatively anaerobic intracellular pathogen that is acquired by ingesting contaminated food. The organism can spread to the bloodstream and the central nervous system (see Chapter 13, Infections of the Nervous System and Senses). It has the capacity to infect a variety of cells, and because it can spread to the circulatory system it is capable of causing infections in a number of different body systems.

The primary source of *Listeria* is believed to be soil and decaying plant matter; the bacterium also can be carried by many animals and may be present in animal feed as well. An estimated 2500 cases are reported annually in the United States, but much larger outbreaks are associated with contaminated food products.

In the 1980s, the U.S. government began to take measures to decrease the occurrence of listeriosis. And in 1999 an outbreak in the United States resulted in a recall of 30 million pounds of meat. At present, processed meats and dairy products are tested for the presence of *Listeria monocytogenes*. The U.S. Food and Drug Administration (FDA) and the U.S. Department of Agriculture Food Safety and Inspection Service (FSIS) monitor food regularly, and if *Listeria* is detected in processed meat and dairy products, the food shipments are halted and food recalls are ordered.

Most infections, whether an individual occurrence and/or a larger outbreak, are associated with the consumption of contaminated or unpasteurized milk; soft cheese; undercooked meat; processed meat such as deli meat, hot dogs, and canned meat; fish; poultry; unwashed vegetables; and cabbage. High-risk populations for this illness are neonates, the elderly, persons with a compromised immune system, and pregnant women because the organism is small enough to cross the placenta. The mortality rate of *Listeria* infections is about 20% to 30%, which is the highest among the foodborne diseases.

After consuming *Listeria*-contaminated food, symptoms of the infection appear anywhere from 11 to 70 days later. Symptoms include fever, muscle aches, and sometimes gastrointestinal symptoms such as nausea or diarrhea. If the infection reaches the nervous system headache, stiff neck, confusion, loss of balance, or convulsions may occur (see Chapter 13, Infections of the Nervous System and Senses). Listeriosis is treated with antibiotics; the duration of treatment depends on the host and the symptoms of the illness.

Bacterial Intoxications

Bacterial food intoxication is an illness caused by the consumption of bacterial toxins. Organisms that are capable of causing this type of toxemia include *Clostridium botulinum*, *Staphylococcus aureus*, *Vibrio cholerae*, *Bacillus cereus*, and possibly other toxin-producing *Bacillus* species.

Botulism

Botulism (see also Chapter 21, Pharmacology) is a rare disease in the United States and healthcare providers report an average of 110 cases per year. Although rare, this mostly foodborne illness can be fatal if not treated quickly. Four forms of botulism have been identified: (1) classic or foodborne botulism, (2) infant botulism, (3) wound botulism, and (4) inhalation botulism. The illness is caused by the toxin produced by *Clostridium botulinum*, an anaerobic organism that flourishes in sealed containers, and is commonly isolated from soil and water samples throughout the world. The organism produces a neurotoxin most commonly acquired by a patient through consumption of contaminated food. Foodborne botulism often can be blamed on home-canned food with low acid content, such as asparagus, green beans, beets, and corn. However, baked potatoes wrapped in aluminum foil but not kept hot have also been blamed for outbreaks. Exposure to the toxin in an aerosolized form can quickly be fatal and is a concern in the defense against its use as a bioweapon (see Bioterrorism in Chapter 24, Microorganisms in the Environment and Environmental Safety).

Symptoms of foodborne botulism generally occur within 18 to 36 hours after ingesting contaminated food, but they can occur as early as 6 hours or as long as 10 days after consumption. The patients become weak and dizzy, and early symptoms also can include blurred vision, dry mouth, constipation, and abdominal pain. With progression of the disease, weakness of the peripheral muscles develops. Death is due primarily to respiratory paralysis.

Staphylococcal Intoxication

Any food prepared and not appropriately chilled or refrigerated after preparation is a potential source of food poisoning. *Staphylococcus aureus* is one of the leading causes of gastroenteritis as a result of contaminated food ingestion, with the illness being caused by the absorption of staphylococcal enterotoxins present in the food. *Staphylococcus aureus* does not form endospores, as do *C. perfringens*, *C. botulinum*, and *B. cereus*. *Staphylococcus* is somewhat heat resistant and even the vegetative organism can tolerate 60° C for up to half an hour. The organism also has high resistance to osmotic changes, allowing it to grow in environments in which other bacteria cannot survive, such as high salt concentrations. *S. aureus* is often present in the normal flora of the nasal cavity; it can also survive on the skin, can be transmitted by hands into food, and, because of its resistance to environmental changes, thrives to produce disease-causing toxins (Figure 12.5). Normally, the infective dose (see Chapter 21, Pharmacology) is reached when the population of *S. aureus* exceeds 100,000 bacteria per gram of food.

The onset of *S. aureus* food intoxication is usually rapid and in many cases acute, but it depends on the individual's susceptibility to the toxin, the amount of contaminated food/toxin ingested, and the general health of the individual. The most common symptoms are nausea, vomiting, retching, abdominal pain, and prostration. They may also include headache, muscle cramping, and changes in blood pressure and pulse rate.

Bacillus Intoxication

Food poisoning caused by *Bacillus cereus* can occur when prepared foods are held without adequate refrigeration for several hours before serving. *Bacillus cereus* is a gram-positive, spore-forming, aerobic organism capable of producing enterotoxins. It is commonly found in soil, on vegetables, and in many raw as well as processed foods. Consumption of foods containing more than 10^6 *B. cereus* per gram may result in one of two possible types of food poisoning: an emetic illness or a diarrheal illness.

- The diarrheal type of the illness is characterized by abdominal pain and watery diarrhea, starting between 4 and 16 hours after a meal. The symptoms last for 12 to 24

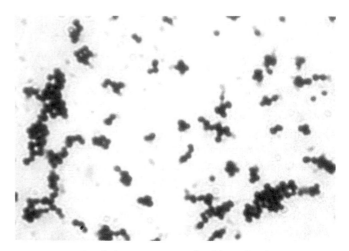

FIGURE 12.5 *Staphylococcus aureus* **food intoxication.** *S. aureus* gram-positive cocci shown in this micrograph are not only responsible for skin and wound infections, but can produce potent enterotoxins that cause serious cases of gastroenteritis.

HEALTHCARE APPLICATION

Organisms Responsible for Food Poisoning

Organism	Transmission	Toxins	Symptoms
Staphylococcus aureus	Ingestion: Mayonnaise and dairy products. Infective dose is 100,000 organisms per gram of food; a toxin dose of less than 1 μg in contaminated food will produce symptoms	Heat-stable enterotoxins (A, B, C, D, and E)	Nausea, vomiting, retching, abdominal cramping, little or no diarrhea, no fever
Bacillus cereus	Ingestion: Meats and cream sauces	Diarrheal: heat-labile enterotoxin	Diarrhea, little vomiting, no fever
	Ingestion: Starchy foods	Emetic: heat-stable enterotoxin	Vomiting, little diarrhea, no fever
Clostridium perfringens	Ingestion of toxin	Single heat-labile protein	Diarrhea, little or no vomiting, no fever
Clostridium botulinum	Ingestion of toxin, or contaminated food (as in cases of infant botulism)	Neurotoxic protein (neurotoxin); lethality from as little as nanogram quantities (1 ng = 10^{-9} g)	Botulism: A progressive, descending, flaccid paralysis of skeletal muscles, beginning at the head (i.e., ptosis of eyelids, facial muscle paralysis; death from diaphragmatic muscle paralysis)

hours. Although nausea may occur, vomiting is extremely rare with this type of intoxication. The enterotoxin associated with this illness is heat and acid labile; it can be inactivated at 56° C in 5 minutes.

- The emetic illness occurs 30 minutes to 6 hours after eating contaminated food as a result of ingestion of preformed toxins, and is characterized by an acute attack of nausea and vomiting. In general, the symptoms persist less than 24 hours. Because of the rapid onset of symptoms, this type of food poisoning is diagnosed quickly, especially with additional evidence of contamination in the food. The toxin associated with the emetic type of illness is a highly heat-stable toxin capable of surviving high temperatures (90 min at 126° C), exposure to trypsin, pepsin, and extreme pH (2–11) changes.

Outbreaks of the illnesses have been associated with cooked meat and vegetables, boiled or fried rice, vanilla sauce, custards, soups, and raw vegetable sprouts. Moreover, raw foods of plant origin are the major source of *B. cereus*. It is widely distributed because the spores can survive drying and are heat resistant. Most ready-to-eat foods can contain *B. cereus* and require various measures to prevent growth. Strains that produce emetic toxin grow well in rice dishes and other starchy foods; strains producing the diarrheal toxin grow in a wide variety of foods, such as vegetables, salads, meats, and casseroles.

Other *Bacillus* species that have been implicated in food poisoning episodes are *B. subtilis* and *B. licheniformis*, both of which can produce a highly heat-stable toxin similar to the emetic type produced by *B. cereus*.

Cholera

One of the most serious gastrointestinal infections is an acute, diarrheal illness caused by the bacterium *Vibrio cholerae*. Although the infection can be mild or without symptoms, about 1 in 20 infected people develop profuse watery diarrhea, vomiting, and leg cramps. The resulting rapid loss of body fluids leads to dehydration and shock, and without treatment death can follow within hours, when approximately 10% to 15% of the total body weight is lost.

V. cholerae is a gram-negative, vibrioid or rod-shaped, facultatively anaerobic bacterium that produces cholera toxin and enterotoxin, acting on the mucosal epithelium of the small intestine, which is responsible for the characteristic massive diarrhea.

Although cholera can be life-threatening it is easily prevented by appropriate water treatment and sanitation systems and is rare in industrialized nations. Still, more than 60 countries report outbreaks of the disease each year. In the United States cholera epidemics presented a major problem in the 1800s but basically have been eliminated through the use of modern sewage and water treatment systems. However, U.S. travelers to parts of Africa, Asia, or Latin America may be exposed to the pathogen and can bring contaminated seafood back to the States, causing foodborne outbreaks.

Infections are usually acquired by ingesting contaminated water or food, although person-to-person transmission is pos-

sible. Persons infected with cholera have massive diarrhea, often described as "rice water stools," which is loaded with the pathogen and can spread under unsanitary conditions. Any contaminated water, food washed in contaminated water, or shellfish living in contaminated water can cause an outbreak of cholera. Furthermore, *V. cholerae*, both toxic and nontoxic strains, are present in zooplankton of fresh, brackish, and salt water. Often coastal cholera outbreaks occur after zooplankton blooms.

The main treatment for cholera is aggressive rehydration and replacement of electrolytes. Antibiotics may play a role in reducing the duration and severity of the disease; however, drug resistance has been reported.

Viral Infections

The rotavirus and norovirus families of viruses are the leading causes of viral gastroenteritis. In addition, a number of other viruses have been implicated in outbreaks of gastroenteritis, including astroviruses, caliciviruses, and enteric adenoviruses. Viral gastroenteritis is usually a mild illness, but it can be lethal if rehydration is not maintained. As with other cases of gastroenteritis, it is transmitted by the fecal–oral route, by

LIFE APPLICATION

Dr. John Snow: Getting a Handle on Cholera

In the mid-1800s people in the Soho district of London were suffering a cholera epidemic. The dominant medical theory at the time was that cholera and other diseases such as the plague were caused by some sort of pollution or "bad air," referred to as *miasma*. The germ theory of disease was not widely accepted. The physician Dr. John Snow (1813–1858) believed that "bad air" was not responsible for the spread of disease but that water from a single pump on Broad Street was responsible for the numerous cholera cases clustered in this geographic area. Snow was not able to conclusively prove his theory, but his studies of the spread pattern of the disease were enough to convince authorities to disable the pump by removing the pump handle. This action reportedly ended the outbreak, although Snow himself admitted that the epidemic itself may have already been on the decline when the handle was removed. In any case, Snow was able to show by a spot map and statistics gathered regarding use of the pump and spread of the disease that the cases were centered around the use of this particular pump. The pump had been dug only a few feet from an old septic pit that began to leak fecal bacteria. Through further research he was able to connect the disease to the quality of the water supply. These events are often regarded as the birth of the science of epidemiology (see Epidemiology and Public Health in Chapter 9, Infection and Disease).

person-to-person contact or ingestion of contaminated foods and water.

Rotaviruses

Rotaviruses are the most common cause of infectious diarrhea in infants and children worldwide and are responsible for more than 50% of hospitalizations of children due to diarrhea. According to the CDC, approximately 55,000 children are hospitalized in the United States each year and more than 600,000 children worldwide die annually from rotavirus infections, with 80% of these occurring in underdeveloped countries.

In general, children obtain at least one rotavirus infection before the age of 5 years. Immunity after infection is incomplete, but repeat infections are less severe, and therefore adults infected with the rotavirus often do not develop symptoms but can be carriers and are able to spread the infection. The incubation period is about 2 days and the gastroenteritis lasts for 3 to 8 days, with fever and abdominal pain being common symptoms.

Several vaccines have been developed and continue to be developed to help countries in which this illness is a major problem. The Rotavirus Vaccine Program (RVP), a partnership between the WHO, PATH (Program for Appropriate Technology in Health), and the CDC, and funded by the Global Alliance for Vaccines and Immunization, has been established to help eliminate deaths from rotavirus infection.

Astroviruses and Caliciviruses

Astroviridae and Caliciviridae are positive-sense single-stranded RNA [(+) ssRNA] viruses and belong to group IV according to the Baltimore classification system. Astroviruses and caliciviruses have been isolated from birds, cats, dogs, pigs, sheep, cows, and humans. They were first described in 1975 with the help of electron microscopy during an outbreak of diarrhea. The viruses are considered to be a major cause of gastroenteritis in children and adults. The infections occur throughout the year with apparent peaks in the winter months. Infections occur worldwide and the symptoms include diarrhea, headache, malaise, and nausea; although vomiting may occur it is not frequent. The incubation period is reported to be 3 to 4 days, with symptoms lasting approximately 5 days if there are no complications.

Noroviruses

Noroviruses (family Caliciviridae), previously described as "Norwalk-like viruses," are a group of related single-stranded RNA, nonenveloped viruses, all of which cause acute gastroenteritis in humans. In addition to diarrhea, nausea, and vomiting, these viruses may cause muscle aches, headache, fatigue, and even a low-grade fever. Noroviruses affect children and adults and often infect families as well as communities, especially in confined, crowded spaces. The illness usually occurs within 18 to 72 hours of exposure, and although symptoms have the tendency to fade within a day or two, infected persons are still contagious for at least 3 days to 2 weeks after recovery from the illness.

Adenoviruses

Adenoviruses (group I double-stranded DNA) are a group of viruses that can infect the membranes of the respiratory tract, the conjunctiva, the gastrointestinal tract, and the urinary tract. Most commonly adenoviruses cause respiratory illness; however, depending on the infecting serotype they can cause different infections and symptoms. Adenoviruses 40 and 41 are a major cause of acute viral gastroenteritis in children, and have been grouped together as enteric adenoviruses (group F). Although the epidemiologic characteristics of adenoviruses vary, they are all transmitted by direct contact, the fecal–oral route, or sometimes through contaminated water.

Hepatitis

Hepatitis is an inflammation of the liver that can be caused by a number of hepatitis viruses, namely A to E. Hepatitis A and E are transmitted by the fecal–oral route and neither one results in a chronic infection. Both infections result in gastroenteritis and can be transmitted through contaminated food or water.

- Hepatitis A, caused by the hepatitis A virus (HAV), can affect anyone and in the United States; infections can be isolated or widespread. Good personal hygiene and appropriate sanitation will curb the spread of the disease. Vaccines are available for long-term prevention among people 12 months of age and older.
- Hepatitis E is rare in the United States. It is caused by the hepatitis E virus (HEV), and is transmitted in the same way as hepatitis A.

Fungal Infections

Mycoses that affect the gastrointestinal system are generally opportunistic and typically do not affect healthy humans. Opportunistic mycoses are limited to people with a compromised immune system, but certain fungi can also cause problems in otherwise healthy people. These species include *Candida albicans, Aspergillus flavus,* and *Claviceps purpurea.*

Candidiasis

Candidiasis is an infection caused by a variety of opportunistic organisms of the genus *Candida. Candida albicans* is part of the normal gastrointestinal flora of about 80% of the human population, and does not usually cause any problems. Only the overgrowth of *Candida* due to changes in the normal environment will cause candidiasis, which can occur in many different body systems. Oral candidiasis, called *"thrush,"* is rare in healthy individuals, occurring in about 5% of newborns and 10% of the elderly, but is common in immunocompromised patients. Thrush presents itself as creamy white or bluish-white patches on the tongue, on the lining of the mouth, and/or in the throat (Figure 12.6). Certain medications such as antibiotics, corticosteroids, and the birth control pill may upset the normal flora

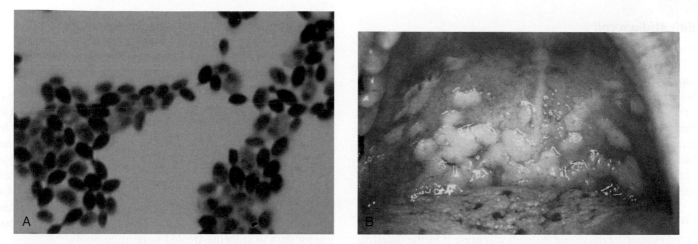

FIGURE 12.6 Thrush. A, Micrograph of the fungus *Candida albicans* in the yeast form (this fungus can also form filamentous mycelia) that is responsible for an oral infection called *thrush*. *C. albicans* can also cause vaginal infections in women. **B,** Thrush or oral candidiasis results in creamy white or bluish-white patches on the tongue, on the lining of the mouth, and/or in the throat. (**B,** Courtesy of J.A. Innes. From Mims C, Dockrell HM, Goering RV, et al: *Medical microbiology,* ed 3, St. Louis, 2004, Mosby.)

of the mouth and allow *Candida* to overgrow. Certain medical conditions such as uncontrolled diabetes, HIV infection, cancer, dry mouth, or pregnancy may also provide a favorable condition for the development of candidiasis. Several antifungal preparations are available for the treatment of this condition (see Chapter 22, Antimicrobial Drugs).

Aspergillosis

Aspergillosis is a term used for illnesses caused by organisms in the genus *Aspergillus*. *Aspergillus* is found in soil, food, compost, agricultural buildings, and air vents of homes and offices worldwide. *Aspergillus flavus* is a mold common on corn and peanuts, and is one of several species of mold known to produce aflatoxin, a carcinogenic substance. Its toxic effects include acute hepatitis, immunosuppression, and hepatocellular carcinoma. Because of these toxic effects, the FDA monitors and regulates the allowable aflatoxin concentration in food and feed.

Aspergillus spp. can be opportunistic pathogens in almost all tissues of the body. They are mainly responsible for three distinct pulmonary diseases (see Chapter 11, Infections of the Respiratory System), but the systemic illness can produce abscesses in the gastrointestinal tract, especially in patients with AIDS.

Ergotism

The fungus *Claviceps purpurea* contaminates rye and wheat and produces substances called *alkaloids*. Ergotism is a result of ingestion of alkaloids (ergotamines) produced by the fungus. In excess, ergotamines can cause symptoms of hallucinations, severe gastrointestinal upset, a type of dry gangrene, and a painful burning sensation in the limbs and extremities that is called "*St. Anthony's fire.*" Because of the effect of alkaloids on the central nervous system, ergotism is discussed in more detail in Chapter 13 (Infections of the Nervous System and Senses).

Parasitic Infections

Although all infectious agents of humans are parasites, parasitic diseases are often defined as those caused by protozoans or helminths, and this section focuses on protozoan and helminthic infections of the human gastrointestinal system.

Protozoans

Protozoans are unicellular eukaryotes (see Chapter 8, Eukaryotic Microorganisms) found in a wide range of habitats; most are free living and not harmful to humans. However, some are parasites and capable of causing debilitating and deadly diseases. They enter the human body either as a trophozoite, the active feeding and reproductive stage, or as a cyst, the dormant stage, becoming active under the appropriate environmental conditions.

Giardia intestinalis (Giardiasis)

Giardiasis is a common waterborne gastrointestinal disease in the United States, with the infective agents present in both drinking and recreational water. The causative agent is *Giardia lamblia,* also known as *G. intestinalis,* an organism that lives in the intestinal tracts of animals and humans worldwide. Once a human or other animal has been infected, the parasite will reside in the intestine and will pass into the feces (see Chapter 8, Eukaryotic Microorganisms). Therefore, *Giardia* is found in soil, food, water, or any surfaces that have been contaminated with infected feces. The symptoms of *Giardia* infection include diarrhea, flatulence, greasy stools, stomach cramps, and nausea, and normally begin 1 to 2 weeks after infection, lasting 2 to 6 weeks. Chronic infections lasting months to years have also been reported. Prescription drugs are available to treat giardiasis, but in addition plenty of fluid intake is necessary to counteract the dehydration due to diarrhea.

Balantidium coli

Balantidium coli is the largest protozoan parasite of humans. It is prevalent in the tropics but is also present in temperate regions. *Balantidium coli* lives in the cecum or colon of pigs and less commonly in monkeys. Transmission occurs by the fecal–oral route and by person-to-person contact via food handlers. Symptoms of the illness include abdominal pain, tenderness, nausea, anorexia, and bloody, watery stools. Risk factors for humans include contact with swine and/or substandard hygienic conditions. For treatment, the drug of choice is tetracycline, or metronidazole and iodoquinol as alternatives.

Entamoeba histolytica (Amebiasis)

Asymptomatic *Entamoeba histolytica* is present in the digestive tracts of about 10% of the human population. These carriers are found predominantly in underdeveloped countries, especially in rural areas where water and sanitation practices are deficient. When the disease develops, it can be fatal and the worldwide annual mortality is about 100,000. Infections most commonly occur through ingestion of water contaminated with human feces that contain cysts. There is no animal reservoir. Another way of transmission is by fecal contamination of hands or food or during any other activities that will allow the organism to be spread from the fecal material of one person to the GI tract of another.

Once ingested, the cysts undergo excystment in the small intestine of the new host. New trophozoites form and migrate to the large intestine to multiply. As a result, both cysts and trophozoites are released to the environment via the feces of an infected person; the trophozoites will die rapidly, but the cysts will remain infective. In as many as 90% of infections the trophozoites reencyst and the infection remains asymptomatic and self-limiting; but disease symptoms may recur. Acute amoebic colitis has a gradual onset of 1 to 2 weeks, involving abdominal pain and diarrhea. Several different antibiotics are available to treat **amebiasis** (see Chapter 23, Human Age and Microorganisms).

Cryptosporidiosis

This parasitic diarrheal disease cryptosporidiosis, also known as *"crypto,"* is caused by the protozoan *Cryptosporidium* and is spread via the fecal–oral route, through contaminated water, and via uncooked or cross-contaminated food. After infection the parasite lives in the intestine of the animal or human and is released with the feces (Figure 12.7). Because of the parasite's outer shell it can survive outside the body of the host for extended periods of time. Furthermore, the organism is rather resistant to chlorine and chlorine-based disinfectants and can live for days in chlorine-treated swimming pools.

According to the CDC, **cryptosporidiosis** is one of the most common waterborne diseases in the United States, because the organism can be found in drinking water and recreational water bodies. In addition to watery diarrhea, the symptoms include dehydration, weight loss, stomach cramps or pain, fever, nausea, and vomiting. Some people do not develop symptoms, but in the rest, the symptoms generally begin 2 to 10 days after infection and in people with a healthy immune system will subside in 1 to 2 weeks.

Helminths

As indicated previously, helminths are not microorganisms, they are macroscopic, multicellular, eukaryotic worms found throughout the globe. What is interesting to microbiologists is the fact that their eggs and larvae are microscopic. The distinguishing traits, life cycle, and classification are described in Chapter 8 (Eukaryotic Microorganisms). This chapter highlights some of the most common human intestinal parasitic helminths.

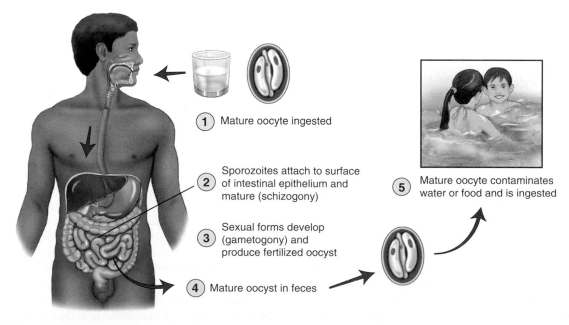

① Mature oocyte ingested

② Sporozoites attach to surface of intestinal epithelium and mature (schizogony)

③ Sexual forms develop (gametogony) and produce fertilized oocyst

④ Mature oocyst in feces

⑤ Mature oocyte contaminates water or food and is ingested

FIGURE 12.7 Life cycle of *Cryptosporidium*.

Taeniasis

Taeniasis, the term for human tapeworm infection, is normally acquired by consuming raw or undercooked meat of infected animals. *Taenia saginata* is common in beef, and *Taenia solium* is common in pigs (Figure 12.8). The larvae present in the infected meat will then grow into an adult tapeworm in the human intestine, where it can live for years and grow very large—longer than 12 feet. Humans are the only definitive host for the two organisms (see Chapter 8) and both species are distributed worldwide. Tapeworm infestation usually does not cause any symptoms, and the infection is normally recognized by the presence of moving worm segments in the stool. Infected individuals can expose other individuals via food handling with contaminated hands, and can also self-infect if personal hygiene is deficient. Tapeworm infestation can be treated and eradication of the tapeworm is expected after treatment.

Pinworm Infection

The best known human pinworm, also known as the *"seatworm,"* is *Enterobius vermicularis,* a small, white intestinal worm (nematode) found in soil, dust, food, and water. It lives in the rectum of humans (Figure 12.9). Pinworm infections are the most common worm infections in the United States, with school-age children and preschoolers being at highest risk. The female pinworm leaves the intestines through the anus, usually during the night, and deposits the eggs on the surrounding skin. This causes itching around the anus, and disturbed sleep in the infected person. Pinworm eggs can survive up to 2 weeks on clothing, bedding, or other objects. Infection can occur after accidentally ingesting pinworm eggs from contaminated surfaces or fingers. Pinworm infections can be treated with either a prescription drug such as mebendazole, or over-the-counter drugs such as pyrantel pamoate, involving a two-dose course.

Ascariasis

Ascaris infection, or **ascariasis,** caused by *Ascaris lumbricoides* (Figure 12.10) is the most common nematode infection of humans worldwide. The infection is most common in tropical and subtropical areas but is also endemic in rural areas of the southeastern United States. *Ascaris* eggs are found in human feces and when soil becomes contaminated, the eggs become infectious after a few weeks. Infection occurs after accidental ingestion of infectious *Ascaris* eggs (see Chapter 8 [Eukaryotic Microorganisms] for its life cycle). The parasite can enter the soil when contaminated with human feces, and the eggs remain viable in the soil for long periods of time. Subsequently, vegetables and fruits grown in this soil become contaminated; when humans consume them they become infected.

Most infected people are asymptomatic, but the illness may cause slower weight gain and growth. In the United States infections are generally treated for 1 to 3 days with antiparasitic medication. The drugs most commonly used against ascariasis are mebendazole, albendazole, and pyrantel pamoate. Heavy infestation may require surgery to repair the intestinal damage and to remove the worms.

Hookworm Infections (Necatoriasis)

Necatoriasis is caused by hookworms, parasitic nematodes that live in the small intestine of mammals such as dogs, cats, and

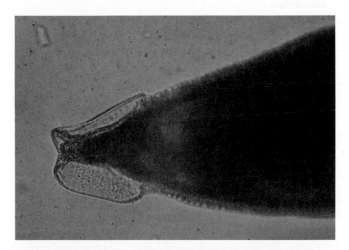

FIGURE 12.9 Pinworm. This micrograph shows the mouth structure of the pinworm *Enterobius vermicularis,* which causes the disease enterobiasis.

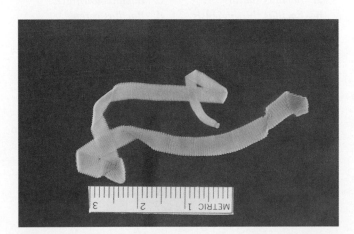

FIGURE 12.8 Tapeworm. Two main features of the tapeworm are the scolex, which has muscular suckers surrounded by hooks for attachment, and the individual body segments called *proglottids.*

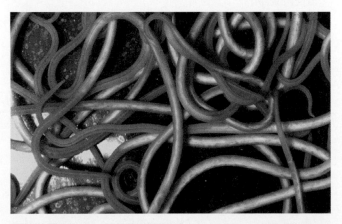

FIGURE 12.10 *Ascaris.* *Ascaris lumbricoides* is a simple roundworm that can cause the disease ascariasis, affecting the digestive tract and/or the lungs. (Courtesy Dr. Richard Martin, Biomedical Science, College of Veterinary Medicine, Iowa State University)

humans. The two species that are capable of causing human infections are *Ancylostoma duodenale* and *Necator americanus*. Once the adult hookworm reaches the intestine (see Chapter 8 [Eukaryotic Microorganisms] for the life cycle) it attaches itself to the villi of the intestinal wall and sucks blood from its host to obtain nutrition. A single *Necator americanus* can take about 30 μl of blood daily; the larger *Ancylostoma duodenale* can take up to 260 μl/day. Slight infections may appear asymptomatic, but others may cause abdominal discomfort, diarrhea, cramps, anorexia, and weight loss. Heavy infections generally lead to iron-deficient anemia. Hookworm can be treated when it is still on the skin, in the migrating stage, and during the intestinal stage.

Summary

- The gastrointestinal tract (GI) is a common and easily accessible portal of entry for microbes or their toxins, and both have the ability to cause illnesses. Therefore, food- and waterborne diseases are a major public health concern worldwide.
- Many different organisms are responsible for infections of the GI tract, ranging from the oral cavity with dental caries and periodontal disease, to the stomach with peptic ulcers, and the intestines with gastroenteritis.
- Salmonellosis, typhoid fever, shigellosis, campylobacteriosis, *Escherichia* spp. gastroenteritis, and yersiniosis are all bacterial infections of different origins but only somewhat different symptoms and outcomes. They all cause a form of gastroenteritis. All these illnesses occur only when the organism is present in the body and has caused an active infection.
- Bacterial gastrointestinal intoxication is a condition caused by the consumption of bacterial toxins. Organisms capable of causing this type of toxemia include *Clostridium botulinum*, the causative agent for botulism, *Staphylococcus aureus*, *Vibrio cholerae*, *Bacillus cereus*, and some other toxin-producing *Bacillus* species.
- In general, bacterial GI tract infections are transmitted through contaminated food, contaminated water supplies, by the fecal–oral route, or by person-to-person contact. Bacterial intoxication, on the other hand, is usually due to faulty food preparation, storage, and/or handling of the food.
- The leading causes of viral gastroenteritis are the rotavirus and norovirus families, but other viruses also have been implicated in outbreaks, including astroviruses, caliciviruses, enteric adenoviruses, and hepatitis viruses.
- Viral gastroenteritis is usually mild, but can become toxic or even lethal if rehydration is not maintained.
- Mycoses that affect the GI tract are generally opportunistic and typically do not affect people with a healthy immune system. However, certain fungi can also cause problems in otherwise healthy people. These include *Aspergillus flavus*, *Claviceps purpurea*, and *Candida albicans*.
- Some protozoans are human parasites capable of causing debilitating and deadly diseases. These include *Giardia intestinalis*, *Balantidium coli*, *Entamoeba histolytica*, and *Cryptosporidium*.
- Helminths are not microorganisms but their eggs and larvae are of microscopic size and capable of causing illnesses in the human GI tract. These infections include taeniasis (tapeworm infection), pinworm infections, ascariasis, and hookworm infections.

Review Questions

1. All of the following are components of the gastrointestinal tract *except*:
   a. Spleen
   b. Pharynx
   c. Esophagus
   d. Stomach

2. Microbial life on teeth was first observed by:
   a. Jenner
   b. Semmelweis
   c. van Leeuwenhoek
   d. Pasteur

3. Many peptic ulcers are due to:
   a. *Salmonella typhi*
   b. *Helicobacter pylori*
   c. *Shigella boydii*
   d. *Salmonella enterica*

4. Bacillary dysentery is also called:
   a. Salmonellosis
   b. Shigellosis
   c. Typhoid fever
   d. Campylobacteriosis

5. There are _____ known forms of gastroenteritis caused by *E. coli*.
   a. Two
   b. Three
   c. Four
   d. Five

6. *Bacillus* intoxication is caused by:
   a. *Bacillus subtilis*
   b. *Bacillus thuringiensis*
   c. *Bacillus anthracis*
   d. *Bacillus cereus*

7. The most common cause of infectious diarrhea in infants and children is by:
   a. Noroviruses
   b. Adenoviruses
   c. Rotaviruses
   d. Caliciviruses

8. A group of (+) ssRNA viruses that have been isolated from birds, cats, dogs, pigs, sheep, cows, and humans, and are a major cause of gastroenteritis, are:
   a. Rotaviruses
   b. Caliciviruses
   c. Adenoviruses
   d. Noroviruses

9. Which of the following organisms produce aflatoxin, a carcinogenic substance?
   a. *Candida albicans*
   b. *Claviceps purpurea*
   c. *Aspergillus flavus*
   d. *Staphylococcus aureus*

10. The human pinworm *Enterobius vermicularis* lives in the _____ of humans.
    a. Duodenum
    b. Ileum
    c. Transverse colon
    d. Rectum

11. A periodontal disease that is restricted to the gums is an inflammation called _____.

12. The term "stomach flu" really refers to _____.

13. Botulism is caused by _____.

14. Staphylococcal intoxication is caused by *Staphylococcus* _____.

15. "Thrush" is caused by _____.

16. Differentiate between bacterial infection and bacterial intoxication.

17. Describe the cause, transmission, symptoms, prevention, and treatment of cholera.

18. Describe rotavirus infections; include prevalence, transmission, prevention, and treatment.

19. Discuss giardiasis; include causative agent, transmission, symptoms, and treatment.

20. Name and discuss the two organisms that cause hookworm infections in humans.

Bibliography

Aas JA, Pater BJ, Stokes LN, et al: Defining the normal bacterial flora of the oral cavity, *J Clinical Microbiology* 43(11):5721–5732, 2005.

Forbes BA, Sahm DF, Weissfeld AS: *Bailey & Scott's diagnostic microbiology*, ed 12, St. Louis, 2007, Mosby/Elsevier.

Mahon CR, Lehman DC, Manuselis G: *Textbook of diagnostic microbiology*, ed 3, St. Louis, 2007, Saunders/Elsevier.

Mims C, Dockrell HM, Goering RV, et al: *Medical microbiology*, ed 3, St. Louis, 2004, Mosby/Elsevier.

Murray PR, Rosenthal KS, Pfaller MA: *Medical microbiology*, ed 5, St. Louis, 2005, Mosby/Elsevier.

Thibodeau GA, Patton KT: *Anatomy and physiology*, ed 6, St. Louis, 2007, Mosby/Elsevier.

Tortora GJ, Funke BR, Case CL: *Microbiology: an introduction*, ed 9, San Francisco, 2007, Benjamin Cummings/Pearson Education.

Internet Resources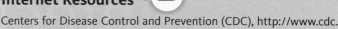

Centers for Disease Control and Prevention (CDC), http://www.cdc.gov/index.htm

Todar's Online Textbook of Bacteriology, http://www.textbookofbacteriology.net/

The Merck Manual of Medical Information—Second Home Edition, Digestive Disorders, Gastroenteritis, http://www.merck.com/mmhe/print/sec09/ch122/ch122a.html

National Digestive Diseases Information Clearinghouse (NDDIC), Bacteria and Foodborne Illness, http://digestive.niddk.nih.gov/ddiseases/pubs/bacteria/

CDC, Norovirus, http://cdc.gov/ncidod/dvrd/revb/gastro/norovirus.htm

FDA Bad Bug Book, Bacillus cereus and Other *Bacillus* spp., http://www.cfsan.fda.gov/~mow/chap12.html

American Dental Association, Periodontal (Gum) Diseases, http://www.ada.org/public/topics/periodontal_diseases.asp

American Academy of Periodontology, http://www.perio.org

American Academy of Periodontology, Tobacco Use and Periodontal Disease, http://www.perio.org/consumer/smoking.htm

CDC, Salmonellosis, http://www.cdc.gov/nczved/dfbmd/disease_listing/salmonellosis_gi.html

Brisabois A, Cazin I, Breuil J, et al: Surveillance of antibiotic resistance in *Salmonella, Euro Surveill* 2(3):pii=181, 1997 (accessed November 17, 2008). Available online: http://www.eurosurveillance.org/em/v02n03/0203-222.asp

CDC Health Information for International Travel 2008, Chapter 4: Prevention of Specific Infectious Diseases, Typhoid Fever, http://wwwn.cdc.gov/travel/yellowBookCh4-Typhoid.aspx

Mayo Clinic, http://www.mayoclinic.com/

Mayo Clinic, *Ascariasis*, http://www.mayoclinic.com/health/ascariasis/DS00688

CDC, *Yersinia enterocolitica*, http://www.cdc.gov/ncidod/dbmd/diseaseinfo/yersinia_g.htm

CDC, Listeriosis, http://www.cdc.gov/nczved/dfbmd/disease_listing/listeriosis_gi.html

13

Infections of the Nervous System and Senses

OUTLINE

Introduction

Bacterial Infections
　Bacterial Meningitis
　Tetanus
　Botulism
　Leprosy
　Conjunctivitis

Viral Infections
　Viral Meningitis
　Poliomyelitis

Rabies
Arboviral Encephalitis

Fungal Infections
　Cryptococcosis

Protozoan Infections
　Cerebral Toxoplasmosis
　Trypanosomiasis

Prion-associated Diseases

LEARNING OBJECTIVES

After reading this chapter, the student will be able to:
- Describe how microorganisms can gain access to the nervous system
- Describe the symptoms of meningitis; discuss the different causes and the different treatment approaches for each type of the illness
- Discuss the different forms of bacterial meningitis; include the cause, symptoms, and treatments
- Describe the four different types of tetanus and the causes, prevention, and treatment
- Discuss botulism and the different types of toxins produced by the different strains
- Explain the causes, symptoms, and treatment of leprosy
- Describe the causes, symptoms, and treatment of conjunctivitis
- Describe the causes, symptoms, prevention, and treatments of poliomyelitis, rabies, and arboviral encephalitis
- Describe the typical fungal infections of the human nervous system
- Differentiate between African and American trypanosomiasis
- Describe prions and the human diseases associated with them

acetylcholine
aseptic
blood–brain barrier
botulism
central nervous system
cerebrospinal fluid
conjunctivitis
encephalitis

inflammatory reflex
meninges
meningitis
meningoencephalitis
motor neuron
neuromuscular junction
neurotoxin
neurotransmitter

otitis media
peripheral nervous
  system
septic
tetany
tetanus

WHY YOU NEED TO KNOW

HISTORY

Polio (poliomyelitis) is an ancient disease, but scientists did not completely identify and name the disease until the twentieth century. The disease is an acute, highly contagious disease caused by the poliovirus. Epidemics have swept across the United States several times in the 1900s, killing thousands and paralyzing even more. Many of the victims were children and the disease became one of the most feared childhood diseases in the first half of the twentieth century. In 1937, the National Foundation for Infantile Paralysis, which became known as the *March of Dimes*, was founded by Franklin Delano Roosevelt, who himself contracted polio in 1921. Funding by the foundation helped Jonas Salk to develop the first vaccine in 1952. Albert Sabin introduced the first oral polio vaccine in 1961, which further reduced the incidence of polio.

Another toxin produced by a microorganism that affects the nervous system is ergot, the product of a fungus *(Claviceps purpurea)* that grows on the rye grain plant. The toxin has been accurately labeled as a pharmaceutical storehouse of biologically active products such as vasoconstrictors, uterine smooth muscle contractors, and substances effective on CNS neurotransmission, just to mention a few. The response following exposure to ergot is ergotism, or long-term ergot poisoning. Ergotism presents a variety of dose-dependent symptoms including vomiting, diarrhea, hallucinations, convulsive seizures, and other irrational behaviors. Some attempts have been made to associate the behaviors of manic melancholia, psychoses, delirium, crawling sensations in the skin of the extremities, dizziness, migraines, vomiting, and diarrhea (all symptoms of ergotism) with similar symptoms seen in the accused "witches of Salem" tried in Salem, Massachusetts in the late 1600s. By 1692, some 20 of these so-called witches of Salem had been convicted and executed for their "crimes."

IMPACT

The knowledge scientists have gained about microorganisms, their toxins, and their effect on the nervous system has led to more and better vaccination regimens, as well as to increased antimicrobial drug development. For example, the success of the tetanus vaccination programs reduced the annual cases of tetanus in the United States to about 100, whereas about 1 million cases are reported worldwide each year.

Unfortunately, the understanding of microorganisms and of their actions on the human body has also led to the threat of their use as bioweapons (see Bioterrorism in Chapter 24, Microorganisms in the Environment and Environmental Safety). Terrorists have tried to weaponize botulinum toxin by refining the toxin and dispersing it in aerosol form. Preparations of the toxins could be used to poison food or beverages, and with a sophisticated delivery system could disseminate the toxin by air. Botulinum toxin spreads throughout the body and affects mostly the nervous system, and has a high mortality rate.

FUTURE

New concepts direct research as much as technological development. An example of such a new concept is the **inflammatory reflex.** It is a response between the nervous system and the immune system via the vagus cranial nerve to create a "neuroimmune axis." The nervous system through the vagus cranial nerve modulates circulating tumor necrosis factor (TNF)-α levels induced by microorganisms or tissue injury. TNF-α is a protein normally present in the body, but its circulating levels are increased by the immune system to mobilize white blood cells in the presence of an infection, with resultant inflammation in the affected area. In general, the inflammation subsides, but if it is caused by certain diseases such as rheumatoid arthritis or Crohn's disease, the inflammation doesn't subside. This draws more white blood cells to the site, which allows TNF-α to increase further, causing additional inflammation, which leads to pain and tissue damage. There are now TNF-α inhibitors that block the effects of TNF-α, reducing their effects of inflammation or other symptoms.

Extensive research is also being conducted in prion-related diseases. Increased attention has been paid to the spread of transmissible spongiform encephalopathies (TSE) in deer populations in the United States. With an increase in the number of deer testing positive for chronic wasting disease (a form of TSE) there is increasing concern regarding the transmission of the prion through consumption of venison by hunters/consumers. Results of this research may have a significant impact on the future of deer hunting and management of natural resources in general.

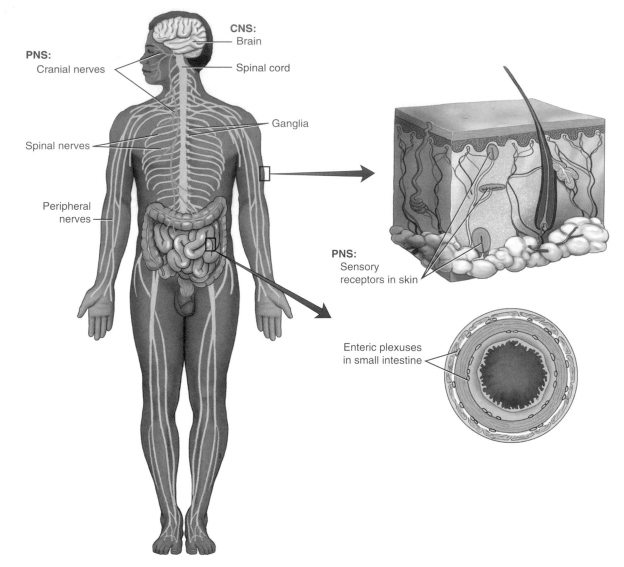

FIGURE 13.1 Overview of the nervous system. The nervous system is divided into two components: the central nervous system composed of the brain and the spinal cord, and the peripheral nervous system containing the cranial and spinal nerves, ganglia, and sensory receptors.

Introduction

The nervous system is divided into two components: the **central nervous system** (CNS) and the **peripheral nervous system** (PNS). The CNS consists of the brain and spinal cord, and the PNS consists of 12 pairs of cranial nerves, 31 pairs of spinal nerves, ganglia, and associated sensory receptors (Figure 13.1).

The brain and the spinal cord are covered by three protective membranes, collectively called **meninges** (Figure 13.2). The outermost membrane is the dura mater, the middle layer is the arachnoid, and the innermost membrane is the pia mater. The space between the pia mater and the arachnoid, referred to as the *subarachnoid space,* contains **cerebrospinal fluid** (CSF), which circulates through the brain ventricles, the central canal

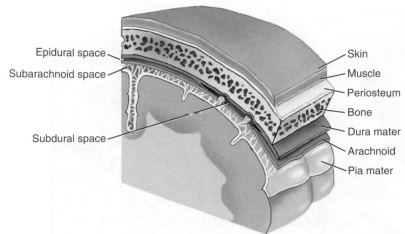

Epidural space
Subarachnoid space
Subdural space
Skin
Muscle
Periosteum
Bone
Dura mater
Arachnoid
Pia mater

FIGURE 13.2 The meninges. The brain and the spinal cord are covered by three protective membranes, collectively called *meninges*. The outermost membrane is the dura mater, the middle layer is the arachnoid, and the innermost membrane is the pia mater.

TABLE 13.1 Cerebrospinal Fluid (CSF) Changes During CSF Infections

	Cause	Cells/ml	Protein (mg/dl)	White Blood Cells
Normal		0–5	15–45	
Aseptic meningitis or meningoencephalitis	Viruses, tuberculosis, leptospira, fungi, brain abscess	100–1000	50–100	Elevated lymphocytes and monocytes
Septic meningitis	Bacteria, amoebae, brain abscess	200–20,000	High (>100)	Elevated granulocytes

of the spinal cord, and the subarachnoid space. The CSF has a low level of complement proteins, circulating antibodies, and some phagocytotic cells; if bacteria get access to the CSF they can multiply with little immune reaction by the body.

A collective inflammation of these protective membrane coverings is called **meningitis** and may be caused by microorganisms, or it may be noninfectious and the result of physical injury, cancer, or certain drugs dosages. Regardless of the cause, meningitis is a serious condition that requires immediate medical attention. The various pathogens causing meningitis include bacteria, viruses, fungi, and protozoans.

During a CNS infection specific changes occur within the CSF. The response in the CSF to a viral infection is generally reflected by an increase in lymphocytes, monocytes, and a slight increase in proteins, and the CSF remains clear. This condition is called **aseptic** meningitis. In the case of a bacterial infection a rapid increase in granulocytes and proteins occurs and the CSF becomes visibly turbid. This condition is called **septic** meningitis (Table 13.1).

The CNS is remarkably resistant to infection, largely because of a barrier between the blood circulation and the nervous tissue, referred to as the **blood–brain barrier.** The capillaries of the blood–brain barrier permit only selected substances to pass from the blood into the brain, with all others being restricted. In essence, only lipid-soluble substances can cross the barrier; the exception is glucose and certain amino acids, none of which are lipid soluble, but that have specific carrier mechanisms transporting them across the barrier. Unless they are lipid soluble, drugs cannot cross the blood–brain barrier. For example, chloramphenicol, a lipid-soluble antibiotic (see Chapter 22, Antimicrobial Drugs), can readily enter the brain whereas penicillin, only slightly lipid soluble, is effective only if taken in large doses.

Although not common, if inflammation of the brain occurs it alters the blood–brain barrier, often allowing drugs to cross that normally cannot. The most common routes of CNS invasion are the bloodstream and the lymphatic system, when an inflammation alters the blood–brain barrier. Invasion of the CNS via the peripheral nerves is a feature of some viruses discussed later in this chapter. An inflammation of the brain is called **encephalitis,** and if both the brain and the meninges are inflamed the condition is referred to as **meningoencephalitis.**

Another structure that can be affected by microorganisms or their toxins is the neuromuscular junction. The **neuromuscular junction** (Figure 13.3) is the connection between the synaptic end bulb (axon terminal) of a **motor neuron,** located in the spinal cord, and a muscle fiber. This junction is essential for muscle contraction. The two cells do not touch each other but are separated by a small space called the *synaptic cleft.* The electrical message from the motor neuron is translated into a chemical message via the **neurotransmitter (acetylcholine)** located in the presynaptic terminal. Once the neurotransmitter is released into the synaptic cleft it diffuses to the receptors on the muscle fiber and generates another electrical event that leads to muscle contraction. Any interference with this delicate structure will lead to problems with muscle contraction.

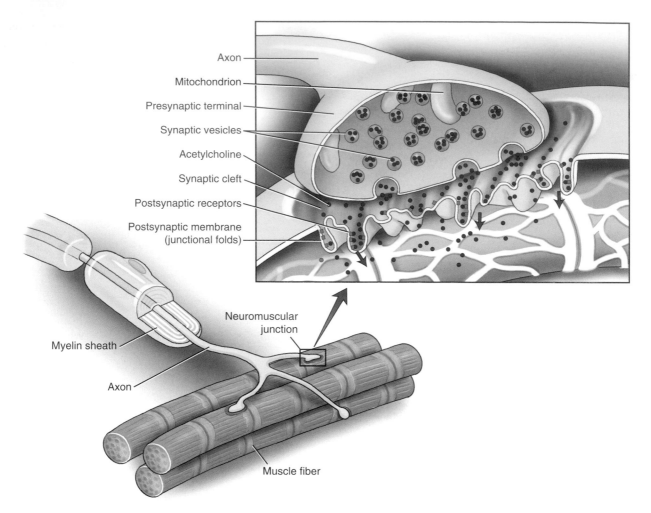

FIGURE 13.3 The neuromuscular junction. The neuromuscular junction is the connection between the synaptic end bulb (axon terminal) of a motor neuron, located in the spinal cord, and a muscle fiber.

Bacterial Infections

Although bacterial infections of the nervous system are rare, they are serious with sometimes lethal outcomes. Before the discovery of antibiotics, bacterial central nervous system infections were almost always fatal.

Bacterial Meningitis

The general symptoms of meningitis initially are nausea, vomiting, fever, headache, and a stiff neck. These symptoms may develop over several hours, but can take from 1 to 2 days. Although the symptoms vary from patient to patient, the initial symptoms may be followed by

- Confusion
- Sleepiness
- Light sensitivity
- Possible progression to convulsions and coma

Bacterial meningitis is less common than viral meningitis but is more severe in nature, because of the production of toxins by the bacteria. The mortality rate for bacterial meningitis varies with the causative agent, and vaccination is available for some. Early diagnosis and treatment of bacterial meningitis are essential to prevent permanent neurological damage. Antibacterial drugs used to treat bacterial meningitis include penicillin G, ampicillin or amoxicillin, chloramphenicol, cefotaxime, vancomycin, and ceftriaxone (see Chapter 22, Antimicrobial Drugs).

Before the 1990s the most common cause of bacterial meningitis was *Haemophilus influenzae* type b (Hib), but vaccine development and the vaccination of children as part of their routine immunization have drastically decreased the number of cases due to *H. influenzae.* At present, the leading causes of bacterial meningitis are *Streptococcus pneumoniae* and *Neisseria meningitidis.* Other bacteria that can cause meningitis include *Listeria monocytogenes,* responsible for about 10% of cases of bacterial meningitis, *Escherichia coli, Klebsiella,* and *Mycobacterium tuberculosis. E. coli* and *Klebsiella* infections usually develop subsequent to a head injury, brain or spinal cord surgery, sepsis, or a nosocomial infection. Furthermore, these infections are more common among people with a compromised immune system, premature infants, and children.

Meningococcal Meningitis

Meningococcal meningitis is caused by *Neisseria meningitidis,* a gram-negative, aerobic diplococcus with an antigenic polysaccharide capsule, responsible for the virulence of the organism. Depending on the geographic location, up to 20% of the population are asymptomatic carriers of the organism in their nose and throat, and therefore represent a reservoir of the infection.

Those most often infected are children under the age of 2 years, who have lost their maternal antibodies, usually after 6 months of age, which leaves them more susceptible to the infection. The bacterium is spread by person-to-person contact or by respiratory droplets. Carriers with other respiratory infections, such as the common cold, have an increase in respiratory secretions and can more readily spread the pathogen. Overcrowded conditions or confinement contribute to the spread of the infection and the likelihood of a disease outbreak.

The onset of meningococcal meningitis is sudden after an incubation period of 1 to 3 days. The symptoms include the following:

- A sore throat
- Headache
- Drowsiness
- Fever
- Neck stiffness
- Photosensitivity

In some patients the bacteria can proliferate in the bloodstream and a hemorrhagic skin rash reflecting septicemia can occur. This gram-negative sepsis is a life-threatening condition; if untreated it can lead to extensive tissue destruction and a need for amputations, and death can occur a few hours after the onset of fever. Antibiotic therapy reduces the mortality rate by 9% to 12%.

Neisseria meningitidis occurs in five capsular serotypes (A, B, C, Y, and W-135); their predominant occurrence varies with the geographic location. In the United States and other developed countries, meningococcal meningitis has been caused predominantly by serotypes B, C, and Y, whereas serotypes A and W-135 are more common in less developed countries. Polysaccharide vaccines are available against serotypes A, C, Y, and W-135, but not against serotype B.

Outbreaks of meningococcal meningitis occur globally. It is endemic in temperate climates, with sporadic cases or small clusters of cases exhibiting seasonal increases in winter and spring. In the United States sporadic outbreaks occur among college students who live in dormitories. Epidemics of meningococcal meningitis have occurred in Africa in periodic waves. In 2002 outbreaks occurred in the Great Lakes region of Central Africa in villages and refugee camps. More than 2200 cases were reported, including 200 deaths (Table 13.2). More recently, during 2007, 54,676 suspected cases of meningitis and 4062 deaths were reported from the "meningitis belt" region in Africa. This region covers 21 sub-Saharan African countries with a population of about 350 million people.

Haemophilus influenzae Meningitis

Haemophilus influenzae is an aerobic, gram-negative coccobacillus, commonly present in the normal flora of the throat. There are six serotypes of *H. influenzae,* differentiated by their capsular polysaccharide. Uncapsulated strains are common in the throat of most healthy people. Capsulated strain b (Hib) is a common inhabitant of the respiratory tract of infants and children. It occasionally enters the bloodstream and causes invasive diseases such as pneumonia, otitis media, epiglottitis, and meningitis.

Before the availability of the Hib conjugate vaccine in the United States and other industrialized countries, the leading cause of bacterial meningitis was *Haemophilus influenzae* serotype b in children under the age of 5 years. Because of the use

---

TABLE 13.2 Recent Outbreaks of Meningococcal Meningitis Worldwide

Time	Place	Number of Cases	Number of Deaths
Until May 12, 1999 (10.7 million doses of vaccine were distributed to the affected states)	19 states of Sudan	22,000	1600
August–September 1999	Angola (Yambala area)	253	147
September–October 1999	Rwanda	No reported numbers	
October 1999 to January 2000	Central African Republic	86	14
December 1999	Hungary	30	4
January to March 2000	Ethiopia		
	Kobo District of Amhara Region	81	3
	Alamata District of Tigray Region	48	6
2002	Great Lakes region (Africa)	2200	200
2002	Burkina Faso (W-135 emerged)	130,000	1500
2007	"Meningitis belt" (Africa)	54,676	4062

Meningitis: The Dorm Disease?

Bacterial meningitis, the swelling of the membranes surrounding the brain and spinal cord, can be caused by a number of different microorganisms. Most of the meningitis cases seen in children or young adults have been attributed to the bacterium *Neisseria meningitidis*. It affects 1400 to 3000 persons in the United States each year and is responsible for 150 to 300 deaths. Among young adults going to college there are 100 to 125 cases occurring on campuses each year, with 5 to 15 deaths. Because the organism is spread through the air by respiratory droplets or by direct contact such as oral contact with shared items such as a drinking glass or by kissing, this disease can be spread rapidly in areas where persons are living in crowded conditions, such as college dorms. Because of the unique conditions in the dorm environment, such as close contact, sharing of personal items, bar patronage, and irregular sleep patterns, college students living in residence halls are much more likely to acquire meningitis than is the rest of the college population. In 2005 the Centers for Disease Control and Prevention voted to recommend that all incoming college freshmen living in residence halls be vaccinated against meningitis. The American College Health Association (ACHA) further recommended that all first-year students living in dorms should be immunized and that all students under the age of 25 years should consider receiving the vaccination.

of the vaccine the incidence of this type of meningitis in young children has declined by more than 95%, but it still causes between 5% and 10% of bacterial meningitis cases in adults.

Transmission occurs by direct contact with respiratory droplets from a carrier or a patient. At-risk groups include infants and young children, persons in the same household as the patient, and day care center classmates. Treatment should be started as soon as disease is suspected and should be via intravenous (IV) antibiotics. Steroids are sometimes used, especially in children to reduce hearing loss, a common complication of meningitis. Preventive therapy is recommended for individuals who have had close contact with an infected individual. This type of contact includes sharing living space, kissing, sharing food and eating utensils, or other contact with oral secretions.

Prevention can be provided by several types of Hib vaccines available for children 2 months of age or older. Immunization is recommended for infants and children by the American Academy of Pediatrics, the National Institutes of Health, and other health agencies. Ideally, the first dose of the vaccine should be administered at the age of 2 months, followed by three or four booster vaccinations (see Chapter 20, The Immune System), depending on the brand of vaccine used.

Pneumococcal Meningitis

Pneumococcal meningitis is caused by *Streptococcus pneumoniae,* a gram-positive, encapsulated, facultatively anaerobic

diplococcus, carried in the throat of many healthy individuals. Differences in the composition of the polysaccharide capsule accounts for approximately 90 different serotypes, some of which are frequently associated with pneumococcal disease, others only rarely. With the decline in Hib meningitis, *Streptococcus pneumoniae* has become the most common cause of meningitis in adults, especially the elderly, and children between the ages of 1 month and 4 years.

Pneumococci are also the cause of millions of cases of acute **otitis media** (middle ear infection) annually (Figure 13.4), and approximately 500,000 cases of pneumonia per year in the United States (see Chapter 11, Infections of the Respiratory System). Middle ear infections are one of the most common reasons for physician's office visits in the United States, resulting in more than 20 million visits annually. In general, by the age of 12 months 60% of children have had at least one episode of acute otitis media. Complications of pneumococcal otitis media include mastoiditis and meningitis.

The immune response to a pneumococcal infection is directed primarily against the capsular serotype involved in a given infection. A conjugate vaccine has been developed and vaccination is recommended for all children less than 24 months old and others at risk. In general, vaccination is recommended for:

- High-risk persons age 2 years and over
- Everyone age 65 years and older
- Patients with sickle cell anemia
- Patients with splenectomy
- Patients with chronic organ failure
- Residents of nursing homes and other long-term care facilities
- People who live in institutions with residents who have chronic health problems
- People with a compromised immune system such as patients with HIV, patients with cancer, or patients who have received an organ transplant
- Persons who receive long-term immunosuppressive drugs, including steroids
- Alaskan natives and certain Native American populations who are genetically predisposed

A serious problem with pneumococcal diseases including meningitis is the increasing emergence of antibiotic-resistant strains of *S. pneumoniae* (also see Chapter 11, Infections of the Respiratory System). Antibiotic-resistant strains are most likely to emerge in settings where antibiotics are commonly prescribed such as in hospitals, nursing homes, and day care centers. At present between 10% and 40% of all infections caused by *S. pneumoniae* are resistant to at least one antibiotic, but more and more multidrug-resistant strains are emerging in the United States. Therefore, vaccination of at-risk groups will play an even more important role in preventing pneumococcal disease in the near future.

Listeria Meningitis

Listeria monocytogenes is a gram-positive coccobacillus and is the causative agent of listeriosis (see Chapter 12, Infections of

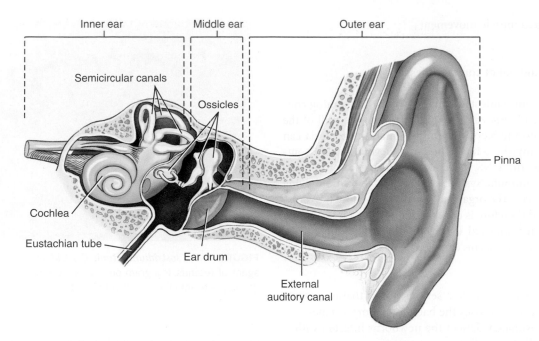

FIGURE 13.4 Anatomy of the human ear. The human ear consists of the outer ear, middle ear, and inner ear.

HEALTHCARE APPLICATION

Bacterial Meningitis

Pathogen	Transmission/Symptoms	Treatment	Prevention
Neisseria meningitidis	Person to person, contact with respiratory droplets or oral secretions Acute onset (6–24 h); skin rash	Penicillin, ampicillin, chloramphenicol, ceftriaxone	Polysaccharide vaccine; prophylaxis with rifampin for close contact
Haemophilus influenzae	Person to person, contact with respiratory droplets, body fluid Onset: 1–2 d	Ampicillin, ceftriaxone, or chloramphenicol	Polysaccharide vaccine against type b (Hib)
Streptococcus pneumoniae	Mostly through respiratory droplets Acute onset: May follow pneumonia and/or septicemia in elderly	Penicillin, ceftriaxone, or chloramphenicol	Prompt treatment of otitis media and respiratory infections; polysaccharide vaccine
Listeria monocytogenes	Foodborne Personality change, fever, uncoordinated muscle movement, tremors, seizures, loss of consciousness	Penicillin or ampicillin plus gentamicin	Avoidance of contaminated food products; complete cooking of all foods
Mycobacterium tuberculosis	Respiratory droplets Onset: Variable	Isoniazid and rifampin	BCG vaccination; isoniazid prophylaxis for contacts (recommended in the United States)
Escherichia coli and other coliforms	Newborns: During delivery at hospital, or at home	Antibiotics	

the Gastrointestinal System), a foodborne illness. This organism can spread from the bloodstream to the central nervous system, causing meningitis, especially in the elderly and in immuno-compromised patients, especially patients with cancer. *Listeria* meningitis is often fatal, and occurs in approximately half the cases of adult listeriosis. The more serious symptoms appear about 4 days after the initial symptoms of slight fever, headache, nausea, vomiting, diarrhea, and tiredness. The symptoms of *Listeria* meningitis include the following:

- Fever
- Personality change

- Uncoordinated muscle movement
- Tremors
- Seizures
- Slipping in and out of consciousness

A person becomes infected with *Listeria* by consuming contaminated food. *Listeria* can then pass through the wall of the intestine and into the bloodstream, by which the bacteria can be transported anywhere in the body; however, they are commonly found in the CNS. *Listeria* lives inside macrophages, hiding from the immune system, and is capable of multiplying in the macrophages. The organism is also small enough to cross the placenta, and therefore is capable of infecting a fetus. When an infant becomes infected before or during childbirth, two types of listeriosis may occur: early-onset disease and late-onset disease.

- *Early-onset disease* refers to a serious illness that is present at birth and usually causes the baby to be born prematurely. Approximately 50% of the newborns infected with *Listeria* will die of the illness.
- *Late-onset disease* occurs when a full-term baby becomes infected with *Listeria* during childbirth, and symptoms generally appear about 2 weeks after birth. These babies typically have meningitis, but have a better chance of survival than those with early-onset disease.

Listeriosis is treated with antibiotics; the duration of treatment varies and is dependent on the physiological state of the patient. The overall fatality rate for the disease is 26% because of the seriousness of the illness in newborns, the elderly, and immunocompromised patients.

Tetanus

Tetanus is an acute, often fatal illness, characterized by prolonged contraction of skeletal muscle fibers, resulting in generalized rigidity and convulsive spasms of the skeletal muscles. The symptoms are caused by tetanospasmin, a neurotoxin (exotoxin) produced by *Clostridium tetani,* a gram-positive, anaerobic rod that may develop a terminal spore, giving it a drumstick-like appearance (Figure 13.5). Whereas the vegetative organism is sensitive to heat and cannot survive the presence of oxygen, the spores are extremely resistant to heat as well as to the usual antiseptics. The spores are also relatively resistant to phenol and other chemical antimicrobial agents.

Spores of *Clostridium tetani* can be found in soil and in the intestines and feces of horses, sheep, cattle, dogs, cats, rats, guinea pigs, and chickens. As a result, manure-treated soil contains an especially large number of *Clostridium* spores. These spores can enter the human body through an anaerobic wound, as small as a scratch or cut, or through a much larger injury. Once spores gain entrance and get to an anaerobic environment, they germinate into the vegetative form. *C. tetani* then produces two types of exotoxins: tetanolysin and tetanospasmin. Although the function of tetanolysin is not completely understood, it is clear that tetanospasmin is the neurotoxin that causes the clinical manifestations of tetanus, and is one of the

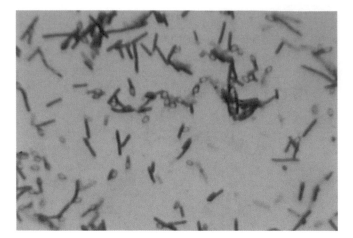

FIGURE 13.5 *Clostridium tetani.* *Clostridium tetani,* the causative agent of tetanus, is a gram-positive anaerobic rod that may develop a terminal spore, giving it a drumstick-like appearance.

most potent toxins known to humans. The estimated minimal lethal dose to humans is 2.5 nanograms (ng) per kilogram of body weight—1 ng is 1 billionth (10^{-9}) of a gram.

Clostridium tetani itself does not spread from the site of infection, and there is no accompanying inflammation. The organism releases its toxins, which are then carried via the peripheral nerves and probably also by the bloodstream to the central nervous system. The toxin then inhibits the release, by the spinal cord neurons, of inhibitory neurotransmitters that normally regulate the relaxation of muscle fibers, resulting in abnormal sustained muscle contraction known as **tetany** (a muscle spasm), which is unrelated to the physiological sustained controlled muscle contraction also called *tetanus*.

The incubation period of tetanus ranges from 3 to 21 days; the farther the injury occurs from the CNS the longer the incubation period. With shorter incubation periods the chance of a fatal outcome increases. On the basis of clinical findings, four different types of **tetanus** are described:

- *Local tetanus* occurs when patients have persistent contractions of muscles at the site of injury. This is an uncommon form of the illness and may persist for many weeks before gradually subsiding. Local tetanus is generally a milder condition and only about 1% of cases are fatal; however, the condition may precede the onset of generalized tetanus.
- *Cephalic tetanus* is a rare form of the disease, which can occur when *C. tetani* is present in the flora of the middle ear or following head injuries. This condition involves the cranial nerves, especially those innervating the facial area.
- *Generalized tetanus* is the most common type of tetanus, responsible for about 80% of reported cases. The first sign of this condition is trismus or lockjaw, followed by stiffness of the neck, difficulty in swallowing, and rigidity of the pectoral and calf muscles. Spasms may occur frequently and last for several minutes. These spasms may continue for 3 to 4 weeks and approximately 11% of reported cases have been fatal.

- *Neonatal tetanus* is a form of tetanus that occurs in newborns who have not acquired the necessary passive immunity from the mother, because she has never been immunized. The condition can occur through infections of an unhealed umbilical stump. This type of tetanus most commonly occurs in developing countries and is responsible for approximately 14% of all neonatal deaths. Neonatal tetanus is rare in the United States and other developed countries.

Botulism

Botulism is a rare, serious illness caused by *Clostridium botulinum,* an anaerobic, gram-positive, spore-forming rod that produces a potent neurotoxin (see also Chapter 12, Infections of the Gastrointestinal System). The organism and its spores are widely distributed in nature. They are present in cultivated and forest soils; the bottom sediment of streams, lakes, and coastal waters; and also in the intestinal tract of fish and mammals and in the gills and viscera of crabs and other shellfish. Seven serotypes of botulism are documented (A, B, C, D, E, F, and G), based on the antigenic specificity of the toxin produced by each strain. Only types A, B, E, and F cause human botulism; types C and D are the cause of most cases of botulism in animals. The toxins produced by the different strains vary considerably in their virulence factors.

- Type A toxin is probably the most virulent of all the botulinum toxins, with lethality occurring at 10^{-9} g levels of exposure. Death can occur when contaminated food is only tasted, not even swallowed. Lethal doses can also be absorbed by small breaks in the skin. If untreated, intoxication with type A toxins results in a 60% to 70% mortality rate. In the United States the strain producing type A toxin is found predominantly in California, Washington, Colorado, Oregon, and New Mexico.
- Type B toxin is responsible for most European outbreaks of botulism and also is the most common type in the eastern United States. The mortality rate is about 25% if left untreated.
- Type E toxin is produced by a *Clostridium* species commonly found in marine or lake sediments, and therefore outbreaks are usually associated with seafood, especially in the Pacific Northwest, Alaska, and the Great Lakes area of the United States.
- Type F toxin is also produced by *C. baratii* and has been shown to cause infant botulism. Type F toxin is also used in the treatment of spasmodic torticollis, a painful and debilitating neurological movement disorder.

Four types of botulism are recognized (also see Chapter 12, Infections of the Gastrointestinal System):

1. Foodborne botulism
2. Infant botulism
3. Wound botulism
4. Inhalation botulism

As stated previously, the botulinum toxin is a **neurotoxin,** a protein that is toxic to nerve cells and is one of the most poisonous naturally occurring substances known. The infective dose is a very small amount, with illness occurring on exposure to only a few nanograms.

Once the botulinum toxin enters the body, the toxin binds to nerve endings at the neuromuscular junction, which stops the release of the neurotransmitter acetylcholine and thereby inhibits muscular contraction. Thus, exposure of the neuromuscular junction to these neurotoxins results in a flaccid paralysis. The common symptoms of all forms of botulism include the following:

- Dry mouth
- Difficulty swallowing
- Slurred speech
- Drooping eyelids

MEDICAL HIGHLIGHTS

Tetanus: The Tale of the Rusty Nail

Tetanus is a disease caused by the toxin produced by the organism *Clostridium tetani,* an anaerobic, spore-forming rod. *C. tetani* is a ubiquitous organism readily found in the soil. The toxin produced causes the skeletal muscles to contract and remain in the contracted state, with the victim being unable to relax the muscles. These muscles include the muscles that facilitate and support breathing. Unable to inhale or exhale, a victim will be unable to breathe and suffocation is the lethal result. One of the typical misconceptions of many is that rust in a puncture wound from a rusty nail can cause tetanus. The environment or conditions in which a person might encounter a rusty nail injury is actually what makes this type of injury a potentially dangerous one. A rusty nail would most typically be found in the outdoors, in contact with the soil. Because *C. tetani* is a natural inhabitant of the soil, there is a good chance that if the organism is near the nail, the spores produced would find the rough, rusty surface of the metal a convenient place to become "attached." Although the spores do not have the ability to actively attach themselves to the surface, the rough physical nature of the nail surface may allow the spores to be deposited in the "nooks and crannies" of the corroded metal. When the nail penetrates the skin and the underlying tissue, a deep puncture hole may be created. When the nail is removed and the blood clots over the small entry wound, a potentially anaerobic environment is created. In this miniature anaerobic growth chamber of the wound channel, the spores are able to revert back to the vegetative state. It is during this transition from spore to vegetative cell that the toxin is produced. Ironically, it's when the nail is removed and the healing process begins that the potential danger of *C. tetani* also begins.

- Muscle weakness
- Double and/or blurred vision
- Vomiting, and sometimes diarrhea

The muscle weakness and paralysis descend from the cranium, affecting all muscles including the muscles that regulate breathing (diaphragmatic and intercostal muscles). Botulism is not an infection; it is an intoxication, caused by the botulinum toxin.

Although the incidence of the disease is low, the mortality rate is high if not treated immediately and properly. Death from botulinum intoxication is generally due to respiratory failure caused by paralysis of the diaphragmatic and intercostal muscles. Therefore, the treatment required is botulinal antitoxin administration and artificial ventilation. The functional recovery time may take several weeks to months.

Leprosy

Leprosy (Hansen's disease) is a chronic, slowly progressive disease caused by *Mycobacterium leprae,* an intracellular, pleomorphic, acid-fast, gram-positive, aerobic bacillus that is surrounded by the characteristic waxy coating unique to mycobacteria. The illness affects the following:

MEDICAL HIGHLIGHTS

Vanity: Thy Name is Botulism

Botulism is a dangerous, potentially deadly disease caused by neurotoxins produced by the gram-positive, spore-forming, anaerobic organism called *Clostridium botulinum.* The neurotoxin blocks the release of acetylcholine at the nerve synapse, which prevents the signal from reaching the skeletal muscle. The victim will suffer paralysis, which in turn results in respiratory failure and, if untreated, death. The same action of the neurotoxin that can cause death can also be used for a number of useful applications. One of the applications in vogue today is Botox. Botox is the registered trademark for botulinum toxin and is used today as a cosmetic treatment to eliminate the wrinkles of aging. When injected into the superficial muscles of the face and neck the toxin causes localized paralysis, thus relaxing the muscles under the skin and eliminating surface wrinkles, resulting in a smooth skin surface. The treatment is not permanent and as the toxin degrades, new toxin must be injected. This procedure has been deemed safe by the U.S. Food and Drug Administration (FDA); however, it is not without potential consequences. Because the superficial muscles of the face are essential for facial expression, aggressive injections of Botox can result in an expressionless, masklike appearance of the face. There are also a few cases in which improper use of the cosmetic toxin produced the onset of full-blown botulism, resulting in widespread paralysis and death.

- The skin (see Chapter 10, Infections of the Integumentary System, Soft Tissue, and Muscle)
- The peripheral nerves, primarily those in the hands and feet
- The mucous membranes of the nose, throat, and eyes (Figure 13.6).

Leprosy was one of the most common infectious diseases of ancient times, and is still a significant health problem in parts of Africa, Asia, the South Pacific, and in some South American countries. Although the disease was thought to be transmissible even by the slightest contact, it is actually less communicable than most other infectious diseases. Most cases of leprosy in the United States involve people who have emigrated from developing countries.

About 95% of people exposed to *Mycobacterium leprae* do not develop the disease because of their intact immune system. The infection can start at any age, but most often starts with people in their 20s and 30s. The incubation period varies from 6 months to 10 years. Patients with the disease are classified as having paucibacillary (tuberculoid) or multibacillary (lepromatous) Hansen's disease. Death from leprosy is rare and is usually a result of infections of the leprous lesions, and not the pathogen itself.

Paucibacillary Hansen's disease is characterized by one or more hypopigmented cutaneous lesions and damaged peripheral nerves that have been attacked by the host's immune system. This causes a loss of sensation in the affected nerves and people with peripheral nerve damage may unwittingly damage and harm the affected areas. Repeated damage may eventually result in loss of fingers and toes. Furthermore, damage to the peripheral nerves may also cause muscle weakness, resulting in a clawing posture of the fingers ("claw hand") and a "drop foot" deformity.

Multibacillary Hansen's disease is the more virulent form of the disease and is manifested by the following:

- Symmetric skin lesions
- Nodules

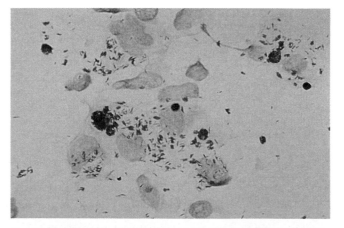

FIGURE 13.6 *Mycobacterium leprae. Mycobacterium leprae,* the causative agent of leprosy, is seen here in nasal scrapings. (Courtesy I. Farrell. From Mims C, Dockrell HM, Goering RV, et al.: *Medical microbiology,* ed 3, St. Louis, 2004, Mosby.)

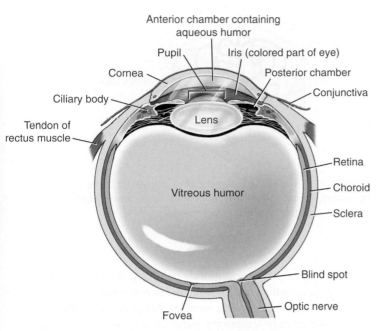

FIGURE 13.7 Human eye. The conjunctiva is the transparent membrane that lines the eyelid and part of the eyeball. It is a portal of entry for many microorganisms.

- Plaques
- Thickened dermis that may also involve the nasal mucosa, resulting in nasal congestion and nose bleeds. In general, there is no nerve damage with this condition.

Transmission of the disease is still not completely understood, but most studies indicate that the disease is transmitted by close and extended contact from person to person via respiratory droplets. Although antibiotic treatment can stop the progression of leprosy it does not reverse any nerve damage or deformity. Early detection and treatment are essential. Because of the development of antibiotic resistance the World Health Organization (WHO, Geneva, Switzerland) recommends a multidrug treatment consisting of dapsone, rifampin, and clofazimine. However, because of the considerable expense of this treatment it has not been implemented in many of the endemic areas of the world.

Conjunctivitis

Conjunctivitis (pink eye) can be caused by bacteria, viruses, allergies, chemicals, or a foreign object. Both the bacterial and viral forms of conjunctivitis are contagious. Because bacterial conjunctivitis is the most common type of ocular infections it is discussed in this section. Conjunctivitis is the inflammation or infection of the conjunctiva, the transparent membrane that lines the eyelid and part of the eyeball (Figure 13.7). The inflammation causes small blood vessels to become more prominent, causing the pink or red appearance of the eye. The most common symptoms of conjunctivitis include the following:

- Redness
- Itchiness
- Roughness
- Discharge
- Tearing

Bacteria that can cause conjunctivitis include but are not limited to *Streptococcus pneumoniae, Haemophilus influenzae, Staphylococcus aureus, Haemophilus* spp., *Chlamydia trachomatis, Neisseria gonorrhoeae, Streptococcus pyogenes, Moraxella* spp., and *Corynebacterium* spp. In newborns, neisserial and chlamydial infections are frequent and acquired during passage through an infected birth canal. Because of the application of antibiotic drops into the eyes of newborns, the incidence of conjunctivitis in newborns in the United States has dropped dramatically. *Chlamydia trachomatis* is one of the leading causes of blindness in the world, mainly in underdeveloped countries.

The infection can be treated with antibiotic eyedrops or eye ointment and should clear within several days. Practicing good hygiene is the best way to control the spread of pink eye.

Viral Infections

Viruses are transmitted by person-to-person contact, respiratory droplets, the fecal–oral route, trauma, injection with contaminated objects or needles, transplants and blood transfusions, insects or animal bites, during gestation, and sexually. Most viruses enter the central nervous system via the circulatory system; however, some can gain access by other pathways such as the peripheral nerves. Several viral infections can be prevented by vaccination; many others can be treated with specific antiviral drugs. In addition, most viral infections need to be treated by supportive therapy such as rehydration and pain control.

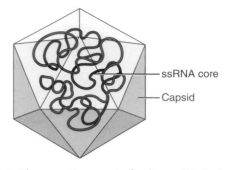

FIGURE 13.8 The causative agent of poliomyelitis is the poliovirus, a small, nonenveloped, ssRNA virus, and human enterovirus of the family of *Picornaviridae*.

Viral Meningitis

Viral meningitis is relatively common but, in contrast to bacterial meningitis, is usually not serious. Viral meningitis is called *aseptic meningitis* (see Table 13.1) and can be caused by any number of viruses, most of which are associated with another disease. Most often it is spread by direct contact with infected feces or nose and throat secretions. Moreover, mosquitoes can be a vector and transmit viral meningitis, usually in the summer and fall. Viral meningitis in the winter months is usually due to another underlying disease. It spreads most rapidly among young children and also in group living environments where running water is in short supply. Although anyone can get the illness, most people over 40 years of age seem to be immune.

Symptoms of viral meningitis include fever, headache, stiff neck, and tiredness. A rash, sore throat, and vomiting may also occur. Appropriate hand washing and avoidance of mosquito bites help prevent the illness. There is no treatment for viral meningitis, and in most cases the immune system will produce the antibodies necessary to destroy the virus. Usually viral meningitis starts suddenly; however, babies may have a gradual illness manifested by refusal to eat, being more sleepy than usual, and fussy. Although rare, bulging of a fontanelle (soft spot) may occur and usually is a late sign of the infection. Most children and adults recover completely within 10 to 14 days.

Poliomyelitis

The causative agent of poliomyelitis is the poliovirus, a small, nonenveloped, single-stranded RNA (ssRNA) virus, a human enterovirus of the family Picornaviridae (Figure 13.8). Usually poliovirus replicates within the gastrointestinal tract and is shed with the feces, and therefore it is spread from person to person via the fecal–oral route. The incubation period varies from 6 to 20 days. Approximately 95% of all infections are asymptomatic and about 4% to 8% of the infections result in a minor, nonspecific illness without clinical or laboratory evidence of central nervous system invasion. This condition is referred to as *abortive poliomyelitis* and complete recovery occurs in less than 1 week.

In approximately 1% to 2% of all poliovirus infections the virus enters the CNS and replicates within the motor neurons of the spinal cord, brainstem, or motor cortex, all of which lead to temporary or permanent muscle paralysis, and overall 5% to 10% of patients with paralytic polio die of respiratory arrest, due to paralysis of the intercostal muscles. Many cases of poliomyelitis result in only temporary paralysis and within 1 month nerve impulses return to the temporarily paralyzed muscles and recovery can be complete within 6 to 8 months.

The virus is transmitted primarily by ingestion of water contaminated with fecal material containing the virus. The infection is initiated by ingestion and the areas of multiplication are the throat and the small intestine, accounting for the initial sore throat and nausea. The neurological phase of the infection seems to be an accidental result of the normal gastrointestinal infection. Once the virus infects the throat, it then enters the tonsils and the lymph nodes and via this route then can enter the bloodstream, causing viremia. In the majority of cases the infection does not go beyond the lymphatic system, but occasionally the virus passes through the capillary endothelium and enters the CNS, where it infects predominantly motor neurons. As a result of viral multiplication the motor neurons die, and paralysis results.

Several factors increase the risk for infection or affect the severity of the disease and these include the following:

- Immune deficiency
- Malnutrition
- Tonsillectomy
- Physical activity immediately after the onset of paralysis
- Intramuscular injection
- Pregnancy

Maternal antibodies to the poliovirus do cross the placenta and provide passive immunity (see Chapter 20, The Immune System) to the infant during the first few months of life.

Three different serotypes of the poliovirus exist, each with a slightly different capsid: PV1 (Mahoney), PV2 (Lansing), and PV3 (Leon). All three serotypes are extremely infectious, but PV1 is the most common form found in nature. Notably, infection with one type of poliovirus does not provide immunity against the other types, and therefore prevention via vaccines must be provided for all three types. At present two vaccines are used to combat polio: the Salk vaccine or inactivated poliovirus vaccine (IPV), first developed in 1952, and the

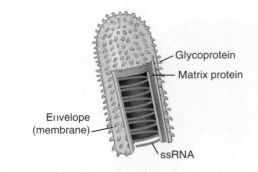

FIGURE 13.9 Rabies virus. The rabies virus is a nonsegmented, negative-sense ssRNA virus with a distinct "bullet" shape.

Sabin or oral polio vaccine (OVP), licensed in 1962. Starting in 1988 the extensive use of poliovirus vaccines in an effort to eradicate polio resulted in a 99% reduction of annually diagnosed cases worldwide. This global effort was led by the WHO, United Nations Children's Fund (UNICEF), and Rotary Foundation.

In the United States only IPV is available for routine polio vaccination of children. In 2002, a five-component vaccine (Pediarix) was approved for use in the United States. The vaccine contains IPV, DTaP (diphtheria, tetanus, and pertussis), and a pediatric dose of hepatitis B vaccine.

About 25% to 40% of individuals who have survived paralytic polio during childhood experience new muscle pain and exacerbation of existing weakness, or develop new weakness or paralysis 30 to 40 years after the initial illness. This condition is referred to as *postpolio syndrome* (PPS). The pathogenesis of the syndrome seems to involve the failure of oversized motor units that were generated during recovery from the original paralytic poliomyelitis, and/or the overuse and disuse of neurons. Postpolio syndrome is not infectious and the poliovirus cannot be shed by persons with the syndrome.

Rabies

Rabies is a preventable zoonotic disease caused by the rabies virus, which belongs to the order Mononegavirales, family Rhabdoviridae, and genus *Lyssavirus*. It is a nonsegmented, negative-sense ssRNA virus with a distinct "bullet" shape (Figure 13.9), and is capable of causing acute encephalitis in all warm-blooded hosts. Although all species of mammals are susceptible to the rabies virus, only a few species are the reservoir of distinct rabies virus variants of the disease in the United States. These variants can be detected in raccoons, skunks, foxes, and coyotes, as well as in some insectivorous bats. Rabies can also spread to domestic farm animals, groundhogs, weasels, dogs, and cats. Most animals that can be infected by the virus can also transmit the disease to humans.

Transmission of the virus commonly begins when infected saliva enters an uninfected host. Different routes of entry have been reported, including mucous membranes such as those of the eyes, nose, and mouth; aerosol transmission; and corneal transplantation. However, the most common mode of transmission is through a bite or scratch of an infected animal (host).

Less than 10% of reported rabies cases involve domestic cats, dogs, and cattle.

Symptoms of rabies are usually vague but they include the following:

- Fatigue
- Muscle aches
- Anxiety
- Irritability
- Agitation
- Insomnia
- Headache
- Nausea
- Vomiting
- Abdominal pain

Early symptoms manifest themselves with pain, itchiness, and numbness at the site of the bite or scratch, and occur in about 55% to 60% of patients. Untreated rabies can lead to coma and death. There is no treatment for rabies after the symptoms of the disease occur. However, immunization given within 2 days of a bite or scratch usually prevents the onset of rabies, and generally rabies does not develop if the vaccine is given promptly. Preexposure vaccination does not eliminate the need for additional treatment, but is recommended for persons in high-risk environments, such as veterinarians, animal handlers, and laboratory personnel, or other individuals whose daily activities puts them at risk to contract rabies.

Postexposure prophylaxis (PEP) is necessary for people possibly exposed to a rabid animal. This includes animal bites, or mucous membrane contamination with infectious tissue, or exposure to saliva. In the United States, PEP consists of a regimen of one dose of immunoglobulin, given as soon as possible after exposure, and five doses of rabies vaccine over a 28-day period. The CDC recommends that any dog, cat, or ferret that bites a person should be confined and observed for 10 days if vaccination of the animal cannot be proven.

To prevent the spread of rabies, pet owners should do the following:

- Keep vaccinations up-to-date for all dogs, cats, ferrets, and other pets
- Keep pets under direct supervision so that they do not come in contact with wild animals
- Inform the local animal control agency to remove any stray animals from the neighborhood
- Spay or neuter pets to help reduce the number of unwanted pets, which may not be properly cared for or vaccinated on a regular basis
- Avoid contact with wild animals

Arboviral Encephalitis

Arthropod-borne viruses, or arboviruses, are transmitted and maintained through biological transmission between a susceptible vertebrate host and mosquitoes, psychodids, ceratopogonids, and ticks. Vertebrate infection occurs due to arthropods that take a blood meal. Encephalitis caused

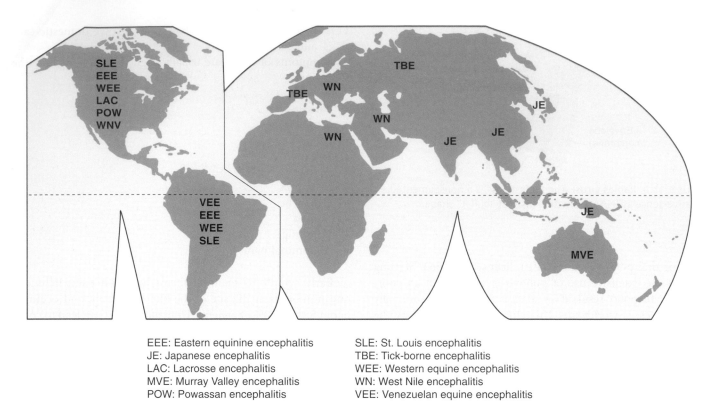

EEE: Eastern equinine encephalitis
JE: Japanese encephalitis
LAC: Lacrosse encephalitis
MVE: Murray Valley encephalitis
POW: Powassan encephalitis

SLE: St. Louis encephalitis
TBE: Tick-borne encephalitis
WEE: Western equine encephalitis
WN: West Nile encephalitis
VEE: Venezuelan equine encephalitis

FIGURE 13.10 Arboviral global distribution.

by these arthropods is fairly common in the United States. Arboviruses that cause human encephalitis belong to the families Togaviridae, Flaviviridae, and Bunyaviridae (see Chapter 7, Viruses).

Arboviral encephalitides have a global distribution (Figure 13.10), but the viral agents currently present in the United States include the following: eastern equine encephalitis (EEE), western equine encephalitis (WEE), St. Louis encephalitis (SLE), La Crosse (LAC) encephalitis, and more recently West Nile virus (WNV) encephalitis, all transmitted via mosquitoes. WNV infects a large number of bird species such as crows and blue jays and has now spread throughout the United States.

- *Eastern equine encephalitis (EEE):* EEE virus is a member of the family Togaviridae, genus *Alphavirus* and causes illness in humans, horses, and some bird species. Transmission of the virus to humans occurs via an infected mosquito and symptoms develop 3 to 10 days after the bite occurred.
- *Western equine encephalitis (WEE)* is caused by an *Alphavirus* species, transmitted by mosquitoes. The infection can cause a range of illnesses from no symptoms to a fatal condition. Mild illness manifests itself as a headache and fever, whereas more severe disease can show the following:
  - Sudden high fever
  - Headache
  - Drowsiness
  - Irritability
  - Nausea

- Vomiting
- Confusion
- Weakness
- Coma

Symptoms usually occur by 5 to 10 days after being bitten by an infected mosquito. At present no licensed vaccine is available for human use and no specific treatment is available for this infection.

- *St. Louis encephalitis (SLE):* The St. Louis encephalitis virus is mosquito borne, a *Flavivirus* species that can cause aseptic meningitis or encephalitis. The fatality rate ranges from 3% to 30%, mostly in the at-risk groups including the elderly and people with an outdoor occupation. However, the majority of infections are subclinical or a mild illness, including fever and headache. The majority of cases in the United States occur in the late summer or early fall, but in milder climates the illness can occur year round. At present no treatment or vaccine is available for the St. Louis encephalitis virus.
- *La Crosse (LAC) encephalitis* is a rare viral infection spread by mosquitoes and usually affects children. The infection is found primarily in the upper Midwestern United States and in the Appalachian region. The majority of infections are subclinical or result in mild illness; symptoms include nausea, headache, and vomiting and severe cases can cause seizures, coma, paralysis, and brain damage. At present no therapy is available and management of the condition is limited to treatment of the symptoms.
- *West Nile virus (WNV) encephalitis* is another arbovirus transmitted by mosquitoes and is common in areas such as

Africa, western Asia, and the Middle East. Symptoms of infection include the following:

- Skin rash
- Headache
- Fever
- Diarrhea
- Nausea
- Vomiting
- Back and muscle aches
- Lack of appetite
- Swollen lymph glands

In less than 1% of cases the virus can cause a serious neurological infection including encephalitis, meningitis, and a condition called *West Nile poliomyelitis* (an inflammation of the spinal cord). Most victims of West Nile virus recover without treatment and even those patients with neurological infections usually need only supportive therapy such as intravenous fluids and pain relievers. The best prevention for West Nile virus infections is to avoid exposure to mosquitoes and to eliminate breeding sites.

Fungal Infections

Fungal infections of the nervous system are far less common than bacterial and viral infections. Most fungal infections are opportunistic, and therefore they take on more importance in all immunocompromised persons, including cancer patients undergoing chemotherapy, patients with AIDS, or patients receiving immunosuppressive therapy for organ transplantation.

Cryptococcosis

Cryptococcosis is a rare infection caused by the fungus *Cryptococcus neoformans,* an encapsulated yeast present worldwide. The fungus is found in soil, especially in soil contaminated with bird droppings. Once the fungus enters the body through inhalation or through a wound it can cause the following:

- Wound or cutaneous cryptococcosis
- Pulmonary cryptococcosis
- Cryptococcal meningitis

Cryptococcal meningitis most often affects immunocompromised persons including patients with AIDS, cancer, and/or diabetes. Initial symptoms of the infection may be vague including mild headache, fever, and nausea. As the infection progresses the following symptoms may appear:

- Severe headache
- Nausea with vomiting
- Blurred vision and light sensitivity (photophobia)
- Stiff neck
- Seizures
- Confusion

- Change in behavior
- Coma

Antifungal intravenous medications are typically used to treat this condition; however, long-term oral medication is suggested for patients with AIDS, to prevent recurrence of the infection.

Protozoan Infections

Although many infectious diseases are caused by endogenous organisms, diseases caused by protozoan and helminthic parasites are being caused by an exogenous source. Many of these infections are acquired via the bites of an arthropod vector, others by ingestion or inhalation of contaminated material from animal or human wastes, or through a break in the skin.

Cerebral Toxoplasmosis

Toxoplasmosis is caused by *Toxoplasma gondii,* an obligate intracellular protozoan parasite. Most infected individuals do not show any symptoms, but the infection can be serious, even fatal in individuals with a compromised immune system. In general, human infections occur via the oral or transplacental route, through the consumption of undercooked meat contaminated with viable cysts, or by direct ingestion of oocytes from contaminated soil or water.

A pregnant woman who contracts toxoplasmosis has a more than 30% chance of passing the infection to her fetus (see Congenital Toxoplasmosis in Chapter 23, Human Age and Microorganisms). Typical symptoms are speech difficulties, seizures, confusion, and lethargy, usually over a period of days to weeks. Treatment includes the use of corticosteroids to reduce cerebral edema and a regimen of trimethoprim-sulfamethoxazole.

Trypanosomiasis

Hemoflagellates of the genus *Trypanosoma* are the causative agents of African trypanosomiasis (sleeping sickness) and Chagas' disease (American trypanosomiasis).

African Trypanosomiasis

African trypanosomiasis, also referred to as *sleeping sickness,* is caused by the protozoan *Trypanosoma brucei.* It is spread by the bite of the tsetse fly. The organism enters the bloodstream and then travels to the CNS, where it can cause meningitis or encephalitis. The main symptom of the disease is coma, which is why it is called *sleeping sickness.* One of the difficulties in treating the infection is the fact that the organism is able to change its surface proteins, challenging the immune system to keep making new antibodies to respond to the new surface antigens. Thus far, there is no effective treatment available and there is no vaccine because of this ability of the organism to keep changing antigens. The best measures to prevent the disease are through the use of insect netting and insecticides.

Chagas' Disease

Chagas' disease, also referred to as *American trypanosomiasis*, is caused by the protozoan *Trypanosoma cruzi*. It is typically spread by the bite of a reduviid ("kissing bug"), which bites around the mouth and other facial sites. They will bite, feed on the blood and tissue juices, and then defecate into the wound, giving the organisms in the feces a portal of entry. If the organism invades the CNS it may produce granulomas in the brain with cyst formation and meningoencephalitis. In extreme cases, in which the disease causes significant tissue damage in the brain, death can result. At present the drug of choice for treating Chagas' disease is nifurtimox, but the most effective measures in controlling the disease are preventive in nature. Insect control, eradication of nests, and even the limited use of dichlorodiphenyltrichloroethane (DDT) in bug-infested homes will contribute significantly to the prevention of this disease.

Prion-associated Diseases

Prion diseases or transmissible spongiform encephalopathies (TSEs) are a related group of rare, infectious, fatal, and progressive neurodegenerative diseases that affect various animals and humans. The causative agents for these diseases are believed to be prions, molecules that begin as a normal protein in animal tissue but abnormally fold and become infectious particles (see Chapter 7, Viruses). Prion diseases have a long incubation time, usually years; however, once the disease process starts they are usually rapidly progressive and always fatal. In humans, prion diseases impair brain function, causing memory changes, personality changes, dementia, and movement disorders that worsen with time. At present, there are no known ways to cure TSE diseases. Prion diseases identified to date include the following:

- Human prion diseases
  - Creutzfeldt-Jakob disease (CJD) is a rare, degenerative, fatal brain disorder. Symptoms generally occur around age 60 years. The only confirmed diagnosis of CJD is biopsy or autopsy. Three major categories of CJD are currently known: sporadic CJD, hereditary CJD, and acquired CJD. There is no treatment to cure or control CJD. Current treatment is to alleviate symptoms of pain and to relieve involuntary muscle movements.
  - Variant Creutzfeldt-Jakob disease (vCJD) is also a rare and fatal human neurodegenerative condition and a new disease that was first described in 1996. In contrast to the traditional forms of CJD, vCJD affects younger persons with the average age of 29 years and has a longer duration of illness. It is strongly linked to exposure, and is most likely foodborne through TSE of cattle (bovine spongiform encephalopathy).
  - Gerstmann-Sträussler-Scheinker syndrome (GSSS) is a particularly rare form of human TSE due to a defective gene encoding the prion protein (PRNP gene) and is identified by particular multicentric amyloid plaques (predominantly in the frontal lobe) in the brain. There is currently no treatment of the underlying pathological mechanisms of the disease.
  - Fatal familial insomnia is also a rare prion disease that interferes with sleep and leads to the deterioration of mental and motor functions; death occurs within a few months to a few years. Fatal insomnia is usually inherited (autosomal dominant) or can also occur sporadically without genetic mutation. No treatment is available at this time.
  - Kuru is an endemic, fatal disease among the Fore tribe of Papua New Guinea, caused by the practice of cannibalism, specifically the eating of brain tissue. As with other TSEs, kuru has a long incubation period and it might even take decades before an infected individual shows symptoms. Symptoms include headaches, joint pains, slurred speech, and shaking of the limbs, because the disease affects mainly the cerebellum (responsible for coordination).
- Animal prion diseases
  - Bovine spongiform encephalopathy (mad cow disease)
  - Chronic wasting disease
  - Scrapie
  - Transmissible mink encephalopathy
  - Feline spongiform encephalopathy
  - Ungulate spongiform encephalopathy

Historically, many of these diseases were called *"slow virus infections,"* a poorly defined group of proposed viral diseases, later found to be caused by prions. Many questions about the prion biosafety of food and drugs remain and many aspects of the basic mechanisms of prions remain unclear. At present no test is available to detect prion infectivity in human blood.

Summary

- The nervous system is divided into the central and peripheral nervous systems and is generally protected from microbial invasion by the meninges and the blood–brain barrier. Infection of the protective CNS membranes (meninges) is referred to as *meningitis*; if the brain tissue itself becomes inflamed the condition is call encephalitis. A variety of microorganisms can cause one or both of these conditions.
- Meningitis manifests itself as fever, headache, and a stiff neck, followed by nausea, vomiting, confusion, sleepiness, and light sensitivity. If untreated, meningitis can lead to convulsions and coma. Bacterial meningitis is less common than viral meningitis but is generally much more severe in nature.
- Tetanus, an acute and often fatal illness, is caused by *Clostridium tetani*, a bacterium that produces a neurotoxin responsible for the symptoms of tetanus. On the basis of clinical findings, four different forms of tetanus are known: local tetanus, cephalic tetanus, generalized tetanus, and neonatal tetanus.

- Botulism is a rare but serious illness caused by various strains of *Clostridium botulinum,* which is capable of producing neurotoxins of different degrees of virulence. Botulinum toxin is one of the most poisonous naturally occurring substances known.
- Leprosy is a chronic, slowly progressive disease that affects the skin and peripheral nerves, primarily in the hands and feet. It is less communicable than most other infectious diseases.
- Poliomyelitis is an acute viral infectious disease spread from person to person, usually by the fecal–oral route. Most infections are asymptomatic but if the virus enters the central nervous system it infects and destroys motor neurons.
- Rabies is a preventable zoonotic disease capable of causing acute encephalitis in all warm-blooded hosts. Transmission begins when infected saliva enters the host, usually through a bite or scratch by an infected animal.
- Fungal infections of the nervous system are less common than bacterial or viral infections. Most fungal infections are opportunistic, capable of causing severe problems for immunocompromised persons.
- Protozoan and helminthic infections of the nervous system are acquired via bites of an arthropod, a break in the skin, or by ingestion or inhalation of contaminated materials from animal or human wastes. These infections include cerebral toxoplasmosis and trypanosomiasis.
- Prion diseases or transmissible spongiform encephalopathies (TSEs) are a related group neurodegenerative disorders caused by abnormally folded proteins, called *prions.*

Review Questions

1. An inflammation of the brain is called:
   a. Meningitis
   b. Meningoencephalitis
   c. Encephalitis
   d. Bacteremia

2. Routine vaccination against meningitis in the United States is provided against:
   a. *Neisseria meningitidis*
   b. *Haemophilus influenzae*
   c. *Mycobacterium tuberculosis*
   d. *Listeria monocytogenes*

3. Meningococcal meningitis is caused by:
   a. *Neisseria meningitidis*
   b. *Haemophilus influenzae*
   c. *Mycobacterium tuberculosis*
   d. *Listeria monocytogenes*

4. Otitis media is commonly caused by which microorganism?
   a. *Staphylococcus epidermidis*
   b. *Listeria monocytogenes*
   c. *Haemophilus influenzae*
   d. *Streptococcus pneumoniae*

5. The most virulent of all botulinum toxins is considered to be:
   a. Type A
   b. Type B
   c. Type E
   d. Type F

6. Hansen's disease is also called:
   a. Tetanus
   b. Leprosy
   c. Kuru
   d. *Listeria* meningitis

7. Poliomyelitis is caused by a virus belonging to the family:
   a. Rhabdoviridae
   b. Reoviridae
   c. Picornaviridae
   d. Bunyaviridae

8. Which of the following is the causative agent for fungal meningitis, mostly in immunocompromised patients?
   a. *Trypanosoma brucei*
   b. *Listeria meningitis*
   c. *Cryptococcus neoformans*
   d. *Trypanosoma cruzi*

9. The organism causing West Nile encephalitis belongs to which of the following?
   a. Arboviruses
   b. Parvoviruses
   c. Flaviviruses
   d. Paramyxoviruses

10. "Sleeping sickness" is caused by which type of microorganism?
    a. Bacterium
    b. Virus
    c. Protozoan
    d. Prion

11. When both the brain and the meninges are inflamed the condition is referred to as _____.

12. Pneumococcal meningitis is caused by _____.

13. African trypanosomiasis is caused by _____.

14. American trypanosomiasis is also referred to as _____ disease.

15. Chemically, prions are _____.

16. Compare and contrast bacterial and viral meningitis.

17. Elaborate on the four clinically different types of tetanus.

18. Describe the steps a pet owner should take to prevent the spread of rabies.

19. Discuss botulism, the different types of toxins, and the geographic prevalence.

20. Describe two prion-associated diseases of humans.

Bibliography

Aguzzi A, Heikenwalder M, Polymenidou M: Insights into prion strains and neurotoxicity, Nature Reviews, *Molecular Cell Biology* 8:552–561, 2007.

Forbes BA, Sahm DF, Weissfeld AS: *Bailey & Scott's diagnostic microbiology*, ed 12, St. Louis, 2007, Mosby/Elsevier.

Mahon CR, Lehman DC, Manuselis G: *Textbook of diagnostic microbiology*, ed 3, St. Louis, 2007, Saunders/Elsevier.

Mastny L: *Eradicating polio: a model for international cooperation*, Washington DC, 1999, Worldwatch Institute.

Mims C, Dockrell HM, Goering RV, et al: *Medical microbiology*, ed 3, St. Louis, 2004, Mosby/Elsevier.

Murray PR, Rosenthal KS, Pfaller MA: *Medical microbiology*, ed 5, St. Louis, 2005, Mosby/Elsevier.

National Institute of Communicable Diseases: Meningococcal disease, CD*Alert* 2005;9:1–8. Available at http://nicd.nic.in/cdalert/April-05.pdf).

Neumann D: *Polio: its impact on the people of the United States and the emerging profession of physical therapy*, J Orthop Sports Phys Ther 34(8):479–492, 2004.

Thibodeau GA, Patton KT: *Anatomy and physiology*, ed 6, St. Louis, 2007, Mosby/Elsevier.

Trojan D, Cashman N: *Post-poliomyelitis syndrome*, Muscle Nerve 31(1):6–19, 2005.

Internet Resources

Barash JR, Tang TWH, Arnon SS: First case of infant botulism caused by *Clostridium baratii* type F in California, *J Clin Microbiol* 43(8):4280–4282, 2005 (accessed November 19, 2008). Copyright © 2005, American Society for Microbiology, available at http://www.pubmedcentral.nih.gov/articlerender.fcgi?artid=1233924

Centers for Disease Control and Prevention (CDC), http://www.cdc.gov/index.htm

CDC, Division of Foodborne, Bacterial and Mycotic Diseases (DFBMD), Leprosy (Hansen's Disease), http://www.cdc.gov/nczved/dfbmd/disease_listing/leprosy_ti.html

CDC, Division of Vector-borne Infectious Diseases, Information on Arboviral Encephalitides, http://www.cdc.gov/ncidod/dvbid/arbor/arbdet.htm

CDC, Division of Vector-Borne Infectious Diseases, St. Louis Encephalitis Fact Sheet, http://www.cdc.gov/ncidod/dvbid/sle/Sle_FactSheet.html

CDC, *Haemophilus influenzae* Serotype b (Hib) Disease, http://www.cdc.gov/ncidod/dbmd/diseaseinfo/haeminfluserob_t.htm

CDC, Meningococcal Disease: Frequently Asked Questions, http://www.cdc.gov/meningitis/bacterial/faqs.htm

CDC, Prion Diseases, http://www.cdc.gov/ncidod/dvrd/prions/

CDC, Rabies, http://www.cdc.gov/ncidod/dvrd/rabies/Introduction/intro.htm

CDC, Vaccines & Immunizations, Vaccines and Preventable Diseases: Pneumococcal Vaccination, http://www.cdc.gov/vaccines/vpd-vac/pneumo/default.htm

CDC, Vaccines & Immunizations, Vaccines and Preventable Diseases: Polio Vaccination, http://www.cdc.gov/vaccines/vpd-vac/polio/default.htm

FDA, Center for Biologics Evaluation and Research, Bovine Spongiform Encephalopathy (BSE), http://www.fda.gov/cber/bse/bseqa.htm

Medline Plus, Medical Encyclopedia, DTaP immunization (vaccine), http://www.nlm.nih.gov/medlineplus/ency/article/002021.htm

Medline Plus, Medical Encyclopedia, Meningitis, http://www.nlm.nih.gov/medlineplus/ency/article/000680.htm

Medline Plus, Medical Encyclopedia, Pneumococcal polysaccharide vaccine, http://www.nlm.nih.gov/medlineplus/ency/article/002029.htm

Merck Manuals Online Medical Library, Central Nervous System Infections, http://www.merck.com/mmhe/sec23/ch273/ch273b.html

MMWR: Meningococcal Disease and College Students, Recommendations of the Advisory Committee on Immunization Practices (ACIP), *MMWR* 49(RR07):11–20, 2000. Available at http://www.cdc.gov/mmwr/preview/mmwrhtml/rr4907a2.htm

National Institute of Neurological Disorders and Stroke, Creutzfeldt-Jakob Disease Information Page, http://www.ninds.nih.gov/disorders/cjd/cjd.htm

National Institute of Neurological Disorders and Stroke, Kuru Information Page, http://www.ninds.nih.gov/disorders/kuru/kuru.htm

National Institute of Neurological Disorders and Stroke, Post-Polio Syndrome Fact Sheet, http://www.ninds.nih.gov/disorders/post_polio/detail_post_polio.htm

The Merck Manual of Medical Information—Second Home Edition, Acute Bacterial Meningitis, http://www.merck.com/mmhe/print/sec06/ch089/ch089b.html

Todar's Online Textbook of Bacteriology, http://www.textbookofbacteriology.net/

U.S. National Library of Medicine, Genetics Home Reference, Genetic Conditions, Prion Diseases, http://ghr.nlm.nih.gov/condition=priondisease

World Health Organization, Variant Creutzfeldt-Jakob disease, http://www.who.int/mediacentre/factsheets/fs180/en/

World Health Organization, World Health Statistics, 2008, Part 1, Ten Highlights in Health Statistics, http://www.who.int/whosis/whostat/EN_WHS08_Part1.pdf

14

Infections of the Circulatory System

OUTLINE

Introduction
Endocarditis
Myocarditis
Pericarditis
Blood-borne Infectious Diseases
Microbemia

Bacterial Infections
Bacteremia
Septicemia
Rheumatic Fever
Gangrene
Zoonotic Diseases
Vector-transmitted Diseases

Viral Infections
Infectious Mononucleosis
Cytomegalovirus Infections
Viral Hemorrhagic Fevers

Fungal Infections
Systemic Mycoses

Protozoan Infections
Malaria
Babesiosis
Toxoplasmosis
Chagas' Disease
Leishmaniasis

LEARNING OBJECTIVES

After reading this chapter, the student will be able to:
- Identify the causes and symptoms of endocarditis, myocarditis, and pericarditis
- Describe blood-borne infectious diseases and microbemia
- Differentiate between bacteremia and septicemia
- Describe the transmission, symptoms, and treatment of rheumatic fever and gangrene

- Discuss zoonotic bacterial infections
- Describe the vector-transmitted bacterial diseases affecting the circulatory system
- Describe the cause, transmission, symptoms, and treatment for infectious mononucleosis
- Describe the causes and symptoms of viral hemorrhagic fevers
- Discuss the causes, symptoms, and treatment of systemic mycoses
- Describe the origin and transmission of the different protozoan infections that affect the circulatory system

KEY TERMS

bacteremia
brucellosis
ehrlichiosis
endocarditis
endocardium
gametocytes
gangrene
ischemia
Lyme disease
merozoites

microbemia
myocarditis
myocardium
pericarditis
pericardium
plague
rheumatic fever
Rocky Mountain spotted
 fever
sepsis

septicemia
septic shock
sporozoites
tularemia
vector
viral hemorrhagic fevers
zoonosis

WHY YOU NEED TO KNOW

HISTORY

Throughout ancient times various civilizations have recognized the importance of blood and understood its role in overall human health. Although blood was recognized as one of the four basic humors of the body, its exact role, composition, and how it moved throughout the body remained mysteries for the ancient physicians. As early as 4 BCE physicians discovered the valves of the heart but did not understand their function. From the second century AD to the mid-1200s there had been a series of discoveries that slowly began to clear up the picture about the functioning of the circulatory system. During this time practices such as leeching or bloodletting were practiced in an attempt to "maintain a balance of the body humors." Imbalances in the humors were believed to be the source of virtually all illnesses and diseases. Ibn al-Nafis in 1242 was the first to describe the process of blood circulation in the human body. Early experimentation in blood transfusion was being conducted as early as the late 1490s, with the first successful transfusion being recorded in the mid-1600s. The 1600s also saw the microscopic examination of blood by Antony van Leeuwenhoek and the subsequent discovery of red blood cells. It was not until William Harvey published his works in 1628 that the modern understanding of the circulatory system was established. Since then our knowledge of the circulatory system has advanced considerably.

IMPACT

Adding to the knowledge that the circulatory system is responsible for carrying nutrients and oxygen to the tissues and cells of the body as well as for taking wastes away from the cells, the importance of the immune system was recognized. The blood and lymph are the delivery systems responsible for transporting various cellular and molecular components throughout the body. In addition, this system is capable of transporting pathogens throughout the body. Therefore, a localized infection can spread and cause a systemic infection affecting multiple organ systems. Such an infection can lead to potentially deadly conditions such as toxic shock syndrome, a condition that can be caused by a number of different bacteria. The damage to heart valves due to bacterial infections that originated in the oral cavity is another example of the complexity of an infection in the circulatory system. The potential for the spread of HIV through blood transfusions also provides a clear example of the impact of circulatory system infections on human health.

FUTURE

Research on organisms responsible for toxic shock syndrome continues as the list of potential pathogens is growing and the "at-risk" group is being expanded. Development of more efficient and effective processes of blood collection, testing, and transfusion screening continues in an effort to minimize the risks involved in the spread of blood-borne diseases. Furthermore, efforts are being made to develop artificial blood to prevent blood-borne diseases. If and when successful, this will have major implications throughout human medicine/healthcare. Whether at the center of an infection or a mere participant in transporting a pathogen through the bloodstream to a target in another body system, the circulatory system remains a central player in the majority of microbial attacks on the body and the subsequent responses.

Introduction

The circulatory system includes the cardiovascular system and the lymphatic system. The lymphatic system consists of the lymph, lymphatic vessels, lymphatic tissue, and lymphatic organs, and is discussed in Chapter 20 (The Immune System). The cardiovascular system consists of the heart, blood, and blood vessels (Figure 14.1). Infection and inflammation of the cardiovascular system frequently cause cardiac and vascular disease. The lymphatic system returns excess tissue fluid back to the cardiovascular system and therefore has direct access to the cardiovascular system. The relationship between the cardiovascular and lymphatic systems is illustrated in Figure 14.2. Once microorganisms gain access to either one of the systems they can spread throughout the body and therefore have the potential to infect any organ system. In general, bacterial and fungal infections will affect the **endocardium** (tissue lining of the heart chambers), causing **endocarditis,** whereas viral and parasitic infections affect the **myocardium** (heart muscle), resulting in **myocarditis.** Inflammation and infection of the **pericardium** (membrane surrounding the heart), called **pericarditis,** can be caused by bacteria, viruses, and rarely by fungi.

Endocarditis

Endocarditis is an inflammation of the endocardium, the lining of the heart or the heart valves (Figure 14.3). The condition can be classified as infective if a microorganism is involved, or as noninfective. Noninfective endocarditis involves the formation of platelet and fibrin thrombi on heart valves and the surrounding endocardium, in response to trauma, circulating immune

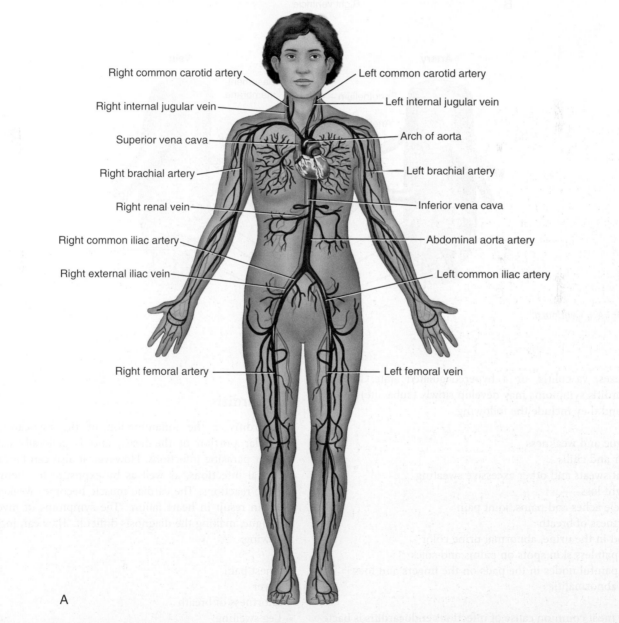

Right common carotid artery	Left common carotid artery
Right internal jugular vein	Left internal jugular vein
Superior vena cava	Arch of aorta
Right brachial artery	Left brachial artery
Right renal vein	Inferior vena cava
Right common iliac artery	Abdominal aorta artery
Right external iliac vein	Left common iliac artery
Right femoral artery	Left femoral vein

A

FIGURE 14.1 Cardiovascular system overview. **A,** The cardiovascular system consists of the heart **(B)** and the blood and blood vessels **(C).**

Continued

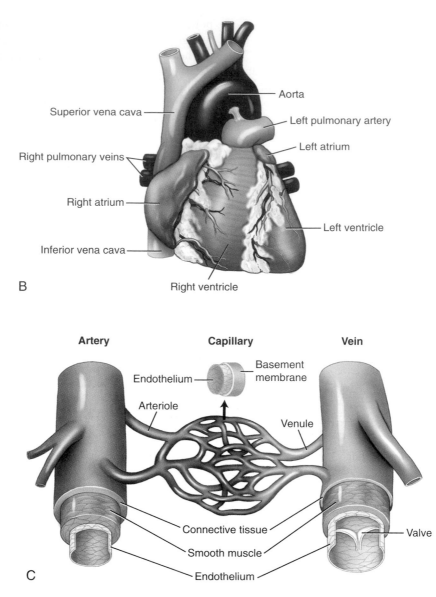

FIGURE 14.1 *Continued.*

complexes, vasculitis, or a hypercoagulated state. Infective endocarditis symptoms may develop slowly (subacute) or suddenly and they include the following:

- Fatigue and weakness
- Fever and chills
- Night sweats and other excessive sweating
- Weight loss
- Muscle aches and pains, joint pain
- Shortness of breath
- Blood in the urine, abnormal urine color
- Red painless skin spots on palms and soles
- Red painful nodes in the pads on the fingers and toes
- Nail abnormalities

The most common cause of infectious endocarditis is bacterial, but it also can be caused by fungi. In some cases, no causative organism can be identified.

Myocarditis

Myocarditis is the inflammation of the myocardium, the muscular portion of the heart, and is generally caused by viral or parasitic infections. However, it also can be caused by bacterial infections, as well as by exposure to chemicals, or allergic reactions. The cardiac muscle becomes weakened and this can result in heart failure. The symptoms of myocarditis are vague, making the diagnosis difficult. They can include the following:

- Chest pain
- Fever
- Shortness of breath
- Leg swelling
- Arrhythmias
- Congestive heart failure

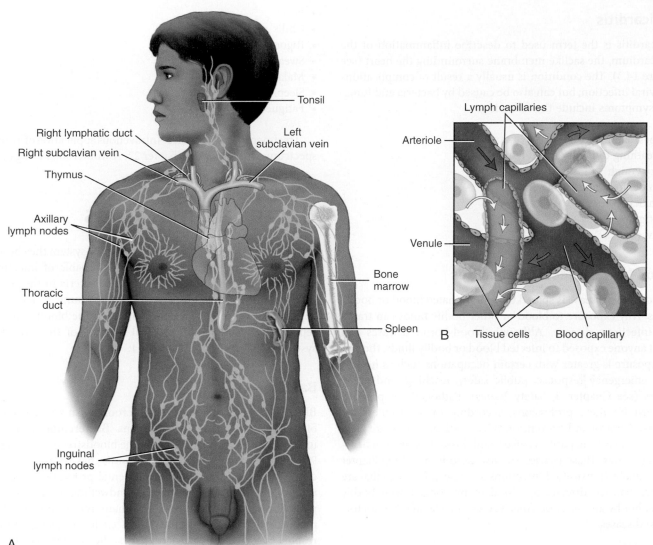

FIGURE 14.2 Relationship between the cardiovascular and lymphatic system. A, The lymphatic vessels drain excess fluid from the tissues and return it to the cardiovascular system. **B,** The inset shows the relationship between the blind-ended lymphatic capillaries and the blood capillaries.

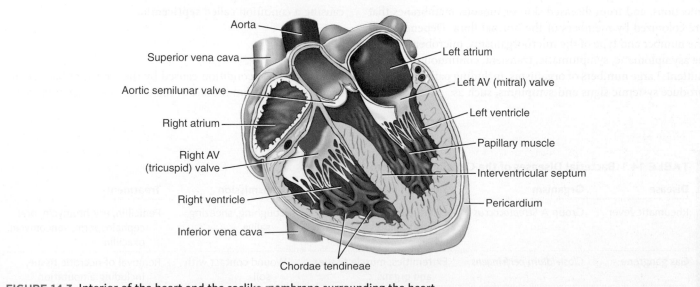

FIGURE 14.3 Interior of the heart and the saclike membrane surrounding the heart.

Pericarditis

Pericarditis is the term used to describe inflammation of the pericardium, the saclike membrane surrounding the heart (see Figure 14.3). The condition is usually a result of complications of a viral infection, but can also be caused by bacteria and fungi. The symptoms include the following:

- Chest pain
- Breathing difficulty when lying down
- Dry cough
- Ankle, foot, and leg swelling
- Anxiety
- Fatigue
- Fever

Blood-borne Infectious Diseases

Blood-borne disease is spread by contaminated blood or bodily fluids. Any exposure to blood or other bodily fluids can transmit infectious disease. Although blood-borne diseases can affect anyone exposed to infected blood or bodily fluids, the risk of exposure is greater with certain occupations such as healthcare, emergency response, public safety, teaching, and many others (see Chapter 5, Safety Issues). Pathogens of primary concern for these professions, according to the Centers for Disease Control and Prevention (CDC, Atlanta, GA), are HIV, hepatitis B virus, hepatitis C virus, and those causing viral hemorrhagic fever. These viruses are discussed in detail in Chapter 17 (Sexually Transmitted Infections/Diseases). Diseases that are not transmitted directly by blood or by contact with bodily fluids, but by an insect or other **vector,** are classified as vectorborne diseases.

Microbemia

Microbemia is the term used to describe infections caused by microorganisms that enter the circulatory system through the lymphatic drainage. This entry occurs from areas of localized infections, and from diseased skin or mucous membranes that are colonized by members of the normal flora. Depending on the number and type of the microorganisms, microbemias may be asymptomatic, symptomatic, transient, continuous, or intermittent. Large numbers of organisms, including pathogens, may produce systemic signs and symptoms, such as:

- Fever
- Chills
- Rigors
- Sweating
- Malaise
- Sleepiness
- Fatigue

Treatment usually involves intravenous application of a broad-spectrum antibiotic (see Chapter 22, Antimicrobial Drugs).

Bacterial Infections

Once bacteria have access to the circulatory system they become widely dispersed (bacteremia) and are capable of infecting a wide range of tissues and organs. If the bacteria in the circulatory system are not destroyed by the immune system or by antibiotic treatment, they can multiply in the blood and cause septicemia. Examples of bacterial diseases of the circulatory system are illustrated in Table 14.1.

Bacteremia

Blood is normally sterile, but microorganisms can enter the blood under a variety of conditions. **Bacteremia** is the term used when bacteria are present in the bloodstream (see Chapter 9, Infection and Disease). Bacteremia has various possible causes including infection during dental procedures, catheterization and the placement of other indwelling devices, surgical procedures, wound infection, and many more. In general, the presence of bacteria in the blood elicits a strong immune response by circulating macrophages, the complement system, and lymphocytes (see Chapter 20, The Immune System), thus preventing bacteria from multiplying. In addition, the blood is relatively low on iron, a requirement for most bacterial growth. If the defenses of the immune and circulatory systems fail microbes can undergo uncontrolled proliferation in the blood, causing a condition called **septicemia.**

Septicemia

Sepsis is a toxic condition caused by the spread of bacteria or bacterial toxins from the site of infection (see Chapter 9, Infec-

---

TABLE 14.1 Bacterial Diseases of the Circulatory System

Disease	Organism	Target of Infection	Transmission	Treatment
Rheumatic fever	Group A *Streptococcus*	Heart, joints, brain, spinal cord, skin	Coughing, sneezing, saliva	Penicillin, erythromycin, oral cephalosporin, vancomycin, oxacillin
Gas gangrene	*Clostridium perfringens*	Extremities, muscle tissues, and organs	Wound contact with soil	Removal of necrotic tissue, including amputation

tion and Disease). Septicemia is sepsis that occurs when bacteria multiply in the bloodstream. Septicemia is a medical emergency that requires immediate medical treatment. If the condition progresses to septic shock the death rate is as high as 50%, depending on the type of organism involved. **Septic shock** is the result of hypotension (low blood pressure) despite adequate fluid substitution. Septicemia develops quickly and the patient becomes extremely ill. Although each individual may experience symptoms differently the most common symptoms include the following:

- Loss of appetite
- Fever
- Chills
- Lethargic, anxious, or agitated behavior
- Accelerated breathing
- Accelerated heart rate

Rheumatic Fever

Rheumatic fever is an inflammatory disease that can develop as a rare complication after a group A streptococcal infection such as strep throat or scarlet fever (see Chapter 11, Medical Highlights: Complications of "Strep Throat"). The condition commonly involves the heart, joints, brain, spinal cord, and skin. In general, rheumatic fever occurs in children between the ages of 4 and 18 years. Symptoms normally begin several weeks after the disappearance of localized throat symptoms and vary greatly between individuals, depending on the parts of the body inflamed. The most common symptoms include the following:

- Joint pain
- Fever
- Chest pain
- Carditis
- Rash
- Nodules under the skin

In some children carditis may not be evident, and the inflammation of the heart is recognized only years later, when heart damage is discovered. Treatment involves long-term antibiotic administration to eliminate any residual streptococcal infection, antiinflammatory medication to reduce inflammation, and also the limiting of physical activity that might aggravate the inflamed structures. People who do not take low-dose antibiotics continually, especially during the first 3 to 5 years after the first episodes of the disease, will likely experience recurrence of the condition, resulting in severe heart complications.

Gangrene

Gangrene is a complication of necrosis, the decay and death of tissue, that is often related to wounds. If the blood supply to a tissue is interrupted by an infection or **ischemia** (restriction of blood supply) gangrene can occur. Gangrene most commonly affects the extremities (Figure 14.4); however, it can also occur in muscle tissue and organs. Enzymes released from the dying cells and tissue will further destroy the surrounding tissues and

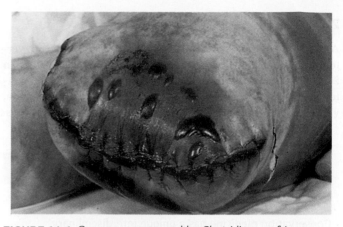

FIGURE 14.4 Gas gangrene caused by *Clostridium perfringens*. (Courtesy J. Newman. From Mims C, Dockrell HM, Goering RV, et al: *Medical microbiology,* ed 3, St. Louis, 2004, Mosby.)

thus provide a perfect nutrient environment for many bacterial species. Tissues devoid of blood supply become ischemic and provide an environment for anaerobic bacteria. Several species of the genus *Clostridium,* gram-positive, endospore-forming anaerobes, grow easily under these conditions. *Clostridium* is commonly found in soil as well as in the intestinal tracts of humans and domestic animals. The most frequent species involved in gangrene is *C. perfringens,* but other species and several other genera of bacteria can also grow under the conditions mentioned.

Treatment of gangrene usually entails the removal of necrotic tissue, and in many cases amputation may be necessary. Because antibiotics cannot reach the ischemic tissue, antibiotics alone are not effective. In addition to surgery and antibiotics, hyperbaric oxygen therapy can be used to kill the anaerobic *Clostridium* causing the condition.

There are different types of gangrene, including the following:

- *Dry gangrene,* due to ischemia and generally beginning at the distal portions of a limb such as in the feet. This condition often occurs in elderly patients with arteriosclerosis, and other persons with impaired peripheral blood flow, such as diabetic patients.
- *Internal gangrene,* also called *white gangrene,* is noticeable by the bleaching of internal tissue, and is generally contracted after surgery or trauma.
- *Wet gangrene* occurs in organs lined by mucous membranes such as the mouth, lower intestinal tract, lungs, and cervix. Although not necessarily associated with moist tissue, bedsores are also categorized as wet gangrene infections. Toxic products formed by the infecting bacteria can be absorbed if the affected tissue is not removed, resulting in septicemia or toxemia, and eventually death.
- *Gas gangrene* is caused by bacteria that produce gas within the infected tissue. Toxins produced by the bacteria will cause necrosis of more tissue, thereby providing further bacterial growth. If untreated, the condition is fatal.

Zoonotic Diseases

Any disease and/or infection that can be transmitted from vertebrate animals to humans is classified as a **zoonosis.** More than 200 zoonoses have been described, but not all affect the circulatory system (Table 14.2). Zoonoses may be caused by bacteria, viruses, parasites, and unconventional agents such as prions.

LIFE APPLICATION

Conservation Medicine

Conservation medicine has a unique interdisciplinary approach that focuses on human and animal health as well as on environmental conditions and the health of the ecosystem. In essence, conservation medicine is an emerging field that deals with the relationship between humans, animals, nonhuman hosts, and pathogens within the environment. This new field requires that multidisciplinary teams tackle emerging diseases or diseases already having an impact on human and animal lives, and the environment. The teams may involve physicians, veterinarians, microbiologists, pathologists, marine biologists, toxicologists, epidemiologists, anthropologists, and many more.

The emerging field of conservation medicine integrates human medicine, veterinary medicine, and environmental services and is largely concerned with zoonoses.

Brucellosis (Undulant Fever)

Brucellosis is an infectious disease that occurs worldwide and is caused by various *Brucella* species. Although the condition is found worldwide, it is most common in areas with insufficient standards for public health and domestic animal health programs. Brucellas are small, gram-negative, aerobic (or capnophilic) coccobacilli that are adapted to intracellular replication. These bacteria affect primarily sheep, goats, cattle, deer, elk, pigs, dogs, and other animals. It is zoonotic and humans become infected by contact with animals or animal products contaminated with the bacteria. Person-to-person spread of brucellosis is extremely rare, but may occur when an infected woman is breastfeeding. High-risk groups include abattoir workers, meat inspectors, animal handlers, veterinarians, and laboratory technicians. In the general United States population, the most common cause of infection is the ingestion of unpasteurized milk or other dairy products.

Clinically, the acute form of brucellosis is nonspecific and represents itself with flulike symptoms including chills, excessive sweating, fever, sweats, weakness, malaise, anorexia, headache, abdominal pain, back pain, and joint pain. Severe infections of the central nervous system or the lining of the heart (endocardium) may occur. Brucellosis can also be

TABLE 14.2 Zoonotic Infections of the Circulatory System

Disease	Organism(s)	Target of Infection	Transmission	Treatment
Brucellosis (undulant fever)	Species of *Brucella*	Systemic infection with symptoms manifested in the gastrointestinal and respiratory systems	Direct contact with sheep, goats, cattle, deer, elk, pigs, dogs, and other animals; contact with animal products contaminated with the bacteria; ingestion of unpasteurized milk or dairy products	Doxycycline plus rifampin for nonpregnant adults Trimethoprim-sulfamethoxazole for pregnant women and children under age 8 yr
Tularemia	*Francisella tularensis*	Blood and lymph nodes	Direct contact with rabbits, ground squirrels and/or through the bite of an infected tick, deerfly, or other insect	Streptomycin, gentamicin fluoroquinolones, and doxycycline
Cat scratch fever	*Bartonella henselae*	Lymph nodes, overall systemic infection	Cat bites, exposure of eye or lesion to infected saliva	Antibiotic therapy is usually not effective but in serious cases cephalosporins, erythromycin, or doxycycline can be used with some success
Rat-bite fever	*Streptobacillus moniliformis* (in United States)	Systemic infection with fever, vomiting, joint pain, headaches, and rash	Bite or scratch from infected rat, handling infected rat, or ingesting contaminated food or water	Penicillin, doxycycline

chronic, with symptoms that include undulant fevers, arthritis, chronic fatigue syndrome, and depression. Treatment with antibiotics is possible but may be difficult, depending on the timing of the treatment and the severity of the disease. The mortality rate of the disease is low and is usually associated with endocarditis.

Tularemia

Tularemia, also known as *"rabbit fever,"* is a zoonotic disease caused by *Francisella tularensis,* a gram-negative bacillus. The organism infects the blood and lymph nodes. The disease is transmitted by contact with infected animals, most commonly rabbits and ground squirrels. People can also contract the illness through an infected tick, deerfly, or other insects. Persons with tularemia do not need to be isolated because the illness is not known to spread from person to person. Although the bacterium can enter the human body at various sites the most common is through a minor abrasion of the skin, where an ulcer will occur. Symptoms of the illness appear 3 to 5 days after exposure, but may take up to 14 days. These symptoms include the following:

- Fever
- Chills
- Headache
- Fatigue
- Dizziness
- Muscle aches
- Joint pain
- Dry cough
- Loss of appetite
- Nausea

The infective dose is very low; only about 10 to 50 organisms are necessary to cause an infection. If not contained the proliferation of *F. tularensis* can lead to sepsis. Tularemia occurs in many parts of the United States and is on the list for nationally notifiable diseases. Because of the highly infectious nature of the organism, the concern rose that it could be used as a biological weapon and is now included in the bioterrorism preparedness response by the CDC.

Cat Scratch Disease

Cat scratch disease is caused by *Bartonella henselae,* an aerobic, gram-negative, rod-shaped bacterium that is found in all parts of the world. The disease is transmitted by cat scratches, bites, or even by exposure to saliva on broken skin or contact with the eye. About 40% of cats carry the organism at some point in their lives, without showing symptoms. Kittens are more likely to be infected and pass the bacterium to humans. Because *Bartonella* is present in the saliva of cats, petting an infected cat with a skin lesion, or touching the eye after contact with the cat's fur, can also be the point of transmission. Initially a blister or bump may be found at the site of a scratch or bite, which often is mistaken for an insect bite. Within 2 to 3 weeks of the infection lymph nodes close to the area of inoculation will swell. Other than the initial bump and swelling of the lymph nodes, symptoms of infection may include the following:

- Fever
- Fatigue
- Malaise
- Headache

Although medical treatment is usually not necessary, in immunocompromised persons and in severe cases of infection antibiotic treatment may be needed. Cat scratch disease does not pass from person to person and can be prevented by avoiding rough play with cats, especially kittens, and by not allowing cats to lick open wounds on a human.

Rat-bite Fever

Rat-bite fever is a rare systemic infectious disease that develops after an individual has been bitten or scratched by an infected rat, has handled an infected rat, or has ingested food or water contaminated with infected rat excreta. Two different organisms can be responsible for the condition. *Streptobacillus moniliformis,* a facultative anaerobic, pleomorphic, gram-negative bacterium is the most common cause of rat-bite fever in the United States. *Spirillum minus,* a gram-negative, spiral-shaped bacterium, is the most common cause of the disease in Asia and Africa. The disease cannot be transmitted from person to person. Symptoms of the disease occur 2 to 10 days after exposure and include the following:

- Abrupt onset of chills and fever
- Vomiting
- Pain in the back and joints
- Headache and muscle pain

Approximately 2 to 4 days after the onset of the fever a rash develops on the hands and feet, and one or more large joints may become swollen, red, and painful. The condition is treatable with antibiotics, usually penicillin, erythromycin, or tetracycline. Possible complications include pericarditis, endocarditis, parotitis (inflammation of the parotid glands), and abscesses in the brain or soft tissue. If the disease is untreated these complications can potentially be fatal.

Vector-transmitted Diseases

Vectors are animals that are capable of transmitting infectious diseases. These vectors include, but are not limited to, flies, mites, fleas, ticks, and rats. Insects are a major cause of human mortality and morbidity due to the transmission of infectious pathogens by blood-feeding species. The transmission of vector-borne diseases is based on a complex relationship between a parasite, the vector, and humans. Vectors are mobile and add an additional dimension to the range of transmission of infectious diseases. This particular section addresses bacterial vector-borne diseases (Table 14.3).

Plague

The **plague** is an infectious disease caused by *Yersinia pestis,* a gram-negative, rod-shaped bacterium. People usually become infected when bitten by a flea that carries the bacteria from an infected rodent or by handling an infected animal. After the flea

TABLE 14.3 Vector-transmitted Diseases of the Circulatory System

Disease	Organism	Target of Infection	Transmission	Treatment
Plague	*Yersinia pestis*	Systemic infection beginning in lymph nodes	Flea bite from infected rodent	Antibiotic therapy as determined through *in vitro* susceptibility testing
Rocky Mountain spotted fever	*Rickettsia rickettsii*	Systemic infection	Tick bite	Tetracycline, chloramphenicol
Lyme disease	*Borrelia burgdorferi*	Systemic infection	Bite of infected blacklegged tick	Early treatment: Amoxicillin, doxycycline, cefuroxime Late treatment: Amoxicillin, doxycycline, ceftriaxone, penicillin G
Ehrlichiosis	*Ehrlichia chaffeensis*	Systemic infection	Bite of infected Lone Star tick	Doxycycline, rifampin
Typhus	Rickettsias	Endothelial cells of the vascular system, systemic infections	Arthropods	Doxycycline, tetracycline, chloramphenicol
Relapsing fever	*Borrelia recurrentis*	Systemic infection	Human body lice, *Ornithodoros* tick	Tetracycline, doxycycline, penicillin

bite, the bacteria enter the bloodstream and proliferate in the lymph and blood. *Y. pestis* can reproduce within cells; therefore even if phagocytosed, they still survive. Once the organism enters the lymph it causes swelling of the lymph nodes, especially in the groin and armpits. These swellings are referred to as *buboes*, and the term *buboes* led to the disease's name, bubonic plague (Figure 14.5). Because the lymph is delivered to the subclavian veins via the right lymphatic duct and the thoracic duct, it ultimately enters the bloodstream and the bacteria within the lymph are now capable of multiplying in the blood, causing septicemic plague, which is followed by septic shock. Septicemic plague can occur when the bacteria enter the bloodstream directly through a flea bite, or as a complication of the bubonic or pneumonic plague. All forms of the plague can be treated with antibiotics in the early stages, but if untreated, septicemic plague is universally fatal.

The least common form of the plague is the pneumonic plague, which occurs if the bacteria are carried to the lungs. The disease can then be spread from human to human by air droplets. Epidemics can be started this way, as happened in the Middle Ages. Even now the mortality rate for this particular type of the plague is nearly 100% if not diagnosed and treated within the first 12 hours of the onset of fever.

Recovery from the plague provides reliable immunity. Vaccines are available for persons who are likely to come in contact with infected fleas, either during field experiments or operations, or for laboratory workers who may have contact with the pathogen. Elimination of the plague is not realistic because it would require the elimination of its reservoir, namely rodents and other wild animals. As a preventive measure, periodic application of rodenticides is advised for ships, airplanes, and buildings or other places with a high population of rodents.

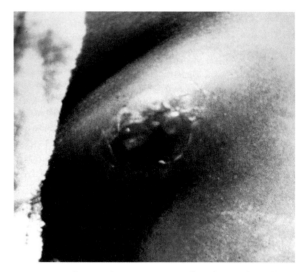

FIGURE 14.5 Bubonic plague, causing the classical swelling of lymph nodes in the groin area. (From Bergquist L, Pogosian B: *Microbiology,* St. Louis, 2000, Saunders.)

Rocky Mountain Spotted Fever

Rocky Mountain spotted fever is caused by *Rickettsia rickettsii,* an obligate intracellular pleomorphic gram-negative bacterium, and is transmitted to humans by ticks. In contrast to its name it occurs throughout the United States; it is a severe disease and the most frequently reported of the rickettsial illnesses. The incubation period varies from 5 to 10 days after the tick bite, with nonspecific symptoms that may resemble a variety of other infectious diseases. These initial symptoms may include the following:

Types of the Plague

Type	Site of Infection	Symptoms	Transmission	Treatment
Bubonic	Lymph nodes	Appears suddenly, usually 2–5 d after exposure; high fever, smooth painful lymph nodes—buboes; chills, malaise, muscle pain, severe headache, seizures	Rodent to rodent; rodent to fleas; fleas to humans	Antibiotics if diagnosed in a timely manner
Pneumonic	Lungs	Symptoms occur 1–4 d after exposure and include severe cough, bloody sputum, difficulty in breathing	Inhalation of the organism by face-to-face contact, coughs, or sneezes	Isolation from other patients; early treatment with appropriate antibiotics is essential—the pneumonic form is almost always fatal
Septicemic	Blood	Abdominal pain, blood-clotting problems, diarrhea, fever, low blood pressure, nausea, vomiting, organ failure	Bacteria enter the bloodstream	Early antibiotic treatment, respiratory support, intravenous fluids; usually fatal

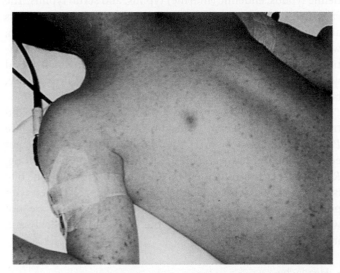

FIGURE 14.6 Typical rash that occurs in Rocky Mountain spotted fever. (Courtesy T.F. Sellers, Jr. From Mims C, Dockrell HM, Goering RV, et al: *Medical microbiology,* ed 3, St. Louis, 2004, Mosby.)

- Fever
- Nausea
- Vomiting
- Severe headache
- Muscle pain
- Lack of appetite
- Rash developing 2 to 5 days after the onset of the fever

  Later signs include the following:

- Rash (Figure 14.6)
- Abdominal pain
- Joint pain
- Diarrhea

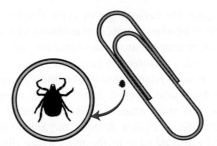

FIGURE 14.7 A bite from an infected blacklegged tick transmits *Borrelia burgdorferi,* **which causes Lyme disease.**

The characteristic rash of the illness is usually not seen until day 6 or later after the onset of the initial symptoms. Only 35% to 60% of patients with the condition develop the characteristic rash, and 50% to 80% of these show the rash on the palms or soles.

Diagnosis of Rocky Mountain spotted fever is based on a combination of clinical signs, symptoms, and laboratory tests. Antibiotic treatment should be given immediately if there is a suspicion of Rocky Mountain spotted fever, even before laboratory confirmation is obtained. At present the most commonly used antibiotics are tetracycline and chloramphenicol. Despite treatment, about 3% to 5% of persons developing the fever still die from the condition.

Lyme Disease

Lyme disease is caused by *Borrelia burgdorferi,* a gram-negative, motile spirochete that is transmitted to humans by the bite of an infected blacklegged tick (Figure 14.7). The infection in humans presents itself in three stages. Typical early symptoms include the following:

- Skin rash, often resembling a bull's-eye (Figure 14.8)
- Fever and fatigue
- Headache and stiff neck
- Muscle pain

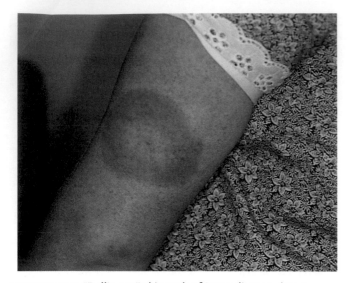

FIGURE 14.8 "Bull's-eye" skin rash of Lyme disease. (From Murray PR, Rosenthal KS, Pfaller MA: *Medical microbiology,* ed 5, St. Louis, 2005, Mosby.)

In most cases the early stages of Lyme disease can be successfully treated by administration of antibiotics for a few weeks. The second stage may occur weeks to months later if the condition is untreated. The infection then can spread to the joints, heart, and nervous system causing symptoms including severe fatigue, myalgia, skin lesions, heart failure, meningitis and encephalitis. The third stage results in repeated and severe attacks of arthritis over years. *Borrelia burgdorferi* can cross the placenta and cause damage to the fetus. Once diagnosed, the disease is a reportable disease for the purpose of surveillance.

Ehrlichiosis

Ehrlichiosis is caused by several species of the genus *Ehrlichia* (family Rickettsiaceae), members of which are gram-negative, obligatory intracellular bacteria. The pathogenic organisms primarily invade leukocytes. At first the pathogens were identified as causing disease in dogs, cattle, sheep, goats, and horses. Some species have now been shown to cause disease in humans. Human ehrlichiosis, caused by *Ehrlichia chaffeensis,* was first reported in 1987, and in the United States transmission occurs primarily by the Lone Star tick, *Amblyomma americanum.* Early signs of the condition are nonspecific and may resemble the symptoms of various other diseases. At present it is not clear whether all infected persons become ill; the illness might be so mild that individuals may not seek medical attention. The incubation period for the disease is about 5 to 10 days and the initial symptoms include fever, headache, malaise, and muscle aches. Other symptoms may include the following:

- Nausea
- Vomiting
- Diarrhea
- Cough
- Joint pains
- Confusion
- On occasion a rash

Severe cases of the disease, especially if untreated, may result in:

- Prolonged fever
- Renal failure
- Disseminated intravascular coagulopathy
- Meningoencephalitis
- Respiratory distress
- Seizures
- Coma

The severity of ehrlichiosis may in part be correlated to the status of the immune system of the patient. Treatment with the appropriate antibiotics should be started immediately when there is a strong suspicion of ehrlichiosis based on clinical and epidemiologic findings.

Typhus

Various, similar typhus diseases exist, all caused by rickettsias, obligate intracellular parasites. The types of typhus include epidemic typhus, endemic (murine) typhus, and scrub typhus. The causative agent of the diseases is spread by arthropod vectors and infects mostly endothelial cells in the vascular system, where it multiplies. The infection then results in an inflammation causing local blockage and rupture of the small blood vessels. The recommended antibiotic treatment is doxycycline, but tetracycline or chloramphenicol is also used.

Epidemic typhus is caused by *Rickettsia prowazekii* and transmitted from person to person by the human body louse *Pediculus humanus corporis.* The bacteria multiply in the gut epithelium of the louse and are excreted during the act of biting. *Rickettsia prowazekii* then enters the human skin when the bite is scratched. The disease is self-limiting and is associated with poverty and war, when human bodies and clothes are not washed frequently. Symptoms of the illness occur quickly and include the following:

- Headache
- Backache
- Arthralgia
- Extremely high fever
- Red rash on the middle of the body that spreads
- Nausea
- Vomiting
- Hacking dry cough
- Abdominal pain
- Sometimes meningoencephalitis
- Coma

In untreated cases the mortality rate for healthy individuals is about 20%, but among the elderly or immunocompromised persons it can be as high as 60%.

Endemic typhus is caused by *Rickettsia typhi,* and is transmitted to humans by the rat flea. Although the symptoms are similar to epidemic typhus, the disease is less severe and most people recover fully. Death may occur among the elderly or patients with a compromised immune system.

Scrub typhus is caused by *Orientia tsutsugamushi* and is transmitted by chiggers found in areas of heavy scrub vegetation in the Far East. The symptoms include the following:

- Fever
- Headache
- Muscle pain
- Cough
- Gastrointestinal symptoms

More virulent strains of the organism can cause hemorrhaging and intravascular coagulation.

Relapsing Fever

Relapsing fever is caused by *Borrelia recurrentis,* a gram-positive spirochete, and is most often transmitted by human body lice, but also by ticks. It is a systemic febrile disease occurring worldwide, but epidemics are more prevalent in overcrowded populations with poor hygiene. The two forms of the disease are either tick-borne or louse-borne.

1. *Louse-borne relapsing fever* is transmitted by the human body louse and causes the epidemic form of the disease.
2. *Tick-borne relapsing fever* is transmitted by the *Ornithodoros* tick and represents the endemic form of the disease.

Relapsing fever is characterized by recurrent febrile episodes occurring at intervals of 2 to 14 days. The febrile periods last 2 to 9 days with alternate afebrile periods of 2 to 4 days. Treatment of the disease involves antibiotics, most likely tetracycline, doxycycline, or penicillin.

Viral Infections

Viruses can cause a number of cardiovascular and lymphatic system diseases, and with a few exceptions most of them are prevalent in tropical areas (Table 14.4).

Infectious Mononucleosis

Mononucleosis (mono) or glandular fever is usually caused by Epstein-Barr virus (EBV). EBV, also called *human herpesvirus 4,* is a member of the herpesvirus family, one of the most common human viruses occurring worldwide. The virus infects B lymphocytes and the disease name refers to the lymphocytes with unusual lobed nuclei that proliferate during the acute infection. Many children become infected with the virus and the symptoms are indistinguishable from those of other mild illnesses of childhood. When an infection with EBV occurs during adolescence it causes infectious mononucleosis 35% to 50% of the time. Symptoms include the following:

- Sore throat
- Fever
- Fatigue
- Swollen lymph glands

On occasion, a swollen spleen or liver problems may develop.

Although most patients recover within 2 to 4 weeks, some will experience fatigue for up to 2 months, and EBV remains dormant or latent in a few cells in the throat and blood for the rest of the person's life. It is essential to avoid sports during the

Examples of Tick-related Infections

Infection/Disease	Tick Vector	Organism	Reservoir
Lyme disease	*Ixodes scapularis* *Ixodes pacificus*	*Borrelia burgdorferi* (gram-negative spirochete)	White-footed mouse
Ehrlichiosis	*Amblyomma americanum* (Lone Star tick); *Ixodes scapularis;* *Ixodes pacificus*	*Ehrlichia chaffeensis, Ehrlichia ewingii, Anaplasma phagocytophila* (pleomorphic, gram-negative bacteria)	White-footed mouse, whitetail deer, coyotes, rats
Rocky Mountain spotted fever	*Dermacentor variabilis* *Dermacentor andersoni*	*Rickettsia rickettsii* (obligate intracellular pleomorphic gram-negative bacteria)	Primary reservoir is ticks, but also mice, deer, wild rodents, dogs
Babesiosis	*Ixodes scapularis,* *Ixodes pacificus;* *Amblyomma americanum* (Lone Star tick)	*Babesia microti, Babesia divergens* (protozoan)	White-footed mouse; whitetail deer, coyotes, rats
Tularemia	*Dermacentor* and *Amblyomma*	*Francisella tularensis* (gram-negative coccobacillus)	Rodents, rabbits, hares
Relapsing fever	Soft ticks, genus *Ornithodoros*	*Borrelia duttonii* *Borrelia hermsii* (gram-negative helical bacteria)	Ground or tree squirrels, chipmunks, prairie dogs

TABLE 14.4 Viral Diseases of the Circulatory System

Disease	Organism	Target of Infection	Transmission	Treatment
Infectious mononucleosis	Epstein-Barr virus	B lymphocytes	Contact with infected saliva	No specific treatment available
Cytomegalovirus infections	Human herpesvirus 5	Monocytes, neutrophils, T lymphocytes	Direct body-to-body contact	No specific treatment available
Viral hemorrhagic fevers	Arenaviridae, Filoviridae, Bunyaviridae, Flaviviridae	Primarily the vascular system	Usually from direct contact with insect host or infected rodents; can be transmitted by direct human-to-human contact	Ribavirin for Arenaviridae infections Antibody-containing serum and interferon therapies for *Filovirus* infections

"Kissing Disease"

A kiss is just a kiss, unless the Epstein-Barr virus is in one of the people's saliva. This is the reason why mononucleosis (mono) is often referred to as the *"kissing disease."* However, transmission also commonly occurs by sharing water bottles (often between athletes), eating utensils, drinking glasses, and anything that gets in contact with infected saliva. The condition is most commonly seen in high school and college students but is certainly not limited to them.

time of the illness, because complications due to exhaustion may lead to rupture of the spleen. Although no specific treatment is available, symptoms may be treated, and bed rest and adequate fluids are recommended. Transmission of infectious mononucleosis requires contact with the saliva of an infected person. From the time of infection to the appearance of symptoms ranges from 4 to 6 weeks in adults and around 10 days in children. The virus is often found in the saliva of healthy people, and therefore transmission of the virus cannot be prevented.

Cytomegalovirus Infections

Cytomegalovirus (CMV), also known as *human herpesvirus 5,* is a large herpesvirus that remains mostly latent in leukocytes, such as monocytes, neutrophils, and T lymphocytes, and replicates very slowly. CMV is spread from person to person by direct contact. The infection is usually harmless but can cause severe disease in people with a compromised immune system. The virus can be present in several bodily fluids including urine, blood, saliva, semen, cervical secretions, and breast milk. Most people have been exposed to the virus, but a healthy immune system keeps the virus in check. Active infections are often associated with salivary glands, but also may be found throughout the body. Symptoms include the following:

- Prolonged high fever
- Chills
- Severe tiredness
- Generally ill feeling
- Headache
- Enlarged spleen

Most people infected with the virus do not develop symptoms; in those who do, the symptoms will appear 3 to 12 weeks after exposure. CMV is common worldwide and an estimated 80% of adults in the United States are infected with the organism. There is no specific cure or treatment for CMV.

Viral Hemorrhagic Fevers

Viral hemorrhagic fevers (VHFs) are a group of febrile illnesses that range in severity from relatively mild to life-threatening, and can result in severe multisystem problems. They are caused by four distinct families: the Arenaviridae, Filoviridae, Bunyaviridae, and Flaviviridae. These viruses share a number of features, including the following:

- They are RNA viruses, covered or enveloped.
- They need a natural reservoir such as an insect host or other animal.
- They are geographically restricted, depending on the host species.
- Humans are not the natural reservoir; however, by accidental contact the viruses can be transmitted from human to human.
- Human cases during outbreaks caused by these viruses are sporadic and cannot be easily predicted.
- With a few exceptions, there is no cure or treatment for VHFs.

All types of VHFs are characterized by:

- Fever
- Overall vascular system damage
- Bleeding disorders, all of which can progress to extremely high fever, shock, and death

The viruses that cause VHFs are scattered over much of the world. Each virus is associated with one or more specific host

species, and therefore the virus and the associated disease are limited to the area where the host species live. Many of these viruses are present in geographically limited areas and the risk of infection by them is restricted to those areas. Transmission to humans occurs by contact with a host, that is, by handling infected animals, their remains, fecal material, urine, or secretions. Viruses associated with arthropod vectors are generally spread by mosquito or tick bites.

An infected person may transmit the disease to other persons either by person-to-person contact, through bodily fluids, or by contact with contaminated objects, contaminated syringes, and needles. Infected people who travel to other areas of the country or world can then infect people outside of the original geographical area (also see Chapter 18, Emerging Infectious Diseases).

Fungal Infections

Under the right circumstances fungi can enter the human body via the lungs, through the gastrointestinal system, the paranasal

sinuses, or the skin. The fungi then spread via the bloodstream or the lymphatic system to the rest of the body (Table 14.5). Most of the mycoses are discussed in the fungal infection sections of the individual body systems. For details about mycoses, see Fungal Infections in Chapters 1–17.

Systemic Mycoses

Systemic mycoses are fungal infections capable of affecting all internal organs and are becoming more and more common in the hospital environment. The clinical features of systemic mycoses depend on the specific organism causing the illness and the organs affected. Whereas persons with a competent immune system will show only minor or no symptoms at all, immune-compromised patients are at high risk of systemic mycoses. These include people infected with HIV, patients with cancer, people with neutropenia (a low neutrophil cell count), organ transplant recipients, patients after surgery for pancreatitis or splenectomy, persons with poorly controlled diabetes mellitus, patients in intensive care, and the very young or very old. Treatment of systemic mycosis may include reducing or discontinuing immune-suppressing medications or systemic antifungal medications. The prognosis depends on the patient's immune function and unfortunately, despite treatment, the infection may be fatal for many of these patients.

Protozoan Infections

Protozoa causing diseases of the circulatory system generally have complex life cycles (see Chapter 8, Eukaryotic Microorganisms) and present unique challenges for treatment and control. The life cycles of many protozoa include intermediate hosts, which may allow for control by interruption of the infection by elimination of the transmission vectors. Once a protozoan infection has reached the human circulatory system, treatment becomes problematic because many of the drug therapies that target these eukaryotic organisms can also be toxic to human cells (Table 14.6).

Malaria

Malaria is one of the most common vector-borne infectious diseases; it is widespread in tropical and subtropical regions including parts of tropical Asia, Africa, and Central and South America. Most cases reported in the United States are related to

---

MEDICAL HIGHLIGHTS

Special Pathogens Branch (SPB)

The scientists of the Special Pathogens Branch (SPB) of the Centers for Disease Control and Prevention (CDC) study highly infectious viruses, many of which cause hemorrhagic fevers. These viruses include Ebola virus, Marburg virus, Lassa fever virus, Rift Valley virus, Crimean-Congo virus, arenaviruses, hantaviruses, and other emerging viral pathogens (see Chapter 18, Emerging Infectious Diseases). Most of these viruses are classified as Biosafety Level 4 pathogens (see Chapter 5, Safety Issues) and therefore must be handled in special facilities. Viruses causing hemorrhagic fever are present all around the globe and because of increased and open travel patterns can become a problem for the population in the United States within hours. The SPB uses several disciplines and tools to identify, understand, and control diseases caused by these viruses. These include public health practices, molecular biology, molecular evolution of viruses, clinical diagnostics, clinical medicine, epidemiology, immunology, pathogenesis, comparative biology, ecology, and community education.

TABLE 14.5 Fungal Diseases of the Circulatory System

Disease	Organism	Target of Infection	Transmission	Treatment
Systemic mycoses	Histoplasmosis capsulatum, Penicilliosis marneffei, Paracoccidioides brasiliensis, Coccidioides immitis	Systemic infections	Contact with spores—airborne, waterborne, food	Varies with specific organism; antifungal agents often used include itraconazole, fluconazole, and amphotericin B

TABLE 14.6 Protozoan Diseases of the Circulatory System

Disease	Organism	Target of Infection	Transmission	Treatment
Malaria	*Plasmodium vivax, Plasmodium falciparum, Plasmodium ovale, Plasmodium malariae*	Erythrocytes, followed by systemic infection	Bite of *Anopheles* mosquito, blood transfusion of infected blood	Chloroquinone, doxycycline, primaquine, pyrimethamine-sulfadoxine
Babesiosis	*Babesia microti*	Erythrocytes, followed by systemic infection	Bite of ixodid ticks	Clindamycin plus quinine, chloroquine, pentamidine
Toxoplasmosis	*Toxoplasma gondii*	Systemic infection	Contact with infected animals; frequently found in rodents and cats	Dependent on nature of infection: pyrimethamine plus sulfadiazine or clindamycin, spiramycin, trimethoprim-sulfamethoxazole
Chagas' disease	*Trypanosoma cruzi*	Systemic infection	Feces from reduviid bugs	Nifurtimox, allopurinol, benzimidazole
Leishmaniasis	*Leishmania donovani, Leishmania tropica, Leishmania braziliensis*	Systemic infection; each species targets different tissue	Bite of infected sandflies (genus *Phlebotomus* or *Lutzomyia*)	Stibogluconate, fluconazole, miltefosine, amphotericin

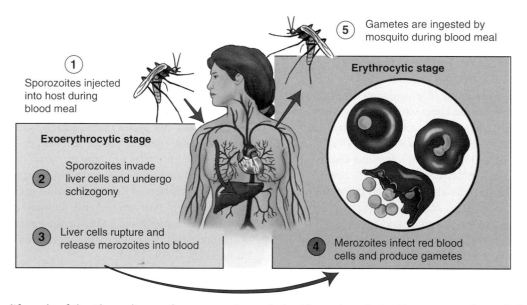

① Sporozoites injected into host during blood meal

Exoerythrocytic stage

② Sporozoites invade liver cells and undergo schizogony

③ Liver cells rupture and release merozoites into blood

⑤ Gametes are ingested by mosquito during blood meal

Erythrocytic stage

④ Merozoites infect red blood cells and produce gametes

FIGURE 14.9 The life cycle of the *Plasmodium* pathogens causing malaria. All are characterized by an exoerythrocytic (extracellular) cycle and an erythrocytic (intracellular) cycle.

exposure through travel or military duty in areas with endemic malaria. The disease is caused by protozoans of the genus *Plasmodium.* Four types of the parasite can infect humans: *Plasmodium vivax, Plasmodium falciparum, Plasmodium ovale,* and *Plasmodium malariae.* All the species are transmitted by female *Anopheles* mosquitoes, but also need to have a human host. The most common form of transmission is through a bite by the mosquito; however, the parasite can also be transmitted by blood transfusion from an infected donor, or by sharing needles.

All species of the malaria parasite have similar life cycles, comprising three distinct stages, and characterized by alternat-

ing extracellular and intracellular forms (Figure 14.9). Malaria parasites are ingested by mosquitoes feeding on an infected human carrier; the mosquitoes then carry *Plasmodium* **sporozoites** in their salivary glands. In humans *Plasmodium* grows and multiplies originally in the liver and then in erythrocytes. Once in the blood the parasites grow inside the erythrocytes and destroy them, releasing daughter parasites referred to as **merozoites,** all of which continue the cycle, invading other red blood cells. It is the blood stage of the parasites that causes the symptoms of malaria. Once the **gametocytes,** a form of the blood stage, are picked up by the mosquito during a blood meal, the parasites start another, different cycle of growth and multiplication in the insect.

Humans infected with the parasite can develop a wide range of symptoms depending on the age and immune status of the patient, and also on the type of the *Plasmodium* species. Malaria can occur as uncomplicated malaria or severe malaria.

Uncomplicated Malaria

Uncomplicated malaria may be asymptomatic (rarely) or show varied combinations of the following symptoms:

- Fever
- Chills
- Sweats
- Headaches
- Nausea and vomiting
- Body aches
- General malaise
- Enlarged spleen

In the case of *P. falciparum,* malaria symptoms may include the following:

- Mild jaundice
- Enlargement of the liver
- Increased respiratory rate

Severe Malaria

Plasmodium falciparum is the most common cause of severe and life-threatening malaria and causes more than 1 million deaths every year. This type of condition occurs when *P. falciparum* infections are complicated by serious organ failures or abnormalities in the blood or metabolism of the patient. The presentation of severe malaria varies with age and geographical distribution, but in general, the manifestations of the disease may include the following:

- Cerebral malaria, impairment of consciousness, seizures, coma, or other neurologic abnormalities
- Severe anemia due to hemolysis (destruction of erythrocytes)
- Hemoglobin in the urine (hemoglobinuria)
- Pulmonary edema or acute respiratory distress syndrome
- Abnormalities in blood coagulation and decrease in platelets
- Cardiovascular collapse and shock

Severe malaria is a medical emergency and occurs most often in people with no immunity or decreased immunity to malaria. These at-risk people include those living in areas with low or no malaria transmission, or young children and pregnant women in areas with high transmission.

Treatment of active malaria infection with *P. falciparum* is a medical emergency and requires hospitalization; infections with *P. vivax, P. ovale,* or *P. malariae* often can be treated on an outpatient basis. Treatment of the disease involves supportive measures as well as antimalarial drugs. The most common and inexpensive drug is chloroquine, but resistance to the drug by

Plasmodium falciparum has spread from Asia to Africa, making the drug ineffective. Other drugs against the parasite form in the blood include the following:

- Sulfadoxine-pyrimethamine
- Mefloquine
- Atovaquone-proguanil
- Quinine
- Doxycycline
- Artemisin derivatives

Babesiosis

Babesiosis is a vector-borne, malaria-like illness caused by the protozoan *Babesia,* and is usually transmitted by ticks. Infections may be asymptomatic or cause a mild nonspecific illness, and cases might go unnoticed. However, the infection can cause severe illness especially in the very young, the very old, or people with immunodeficiency. The symptoms of severe illness include the following:

- High fever
- Chills
- Anemia, possibly resulting in organ failure

Babesia parasites reproduce in red blood cells and can be easily misdiagnosed as *Plasmodium.* The life cycle involves two hosts: a rodent, usually the white-footed mouse, and the definitive host, the deer tick. Deer are the hosts that the adult ticks feed on and therefore are indirectly part of the cycle. If a deer population increases, the tick population increases, and the potential for transmission is heightened. Humans enter the cycle when bitten by an infected tick. Humans are generally considered the dead-end host, and human-to-human transmission can occur only through blood transfusions. The most common treatment is a combination of quinine and clindamycin for 7 to 10 days.

Toxoplasmosis

Toxoplasmosis is a disease caused by the protozoan *Toxoplasma gondii* (Figure 14.10), a single-celled, spore-forming parasite found throughout the world. The organisms carry out their reproductive cycle within the members of the cat family only. The cat is the definitive host. Transmission of toxoplasmosis to humans can occur in the following ways:

- Consumption of raw or undercooked meats, especially pork, lamb, or wild game
- Consumption of untreated water
- Fecal–oral route: After gardening, handling cats, cleaning cat litter boxes, or contaminating hands with anything that has come in contact with cat feces
- Mother-to-fetus, if the mother becomes infected during pregnancy
- Through organ transplant or blood transfusions; however, this mode of transmission is rare

It is estimated that more than 60 million people in the United States carry the *Toxoplasma* parasite, but because of an intact immune system very few ever show symptoms. Newly infected pregnant women and people with a compromised immune system should be aware that toxoplasmosis can have severe consequences for the unborn fetus including brain damage and damage to the eyes and other organs. Toxoplasmosis can be acquired by contact with wastes from an infected cat, consumption of contaminated meat (raw or undercooked), contact with utensils or cutting boards that have been in contact with raw meat, consumption of contaminated drinking water, or by

receiving an organ transplant or blood transfusion from an infected individual. Most people with toxoplasmosis do not require treatment, but it is available for pregnant women and persons with a compromised immune system.

Chagas' Disease

Chagas' disease, also referred to as *American trypanosomiasis,* is caused by *Trypanosoma cruzi,* a flagellated protozoa, and is transmitted to humans and other mammals by insect vectors that are currently found only in the Americas, primarily in the areas of Latin America with widespread poverty. It is estimated that 8 to 11 million people in Mexico, Central America, and South America are infected, with most of them not even knowing that they are infected. The infection is lifelong and if not treated can be life-threatening. There are two phases of the disease: an acute phase and a chronic phase.

The acute phase of the disease lasts for the first few weeks or months after infection and is often unnoticed because the symptoms are mild and not necessarily unique to Chagas' disease. These symptoms may include the following:

- Fever
- Fatigue
- Body aches
- Headache
- Rash
- Loss of appetite
- Diarrhea
- Vomiting

There also may be a mild enlargement of the spleen or liver and swollen glands at the site of parasite entry.

The chronic phase may remain silent for decades or even for life. Some people develop cardiac complications including an enlarged heart, heart failure, altered heart rate or rhythm, and cardiac arrest. Furthermore, intestinal complications can occur, including an enlarged esophagus or colon, and also can lead to difficulties with eating and/or defecation. Treatment of the condition includes antiparasitic and symptomatic treatment; no vaccines are currently available to prevent the infection.

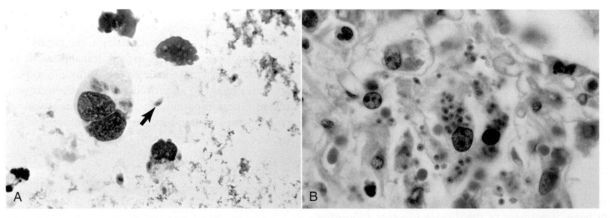

FIGURE 14.10 **A,** *Toxoplasma gondii* tachyzoites; **B,** *T. gondii* tachyzoites in lung tissue. (From Mahon CR, Lehman DC, Manuselis G: *Textbook of diagnostic microbiology,* ed 3, St. Louis, 2007, Saunders.)

Leishmaniasis

Leishmaniasis is a widespread complex disease caused by protozoan parasites of the genus *Leishmania,* with about 20 different species involved. The disease exhibits several clinical forms including the following:

- *Visceral leishmaniasis:* A serious form and potentially fatal if untreated
- *Cutaneous leishmaniasis:* The most common form, causing a sore at the bite site that will heal in a few months to a year
- *Diffuse cutaneous leishmaniasis:* Causes widespread skin lesions and is difficult to treat
- *Mucocutaneous leishmaniasis:* Causes skin ulcers that spread and can cause tissue damage to the nose and mouth

The infection is transmitted by female sandflies found in the tropical world and around the Mediterranean. Although most forms of the disease are transmitted only by insects to humans, some can be spread between humans. The illness is commonly found in Mexico, Central America, and South America. Cases also have been reported in southern Texas, southern Europe, Asia, the Middle East, and Africa. Although treatment is available, some species have developed drug resistance.

Summary

- The circulatory system consists of the cardiovascular system (including the heart, blood, and blood vessels) and the lymphatic system (consisting of the lymph, lymphatic vessels, lymphatic tissues, and lymphatic organs).
- Endocarditis is generally caused by bacteria and fungi; myocarditis is most often caused by viruses and parasites; and pericarditis can be caused by bacteria, viruses, and sometimes by fungi.
- Exposure to blood or other bodily fluids can transmit infectious disease and present a problem to a wide range of occupations, specifically to healthcare workers, emergency response teams, public safety personnel, and teachers.
- Bacteremia is the presence of bacteria in the blood; septicemia is the multiplication of bacteria in the blood.
- Rheumatic fever can occur as a complication after a streptococcal infection. Gangrene is a complication of necrosis due to tissue death.

- Zoonotic diseases are transmitted from vertebrate animals to humans, and are an emerging field of conservation medicine.
- Vectors are animals that are capable of transmitting diseases, and include flies, mites, fleas, ticks, and rodents.
- Viruses cause a variety of circulatory diseases, and with the exception of infectious mononucleosis are most prevalent in tropical areas.
- Fungi can enter the human body through the lungs, gastrointestinal system, paranasal sinuses, or the skin. After entry the fungi spread via the bloodstream or the lymphatic system, at which time the infection becomes difficult to treat.
- Protozoa that cause disease in the circulatory system of humans have a complex life cycle and include species causing malaria, babesiosis, toxoplasmosis, Chagas' disease, and leishmaniasis.

LIFE APPLICATION

Sandflies: A Tiny Enemy

In both the Desert Storm and Iraqi Freedom conflicts military personnel have been fighting a tiny, mostly unseen enemy—sandflies. These tiny insects are particularly important as they are the vector for the spread of the protozoan that causes the disease leishmaniasis. The form of the disease most frequently being treated by military medical personnel is the cutaneous form, which can be as simple as a sore at the site of the bite; in some cases it can spread, causing significant tissue damage. When diagnosed early and treated with antimony-containing compounds, pentamidine, or amphotericin B, the cure rate is high. Depending on the amount of tissue damage, recovering patients may need corrective surgery to repair the disfigurement that is sometimes caused by the disease. A small number of visceral forms have been found among service members in Iraq. The visceral form typically produces a much more serious form of the disease than the cutaneous form. All military and civilian personnel serving in Iraq are given factsheets and briefings to inform and educate them regarding leishmaniasis. The military uniforms are being treated with a repellant and personnel are provided with DEET repellant to keep the flies from spreading this disease.

Review Questions

1. All of the following are symptoms of endocarditis *except:*
   - **a.** Fever and chills
   - **b.** Weight loss
   - **c.** Leg swelling
   - **d.** Muscle aches

2. The toxic condition caused by the multiplication of bacteria in the blood is referred to as:
   - **a.** Bacteremia
   - **b.** Septicemia
   - **c.** Shock
   - **d.** Blood-borne infection

3. When microorganisms enter the circulatory system through lymphatic drainage and cause an infection the condition is called:
   - **a.** Bacteremia
   - **b.** Septicemia
   - **c.** Microbemia
   - **d.** Viremia

4. Rheumatic fever is an inflammatory disease and rare complication due to:
   a. Strep throat
   b. Gangrene
   c. Brucellosis
   d. Tularemia

5. All of the following are considered to be zoonotic diseases *except:*
   a. Brucellosis
   b. Undulant fever
   c. Plague
   d. Tularemia

6. "Rabbit fever" is a zoonotic disease is caused by:
   a. *Bartonella henselae*
   b. *Spirillum minus*
   c. *Francisella tularensis*
   d. *Yersinia pestis*

7. Rocky Mountain spotted fever is caused by:
   a. *Borrelia burgdorferi*
   b. *Rickettsia rickettsii*
   c. *Rickettsia prowazekii*
   d. *Ehrlichia chaffeensis*

8. Cytomegalovirus infections are caused by the human herpesvirus:
   a. 2
   b. 3
   c. 4
   d. 5

9. Malaria is caused by a:
   a. Virus
   b. Bacterium
   c. Helminth
   d. Protozoan

10. Which of the following is a disease caused by a protozoan?
    a. Cat scratch disease
    b. Toxoplasmosis
    c. Relapsing fever
    d. Plague

11. A common complication of necrosis, often related to wounds, is referred to as _____.

12. Any infectious disease or infection that can be transmitted from vertebrate animals to humans is classified as _____.

13. When bacteria are found in the blood the condition is referred to as _____.

14. The toxic condition caused by the spread of bacteria or bacterial toxins from the site of infection is called _____.

15. Chagas' disease is caused by _____.

16. Describe the different types of gangrene.

17. Describe the general principles of viral hemorrhagic fevers.

18. Discuss systemic mycoses.

19. Describe the life cycle of the protozoan causing malaria.

20. Describe the four different types of leishmaniasis.

Bibliography

Forbes BA, Sahm DF, Weissfeld AS: *Bailey & Scott's diagnostic microbiology*, ed 12, St. Louis, 2007, Mosby.

Mahon CR, Lehman DC, Manuselis G: *Textbook of diagnostic microbiology*, ed 3, St. Louis, 2007, Saunders.

Mims C, Dockrell HM, Goering RV, et al: *Medical microbiology*, ed 3, St. Louis, 2004, Mosby.

Murray PR, Rosenthal KS, Pfaller MA: *Medical microbiology*, ed 5, St. Louis, 2005, Mosby.

Talaro KP: *Foundations in microbiology*, ed 6, 2005, McGraw-Hill.

Totora GJ, Funke BR, Case CL: *Microbiology: an introduction*, ed 9, 2007, Pearson, Benjamin Cummings.

Internet Resources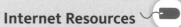

Centers for Disease Control and Prevention, http://www.cdc.gov/

The Merck Manuals Online Medical Library, Bacteremia, http://www.merck.com/mmpe/sec14/ch167/ch167g.html

NIOSH Safety and Health Topic: Bloodborne Infectious Diseases: HIV/AIDS, Hepatitis B Virus, and Hepatitis C Virus, http://www.cdc.gov/niosh/topics/bbp/

The Merck Manuals Online Medical Library, Noninfective Endocarditis, http://www.merck.com/mmpe/sec07/ch077/ch077c.html

Baron S: Medical Microbiology, ed 4, © The University of Texas Medical Branch at Galveston. Clinical Syndromes: Microbemia, http://www.ncbi.nlm.nih.gov/books/bv.fcgi?indexed=google&rid=mmed.section.5077

Pelletier LL Jr: Microbiology of the Circulatory System, Microbemia, http://www.gsbs.utmb.edu/microbook/ch094.htm

MayoClinic.com, Rheumatic Fever, http://www.mayoclinic.com/print/rheumatic-fever/DS00250/DSECTION=all&METHOD=print

CDC, National Center for Infectious Diseases, Brucellosis, http://www.cdc.gov/ncidod/diseases/submenus/sub_brucellosis.htm

CDC, Tularemia Fact Sheet, http://www.cdc.gov/ncidod/dvbid/tularemiafacts.pdf

Wikipedia, Bubonic Plague, http://en.wikipedia.org/wiki/Bubonic_plague

Consortium for Conservation Medicine, http://www.conservation-medicine.org/

CDC, Plague Information, http://www.bt.cdc.gov/agent/plague/

CDC, Rocky Mountain Spotted Fever, http://www.cdc.gov/ncidod/dvrd/rmsf/overview.htm

CDC, Cat Scratch Disease, http://www.cdc.gov/healthypets/diseases/catscratch.htm

Public Health Agency of Canada, Material Safety Data Sheets (MSDS) for Infectious Substances, http://www.phac-aspc.gc.ca/msds-ftss/msds144e.html

CDC, Special Pathogens Branch (Hemorrhagic Fevers), http://www.cdc.gov/ncidod/dvrd/spb/index.htm

MMWR: Fatal Rat-bite Fever—Florida and Washington, 2003, *MMWR* 53(51 & 52):1198–1202, 2005, http://www.cdc.gov/MMWR/preview/mmwrhtml/mm5351a2.htm

CDC, Tickborne Rickettsial Diseases: Ehrlichiosis, http://www.cdc.gov/ticks/diseases/ehrlichiosis/

Taege A: Tick-related Infections, Cleveland Clinic, http://www.clevelandclinicmeded.com/medicalpubs/diseasemanagement/infectiousdisease/ticks/ticks.htm

CDC, Tickborne Rickettsial Diseases, Rocky Mountain Spotted Fever, http://www.cdc.gov/ticks/diseases/rocky_mountain_spotted_fever/

CDC, Emergency Preparedness and Response, Tularemia FAQ, http://www.bt.cdc.gov/agent/tularemia/faq.asp

CDC, Tick Borne Relapsing Fever, http://www.cdc.gov/ncidod/dvbid/relapsingfever/index.htm

American Lyme Disease Foundation, Other Tick-borne Diseases, http://www.aldf.com/majorTick.shtml

CDC, National Center for Infectious Diseases, Epstein-Barr Virus and Infectious Mononucleosis, http://www.cdc.gov/ncidod/diseases/ebv.htm

CDC, Special Pathogens Branch, http://www.cdc.gov/ncidod/dvrd/spb/mnpages/whoweare.htm

CDC, Malaria, http://www.cdc.gov/malaria/disease.htm

CDC, Malaria, Schema of the Life Cycle of Malaria, http://www.cdc.gov/malaria/biology/life_cycle.htm

Healthline, Medicine for the Outdoors, Artesunate for Falciparum Malaria, http://www.healthline.com/blogs/outdoor_health/2008/06/artesunate-for-falciparum-malaria.html

CDC, Toxoplasmosis, http://www.cdc.gov/toxoplasmosis/

CDC, Chagas Disease Fact Sheet, http://www.cdc.gov/chagas/fact-sheets/detailed.html

15

Infections of the Urinary System

OUTLINE

Introduction
    Urinary Tract Infections (UTIs)
    Diagnosis of UTIs
    Risk Factors for UTIs
    Prevention and Treatment of UTIs

Bacterial Infections

Viral Infections
    Polyomaviruses JC and BK
    Cytomegalovirus
    Adenovirus

Fungal Infections

Parasitic Infections

LEARNING OBJECTIVES

After reading this chapter, the student should be able to:

- Identify the parts of the urinary system that are the sites of the most common urinary tract infections (UTI)
- Identify the microorganisms that are the most common causes of UTIs
- Describe typical symptoms of a UTI
- Identify and describe the three most common types of UTIs
- List common risk factors for a UTI
- Identify the patient group with the highest risk for a UTI and give reasons why
- Describe the typical diagnosis process to identify a UTI
- Identify and discuss various methods of treatments for UTIs
- List and discuss prevention factors for UTIs in men, women, children, the elderly, and individuals who are immunocompromised
- Identify some of the major groups of antibiotics specifically used in treating a UTI

bacteriuria
Chlamydia
colony-forming units
(CFU)
cystitis
glomerulonephritis
hematuria

homeostasis
kidneys
leptospirosis
Mycoplasma
nephrons
nephrostomy
pyelonephritis

ureters
urethra
urethritis
urinary bladder
urinary system

WHY YOU NEED TO KNOW

HISTORY

As far back as 3000 BCE, the Chinese recognized infections and diseases involving the urinary tract and developed an extensive list of herbal remedies. One of the most comprehensive ancient documents dealing with urinary tract infections and potential cures was the Ebers papyrus written in Egypt at about 1550 BCE. This document identified the illness and potential herbal cures but did not offer any attempts to explain the actual causes of these infections. In ancient Greece, Hippocrates (460–375 BCE) offered an explanation for urinary tract infections that involved an imbalance in the four humors of the body. He noted the presence of sand in urine that came from the consumption of contaminated water by the individual, which eventually led to the formation of stones, blocking the elimination of urine. This blockage caused the imbalance in the humors and the resultant disease. It was not until the mid-nineteenth century that Pasteur documented that microorganisms were responsible for the contamination of urine associated with urinary tract infections. Treatments at this time primarily involved the use of chemicals that altered the pH of the urinary bladder and the lower urinary tract. The development of antibiotics in the twentieth century resulted in modern regimens for effective treatment of urinary tract infections.

IMPACT

Today, in the United States urinary tract infections (UTIs) account for more than 8 million doctor visits each year. Women are especially prone to these infections; one in five to one half of women will develop one or more UTIs in their lifetime. Although UTIs occur with less frequency in men, they can be very serious.

FUTURE

Research is being conducted to develop a vaccine that can prevent the recurrence of UTIs in patients. Thus far there appear to be data indicating that women and children who experience repeated infections are likely to lack certain immunoglobulins to fight off infections. The vaccine stimulates the immune system to produce antibodies that fight the pathogen (see Chapter 20, The Immune System).

Introduction

The **urinary system** consists of the **kidneys, ureters, urinary bladder,** and **urethra** (Figure 15.1). The kidneys are the central organ of the system and are responsible for filtering wastes from the blood as well as for removing any excess liquid, thus forming urine. The functional units in the kidneys are the **nephrons** (Figure 15.2) and in addition to their filtering capacity they also keep a stable balance of minerals, salts, and other substances to maintain the **homeostasis** (the maintenance of a relatively stable environment of the body) of the blood. Furthermore, the kidneys produce erythropoietin, the hormone that aids in the formation of red blood cells. The ureters are narrow tubes that carry the urine from the kidneys to the urinary bladder, which stores the urine for later expulsion from the body. The urine stored in the urinary bladder is emptied through the urethra, whose length varies between male and female. The male urethra is longer than the female and the opening is located on the penis. Normally urine is sterile, free of any microorganisms; however, an infection can occur when infectious organisms, usually bacteria from the gastrointestinal tract, gain access to the opening of the urethra and multiply. The urinary tract is one of the most common sites of bacterial infection, particularly in females.

Urinary Tract Infections (UTIs)

There are a number of organisms that can be responsible for a urinary tract infection (UTI) infection but the most common is *Escherichia coli*, a gram-negative, facultatively anaerobic rod that can thrive in a relatively wide range of pH. The infection may remain localized in the urethra, but the organisms can also travel up the urethra and infect the urinary bladder. When a urinary bladder infection is not treated, it may spread to the kidneys. In a small number of cases, UTIs have been caused by organisms that originated in oral/gum infections. In these cases the organisms traveled through the bloodstream to the kidneys, where they gave rise to a kidney infection. In healthy individuals the urinary system is designed to prevent urine from backing up from the urinary bladder to the ureters and kidneys, and the flow of urine from the bladder typically helps wash away any microorganisms. The prostate gland in men also produces slightly acidic secretions that tend to slow bacterial growth. These structural and chemical mechanisms, along with the actions of a healthy immune

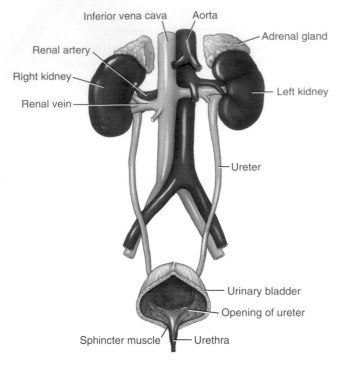

FIGURE 15.1 Diagram of the human urinary system. The urinary system consists of the kidneys, ureters, the urinary bladder, and the urethra.

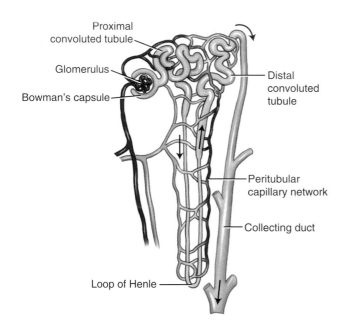

FIGURE 15.2 Nephrons are the functional units of the kidneys. Each nephron has a glomerulus, a Bowman's capsule, and a tubular portion that consists of the proximal convoluted tubule, the loop of Henle, the distal convoluted tubule, and a collecting duct.

system, are normally effective at preventing UTIs. The type of infection is typically defined by the organ or structure where the infection is located.

Organisms that cause UTIs may be sexually transmitted and the infections usually remain limited to the urethra and the organs of the reproductive system. Not all individuals with a

UTI show easily recognizable symptoms, but most cases include the following:

- Urgency to urinate
- Burning/painful sensation when urinating (dysuria)
- Frequency of urination, passing only small amounts each time
- Presence of blood or pus in the urine, or a cloudy, strong-smelling urine

Other symptoms may vary among individuals and depend on the specific type of infection. These symptoms may include the following:

- Uncomfortable pressure above the pubic bone in women
- A fullness of the rectum in men
- Pain in the back or side below the ribs
- Nausea
- Vomiting
- Fever
- Irritability
- Loss of appetite in children

Urinary tract infections are identified by the specific location or organ being affected by the microorganisms. The most common infections are urethritis, cystitis, pyelonephritis, leptospirosis, and glomerulonephritis.

Urethritis

Urethritis is a localized infection usually limited to the urethra. It can be caused by *E. coli* but also by **Chlamydia** or **Mycoplasma,** because the urethra is also associated with organs of the reproductive system. A common source of this infection for older or hospitalized patients is a catheter. If not treated early, the infection can travel up the catheter and spread the infection to the urinary bladder. *Trichomonas vaginalis,* a protozoan, has also been associated with urethritis as well as vaginitis (see Chapter 16, Infections of the Reproductive System). Enterococci and *Candida albicans* are other organisms that occasionally can cause urethritis.

Cystitis

Cystitis is an infection that occurs in the urinary bladder and is sometimes simply referred to as a *bladder infection.* *E. coli* is the primary cause of this infection but others, such as *Staphylococcus* species, and members of *Proteus, Enterobacter, Klebsiella,* and *Candida,* have also been identified as organisms causing urinary bladder infections. The bacteria travel up the urethra, sometimes via a catheter, into the bladder, where they multiply and cause inflammation. If the infection remains untreated, it can spread to the kidneys, causing an even more serious infection. The helminth *Schistosoma haematobium* has been associated with urinary bladder infections and the human polyomaviruses JC and BK can cause hemorrhagic cystitis.

Pyelonephritis

Pyelonephritis is often referred to simply as a *kidney infection,* and this serious infection can cause extensive and permanent damage to the kidneys. The same organisms responsible for most cases of cystitis are also responsible for most kidney infections, with *E. coli* alone being responsible for more than 80% of these infections.

Leptospirosis

The spirochete *Leptospira interrogans* is a zoonotic organism that can cause a kidney infection or other nonspecific illnesses. Many mammals such as dogs, cats, and rats carry the organism, which can come in contact with humans through contaminated urine, direct contact with the animal, or through water or soil. Many cases of **leptospirosis** are asymptomatic and fewer than 100 cases are reported each year in the United States.

Glomerulonephritis

Glomerulonephritis, also referred to as *Bright's disease,* involves inflammation and damage to the glomeruli of the kidneys. This is actually an immune complex disease that sometimes follows an oral streptococcal or viral infection. Antibody–antigen complexes are eventually filtered out in the kidneys, where they cause inflammation. This infection can cause some permanent damage to the kidneys and can be fatal.

Diagnosis of UTIs

Typically the detection/diagnosis process occurs in two stages. The first stage involves gathering a sample of urine for evaluation and the second stage involves testing the antibiotic sensitivity of any microorganisms that may be present. The collection of urine involves a procedure called a *"clean catch,"* wherein the patient thoroughly washes the genital area and then collects a midstream sample in a sterile container. The sample can then be both cultured for microbial growth as well as examined microscopically to determine the presence of microbes, pus, or blood. Typically the urine sample is streaked on a blood agar plate, using a special pattern to provide a semiquantitative analysis of the sample (Figure 15.3). If microbial growth occurs on the growth medium, the organisms can be tested with various antibiotics to identify the most effective one against a specific pathogen. This step is called a *sensitivity test.* The general term for the presence of bacteria in the urine is **bacteriuria.**

Risk Factors for UTIs

The risk factors for UTIs vary from individual to individual and from situation to situation; however, there appear to be certain factors that are common in many patients. The following groups exhibit unique risk factors:

- *Diabetics:* Patients with diabetes often have a higher risk for UTIs because of changes in the immune system that make them more vulnerable to infection.
- *Patients with catheters:* Patients with catheters in place for extended periods of time have an increased risk of infection of the urethra and ultimately the urinary bladder. About 20% of patients catheterized for more than 30 days will develop UTIs. The catheter itself can act as a location for the development of a biofilm (see Chapter 3, Cell Structure

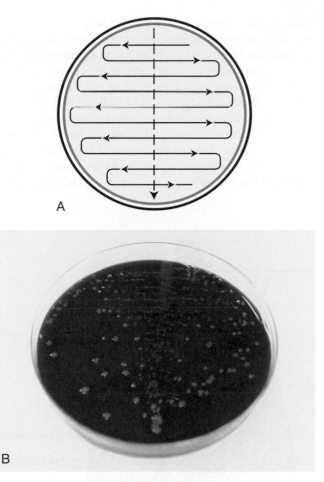

FIGURE 15.3 Method for streaking blood agar plates with a calibrated urine loop to produce isolated colonies with countable units. **A,** The drawing shows a streak pattern; **B,** the photograph shows a completed/incubated plate.

and Function), resulting in a greater diversity of species than may normally be found in the urinary bladder.

- *Infants/children with abnormalities of the urinary tract:* In boys the infections usually occur before the first birthday, and in girls the infections are common around the age of 3 years, overlapping with the period of toilet training. Infections in girls at a young age are especially dangerous because chronic infections over a long time period can lead to serious kidney damage. Some abnormalities that may lead to UTIs in children include vesicoureteral reflux (VUR), urinary obstruction, and dysfunctional voiding. VUR involves the reverse flow of urine from the bladder up the ureters and back to the kidneys. This condition can be corrected by surgical repositioning of the connection between the ureters and the urinary bladder in order to prevent the reverse flow. Urinary obstructions can include narrow ureters, kidney stones, or improper connection of the ureters to the kidneys or urinary bladder. Obstructions are typically solved by corrective surgical procedures or dissolving of the stones. Dysfunctional voiding is often a behavioral problem wherein children may intentionally delay voiding the bladder. This problem involves a simple process of behavior modification.

- *Women:* The largest group of patients who suffer with UTIs are adult women. Anatomically, women have a higher risk of infection because of the short length of the urethra and the close proximity of the opening to the anus (Figure 15.4), thus presenting a higher risk of fecal bacteria entering the urethra. Statistics also indicate that the incidence of infection increases with age and sexual activity. Rates of infection are particularly high in postmenopausal women because of incomplete urinary bladder emptying, and the loss of estrogen, which results in changes in the vaginal flora. Furthermore, the loss of normal flora such as lactobacilli decreases the level of competition with organisms such as *E. coli*. In addition, the tissues of the urethra become thinner and more fragile due to a decrease in estrogen, providing a good environment for opportunistic organisms. Sexual activity can irritate the urethra, allowing bacteria to more easily penetrate and move to the urinary bladder. The regular use of a diaphragm as a contraceptive measure can also lead to increased risk of infection particularly in premenopausal women.

- *Men:* The occurrence of UTIs in men under the age of 50 years is relatively low. The infections that do occur in this group are largely due to sexual activity that causes irritation of the urethra and subsequent penetration of the bacteria into the urinary bladder (Figure 15.5). There is evidence that uncircumcised men are at higher risk of developing a UTI. Most cases that occur in older men are associated with an obstruction or a medical procedure involving the placement of a catheter. In most cases an obstruction may be the result of kidney stones, blood clots, tumors, scar tissue, or a structural defect such as kinking of the ureters or a compression of the ureters by fibrous connective tissue. Surgical procedures can correct most of these defects. In the case of kidney stones, sound shock waves are commonly used if the stones do not pass through the system naturally; surgery is generally not the first course of treatment. Those older men who have an infection of the prostate gland are also at higher risk for a UTI.

Prevention and Treatment of UTIs

Prevention of UTIs

Specific prevention measures depend on the individuals involved, and the risk factors vary between groups on the basis of sex and age. The preventive measures are outlined according to the groups previously identified.

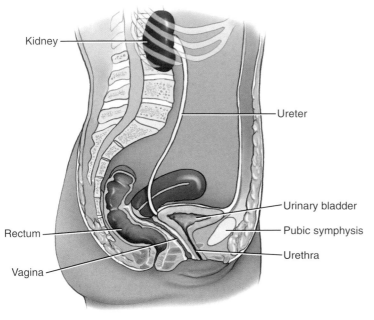

FIGURE 15.4 Structure of the female urinary system.

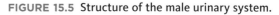

FIGURE 15.5 Structure of the male urinary system.

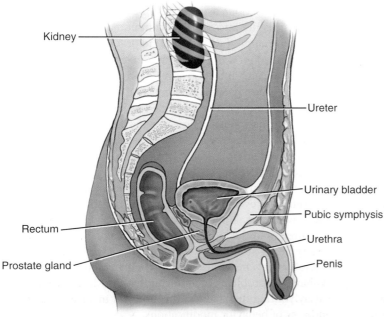

Circumcision

It has been shown that circumcision in the first year of an infant's life will provide significant protection against UTIs, and even in adults circumcision shows protection against UTIs. Infections of the urinary tract in infants can lead to significant morbidity in boys prior to 6 months of age. Complications of UTIs in infants include kidney infections and generally abnormal kidney function that in the future may cause high blood pressure and kidney failure. The lack of circumcision has been shown to be a risk factor for urinary tract infections in newborn boys.

- *Diabetics:* Preventive measures generally involve actions that improve the health of a diabetic, such as careful control of glucose levels and blood pressure. Those measures will ensure a healthy immune system that in turn will help to prevent UTIs.
- *Patients with catheters:* The best measures to prevent a UTI are frequent cleaning of the catheter and associated areas, and its removal, done as soon as it is no longer necessary. Although there is some debate about when a transurethral catheter should be changed, the practice in most health facilities is to do a monthly change. On diagnosis of a UTI, catheters need to be changed immediately. Because of the potential for UTIs and other complications, federal regulations mandate that indwelling catheters should be used only when there is valid medical justification.
- *Infants/children with abnormalities of the urinary tract:* The most effective measure is early identification of the problem followed by corrective surgery or procedures done as soon as possible.
- *Women:* The following measures have been suggested to help prevent infections in women:
  - Don't resist the urge to urinate.
  - Wipe from front to back to prevent bacteria around the anus from being spread to the area of the urethra.
  - Take showers instead of tub baths.
  - Cleanse the genital area before sexual intercourse.
  - Urinate after intercourse.
  - Avoid using feminine hygiene products, which may irritate the urethra.
  - Drink plenty of water every day.
- *Men:* Basic measures for men include the following:
  - Drink plenty of water every day.
  - Cleanse the genital area before intercourse.
  - Don't resist the urge to urinate; urinate when you feel the need.
  - Urinate after intercourse.

Treatment of UTIs

Once the causative pathogen has been identified, the treatment regimen with specific antibiotics may be determined. Determination of the specific drug to be used and the length of treat-

UTI Prevention: The Promise of New Vaccines

Statistically, UTIs are becoming almost as common as the common cold. *E. coli* continues to be the bacterium primarily responsible for most UTIs and although the majority of these infections are not life-threatening, they result in more than 7 million visits to the doctor annually. Recent research in vaccines to prevent UTIs has been showing promise on a number of fronts. One of the areas involves preventing the physical attachment of *E. coli* to the surface of the epithelium that lines the regions of the urinary tract. Without the attachment to tissue, bacteria are not able to colonize and cause infection. The vaccines being developed target the pili protruding from the surface of *E. coli;* the pili are the structures responsible for attachment. Other areas of research are also investigating the use of vaccines to enhance the effectiveness of dendritic cells—part of the body's immune system—to more effectively identify and destroy *E. coli* within the urinary tract. At this time most of these vaccines are in the clinical testing stage of development, but it does not appear that it will be too long before they should be readily available to the general public.

ment depends on the pathogen involved. The general health of the patient is also a major component of the treatment. For example, specific treatment may be based on the category to which the patient belongs: diabetic, pediatric, hospitalized/non-hospitalized, male, or female (further subdivided into pregnant and nonpregnant). The following is a list of drugs commonly used for simple UTIs:

- Amoxicillin
- Nitrofurantoin
- Trimethoprim
- Combination of trimethoprim and sulfamethoxazole
- Gentamicin
- Ciprofloxacin
- Cefadroxil
- Mecillinam
- Fosfomycin
- Cephalosporins

With effective treatment UTI symptoms will clear up within a few days. However, antibiotics may need to be continued for a week or so to prevent recurrence. As with all antibiotics it is important that a patient take the entire course of medication that was recommended to ensure that the infection is completely eliminated and to avoid development of antimicrobial resistance. Recurrent UTIs will require a longer course of antibiotic treatment. In infections caused by sexual activity, such as *Chlamydia* or *Mycoplasma* infections, a single dose of antibiotic may be recommended after sexual intercourse. Severe UTIs may require hospitalization and intravenous administration of antibiotics.

UTI Antibiotics

Antibiotic	Trade Name	Comments
Amoxicillin	Amoxil, Augmentin, Apo-Amoxi	β-Lactam antibiotic, effective against gram-positive bacteria
Cephalosporins	Keflex, Ultracef, Duricef, Velosef, Ceclor, Cefzil, Ceftin, Lorabid, Vantin, Omnicef, Spectracef, Suprax, Cedax, Rocephin	Used in treating resistant infections
Trimethoprim-sulfamethoxazole (TMP-SMX)	Bactrim, Cotrim, Septra	Serious allergic reactions are possible; high rate of resistance in some parts of the United States
Fluoroquinolones	Floxacin, Cipro, Noroxin, Levaquin, Tequin, Zagam	Wide spectrum, expensive, dangerous side effects in pregnant women and children
Nitrofurantoin	Furadantin, Macrodantin, Macrobid	Specifically used for UTIs; not useful for kidney infections; can upset stomach; reacts with other drugs; not to be given to mothers near end of pregnancy, nursing, or with kidney disease
Fosfomycin	Monurol	Resistant rates are low; safe for pregnant women
Tetracyclines Tetracycline Doxycycline Minocycline	Achromycin, Tetracyn, Tetramed, Cyclopar, Tetracycline, Sumycin Doxycycline, Doxycin Periostat, Arestin, Minocin, Dynacin	Effective against UTIs caused by *Mycoplasma* and *Chlamydia;* side effects include skin reactions to sunlight
Aminoglycosides Gentamicin Kanamycin Tobramycin Amikacin	Gentamicin, Alcomicin, Garamycin, Gentacidin Kantrex Tobramycin, Nebrin Amikin	Given only in combination with other antibiotics; serious side effects may include: damage to hearing, sense of balance, and kidney damage
Ertapenem	Invanz	Possible seizures and adverse CNS reactions

TABLE 15.1 Bacterial Diseases of the Urinary System

Infection/Disease	Pathogen	Symptoms	Treatment
Urinary bladder infection (cystitis)	*Escherichia coli, Staphylococcus saprophyticus*	Difficulty and/or pain in urination	Trimethoprim-sulfamethoxazole
Pyelonephritis	Mostly *Escherichia coli*	Fever, back pain	Cephalosporin
Leptospirosis	*Leptospira interrogans*	Headaches, muscle pain, fever, kidney failure	Doxycycline

Bacterial Infections

Most UTIs are caused by bacteria and the primary microorganism responsible for most UTIs is *E. coli;* however, *Chlamydia,* a gram-negative, coccoid obligate parasite, and *Mycoplasma,* a gram-negative, pleomorphic facultative anaerobe, may also cause infections. Some other organisms that have been associated with UTIs are *Klebsiella, Proteus, Enterobacter, Citrobacter, Serratia, Pseudomonas, Enterococcus,* and coagulase-negative *Staphylococcus.* The actual designation as a bacterial UTI is based on the presence of greater than 100,000 **colony-forming units (CFU)**/1 ml of urine. A summary of the most common bacterial infection of the urinary system is shown in Table 15.1.

In some cases, especially in older adults, bacteria may be present in the urine without any indication of infection. This condition is known as *asymptomatic bacteremia* and usually does not require treatment. There has been some research into the possible connection between UTIs in older adults and delirium or dementia. At this time there does not appear to be a consensus in the medical community as to whether a UTI causes diminished mental capabilities or if the UTI is the result for a patient who is exhibiting mental difficulties and not voiding his or her urine regularly.

Viral Infections

Viral UTIs are rare, but certain viruses may be found in urine even in the absence of urinary tract infections/disease. These viruses include human polyomaviruses JC and BK, cytomegalovirus (CMV), adenovirus, hantavirus, and a number of other viruses that can infect the kidneys, including mumps and HIV. Viruses are increasingly recognized as the cause of lower UTIs, especially hemorrhagic cystitis after stem cell and organ transplantation. Early diagnosis and treatment of viral UTIs may prevent the significant morbidity of hemorrhagic cystitis. Diagnosis of viral UTIs is based on molecular techniques including the polymerase chain reaction (see Chapter 25, Biotechnology), which allows quantification of the viral load. The current drug of choice against viral UTIs is cidofovir, because it is active against the most common viral pathogens.

Polyomaviruses JC and BK

Polyomaviruses JC and BK enter the human body via the respiratory route, spread throughout the body, and infect the epithelial cells of the kidney tubules and ureters. The viruses then establish latency, with the viral genome being present but not infectious in healthy people. Approximately one third of healthy individuals show the DNA sequence of these polyomaviruses in their kidneys without experiencing symptoms. Reactivation of these viruses may occur during pregnancy and also in immunocompromised patients, resulting in large amounts of virus in the urine. In some transplant patients the BK virus manifests itself subsequent to the necessary use of immunosuppressant medication and ultimately attacks the kidney via BK nephropathy.

Ureteric stenosis in renal transplant patients has been associated with polyomavirus infections. The viruses induce proliferation of the transitional epithelial cells of the ureters, which can lead to partial obstructions or stricture formation. The BK virus also has been associated with cases of acute hemorrhagic cystitis following bone marrow transplantation.

Cytomegalovirus

Cytomegalovirus infections are widely recognized as potentially serious causes of complications in the lung, spinal fluid, and brain, and also as the cause of graft failure in renal transplantation. Cytomegalovirus can also cause asymptomatic shedding in the urine of congenitally infected infants (see Congenital Infections in Chapter 23, Human Age and Microorganisms).

Adenovirus

Adenoviruses are a group of viruses that typically cause respiratory illnesses (see Chapter 11, Infections of the Respiratory System), but can also cause infections of the urinary and intestinal tracts. Some serotypes of the adenovirus have been implicated as the cause of hemorrhagic cystitis. In immunocompromised patients severe adenoviral infections are serious complications, especially in patients receiving hematopoietic stem cell transplantations. The most critical and fatal for these transplant patients are adenovirus-induced urinary tract infections and acute necrotizing tubulointestinal nephritis.

Fungal Infections

Fungal infections of the urinary tract affect primarily the bladder and the kidneys, with *Candida* species being the most common cause. However, all invasive fungi such as *Cryptococcus neoformans, Aspergillus* species, Mucoraceae species, *Histoplasma capsulatum, Blastomyces* species, and *Coccidioides immitis* may infect the kidneys as a result of a systemic or disseminated mycotic infection. *Candida* infections are usually associated with a urinary catheter, often after bacteriuria and antibiotic therapy. Renal candidiasis spread by the blood commonly originates from the gastrointestinal tract. Other *Candida* infections can occur in patients with **nephrostomy** tubes, other permanent indwelling devices, and stents. At high risk for these infections are patients who are immunocompromised because of chemotherapy, AIDS, or immunosuppressants after transplantation. Fungal pathogens are a cause of the increasing numbers of healthcare-associated (nosocomial) infections (see Healthcare-associated [Nosocomial] Infections in Chapter 9, Infection and Disease).

Parasitic Infections

Few parasites cause UTIs in humans; they include the protozoan *Trichomonas vaginalis* and the helminth *Schistosoma haematobium. Trichomonas vaginalis* can cause urethritis in both males and females, but in females it often also causes vaginitis (see Chapter 16, Infections of the Reproductive System).

Schistosomiasis is one of the most common parasitic infestations in the world, caused by flukes in the genus *Schistosoma* (see Helminths in Chapter 8, Eukaryotic Microorganisms). The organism associated with urinary schistosomiasis is *Schistosoma haematobium,* found in the Middle East, India, Portugal, and Africa; to date it does not exist in the United States. Typically the infection involves the bladder, but ureteral involvement can be found in as many as 30% of the patients. Adult *Schistosoma* is present in the venous plexuses around the urinary bladder, where they release their eggs. The eggs then cross the wall of the bladder, causing **hematuria** and fibrosis of the bladder. Subsequently the bladder becomes calcified, which increases the pressure on the ureters and kidneys. The main cause of schistosomiasis is the contamination of water supplies with human waste.

Summary

- The most common sites of infection in the urinary tract are the urethra, ureters, urinary bladder, and kidneys.
- The microorganism most frequently identified as the cause of a UTI is *E. coli,* with *Mycoplasma* and *Chlamydia* also being significant culprits.
- The most common UTIs are urethritis—infection of the urethra, cystitis—infection of the urinary bladder, and pyelonephritis—infection of the kidneys.
- The detection/diagnosis of a UTI occurs in two stages: gathering a sample of urine for testing and the subsequent testing of any organisms that may be present for antibiotic susceptibility.
- The risk factors associated with UTIs vary from individual to individual, but the largest risk groups are women and the elderly (particularly those with catheters or previous urinary tract problems).
- The primary treatment for UTIs is antibiotics. The specific antibiotic used and the prescribed regimen depends on the target microorganism and the general health/condition of the infected individual.
- Incidences of recurring infections are of particular concern for women, among whom as many as one in three will experience a recurrence within 1 year.
- Preventive measures to avoid a UTI in women include the following: take showers instead of baths, don't resist the urge to urinate, wipe from front to back, clean the genital area before intercourse, urinate after intercourse, drink plenty of water, and avoid feminine hygiene products that may irritate the urethra.
- Preventive measures to avoid a UTI in men include the following: drink plenty of water, clean the genitals before intercourse, don't resist the urge to urinate, and urinate after intercourse.
- The antibiotics commonly used to treat UTIs include amoxicillin, nitrofurantoin, trimethoprim, a combination of trimethoprim and sulfamethoxazole, gentamicin, ciprofloxacin, cefadroxil, mecillinam, fosfomycin, and the cephalosporins.

Review Questions

1. The main organs/structures of the urinary system are:
   a. Large intestine, stomach, esophagus, urinary bladder
   b. Small intestine, liver, urinary bladder, urethra
   c. Urethra, pancreas, liver, kidneys
   d. Kidneys, ureters, urinary bladder, urethra

2. The primary bacterium responsible for most UTIs is:
   a. *Staphylococcus aureus*
   b. *Bacillus subtilis*
   c. *Lactobacillus acidophilus*
   d. *Escherichia coli*

3. Diagnosis of a UTI is a two-stage process that involves:
   a. Collecting a blood sample and conducting a physical examination of the bladder
   b. Exploratory surgery and radiation therapy
   c. Collecting a urine sample and testing for antibiotic susceptibility of the organism
   d. Modifying the diet of the patient and conducting a physical examination of the urethra

4. The group most susceptible to recurring UTIs is:
   a. Teen-aged boys
   b. Women
   c. Teen-aged girl
   d. Normally healthy elderly men

5. Which of the following has not been shown to be a preventive against UTIs in women?
   a. Taking a daily dose of 81 mg of aspirin
   b. Urinating soon after sexual intercourse
   c. Taking showers instead of baths
   d. Urinating when the urge occurs

6. The urinary tract infection involving infection of the urinary bladder is called:
   a. Colitis
   b. Cystitis
   c. Phenylketonuria
   d. Toxoplasmosis

7. The urinary tract infection of the kidneys is called:
   a. Urethritis
   b. Cystitis
   c. Cellulitis
   d. Pyelonephritis

8. An effective method for treating a UTI is:
   a. Flushing the urinary bladder with saline
   b. Low doses of laxatives
   c. Application of a cold pack over the abdomen
   d. Regimen of the antibiotic amoxicillin

9. The following are typical symptoms of a UTI:
   a. Vomiting, blood in the urine
   b. Painful urination, cloudy urine
   c. Swollen abdomen, rapid heart rate
   d. Painful bowel movements, tightness in chest

10. What anatomical features in women can increase the possibility of a UTI?
    a. A shorter urethra, close proximity of the anus to the urethral opening
    b. A longer urethra, smaller urinary bladder
    c. Longer ureters, larger urinary bladder
    d. A longer urethra, close proximity of the anus to the vagina

11. The _____ are the central organs of the urinary system and are responsible for filtering wastes from the blood.

12. _____ is a UTI that occurs in the urinary bladder.

13. The method of collecting urine in which the patient washes the genital area and collects a midstream sample in a sterile container is called the _____ _____ procedure.

14. _____ and _____ are genera of organisms that are usually associated with UTIs related to sexual activity.

15. Glomerulonephritis is also referred to as _____ disease.

16. Describe some of the functions of a normal healthy body that help prevent the occurrence of UTIs.

17. List two reasons why postmenopausal women are at higher risk for UTIs.

18. Briefly describe the steps in the diagnosis of a UTI.

19. Name the typical antibiotic treatment regimen for UTIs.

20. Outline the path of infection that begins as urethritis and eventually becomes pyelonephritis.

Bibliography

Black JG: *Microbiology: principles and explorations*, ed 4, Upper Saddle River, NJ, 1999, Prentice-Hall.

Fishman J: BK virus nephropathy—polyomavirus adding insult to injury, *N Engl J Med* 347(7):527–530, 2002.

Mims C, Dockrell HM, Goering RV, et al: *Medical microbiology*, ed 3, St. Louis, 2004, Mosby.

Murray PR, Rosenthal KS, Phaller MA: *Medical microbiology*, ed 5, St. Louis, 2005, Mosby.

Paduch DA: Viral lower urinary tract infections, *Curr Urol Rep* 8(4):324–335, 2007.

Talaro KP: *Foundations in microbiology*, ed 6, New York, 2005, McGraw-Hill.

Totora GJ, Funke BR, Case CL: *Microbiology: an introduction*, ed 9, San Francisco, 2007, Benjamin Cummings/Pearson Education.

Internet Resources

About.com Heath Topics, Urinary Tract Infection Risk Factors, http://adam.about.com/reports/000036_3.htm

About.com Heath Topics, Urinary Tract Infection Medications, http://adam.about.com/reports/000036_7.htm

eMedicine by WebMD, Urinary Tract Infection, Female, http://www.emedicine.com/EMERG/topic626.htm

Urology Channel, Urinary Tract Infection, http://www.urologychannel.com/uti/

MayoClinic.com, Urinary Tract Infection, http://www.mayoclinic.com/print/urinary-tract-infection/DS00286/DSECTION=all&MET

National Kidney and Urologic Diseases Information Clearinghouse, Urinary Tract Infections in Adults, http://kidney.niddk.nih.gov/Kudiseases/pubs/utiadult/

Boyum DA: BK virus in kidney transplantation: a case study, *Progress in Transplantation*, Sep 2004. http://findarticles.com/p/articles/mi_qa4117/is_200409/ai_n9458266

eMedicine by WebMD, Schistosomiasis, Bladder, http://www.emedicine.com/radio/TOPIC621.HTM

16

Infections of the Reproductive System

OUTLINE

Introduction
Types of Infections
Global Burden

Infections of the Female Reproductive System
Bacterial Infections
Fungal Infections
Protozoan Infections

Infections of the Male Reproductive System
Bacterial Infections
Fungal Infections
Protozoan Infections

LEARNING OBJECTIVES

After reading this chapter, the student will be able to:

- Identify the organs and structures of the female and male reproductive systems
- Discuss the differences and similarities between the female and male reproductive systems regarding structure and function
- Describe the common microbial infections that affect the female reproductive system
- Describe the common microbial infections that affect the male reproductive system
- Discuss the structural and functional interactions between the urinary and reproductive systems and how they contribute to microbial infections
- List the common symptoms of both female and male reproductive system infections
- Identify the common methods for the diagnosis of reproductive system infections
- Discuss preventive measures that can be taken to minimize reproductive system infections
- Identify reproductive system infections that can also be sexually transmitted
- Discuss the different methods of treatment for reproductive system infections

accessory glands
balanitis
candidiasis
endogenous infections
endometritis
epididymitis
fallopian tubes
iatrogenic infections

lysozyme
mastitis
opportunistic
ovaries
pelvic inflammatory
  disease
prostate gland
prostatitis

sexually transmitted
  infections
testes
toxic shock syndrome
trichomoniasis
uterus
vagina
vaginitis

WHY YOU NEED TO KNOW

HISTORY

Written as far back as 1825 BCE, the Kahun gynecological papyrus contains a discourse on the female reproductive system including the diagnosis and treatment of various infections and diseases. In the more recent past, in 1980 an outbreak of toxic shock syndrome (TSS) occurred that was found to originate in the reproductive system. Hundreds of women using a specific brand of tampon were struck with TSS because of defects in the product design. The tampon was causing lesions when inserted, leading to excessive bleeding and irritation. The tampon was also designed with a very absorbent material to allow the woman to leave the tampon inserted for a longer period of time. The combination of bleeding and highly absorbent material created an ideal growth environment for *Staphylococcus aureus*, which produced large amounts of toxin that entered the bloodstream, causing TSS.

IMPACT

After the realization that some superabsorbent tampons increased the risk for developing TSS, Procter & Gamble voluntary recalled these products in September 1980.

With the advent of hormone therapy to help attenuate the negative factors associated with menopause, there is a new potential for vaginal infections in women. When the hormones cause chemical changes in the female reproductive system they can alter the pH in the vagina and also increase vaginal discharge, which keeps the area extra moist, thus favoring the growth of bacteria and/or fungus. The use of oral contraceptives also causes pH changes that favor the growth of certain infectious organisms. Circumcision in males is considered by many health professionals as an important measure to help improve hygiene in men and reduce the chance of infection of the genitalia.

FUTURE

Research today is revealing potential connections between reproductive system infections and the development of certain types of cancer. For example, mastitis, infection of the breast, has been suspected to be associated with the development of noninflammatory breast cancer. Some data appear to indicate a positive correlation, as noninflammatory breast cancer often appears after a severe infection of the breast. In addition, it has been shown that 90% of cervical cancer is linked to infections with human papillomavirus (HPV) and almost 80% of cases occur in low-income countries. Research on the prevalence and prevention of reproductive tract infections in developing countries is and will continue to be a major undertaking to develop more appropriate programmatic and policy responses for governments in low-income/developing countries.

Introduction

The human reproductive system consists of numerous organs and structures that are often closely associated with the urinary system (see Chapter 15, Infections of the Urinary System). Many texts will combine the two systems into the urogenital system. Although different in purpose and function these systems sometimes share the same organs/structures and therefore are susceptible to infections with the same microorganisms. This chapter specifically examines infections of the reproductive systems that are not sexually transmitted, as sexually transmitted infections are addressed in Chapter 17 (Sexually Transmitted Infections/Diseases).

The normal flora of the reproductive system varies greatly between the sexes; however, some typical resident flora in both reproductive systems include *Streptococcus, Bacteroides, Mycobacterium, Neisseria,* and some Enterobacteriaceae. Because of hormonal changes during the life of a woman, changes in the chemical environment in parts of the female reproductive system occur and will affect the resident flora, as well as the potential for infections. With the exception of the lower one third of the urethra, the healthy male reproductive system does not contain any resident flora and is normally sterile. In both the male and female systems, numerous defense mechanisms exist. They are in place to prevent infections within the organs and structures of the reproductive tract. These mechanisms include the following:

- Competition from the normal resident flora
- Chemical conditions such as acidic pH
- High salt concentrations
- Sphincter muscles in the ducts that prevent any backflow
- The flow of urine through parts of the system that wash away bacteria
- Enzymes such as **lysozyme,** found in semen and cervical mucus

In spite of these preventive mechanisms, the reproductive system is rather susceptible to sexually transmitted infections, which are discussed in detail in the next chapter. Because of the unique structures and biochemical factors, the examination of infections of the reproductive system, exclusive of sexually transmitted diseases, is addressed separately for the female and male systems.

Types of Infections

These infections impact the health and reproductive capacity of women, men, their families, and their communities. Consequences of the infections include infertility, ectopic pregnancy, chronic pelvic pain, pelvic inflammatory disease, miscarriage, and increased risk of contracting sexually transmitted infections (see Chapter 17, Sexually Transmitted Infections/Diseases). Reproductive tract infections (RTIs) can be categorized as endogenous, iatrogenic, and sexually transmitted infections.

- **Endogenous infections** are common RTIs worldwide. These infections result from an overgrowth of the normal vaginal flora. They include bacterial vaginosis and candidiasis, both of which can be treated and cured.
- **Iatrogenic infections** are caused by the introduction of microorganisms into the reproductive tract through a medical procedure. These include the following: abortion, menstrual regulation, insertion of an intrauterine device (IUD), unhygienic conditions during childbirth, as well as sterilization procedures and circumcision performed under unhygienic conditions.
- **Sexually transmitted infections** (STIs) are transmitted by sexual activity with an infected partner. STIs are discussed in Chapter 17.

Global Burden

RTIs are recognized by the World Health Organization (WHO, Geneva, Switzerland) and other agencies to be a serious global health problem. Whereas both women and men are affected by RTIs, studies show that women are more susceptible to these infections. In addition, complications can be more serious in women. RTIs can cause pregnancy-related complications, as well as congenital infections. Other consequences of RTIs include pelvic inflammatory disease (PID), infertility, ectopic pregnancy, and chronic pain. Furthermore, studies have shown that certain RTIs can increase the chances of HIV transmission. Signs and symptoms of many infections may not show until damage with serious consequences to the reproductive organs occurs.

Infections of the Female Reproductive System

Because of the differences in structure, function, and systemic biochemical processes between males and females, the mechanisms of infection along with the targets and causative agents

of infections differ considerably. The female reproductive system consists of the **ovaries, fallopian tubes, uterus, vagina,** and the external genitalia (Figure 16.1). The mammary glands are part of the female system but they are not necessary for reproduction; they play a role only after birth.

Bacterial Infections

Several bacterial infections of women's reproductive system may cause pain, irritation, or other symptoms. Some of these infections can lead to infertility or present a serious health risk. It is not uncommon for more than one infection to occur simultaneously. Unfortunately, having any one of the bacterial infections does not provide immunity against a future infection.

Vaginitis

Bacterial **vaginitis** (BV) is a common infection usually caused by an **opportunistic** pathogen within the normal resident flora that multiplies to abnormally high numbers. This overgrowth of a bacterial population normally found in relatively low numbers is due to any number of factors, including the following:

- Use of antibiotics
- A condition that affects the immune system such as diabetes
- Pregnancy
- Use of contraceptives
- Menopause
- Any condition that changes the pH of the vagina

A number of bacteria can account for bacterial vaginitis, none of which produce the infection alone. Typically a number of bacteria, usually anaerobes, interact to produce an infection. The bacterium *Gardnerella vaginalis* in combination with other anaerobic bacteria accounts for about 30% of vaginitis cases. *Gardnerella vaginalis* is a tiny, gram-negative coccobacillus that is normally present in either the urinary or reproductive tract of 20% to 40% of healthy women. In women of reproductive age, the normal vaginal pH is 3.8 to 4.4, with readings in the neutral range in young girls and elderly women. When the vaginal pH reaches the range of 5 to 6, *Gardnerella vaginalis* can interact with anaerobes such as those in the genera *Bacteroides* and *Peptostreptococcus* to cause bacterial vaginitis. This type of infection is sometimes called *nonspecific vaginitis* because different anaerobes are reacting with *Gardnerella* to cause the infection. This type of infection is characterized by a frothy, fishy smelling vaginal discharge that may be small in volume but may contain millions of organisms.

Diagnosis can be made by microscopic examination of wet mounts made from vaginal discharge. Vaginal epithelial cells are referred to as *"clue cells"* and will be covered with many of the coccobacilli in the case of a vaginitis infection. BV can lead to pelvic inflammatory disease and also may increase the risk of transmitting or acquiring HIV.

There are a number of preventive measures that can be taken to help women avoid bacterial vaginitis, and they include the following:

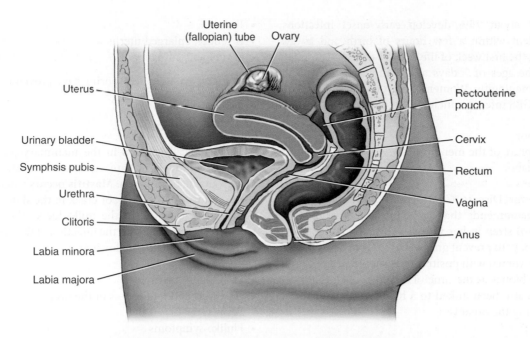

FIGURE 16.1 The female reproductive system consists of the ovaries, fallopian tubes, uterus, vagina, and external genitalia.

Labels in figure:
Uterine (fallopian) tube · Ovary · Uterus · Urinary bladder · Symphsis pubis · Urethra · Clitoris · Labia minora · Labia majora · Rectouterine pouch · Cervix · Rectum · Vagina · Anus

- Avoid frequent douching
- Avoid tampons that irritate the vaginal wall
- Avoid tight pants
- Use of panties or panty hose with a cotton crotch

Treatment of vaginitis usually involves a two-pronged approach: First, the use of antibiotics to bring the infection under control and second, the use of live bacterial cultures such as those found in yogurt as a douche to replace the normal lactobacillus flora that may have been killed by the antibiotics. Antibiotics such as metronidazole, ampicillin, and tetracycline have proven effective against the anaerobes that work with *Gardnerella* to produce the infection.

Toxic Shock Syndrome (TSS)

Toxic shock syndrome (TSS) is usually considered a blood-borne infection and is discussed in detail in Chapter 14 (Infections of the Circulatory System). However, one of the areas of the body especially prone to an infection causing TSS in women is the reproductive tract, specifically the vagina. The bacteria most often associated with TSS originating in the vagina is *Staphylococcus aureus,* and between 5% and 15% of women normally have *S. aureus* among their vaginal microflora. This type of infection normally manifests itself when use of a tampon causes a lesion in the vagina. The menstrual flow blood accumulates in the absorbent material of the tampon, which provides ideal growing conditions for the bacteria. As the bacteria multiply they produce exotoxin C, which can travel into the bloodstream through the lesion in the tissue of the vagina, causing a systemic reaction. Manifestations of TSS include the following:

- Fever
- Low blood pressure
- Rashes

- Peeling of the skin, often on the palms of the hands and plantar surface of the feet

The most effective treatment is the immediate use of the antibiotic nafcillin. In severe cases, death can occur as a result of shock. Recurrence of a TSS infection is possible, especially during subsequent menstrual cycles. To prevent recurring infections, the prophylactic use of antibiotics and the cessation of use of tampons have proven to be effective.

Group B Streptococcal Infection

Streptococcus is a genus of spherical gram-positive bacteria capable of causing infections in many parts of the body, including the reproductive system. Streptococci are also part of the normal flora of the skin, mouth, upper respiratory tract, intestine, and reproductive tract of humans. Numerous strains of *Streptococcus* have been identified, with types A, B, C, D, and G being most likely to cause serious infections. Streptococcal infections are communicable diseases that develop when the organism overgrows, or invades other parts of the body and contaminates blood or tissue.

Group B strep, or GBS, is *Streptococcus agalactiae* and most often affects pregnant women, infants, the elderly, and chronically ill adults. The organism emerged in the 1970s and since then has been the primary cause of life-threatening illness and death in newborns. GBS exists in the reproductive tract of 20% to 25% of all pregnant women, but only 2% of them develop an invasive infection. If the organisms gain access to the amniotic fluid, the results include sepsis, pneumonia, or meningitis in the newborn infant. Unfortunately, 40% to 73% of the women with the organism present will transmit the bacteria to their babies during delivery.

Two or three newborns per 1000 live births will end up with a GBS infection and up to 50% of these infants will die. Of the infants infected about 75% develop early-onset infections, sometimes evident within a few hours of birth and always apparent during the first week of life. Others develop late-onset GBS between the ages of 7 days and 3 months, when these babies develop meningitis. Women at high risk of giving birth to infants with GBS infection include those having:

- Premature labor
- Premature rupture of the membranes
- Fever during labor

The Centers for Disease Control and Prevention (CDC, Atlanta, GA) recommends that pregnant women should be tested for group B strep in her vagina and rectum at 35 to 37 weeks of pregnancy. To prevent group B strep from being passed to the newborn, women with positive tests should receive intravenous (IV) antibiotics at the time of labor or when the water breaks. GBS has also been linked to a history of breast cancer in women carrying the organism.

Endometritis

Endometritis affects the uterus and can be caused by a number of different organisms. *Escherichia coli* and group B streptococci are among those frequently associated with the infection. This particular infection is most likely to occur after childbirth or an abortion because of the trauma to the lining of the uterus, which makes it susceptible to microbial attack. The trauma may occur during a pelvic examination or delivery, when instruments are inserted into the uterus. Symptoms of endometritis include the following:

MEDICAL HIGHLIGHTS

Streptococcus agalactiae: Not Just a Cow's Problem Anymore

For many years the sole member of *Streptococcus* group B organisms, *S. agalactiae,* was known primarily as a pathogen of dairy cows and as only an occasional opportunistic human urogenital pathogen. In dairy cows it was long known to be a frequent cause of mastitis, thus leading to its species name, *agalactiae,* which literally means "no milk." More recently this bacterium has now been identified as a serious human pathogen that has proven to be particularly dangerous to newborns as well as pregnant mothers and even the elderly. About 25% of women have *S. agalactiae* as part of the normal vaginal flora. If passed to the newborn, the organism can cause general bacteremia, pneumonia, or meningitis. It has been shown that once a pregnant woman is identified as a carrier, if antibiotics are administered before birth, the chance of the newborn becoming infected is dramatically decreased. Without antibiotic treatment the chance of a baby becoming infected by a carrier mother is 1 in 200, whereas treatment with antibiotics before birth decreases the chance to 1 in 4000, a 20-fold difference.

- Fever
- A tender, enlarged uterus
- Severe abdominal pain

Treatments with cephalosporins have proven to be effective.

Mastitis

Mastitis typically occurs in the mammary glands of nursing mothers, although in rare circumstances this condition can occur outside of lactation. **Mastitis** occurs when bacteria enter the breast through a break or crack in the skin of the nipple, or through the opening to the milk ducts. The organism most frequently associated with the infection of the breast is *S. aureus.* Symptoms include the following:

- Swelling of the breast
- Hardness and tenderness of the breast
- Fever
- Flulike symptoms

Penicillin is frequently the antibiotic of choice when treating this infection.

Risk factors for developing mastitis include the following:

- Sore or cracked nipples
- Previous bout of mastitis while breastfeeding
- Using only one position to breastfeed, which may not fully drain the breast
- Wearing a tight-fitting bra that may restrict milk flow

Pelvic Inflammatory Disease (PID)

On occasion bacteria from the vagina can travel upward and infect the uterus, fallopian tubes, and ovaries, causing **pelvic inflammatory disease.** PID is a collective term for any extensive bacterial infection of the pelvic organs, including the uterus, fallopian tubes, and/or ovaries. The infection may lead to tissue necrosis with or without abscess formation. Pus may be released into the peritoneum, that is, the abdominal lining. Although normally caused by sexually transmitted pathogens, organisms such as *Mycoplasma hominis,* which is a common component of the vaginal flora, have been known to cause opportunistic infection of the pelvic organs. PID infections may be asymptomatic; however, they often exhibit the following:

- Fever,
- Vaginal bleeding
- Severe abdominal pain

If damage occurs to parts of the pelvic organs such as the fallopian tubes (salpingitis), there is increased risk of infertility or a more dangerous condition called an *ectopic pregnancy,* in which the fertilized egg implants in the fallopian tube instead of the uterus. The administration of tetracyclines and cephalosporins has proven effective in treating these infections.

Fungal Infections

Fungi live in air, soil, plants, and water. Some types of fungi are present on surface structures of the body, in the mouth, vagina, and in the intestines of humans. Although normally harmless, these fungi occasionally cause local infections of the skin and nails, vagina, mouth, or sinuses. In persons with a compromised immune system or in individuals with foreign material (e.g., a catheter) in their body, fungal infections can have serious consequences.

Candidiasis

Vaginal **candidiasis,** or simply vaginal yeast infection, is caused by the organism *Candida albicans.* This organism is a yeastlike fungus that is often part of the normal vaginal flora; however, it can become an opportunistic pathogen when the competing microflora is suppressed by antibiotics or other factors such as the use of oral contraceptives, pregnancy, or menstruation. *C. albicans* is the most common cause of vaginitis in women, with about 75% of all women experiencing at least one episode in their lifetime. Symptoms of the infection are vaginal itching and a thick, white, or yellowish-green, yeasty smelling discharge. Diagnosis of an infection usually involves microscopic examination of scrapings from the infected area and isolation of the fungus in culture. A number of antifungal drugs such as nystatin, clotrimazole, miconazole, and oral administration of ketoconazole are effective at treating vaginal candidiasis.

LIFE APPLICATION

Yeast Infections: The Lurking Opportunist

The environment around us is filled with microbial life including numerous types of fungi. Many fungal cells and spores are on our bodies. Fortunately, the numbers of these organisms are kept in check through competition with the normal bacterial flora as well as inhibitory conditions such as the pH. When these control mechanisms are disrupted, the fungi can become opportunistic pathogens causing an assortment of infections. The reproductive system is especially susceptible to fungal (typically yeast) infections as this system is subject to natural changes over time that affect the normal inhibitory conditions. Women are especially at risk of a yeast infection due to the hormonal changes that occur throughout their lifetimes. The normal vaginal pH of healthy women of reproductive age is 3.8 to 4.4. In young girls and elderly women the pH is close to neutral (pH 7). Yeasts such as *Candida albicans* thrive in the more acidic environment and populations that are usually present in relatively low numbers in a neutral environment will increase dramatically as opportunistic pathogens. These same changes can also occur if a woman uses oral contraceptives, antibiotics, is involved in hormone therapy, or experiences any changes in the normal pH levels of the vagina.

Protozoan Infections

Protozoans are eukaryotic organisms (see Protozoans in Chapter 8, Eukaryotic Microorganisms), some of which can be parasites of humans. The organism may colonize and infect the oropharynx, duodenum, colon, and urogenital tract of humans.

Trichomoniasis

Trichomoniasis is transmitted primarily through sexual intercourse; however, there have been cases of transfer by other means. Although a relatively rare occurrence, there are confirmed cases of children becoming infected due to contact with contaminated linens and toilet seats. The organism that causes the infection is *Trichomonas vaginalis* (Figure 16.2), a large flagellate with an undulating membrane. The organism is thought to be part of the normal microflora, where it feeds on bacteria and cell secretions. The optimal pH for growth of this organism is 5.5 to 6.0, and so it is only when the pH of vaginal secretions is disturbed that conditions favor the growth of this protozoan. Successful competition with the normal flora will result in the overgrowth of *Trichomonas* to an infectious level. Other conditions such as bacterial antibiotic therapy, diabetes, and physical lesions may also favor an infection with this protozoan. Symptoms of infection include the following:

- Intense itching
- Burning pain during urination
- A white-yellow, frothy, foul-smelling discharge

Diagnosis is accomplished by direct microscopic examination of the discharge to identify the presence of the organisms. The organism can also be isolated and grown in laboratory media. The drug of choice for treatment is metronidazole, administered orally.

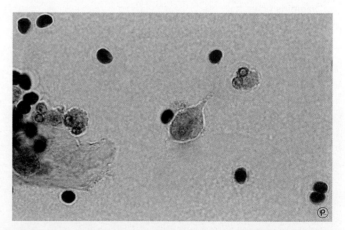

FIGURE 16.2 Trichomonas vaginalis trophozoite with flagella. (From Marler LM, Siders JA, Simpson A, et al: Parasitology image atlas CD-ROM, Indiana Pathology Images, 2003. In Murray PR, Rosenthal KS, Pfaller MA: *Medical microbiology,* ed 5, St. Louis, 2005, Mosby.)

Nonsexually Transmitted Diseases of the Female Reproductive System

Disease	Organism	Target of Infection	Symptoms	Treatment
Bacterial				
Vaginitis	*Gardnerella vaginalis* and other anaerobes normally found in the vagina, typically *Bacteroides* and *Peptostreptococcus*	Vagina	Vaginal irritation and inflammation; frothy, fishy-smelling discharge	Metronidazole (Flagyl), ampicillin, tetracycline
Toxic shock syndrome	*Staphylococcus aureus*	Systemic infection, primarily involving the circulatory system	Fever, low blood pressure, shock, diarrhea, extensive skin rash followed by shedding of the skin (particularly on palms of hands and soles of feet)	Nafcillin (Unipen) Erythromycin (E-Mycin) lincosamide, clindamycin (Cleocin)
Endometritis	*Escherichia coli*, group B streptococci	Uterus	Lower abdominal pain, fever, uterine tenderness, malaise, abnormal or bloody vaginal discharge	Clindamycin (Cleocin), gentamicin (Gentacidin, Garamycin), ampicillin (Omnipen, Marcillin), metronidazole (Flagyl), doxycycline (Vibramycin, Bio-Tab, Doryx), ertapenem (Invanz)
Mastitis	*S. aureus*	Breast	Tenderness and swelling of breast, body aches, fever and chills, fatigue, sometimes abscesses	Erythromycin, cephalexin (Keflex), dicloxacillin (Dycill)
Pelvic inflammatory disease (PID)	Numerous organisms, including *Mycoplasma hominis*, *Bacteroides*, *Enterococcus*, *E. coli*, group B streptococci, *Gardnerella*	Pelvic organs	Fever, vaginal bleeding, severe abdominal or back pain, painful sexual intercourse; sometimes asymptomatic	Tetracyclines, cephalosporins
Fungal				
Candidiasis (fungal vaginitis or yeast infection)	*Candida albicans*	Vagina	Vaginal itching; thick, white, yeasty smelling vaginal discharge	Oral: Fluconazole (Diflucan), ketoconazole (Nizoral), itraconazole (Sporanox) Vaginal application: Butoconazole (Femstat), clotrimazole (Mycelex, Gyne-Lotrimin, FemCare), miconazole (Monistat-7, Femizol-M), nystatin (Mycostatin), terconazole (Terazol), tioconazole (Vagistat-1)
Protozoan				
Trichomoniasis	*Trichomonas vaginalis*	Vagina	Intense itching, burning pain during urination; white-yellow, frothy, foul-smelling vaginal discharge	Metronidazole (Flagyl) For pregnant women: Topical use of clotrimazole (Gyne-Lotrimin, Mycelex-7)

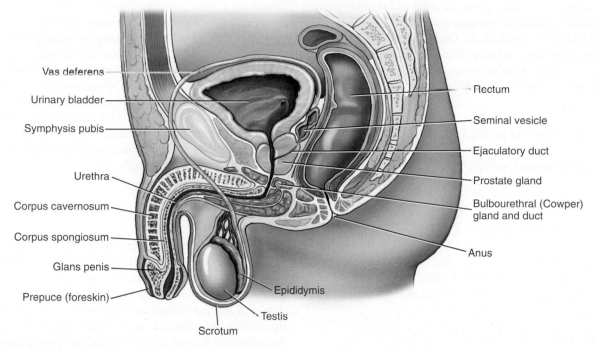

FIGURE 16.3 The male reproductive system consists of the testes, a system of ducts, the accessory glands (prostate, seminal vesicles, and Cowper's gland), and the penis.

Infections of the Male Reproductive System

The male reproductive system consists of the **testes,** a system of ducts, the **accessory glands** (prostate, seminal vesicles, and Cowper's gland), and the penis (Figure 16.3). Differences in structure and function between the female and male reproductive systems result in different types of infections. In general, the male reproductive system is sterile and has no population of normal flora.

Bacterial Infections

Prostatitis

The **prostate gland** is located at the base of the penis and secretes liquid substances into the semen that aid the sperm. This fluid is normally sterile, but bacteria from urine can enter the prostate gland via the urethra. Bacteria that are capable of causing **prostatitis** include the following:

- *Escherichia coli*
- *Klebsiella pneumoniae*
- *Pseudomonas aeruginosa*
- *Proteus* spp.
- *Staphylococcus* spp.
- *Enterococcus* spp.
- *Chlamydia trachomatis*
- *Ureaplasma urealyticum*
- *Mycoplasma hominis*

Once in the prostate gland these bacteria can rapidly multiply and cause an acute infection. Because common structures are involved, prostatitis is almost always accompanied by a urinary tract infection.

Symptoms of prostatitis include the following:

- Fever and chills
- Malaise
- Frequent need to urinate
- Pain in the area between the base of the penis and the rectum
- Painful urination
- Weak urine flow

Diagnosis of prostatitis typically involves actual palpation of the gland through a rectal examination to detect whether the gland is tender or swollen. A urine sample may also be taken to detect high bacterial and white blood cell counts. Prevention of a prostate infection primarily involves complete voiding of urine and treating any blockages that may limit the flow of urine. Acute bacterial prostatitis is treated with antibiotics. Drugs typically used in treatment are as follows:

- Ciprofloxacin
- Levofloxacin
- Norfloxacin
- Ofloxacin
- Trimethoprim-sulfamethoxazole

Epididymitis

Epididymitis, or inflammation of the epididymis, usually represents a complication of urethritis or prostatitis. In a young man this condition is usually a complication of a sexually transmitted infection caused by pathogens such as *Neisseria gonorrhoeae* and *Chlamydia trachomatis*. On the other hand, in older patients the condition is usually caused by uropathogens, and typically is a complication of urinary obstruction or prostate surgery. Symptoms include the following:

- Fever
- Pain that develops over several hours

  Other symptoms may include:

- Chills
- Pain in the groin
- Tender, swollen epididymides

Treatment requires antibiotics and medication for pain relief. Complications of acute epididymitis include abscess formation, testicular infarction, development of chronic pain, and infertility.

Balanitis

Balanitis is the inflammation of the glans penis, and if this infection involves the foreskin and prepuce it is referred to as *balanoposthitis*. The most common complication of this infection is the inability to retract the foreskin from the glans penis. Men at highest risk are uncircumcised men who have poor personal hygiene. In the United States balanitis is a common condition affecting 11% of adult men seen in urology clinics, and 3% of children. Although caused mostly by bacteria, several other microorganisms can cause this condition, including the following:

- *Candida* spp.
- *Gardnerella vaginalis*
- *Treponema pallidum*
- *Borrelia vincentii* and *B. burgdorferi*
- Human papillomavirus (HPV)
- *Trichomonas* spp.

The most common symptoms of balanitis are discharge from the penis, and a red, itchy and moist penis. Treatment depends on the microbe causing the condition and may be an antibiotic or an antifungal agent. Because anaerobic conditions are necessary for the growth of the organisms causing the infection, simple exposure to air and local cleansing is most often effective.

Fungal Infections

Male Yeast Infections

Although usually associated with vaginitis, fungi such as *Candida albicans* can cause infections of the prostate gland. Most male yeast infections are a result of sexual transmission; however, infections can also occur when there is overgrowth due to suppression of competing microflora by antibiotics or other factors. The infection can occur on mucous membranes in the reproductive organs, such as the prostate gland, or on the skin of the external genitalia. Prostatitis can sometimes be caused by a yeast infection; however, internal infections can sometimes be asymptomatic in men. Skin-type infections can cause dry, flaking skin, and itching or burning in the infected area. Diabetics and those who are immunocompromised tend to be more susceptible to yeast infections. Diagnosis of a yeast infection can be accomplished by microscopic examination of scrapings of lesions and/or by culturing the scrapings or discharge from lesions. Treatment for internal infections includes use of the oral antifungal medication ketoconazole. For skin or surface infections, topical application of clotrimazole or miconazole is an effective treatment.

Protozoan Infections

Trichomoniasis

The infection of the male reproductive system is similar to that in the female reproductive system, in that the protozoan *Trichomonas vaginalis* usually overgrows the normal microflora in the genital mucosa. However, in the male, symptoms are only rarely displayed and the individual acts more as a carrier of the infection. When the infection is significant, symptoms may include irritation and itching in the infected area and a purulent discharge, a result of an accompanying bacterial infection. Diagnosis can be accomplished by microscopic examination of the discharge for presence of the organism. The organism can also be found in the semen or urine of males who are infected but asymptomatic, or isolated and grown on laboratory media. Oral metronidazole is an effective treatment that readily clears up the infection.

Summary

- The primary organs/structures of the female reproductive system include the following: ovaries, fallopian tubes, uterus, and vagina (mammary glands can also be included).
- The primary organs/structures of the male reproductive system include the following: testes, prostate gland, urethra, penis, and associated ducts.
- Because of close physical proximity and the sharing of some ducts, infections of the urinary tract often contribute to infections of the reproductive system, particularly in the male system, where infection almost always occurs when infected urine backs up into the urethra.
- Urinary tract infections (UTIs) may be endogenous, iatrogenic, or sexually transmitted (see Chapter 17, Sexually Transmitted Infections/Diseases).
- Common bacterial infections of the female reproductive system that are not strictly sexually transmitted include vaginitis, toxic shock syndrome, endometritis, mastitis, and pelvic inflammatory disease.
- Group B streptococci (*S. agalactiae*) can colonize in the vagina, not causing an infection in the woman, but possibly being transmitted to a newborn, often with devastating results.
- Fungal infections of the female reproductive system are limited to candidiasis; and protozoan infections are limited to trichomoniasis.

Nonsexually Transmitted Diseases of the Male Reproductive System

Disease	Organism	Target of Infection	Symptoms	Treatment
Bacterial				
Prostatitis	Infectious organisms of the urinary system	Prostate gland	Pain in genital area, fever and chills, malaise, frequent need to urinate, painful weak urination	Ciprofloxacin, ofloxacin, norfloxacin, levofloxacin
Epididymitis	*Young adults:* Sexually transmitted *Neisseria gonorrhoeae, Chlamydia trachomatis* *Older adults:* Uropathogens	Epididymides	Fever, pain, chills; tender, swollen epididymides	Antibiotics and pain relievers
Balanitis	Various microbes	Glans penis	Discharge from penis; red, itchy and moist penis	Depends on causative agent; exposure to air and local cleansing
Fungal				
Male yeast infection	*Candida albicans*	Prostate gland, skin of external genitalia	*Internal:* Same symptoms as for prostatitis *External:* Itchy, burning, flaking skin	*Internal:* Ketoconazole *External:* Topical application of clotrimazole or miconazole
Protozoan				
Trichomoniasis	*Trichomonas vaginalis*	Urethra	Asymptomatic; male acts as a carrier	Metronidazole

- Preventive measures that can be taken to minimize the potential for vaginitis include avoiding the following: frequent douching, tampons that irritate the vagina, tight pants, and use of panties/panty hose without cotton crotch material.
- Common microbial infections of the male reproductive system include bacterial prostatitis, epididymitis, balanitis, male yeast infection, and trichomoniasis (protozoan).

- The methods most commonly used to diagnose a reproductive system infection are the microscopic examination of discharge from infected organs and microscopic examination of urine for infection organisms.

Review Questions

1. The female reproductive system includes the following organs/structures:
   a. Ovaries, kidneys, uterus, vagina
   b. Uterus, vagina, bladder, duodenum
   c. Bladder, ureter, vagina, uterus
   d. Uterus, ovaries, vagina, fallopian tubes

2. Bacterial infections of the female reproductive system include:
   a. Vaginitis, toxic shock syndrome, endometritis, salpingitis
   b. Nephritis, endometritis, vaginitis, pelvic inflammation disease
   c. Toxic shock syndrome, nephritis, endometritis, cystitis
   d. Endometritis, vaginitis, cystitis, toxic shock syndrome

3. Bacteria that have been identified as frequently responsible for nonsexually transmitted infections of the reproductive system include:
   a. *Escherichia coli, Gardnerella vaginalis, Staphylococcus aureus*
   b. *Streptococcus faecalis, Klebsiella oxytoca, Serratia marcescens*
   c. *Clostridium tetani, Bacillus cereus, Staphylococcus aureus*
   d. *Neisseria gonorrhoeae, Helicobacter pylori, Pseudomonas aeruginosa*

4. The most common bacterial nonsexually transmitted infection of the male reproductive system is:
   a. Cystitis   c. Mastitis
   b. Prostatitis   d. Nephritis

5. The normal flora present in the healthy male reproductive system is best characterized as:
   a. Primarily gram-positive rods
   b. Acid-fast rods
   c. Sterile, no normal flora
   d. Gram-positive spore formers only

6. Methods typically used to diagnose bacterial infections of the reproductive system include:
   a. Microscopic examination of discharge from infected organ and microscopic examination of urine for organisms
   b. Biopsy of infected tissue and use of selective media
   c. Microscopic examination of fecal sample and protein test of urine
   d. Antibody agglutination test and coagulation test

7. Factors that can increase the chances of vaginitis are:
   a. Urinary blockage, drug use, stress
   b. Use of antibiotics, pregnancy, menopause
   c. Puberty, exposure to HPV, smoking/tobacco use
   d. Menopause, stress, steroid use

8. The organism that is responsible for the vast majority of cases of fungal vaginitis is:
   a. *Escherichia coli*
   b. *Streptococcus agalactiae*
   c. *Klebsiella oxytoca*
   d. *Candida albicans*

9. Symptoms of prostatitis include:
   a. Muscle aches, sore throat, swollen lymph nodes
   b. Painful joints, nausea, painful urination
   c. Painful urination, fever and chills, weak urine flow
   d. Weak urine flow, severe abdominal pains, bloody stool

10. Measures that can be taken to prevent bacterial vaginitis include:
    a. Douching, use of contraceptive pills, exercise
    b. Use of absorbent tampons, frequent douching, avoidance of tight pants
    c. Avoidance of douching, wearing panties with cotton crotch, exercise
    d. Avoidance of tight pants, wearing panties with cotton crotch, infrequent douching

11. Vaginal epithelial cells that can be examined to determine the presence of *Gardnerella vaginalis* are referred to as _____ _____.

12. Enzymes such as _____, found in cervical mucus and semen, are instrumental in providing a chemical defense against bacterial infections of the reproductive organs.

13. The bacterium most frequently responsible for toxic shock syndrome that originates in the reproductive system is _____.

14. Although normally caused by sexually transmitted organisms, pelvic inflammatory disease is sometimes caused by _____, which is a common part of the vaginal microflora.

15. _____ is a collective term for any extensive bacterial infection of the pelvic organs.

16. Identify measures that can be taken to prevent the recurrence of toxic shock syndrome originating in the reproductive organs.

17. List some members of the normal microflora of the reproductive system and discuss the effect they have on bacterial infections of the reproductive system.

18. As women age, discuss the role of changing pH within organs of the reproductive system and how this affects the potential for bacterial infections.

19. Discuss the features of the healthy reproductive system that contribute to the defense of the reproductive system from infections.

20. Discuss factors that may contribute to an abnormal increase in the normal microflora in female organs that could lead to vaginitis.

Bibliography

Black JG: *Microbiology: principles and explorations*, ed 6, Upper Saddle River, NJ, 2004, Prentice Hall.

Damjanov I: *Pathology for the health professions*, ed 3, St. Louis, 2006, Saunders.

Mims C, Dockrell HM, Goering RV, et al: *Medical microbiology*, ed 3, St. Louis, 2004, Mosby.

Murray PR, Rosenthal KS, Phaller MA: *Medical microbiology*, ed 5, St. Louis, 2005, Mosby.

Prescot L, Harley J, Klein D: *Microbiology*, ed 5, New York, 2002, McGraw-Hill.

Talaro KP: *Foundations in microbiology*, ed 6, New York, 2005, McGraw-Hill.

Totora GJ, Funke BR, Case CL: *Microbiology: an introduction*, ed 9, San Francisco, 2007, Benjamin Cummings/Pearson Education.

Internet Resources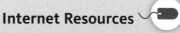

Centers for Disease Control and Prevention, http://www.cdc.gov

Women's Health Information, http://www.womens-health.co.uk

3-RX.com, http://www.3-rx.com

CDC, Group B Strep Prevention, General Public Frequently Asked Questions, http://www.cdc.gov/GroupBStrep/general/gen_public_faq.htm

University Hospitals, http://www.uhhospitals.org

A Health Blog, http://www.living4good.blogspot.com

eMedicineHealth, http://www.emedicinehealth.com

MedicineNet.com, http://www.medicinenet.com

Population Council, Reproductive Tract Infections Fact Sheet, http://www.popcouncil.org/pdfs/RTIFacsheetsRev.pdf

17

Sexually Transmitted Infections/Diseases

OUTLINE

Introduction

Bacterial Infections
Gonorrhea
Syphilis
Chlamydia
Mycoplasmal and Ureaplasmal Nongonococcal Urethritis (NGU)
Chancroid
Donovanosis (Granuloma Inguinale)

Viral Infections
HIV and AIDS
Hepatitis B, C, and D
Genital Herpes
Human Papillomavirus (HPV)
Molluscum Contagiosum

Fungal Infections
Vulvovaginal Candidiasis
Balanitis
Jock Itch

Protozoan Infections
Trichomoniasis

LEARNING OBJECTIVES

After reading this chapter, the student will be able to:
- Explain the difference in the terminology between sexually transmitted infections (STIs) and sexually transmitted diseases (STDs)
- Describe gonorrhea, syphilis, and chlamydia, and their incidence, symptoms, and treatment
- Describe the less common bacterial STIs including NGU, chancroid, and donovanosis
- Discuss the cause, prevention, and treatment of HIV and AIDS
- Discuss the cause, prevention, and treatment of hepatitis B, C, and D
- Describe the cause, prevention, and treatment of genital herpes and human papillomavirus infections

- Describe fungal STIs, their causative agents, and possible treatment
- Discuss the epidemiology of trichomoniasis
- Describe the complications that can occur with STIs and STDs
- Discuss the most common STIs in the US

KEY TERMS

acquired immune
   deficiency syndrome
   (AIDS)
chancroid
chlamydia
donovanosis
enzyme-linked
   immunosorbent assay
   (ELISA)
gonorrhea
hepatitis B (HBV)
hepatitis C (HCV)

hepatitis D (HDV)
human
   immunodeficiency
   virus (HIV)
HIV polymerase chain
   reaction (HIV PCR)
lymphogranuloma
   venereum (LGV)
nongonococcal urethritis
   (NGU)
OraSure

pelvic inflammatory
   disease (PID)
sexually transmitted
   infections/diseases
   (STIs/STDs)
syphilis
toxic shock syndrome
   (TSS)
trichomoniasis
urinanalysis
Western blot

WHY YOU NEED TO KNOW

HISTORY

History is replete with incidents of sexually transmitted diseases/infections (STDs/STIs). Virtually every major civilization and culture has recorded its experiences with sexually transmitted diseases and the effects they have had. In ancient Babylonia it was thought that sexually transmitted diseases were punishments enacted by the gods of love and fertility. In Hammurabi's code there was a specific warning that anyone who opposed him would suffer an "evil disease" that would produce dangerous sores that could not be cured, a disease that physicians could not diagnose, would destroy a person's seed, eliminating the chance to produce future offspring, and one that would inevitably lead to death—a description that perfectly fits STDs.

In more recent history we can see that STIs involve all aspects of a society. The notorious gangster of the 1920s, Al Capone, was able to escape the best efforts of law enforcement to put him away forever for his crimes. Although they finally were able to imprison him on charges of tax evasion, it appeared to many that he was going to escape judgment for his most serious crimes, until biology became the new prosecutor. Capone had contracted syphilis, which acted as judge and executioner, killing him in 1947.

IMPACT

One need not look far in national and international news to see headlines about STIs. The disease that has probably received the most attention in the past few decades is AIDS. The serious problems in dealing with the epidemic, especially in the African nations, have drawn the attention of the world. The United Nations and the United States have committed an enormous amount of money and support to help these nations, which are struggling to survive under the scourge of this sexually transmitted disease. Today AIDS is not limited to the African continent or to third-world nations, but continues to spread and claim lives in virtually every corner of the world and every level of society. Another disease that continues to hold its own is chlamydia, as it is one of most frequently found STIs in the United States. Although curable with antibiotics, many infected individuals do not display obvious symptoms, facilitating the spread of chlamydia. Chlamydia is also a disease that can weaken the body and allow it to become more susceptible to other, more serious STIs. And then there is gonorrhea; the use of oral contraceptives has become commonplace in today's society, and it has been discovered that women using the birth control pill are actually more susceptible to gonorrhea because of chemical changes produced in the body by "the pill."

FUTURE

Extensive research continues in an effort to discover a cure for AIDS; however, the prospects for a cure in the near future are looking bleak. The mutation rate of the HIV virus is high, which means researchers are chasing an elusive and ever-changing pathogen. *Neisseria gonorrhoeae,* in the past considered a fragile and fastidious pathogen, has more recently proven that strains of the pathogen are capable of surviving outside of the body in an infectious form for periods in excess of a month! New antibiotic-resistant strains of this bacterium have also appeared, challenging the present treatment regimens. All viral STIs are presently incurable and only a few vaccines have been developed to prevent viral sexually transmitted infections.

Introduction

Sexually transmitted infections/diseases (STIs/STDs) affect the same organs as the organs and structures covered in Chapter 16 (Infections of the Reproductive System). While affecting the same anatomical structures, the primary difference between infections of the reproductive system and sexually transmitted infections is the method of transmission. Sexual intercourse or any other sexual activity can lead to STIs, and eventually to STDs. Although the terms *sexually transmitted infection* and *sexually transmitted disease* are often used interchangeably, there is a distinction between the two. The term *infection* refers to just that, the presence of pathogenic organisms in a host, and symptoms of infection may be completely absent. The term *disease* refers to the appearance of symptoms and damaging effects as a result of an infection (see Chapter 9, Infection and Disease).

For the purpose of simplicity, STIs and STDs are referred to as STIs throughout this chapter. The organs that are affected by STIs in females are the ovaries, fallopian tubes, uterus, vagina, and external genitalia. In males the affected organs include the testes, prostate gland, urethra, and penis. Although reproductive organs are the primary targets, STIs may affect other organ systems and cause systemic problems. One of the likely reasons that sexual activity can lead to a high probability of STI transmission is the fact that most areas of the reproductive system are lined with mucous membranes, which are more susceptible to the penetration of pathogens than the skin (see Chapter 20, The Immune System). STIs can be caused by a variety of organisms including bacteria, fungi, viruses, and protozoa.

LIFE APPLICATION

Prevalence and Incidence of STIs and STDs

In statistical data, the term "prevalence" generally refers to the estimated population of people managing STIs or STDs at any given time. The term "incidence," on the other hand, refers to the number of new cases of STIs or STDs diagnosed annually. STIs are among the most common causes of infectious diseases in the United States, and they affect men and women of all backgrounds and economic levels. According to the Centers for Disease Control and Prevention (CDC), the incidence of STIs is rising, partly because in the last few decades young people have become sexually active earlier, and marry later. Furthermore, the divorce rate has been increasing, resulting in people who are sexually active having multiple sex partners during their lifetime, thus having an increased risk of acquiring STIs. CDC statistics indicate the following for the United States:

- Prevalence: About 65 million people in the United States are living with an incurable STI (1 in 4, or 25%).
- Incidence: About 15.3 million new cases occur annually (1 in 17, or about 6%)

Bacterial Infections

Bacterial STIs include chlamydia, gonorrhea, syphilis, chancroid, and others. Most of these infections are treatable with antibiotics. However, with any of the bacterial STIs, when not diagnosed and treated early, significant problems including infertility may occur. Some strains of the bacteria causing STIs have also become resistant to certain antibiotics.

Gonorrhea

Gonorrhea is the most reported STI in the United States.* The infection is caused by the bacterium *Neisseria gonorrhoeae*, a gram-negative diplococcus, and humans are the only known natural host. Once thought to be rather fragile and fastidious, not surviving for long periods of time outside of the host, research has recently discovered strains that are capable of surviving in dried pus on a bed sheet for 6 weeks. The organism can be transmitted through vaginal, anal, and oral sexual activity. The typical incubation time for the infection is between 2 and 7 days. Gonorrhea can be transmitted by individuals who are asymptomatic. Up to 40% of males and between 60% and 80% of females may be infected without any symptoms, but they can act as carriers for up to 5 to 15 years. A small number of organisms, in some cases only about 1000, is required to cause an infection. The symptoms of gonorrhea vary between males and females (Box 17.1). Besides infections of the genitals, oral and anal sexual activity can also lead to gonorrheal infections in the pharynx and the rectum, leading to general systemic bacteremia. Symptoms of systemic gonorrheal infections include the following:

- Fever
- Endocarditis
- Skin lesions (Figure 17.1) that can move to the joints, causing arthritis

Gonorrhea increases the risks of other infections, including HIV and chlamydia. Men with prolonged infections may also develop an inflammation of the testicles called *epididymitis*, a condition often leading to infertility. Prolonged infections in women can result in pelvic inflammatory disease (see Chapter

---

BOX 17.1 Symptoms of Gonorrhea

Female
- Vaginal discharge
- Painful burning during urination
- Painful intercourse
- Bleeding between periods

Male
- White, yellow, or green discharge from the penis
- Painful burning during urination
- Swelling of testicles

See http://www.cdc.gov/std/gonorrhea/STDFact-gonorrhea.htm

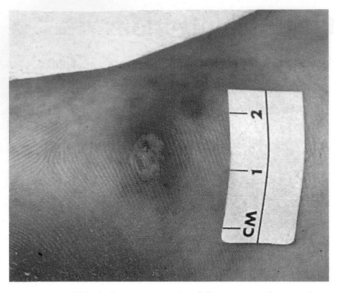

FIGURE 17.1 Skin lesions as a result of disseminated gonorrhea. The lesions start as erythematous papules and often develop into necrotic, grayish central lesions surrounded by an erythematous base. (From Morse S, Ballard RC, Holmes KK, et al: *Atlas of sexually transmitted diseases and AIDS,* ed 3, St. Louis, 2003, Mosby.)

TABLE 17.1 Stages of Syphilis

Stage	Time Frame	Symptoms
Primary	Ten to 90 d after initial infection	Small, red skin sores
Secondary	Two to 10 wk after primary stage	Red-brown rash on palms of hands and soles of feet; fever, swollen lymph nodes, sore throat, muscle and joint pain, loss of patches of hair, malaise, rash on skin and mucous membranes of mouth, throat, and cervix
Latent	After secondary stage	None
Tertiary	Many years from onset of the latent phase	Gummas—rubbery masses of tissue in various organs; memory loss, ataxia, paralysis, insanity, and finally death

16, Infections of the Reproductive System), which may include the uterus and fallopian tubes. Scar tissue in the fallopian tubes can prevent fertilization, and damage to the uterine wall can stop implantation of a fertilized ovum (zygote). Pelvic inflammatory disease also increases the risk of ectopic pregnancy.

During delivery gonorrhea can be passed from the infected mother to the baby as it moves through the birth canal (see Chapter 23, Human Age and Microorganisms). Infection of the newborn often leads to infection of the joints, blood infection (bacteremia), and/or blindness.

Diagnosis of gonorrhea is accomplished by identifying the organism by microscopic examination of discharge samples or in laboratory cultures of swabs from infected tissue. Treatment of gonorrhea originally involved sulfonamides and/or penicillin, but the organism has developed resistance to these antibiotics. Antibiotics currently used include ciprofloxacin, cefixime, ofloxacin, and levofloxacin.

Although treatment with antibiotics has a high success rate in eliminating the infection, any damage done to the organs during the infection is permanent.

At the present time there is no vaccine for gonorrhea but research is underway. Preventive measures to avoid contracting an infection include the following:

- Limiting the number of sex partners
- Informing partners about an infection
- Reporting signs or symptoms to a doctor
- Using condoms during sexual activity
- Abstaining from sexual activity

Syphilis

Syphilis has been in the human population for many years and is documented in many historical writings. Because it causes symptoms that can be associated with numerous other diseases, syphilis is sometimes referred to as the *"great imitator."* It is caused by *Treponema pallidum,* a gram-negative spirochete. Humans are the organism's only natural reservoir and transmission occurs through direct contact with sores of an infected person. Although the bacterium can be passed on through body fluids such as saliva, the primary means of transmission is through any sexual activity—vaginal, anal, or oral. A pregnant woman can also pass the infection on to her child during pregnancy. This infection is known as *congenital syphilis* (see Chapter 23, Human Age and Microorganisms).

Syphilis takes place in three stages, with an incubation time between 10 and 90 days after the initial infection. The initial symptoms may be mild and are sometimes difficult to diagnose because they resemble symptoms of other diseases such as gonorrhea. Many infected persons in the early stages do not realize that they are infected. If treated early, syphilis can be cured without any resulting serious or long-term health problems. Untreated, syphilis manifests itself in three stages: primary, secondary, and tertiary syphilis (Table 17.1).

- Primary syphilis represents itself as small, red sores (chancres) that appear on the body at the site of infection within 10 to 90 days after initial contact. These sores will eventually disappear, leaving a scar on the skin. if untreated, the symptoms will move to the secondary stage.
- Secondary syphilis occurs within 2 to 10 weeks of the primary stage (Figure 17.2). During this stage the organism enters the bloodstream and travels to other organ systems, causing a wide variety of symptoms including the following:
  - A red-brown rash on the palms of the hands and soles of the feet
  - Fever

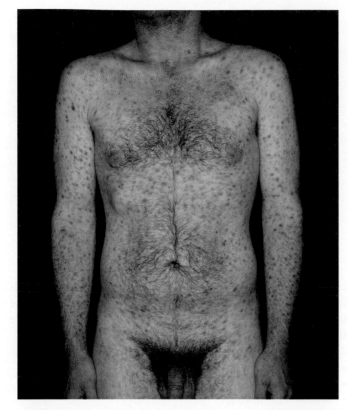

FIGURE 17.2 Rash of secondary syphilis. (From Habif TP: *Clinical dermatology: a color guide to diagnosis and therapy,* St. Louis, 1996, Mosby.)

- Swollen lymph nodes
- Sore throat
- Muscle and joint pain

Without treatment at this point the disease will move into the tertiary stage:

- Tertiary syphilis is the final stage of the disease, characterized by gummas (lesions) that begin to affect vital organs including the eyes, liver, heart, kidneys, and the brain. This stage results in conditions such as:
  - Memory loss
  - Ataxia
  - Paralysis
  - Insanity
  - Loss of muscle control
  - Vision problems followed by blindness
  - Deafness
  - Seizures
  - Dementia
  - Death

Patients with syphilis in the later stages are also at increased risk for HIV infection.

Pregnant women run the risk of passing the infection on to their unborn child and they have an increased risk for miscarriage, premature delivery, and stillbirth (see Chapter 23, Human Age and Microorganisms). Diagnosis of syphilis can be done by a number of different methods. Observing a sample from a lesion for the organism itself, using a dark-field microscope, is typically one of the first methods used for early detection. Along with microscopic examination, a number of blood-screening tests are available to confirm an infection. These include the following:

- Venereal disease research laboratory (VRDL) test
- Fluorescent treponemal antibody absorption (FTA-ABS) test
- Rapid plasma reagin (RPR) test
- *Treponema pallidum* hemagglutination assay (TPHA)

Because of the possibility that a single test may result in a false positive or negative reading during the different stages of the disease or under different circumstances, at least two blood tests are done to determine and confirm an infection. For example, the tests based on detection of antibodies are not useful in diagnosing the infection in a person who has had the disease previously, as the antibodies remain in the body for years.

Treatment for syphilis in the primary and secondary stages is fairly simple and can often be achieved with a single intramuscular dose of penicillin. In a more advanced stage of the infection hospitalization and a daily antibiotic regimen may be required. Tetracycline and erythromycin have proven to be effective for persons allergic to penicillin. At the present time there is no vaccine available; however, research is ongoing. Preventive measures to avoid contracting syphilis include the following:

- Avoiding contact with lesions and body fluids
- Use of condoms during intercourse
- Syphilis testing and treatment early in pregnancy

Chlamydia

Although usually referred to simply as **chlamydia,** the organism *Chlamydia trachomatis,* a gram-negative coccus and an intracellular obligate parasite, is responsible for a number of different infections of the reproductive system. These include **nongonococcal urethritis (NGU), pelvic inflammatory disease (PID),** and **lymphogranuloma venereum (LGV).** Chlamydial infections are now the most prevalent STIs in the United States (Box 17.2). Female carriers of the infection are often asymptomatic, thus increasing the transmission of chlamydial infections. Transmission occurs through exchange of semen or vaginal fluid during vaginal, oral, or anal sexual activity. Pregnant women can also pass the infection on to their child during labor and delivery. The incubation period is between 1 and 3 weeks before symptoms appear. The symptoms of a chlamydial infection tend to be very mild or virtually nonexistent. According to research data, up to 75% to 80% of infected women and up to 50% of infected men show no symptoms at all.

Left untreated, chlamydial infections can cause serious health problems in both men and women. In males the infection can lead to epididymitis, possibly resulting in sterility and other complications. Furthermore, in males an NGU chlamydial infection may manifest itself as urethritis (see Urinary Tract

BOX 17.2 Symptoms of Chlamydial Infections

Nongonococcal urethritis (NGU)

Male
- Discharge from the tip of the penis
- Burning during urination
- Itching sensation at the tip of the penis

Female
- Abnormal vaginal discharge
- Painful intercourse
- Burning sensation during urination

Lymphogranuloma venereum (LGV)

Male
- Lesions at the site of infection
- Fever, malaise
- Nausea, vomiting
- Enlarged, painful lymph nodes
- Rectal infections in homosexual men
- *Rare cases:* Arthritis, meningitis, pericarditis

Female
- Lesions at the site of infection
- Rectal infection
- *Rare cases:* Arthritis, meningitis, pericarditis

Pelvic inflammatory disease (PID)

Female
- Abnormal vaginal discharge
- Painful intercourse
- Burning sensation during urination

chlamydial infections consists of a course of antibiotics including tetracycline, azithromycin, and erythromycin. Preventive measures to avoid contracting a chlamydial infection include the following:

- Use of a condom during sexual activity
- Limiting the number of sex partners
- Annual STD testing
- Seeking immediate treatment if symptoms appear
- If infection is confirmed, notification of all sex partners

Mycoplasmal and Ureaplasmal Nongonococcal Urethritis (NGU)

NGUs can also be caused by *Mycoplasma hominis* and *Ureaplasma urealyticum*. Both organisms are gram-negative pleomorphic bacteria that lack cell walls and are frequently found among the normal urogenital microflora, especially in women. Transmission occurs primarily through vaginal sexual activity. Although usually associated with NGU, *M. hominis* occasionally will cause PID in women and urethritis in men. Outward symptoms are generally not evident, but the effects can be serious, especially in pregnant women. *M. hominis* can colonize the placenta, causing spontaneous abortion, premature births, low birth rates, and ectopic pregnancies.

U. urealyticum is one of the smallest bacteria known to be a human pathogen. Infections caused by this pathogen account for more than half of all infections that eventually result in infertility of couples. Moreover, *U. urealyticum* is a major cause of fetal and neonatal death, premature births, miscarriages, and low birth weight.

Diagnosis is done by culturing the organism from the placenta, or in urethral and vaginal discharge. Serological tests such as complement fixation, enzyme immunoassays, and cold agglutinin tests are helpful in identifying these pathogens. Microscopy is not particularly useful because cell walls are absent and staining is thereby greatly reduced.

Treatment for these infections is typically tetracycline; however, erythromycin, spectinomycin, and clindamycin have also proven to be effective. Because of the lack of a cell wall, penicillin is not effective against these microbes (see Chapter

Infections in Chapter 15, Infections of the Urinary System) and in women as vulvovaginitis or cervicitis (inflammation of the cervix). Women are more likely to experience serious problems associated with a chlamydial infection in the form of PID (see Chapter 16, Infections of the Reproductive System). LGV chlamydial infections are 20 times more common in men than in women. The lesions characteristic of this type of infection usually heal on their own; however, 1 week to 2 months after the lesions heal the organism invades the lymph nodes, causing large, painful buboes. If the buboes are not drained, inflammation can create obstructions in the lymph vessels, causing massive enlargement of the external genitalia in both males and females.

Chlamydial infection can also be detrimental during a pregnancy, as it increases the possibility of a premature birth or ectopic pregnancy. In addition, the infection can be passed to the child during delivery, causing eye infections and pneumonia.

Diagnosis is typically accomplished by special staining and microscopic examination of pus from lymph nodes or discharge/lesion samples. Staining with iodine reveals the bacteria, as they appear as inclusions in the sample. Serological tests are obtainable but they frequently give false-positive results. At present there is no vaccine available for chlamydial infections; however, research is ongoing. Current treatment for all types of

Sexually Transmitted Toxic Shock Syndrome (TSS)

As discussed in Chapter 16, *Staphylococcus aureus* is a gram-positive coccus that produces a potent bacterial toxin capable of causing severe systemic problems. Research shows that certain strains of methicillin-resistant *S. aureus* can be transmitted through sexual activity and cause both local and systemic problems (toxic shock syndrome, TSS). According to the Centers for Disease Control and Prevention (CDC), the most common symptoms of staphylococcal TSS include the following:

- Fever higher than 38.9° C (102° F)
- Chills
- Malaise
- Headache
- Fatigue
- Rash
- Shedding of skin
- Low blood pressure
- Vomiting
- Diarrhea
- Muscle pain
- Increased blood flow to mouth, eyes, and vagina, making them appear red
- Decreased urine output and sediment in urine
- Decreased liver function
- Bruising due to low blood platelet count
- Disorientation and confusion

Antibiotics other than methicillin may be prescribed for the treatment, depending on the specific strain of the bacterium. The antibiotic of choice for the treatment of TSS is usually vancomycin.

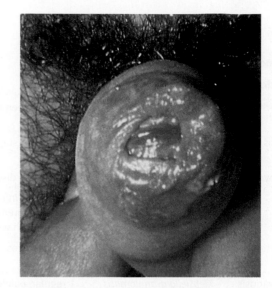

FIGURE 17.3 Chancroid. Several irregular ulcers on the prepuce. (Courtesy L. Parish. From Mims C, Dockrell HM, Goering RV, et al: *Medical microbiology*, ed 3, St. Louis, 2004, Mosby.)

22, Antimicrobial Drugs). Preventive measures against these NGU infections include simply abstinence from sexual activity or use of a condom.

Chancroid

Chancroid infection is relatively rare in the United States but its incidence worldwide may be greater than that of either gonorrhea or syphilis. The soft chancres (Figure 17.3) of this infection distinguish it from the hard lesions that are characteristic of syphilis. The causative agent is *Haemophilus ducreyi*, a short gram-negative bacillus. Humans are the host for this organism, and the method of transmission is vaginal sex. Incubation time between initial infection and the appearance of symptoms is about 3 to 7 days. This infection affects both men and women, with a much higher incidence of infection noted among men. The primary symptom is the appearance of soft, painful lesions or chancres. These chancres bleed easily and usually appear on the genitals or in the genital area 3 to 5 days after exposure. On occasion an infection will be present without the lesions, but a burning sensation after urination occurs. Chancres can also appear in the mouth or on the lips, but regardless of their location, they are highly infective. Simply touching a chancre with bare skin can result in transmission of the infection. In about 30% of cases the infection will move to the groin area, where it will form enlarged masses of lymphatic tissue, called *buboes*. Each bubo will then enlarge greatly and can break through the skin, discharging pus. Untreated lesions can persist for months, but the infection will often resolve without treatment.

Diagnosis involves identifying the presence of the organism in scrapings from a lesion or from fluids from a bubo, by microscopy and subsequent biochemical testing and growth on selective media (specialized gonococcal agar, or GC agar). Treatment includes the use of tetracycline, erythromycin, sulfanilamide, and trimethoprim-sulfamethoxazole. Treatment will heal the lesions but deep tissue scarring may remain. As with most other sexually transmitted infections, preventive measures include abstinence from sexual activity, use of condoms, and protection from contact with lesions (primarily for caregivers). There is no vaccine presently available for this infection.

Donovanosis (Granuloma Inguinale)

Donovanosis is relatively uncommon in the United States, with most cases occurring among homosexual men. The infection is caused by *Klebsiella granulomatis* (the genus was previously called *Calymmatobacterium*), a gram-negative, encapsulated bacillus. The precise epidemiology of this infection is not fully established, but it does appear that many cases are sexually transmitted, whereas others are not. Whatever the method of transmission, the infection rate is relatively low and even with regular sexual contact the infection may not spread. If the disease occurs, the symptoms include the appearance of irregular, painless ulcers on or near the genitals within 9 to 50 days of the initial infection.

Common Bacterial STIs

Infection	Organism	Symptoms	Treatment
Gonorrhea	Neisseria gonorrhoeae	Vary between females and males*	Ciprofloxacin, cefixime, ofloxacin, levofloxacin
Syphilis	Treponema pallidum	Differ with stages†	Benzathine penicillin; azithromycin, doxycycline, tetracycline
Chlamydia	Chlamydia trachomatis	Depend on disease	Tetracycline, azithromycin, erythromycin
NGU	Ureaplasma urealyticum	May cause infertility; fetal and neonatal death; premature births, miscarriages, low birth weight	Tetracycline; erythromycin, spectinomycin, clindamycin
Chancroid	Haemophilus ducreyi	Soft chancres on genitals or genital areas	Tetracycline, erythromycin, sulfanilamide, trimethoprim-sulfamethoxazole
Donovanosis	Klebsiella granulomatis	Irregular, painless ulcers on or near genitals	Ampicillin, tetracycline, erythromycin, gentamicin

NGU, Nongonococcal urethritis.
*See Table 17.1.
†See Table 17.2.

The infection can be spread by touching the ulcers, and subsequently contaminating other parts of the body. The ulcers may heal without treatment, but they do cause loss of skin pigment in the area of the lesion. Furthermore, if untreated, the infection can spread and result in extensive tissue damage.

Diagnosis is performed by staining of scrapings from the lesions and microscopic examination. The infection is confirmed by the presence of encapsulated bacteria inside macrophages. The bacteria themselves resemble the shape of closed safety pins and are called *Donovan bodies.* Antibiotic treatment may include the use of ampicillin, tetracycline, erythromycin, and gentamicin.

Viral Infections

STIs caused by viruses are about as common today as those caused by bacteria. However, unlike bacterial STIs, viral STIs are at the present time incurable. The antiviral drugs available can be used to manage the disease but not to cure the disease.

HIV and AIDS

The **human immunodeficiency virus (HIV)** is the causative agent of **acquired immune deficiency syndrome (AIDS),** a secondary immune deficiency (see Chapter 20, The Immune System). AIDS is not a disease but a syndrome because it has complex signs and symptoms, and a variety of diseases are associated with a common cause. AIDS results in many opportunistic infections due to a severely compromised immune system.

HIV infection in humans is now a pandemic, that is, an infection that occurs worldwide. There are at least two types of the virus, HIV-1 and HIV-2, that are responsible for causing AIDS (discussed in Chapter 20). The HIV virus basically destroys the immune system, thus leaving the body open to various infections that ultimately prove fatal. The virus targets cells of the immune system including helper T cells, macrophages, dendritic cells, and Langerhans cells. As these components of the immune system battle the virus in the early stages of infection the virus survives but may be kept in check, and the result can be almost a draw between the body and the virus. However, over time the body's ability to replace the cells of the immune system will be diminished and unable to keep up with the rapidly replicating, and usually mutating virus. Without the helper T cells and macrophages the B cells will not be stimulated to form plasma cells, which are responsible for producing the antibodies to fight the infection (see Chapter 20). A count of the helper T cells is a good indicator in predicting the progression of the infection and the onset of AIDS-related symptoms. The progression of HIV infections depends primarily on two factors: the actual amount of virus a person was exposed to, and how often repeated exposure occurred. According to the Centers for Disease Control and Prevention (CDC, Atlanta, GA) the stages of HIV infections are classified into four groups or stages (Table 17.2).

Most patients with full-blown AIDS will also develop a malignancy called *Kaposi's sarcoma,* in which blood vessels grow in a tangled mass filled with blood and rupture easily. The masses appear as pink or purple splotches on the skin but can also spread to organs of the digestive tract, the lungs, liver, spleen, and the lymph system.

Transmission of the HIV virus has been an area of contention among medical researchers. Most agree that casual contact will not result in transmission of the virus, that instead it requires more intimate contact with the body fluids of an

Selected Opportunistic Infections: AIDS

The infections listed in this highlight are only a few that are often associated with HIV infections and AIDS due to the compromised immune system. This list only provides samples and links for more information on each of the infections.

Bacterial infections

- *Mycobacterium avium* complex (comprising *M. avium* and *M. intracellulare*): The disease in not a reportable disease, but it has been reported that the incidence is decreasing among HIV-infected patients as a result of new treatment modalities. The symptoms of the disease in HIV patients include night sweats, weight loss, abdominal pain, fatigue, diarrhea, and anemia.
  - http://www.cdc.gov/ncidod/dbmd/diseaseinfo/mycobacteriumavium_t.htm
- Salmonellosis (if recurrent): The frequency of salmonellosis (see Chapter 12) in patients with AIDS is estimated to be 20 times higher than in the general population.
  - http://www.cdc.gov/nczved/dfbmd/disease_listing/salmonellosis_gi.html
- Syphilis: There is an estimated two- to fivefold increase in the risk of acquiring AIDS if exposed to that infection when syphilis is present.
  - http://www.cdc.gov/std/syphilis/STDFact-Syphilis.htm
- Tuberculosis (see Chapter 11): Worldwide TB is one of the leading causes of death among HIV-infected persons.
  - http://www.cdc.gov/tb/pubs/TB_HIVcoinfection/default.htm

Viral infections

- Cytomegalovirus: Infection with CMV is a major cause of disease and death among immunocompromised patients, including HIV-infected patients. In people with HIV, CMV can cause retinitis, which can cause blindness.
  - http://www.cdc.gov/cmv/
- Hepatitis: HIV-positive persons also infected with hepatitis B virus are at increased risk for developing chronic HBV infection and can have serious medical complications, including an increased risk for liver-related morbidity and mortality. About one quarter of HIV-infected persons in the United States are also infected with hepatitis C, causing chronic liver disease and more rapid liver damage in HIV-infected people.
  - http://www.cdc.gov/ncidod/diseases/hepatitis/index.htm
- Herpes: People infected with both HIV and the herpesvirus often have longer lasting, more frequent, and more severe outbreaks of herpes symptoms. Furthermore, it may cause HIV to multiply at a faster rate, causing AIDS.
  - http://www.cdc.gov/std/herpes/STDFact-herpes.htm

Fungal infections

- Aspergillosis: Aspergillosis in patients with AIDS most commonly affects the lungs. Other sites, less commonly affected, include the blood, sinuses, skin, ear, brain, and heart.
  - http://www.cdc.gov/nczved/dfbmd/disease_listing/aspergillosis_gi.html
- Candidiasis: 90% of patients with HIV/AIDS will develop candidiasis.
  - http://www.cdc.gov/nczved/dfbmd/disease_listing/candidiasis_gi.html
- Coccidioidomycosis: Coccidioidomycosis during HIV infections has many different manifestations including diffuse, reticulonodular pneumonia; focal primary pneumonia; and disease disseminated beyond the thoracic cavity. Treatments currently available include polyene antifungal amphotericin B and triazole antifungals.
  - http://health.utah.gov/epi/fact_sheets/cocci.html
- Histoplasmosis: Histoplasmosis in patients with AIDS almost always is manifested by symptoms of progressive disseminated disease. Advancement in antiviral therapy for AIDS has shown a decrease in the incidence of histoplasmosis among people with AIDS.
  - http://www.cdc.gov/nczved/dfbmd/disease_listing/histoplasmosis_gi.html

---

infected person or is transmitted from mother to fetus. The fluids typically involved in transmission of the virus include blood, semen, and vaginal secretions. The portal of entry is usually a break in the skin or mucous membranes that come in contact with the infected fluid. Therefore any contact that involves the exchange of bodily fluids may allow the virus to be transmitted from person to person. These types of contact include the following:

- Sexual contact—all forms of sexual activity: Heterosexual and homosexual intercourse whether vaginal, anal, or oral
- Sharing contaminated needles between intravenous drug users
- Receiving any contaminated blood products

- Transfer from infected mother to infant either during the pregnancy, during delivery, or through breastfeeding

Diagnosis of HIV infections can include the following methods:

- **Enzyme-linked immunosorbent assay (ELISA):** This is typically the first step in HIV testing, which detects the presence of HIV antibodies in a sample of blood. If positive, the second step will be a confirmation test. If negative, testing stops here. This is the U.S. Food and Drug Administration (FDA)-approved method for detecting HIV infections.
- **Western blot** is used to confirm the positive ELISA results. This test involves detection of specific proteins present in

TABLE 17.2 Stages of HIV Infections and AIDS

Stage	Time Frame	Symptoms
1	1–12 mo	HIV antibodies appear; flulike symptoms
2	1–8 yr	Mild anemia, low white blood cell count, some decrease in T cell count, seborrheic dermatitis, shingles, hairy leukoplakia
3	9–15 yr	Moderate anemia, low albumin, low cholesterol, decrease in helper T cell count, severe dermatitis, thrush, weight loss, diarrhea, recurring fever, tuberculosis, various bacterial infections, recurrent shingles
4	Months to years	Death—usually 2 yr after diagnosis in men, 12–18 mo in women. Causes of death vary, but usually involve opportunistic infections, lymphoma, and wasting syndrome

the blood of an HIV-positive patient. Combined with the ELISA, a positive result with the Western blot is 99.9% accurate. This test is FDA approved for detecting an HIV infection.

- **HIV polymerase chain reaction (HIV PCR)** is used to detect the presence of specific DNA and RNA sequences that indicate the presence of HIV as the viral DNA/RNA circulate in the blood after infection has occurred. This test is FDA approved for detecting an HIV infection.
- **OraSure** is a home-type test using secretions from between the cheek and the gums to detect the presence of HIV antibodies; this is in contrast to the blood used in the three previous tests. The principle is essentially the same as with the ELISA, but involves a different sample type. This test is not currently approved by the FDA for a definitive diagnosis of HIV infection.
- **Urinanalysis** is also used to detect an HIV infection but tends to be inaccurate in the present form. This test is not FDA approved for detecting an HIV infection.

The ELISA, Western blot, and PCR methods are discussed in detail in Chapter 25 (Biotechnology). There are a number of testing methods and protocols being developed to improve the speed and accuracy of the tests.

At the present time there is no treatment that can cure an HIV infection. However, the FDA has approved more than 30 different drugs that have shown some success in inhibiting or slowing the infection's progress. These drugs fall into seven categories:

1. Integrase inhibitors
2. Entry inhibitors
3. Nonnucleoside reverse transcriptase inhibitors (NNRTIs)
4. Nucleotide analogs
5. Protease inhibitors
6. Nucleoside reverse transcriptase inhibitors (NRTIs)
7. Combination medications

In addition to treating the HIV infection, a patient in advanced stages of the disease may require other drugs including antibiotics to treat opportunistic infections. These opportunistic infections include (but are not limited to) cytomegalovirus, encephalitis *(Toxoplasma gondii),* yeast infections *(Candida albicans),* and respiratory diseases.

Research in pursuit of a vaccine to prevent HIV infection is ongoing but no vaccine is currently available. Although vaccine research continues, many experts in the study of HIV have stated that because of the high mutation rate of the virus and the nature of the viral action itself, the development of a vaccine may be decades away.

Hepatitis B, C, and D

Hepatitis is an infection of the liver, capable of causing significant destruction of liver cells (see Chapter 9 [Infection and Disease] and Chapter 12 [Infections of the Gastrointestinal System]). Hepatitis B, C, and D viruses can be transmitted during sexual activity and are therefore considered STIs although they do not specifically target or affect organs of the reproductive system.

- Hepatitis B (HBV) transmission occurs when blood from an infected person enters the body of another. It can be transmitted through sexual activities with an infected person, by sharing needles, and from infected mother during birth or by breastfeeding. Transmission has also been documented through artificial insemination with contaminated semen. Furthermore, transmission can occur through needlesticks or exposure to sharps. The incubation time is between 45 and 180 days, with an average of about 90 days. The virus itself replicates in liver cells, lymph tissue, and hematopoietic tissue. The virus may stay in the blood for years and be passed on by the carrier at any time. The symptoms of a HBV infection are not immediately obvious but once they do appear they include the following:
  - Yellowing of the skin
  - Malaise
  - Nausea
  - Diarrhea
  - Abdominal pain
  - Lack of appetite

Hepatitis B infections can be prevented by vaccination, which is required for most healthcare providers or other persons who may be exposed to blood products. Three injections are given over a period of 6 months. This immunization has been shown to be effective in more than 90% of healthy individuals.

- Hepatitis C (HCV) in most cases is transmitted by blood-to-blood contact but may be sexually transmitted, especially among individuals already infected with another STI. Signs and symptoms of the infection are similar to those of hepatitis B infections. Hepatitis C can be either acute, that is, a short-term illness occurring within the first 6 months after exposure to the virus, or chronic. Seventy to eighty percent of acute infections will develop into a chronic infection, a serious disease that can result in long-term health problems, or even death. HCV RNA can be detected in the blood within 1 to 3 weeks of exposure, and antibodies to HCV can be detected in more than 97% of persons by 6 months after exposure. At present there is no vaccine available for hepatitis C and the CDC recommendations for prevention and control of HCV infections include screening and testing of blood donors, viral inactivation of plasma-derived products, risk reduction counseling, screening of persons at risk for HCV infection, and routine practice of infection control in healthcare settings.

- Hepatitis D (HDV) is caused by the hepatitis D virus, a defective virus that needs the hepatitis B virus to exist and therefore is found in the blood of persons infected with the HBV virus. HDV may worsen hepatitis B infection or existing hepatitis B liver disease. Symptoms of the infection are similar to those of HBV infections but may also include the following:
  - Nausea and vomiting
  - Fatigue
  - Joint pain
  - Dark (tea-colored) urine

Tests for the infection include liver enzymes, which are higher than normal; anti-delta agent antibody, which will be positive for HDV; and liver biopsy. Because hepatitis D occurs only in persons with hepatitis B infections, vaccination against HBV is recommended for people who are at high risk for HBV infections. Prompt recognition and treatment of HBV infection can help prevent HDV. Patients with a long-term HDV infection may be treated with interferon-α or a liver transplant.

Genital Herpes

Genital herpes, a highly contagious and common STI in the United States, is caused by the herpes simplex virus HSV-2 or HSV-1. Although most genital herpes is caused by HSV-2, it can also be caused by HSV-1, the organism that most commonly causes "fever blisters" of the mouth and lips (see Chapter 10, Infections of the Integumentary System, Soft Tissue, and Muscle). Genital herpes infections typically result in one or more blisters on or around the genitals or rectum. After the blisters break they leave tender sores that take 2 to 4 weeks to heal. Other outbreaks may occur weeks or months thereafter, with the number of outbreaks generally decreasing over the years. The signs and symptoms of the infection vary greatly and some individuals infected with HSV-2 may not be aware of their infection. Even without clear signs and symptoms of the infection HSV can be detected by the use of blood tests, because of the presence of antibodies.

There is no cure for herpes, but antiviral medications are available to shorten and even prevent an outbreak during the time the medication is taken. Persons with herpes lesions should abstain from sexual activity with an uninfected person. Although daily suppressive therapy for symptomatic herpes

may reduce transmission, it needs to be noted that an infected person without lesion can still transmit the organism.

Neonatal herpes (see Chapter 23, Human Age and Microorganisms) is a condition of concern for women of childbearing age because the virus can cross the placenta and infect the fetus. Serious damage to the fetus may occur, including mental retardation and defective hearing and vision. Spontaneous abortions have also been reported. If the infection is acquired during the late stages of pregnancy a cesarean delivery is usually performed to protect the child.

Human Papillomavirus (HPV)

Genital HPV is one of the most common sexually transmitted diseases, and is caused by a virus that infects the skin and mucous membranes. More than 60 serotypes of the virus exist, 40 of them capable of infecting the genital areas of men and women. According to the CDC most people infected with HPV do not develop symptoms, whereas among others the virus causes genital warts. These can appear as small bumps or groups of bumps. They can be raised or flat, single or multiple, small or large, and may have a cauliflower shape. In women they can materialize on the vulva, in or around the vagina or anus, and on the cervix. In men genital warts may emerge on the penis, scrotum, groin, or thigh. As with other papillomavirus infections the immune system may clear the infection naturally within a few years.

Genital warts are diagnosed by visual inspection. There is no treatment for the virus itself but the visible genital warts can be removed by patient-applied medications such as podofilox solution or gel, or imiquimod cream. Healthcare providers may remove visible genital warts by cryotherapy; treatment with podophyllin resin, trichloroacetic acid, or bichloracetic acid; or by surgical removal.

Some of the HPV strains may not cause warts but are able to cause cervical cancer or less common forms of cancer such as cancers of the vulva, vagina, anus, and penis. In women, routine Pap testing can identify problems before the development of cancer. Cervical cancer is most treatable when diagnosed and treated in the early stages.

MEDICAL HIGHLIGHTS

HPV Vaccination

The first vaccine developed to prevent cervical cancer and genital warts caused by human papillomavirus (HPV) is Gardasil, which was licensed by the FDA in June 2006. The vaccine is given in three doses and is recommended for girls between the ages of 11 and 12 years. The vaccine can also be given to women, 13 through 26 years of age, who did not receive the vaccine or who did not complete the vaccination series. Ideally, the vaccine should be given to girls/women before their first sexual contact, when they could be exposed to HPV. The vaccine does not work as well for those who were exposed to the virus before they are vaccinated. Also, the vaccine does not treat existing HPV infections.

Molluscum Contagiosum

Molluscum contagiosum is caused by molluscum contagiosum virus, a member of the poxvirus family. Infections are common in children but may affect adults also, and involve the genitals. Therefore the infection in adults can be considered a sexually transmitted infection. The infection does spread through direct person-to-person contact and through contact with contaminated objects. Molluscum contagiosum infections result in raised, round, flesh-colored papules (bumps) on the skin and usually disappear within a year even without treatment.

The infection spreads easily and treatment, especially for adults, involves the removal of the papules by curettage, freezing, or laser therapy. Medications that are helpful in the removal of warts also may be helpful in removing the papules. To prevent the spread of the virus is the following are recommended:

- Avoid touching, rubbing, or scratching the papules
- Avoid using the personal items of an infected person
- Avoid sexual contact until the papules are treated and have been completely resolved.

Fungal Infections

The organisms primarily associated with fungal reproductive system infections are *Tinea* sp., *Epidermophyton floccosum,* and *Candida albicans.* They are mostly responsible for infections on the surface of external genitalia; however, *Candida* can also infect various mucous membranes.

Vulvovaginal Candidiasis

Vulvovaginal candidiasis infection can occur if *Candida albicans* is transmitted to the female during sexual activity. The symptom of this type of vaginitis is a curdlike, yellow-white, or yellow-green discharge from the vagina. Diagnosis is difficult because a mixed population of organisms is often found in the infected area and no definitive specific immunological tests exist for identifying *Candida.* Standard sampling of the discharge, culturing on selective media, and then microscopic examination, including a potassium hydroxide (KOH) preparation, may reveal the presence of the organism but not identify it as the sole cause of the infection. Treatment for fungal vaginitis involves the use of oral antifungal agents, including:

- Ketoconazole
- Amphotericin B
- Fluconazole
- Itraconazole
- Flucytosine

Balanitis

Balanitis is a *Candida* infection of the glans penis that can occur in males through transmission of the fungus during sexual activity. This type of infection occurs primarily in uncircumcised males. The infection begins as vesicles on the penis, which then develop into patches that cause severe itching and burning. Diagnosis is the same as for any presumed *Candida* infection, which often will not identify *Candida* as the definitive cause, only its presence. Treatment is often done with topical antifungal medications, including the following:

- Miconazole
- Tolnaftate
- Clotrimazole

Jock Itch

Although the name "jock itch" implies that this is a male infection, females can experience a similar infection in the areas of their external genitalia. The organisms usually involved are *Tinea* spp. and *Epidermophyton floccosum,* which are transmitted by direct contact of genitalia or infected areas such as the groin during sexual activity. The infection typically manifests itself as a skin rash or irritating lesions on the groin or genitalia. If the skin is ruptured through scratching, other opportunistic infections may occur. Diagnosis involves microscopic evaluation of skin samples from the infected area and by further culturing of the sample on selective media (Sabouraud dextrose agar). Treatment typically entails the application of topical antifungal medications including the following:

- Miconazole
- Tolnaftate
- Clotrimazole

In more persistent or serious cases oral medication may be prescribed, including griseofulvin and itraconazole.

Protozoan Infections

The only currently know STI caused by a protozoan is **trichomoniasis,** which affects both men and women; however, symptoms are more common in women.

Trichomoniasis

Trichomoniasis is a common STI that affects both women and men, but is more prevalent in young, sexually active women. The infection is caused by *Trichomonas vaginalis,* a single-celled protozoan. The most common site of infection in women is the vagina, and in men the urethra. Women can be infected by men or women; men usually contract the infection only from infected women. In men the infection often does not have symptoms, but in some cases a slight irritation inside the penis, a mild discharge, or a slight burning sensation after urination or ejaculation may occur. Signs and symptoms in women include frothy, yellow-green vaginal discharge with a strong odor. For diagnosis the healthcare provider needs to perform a physical examination and laboratory tests. In men the parasite is more difficult to detect than in women, in whom a pelvic examination may reveal small red ulcerations on the wall of the vagina or on the cervix. Other tests such as a vaginal culture or DNA test may also be used. Treatment of the infection is either metronidazole or tinidazole.

The incidence of trichomoniasis infections is as high as or higher than those of gonorrhea and chlamydia, but the infection is considered mild and is not reportable. In pregnant women the infection has been associated with preterm delivery and low birth weight.

Summary

- Sexually transmitted infections (STIs) and diseases (STDs) are the result of some type of sexual activity and affect both men and women, but can also affect the unborn child.
- STIs affect mostly the organs of the reproductive system, but depending on the infection can affect all systems of the human body.
- STIs can be caused by bacteria, viruses, fungi, and protozoans.
- The most common bacterial STIs are chlamydia, gonorrhea, and syphilis. Others include chancroid, mycoplasmal and ureaplasmal nongonococcal urethritis, and donovanosis.
- Most bacterial STIs can be treated with antibiotics. Damage to tissues and organs that occurs before treatment generally cannot be reversed.
- Viral STIs are as common as bacterial STIs but at the present time are incurable. Vaccination is available for some.
- The most common viral STIs include HIV, hepatitis B, C, and D, genital herpes, and human papillomavirus infections.
- Fungal STIs include candidal vaginitis, balanitis, and jock itch. These infections are not always sexually transmitted.
- Trichomoniasis is the only known STI transmitted by a protozoan.
- STIs are preventable but remain a major public health challenge worldwide and in the United States.

Review Questions

1. Which of the following organisms is the causative agent for gonorrhea?
   a. *Treponema*
   b. *Neisseria*
   c. *Mycoplasma*
   d. *Ureaplasma*

2. Which of the following STIs is also referred to as the "great imitator"?
   a. Gonorrhea
   b. Chlamydia
   c. Syphilis
   d. Chancroid

3. Gummas are characteristic lesions of:
   a. Gonorrhea
   b. Chlamydia
   c. Syphilis
   d. Chancroid

4. The secondary stage of syphilis includes which of the following time periods after the primary stage:
   a. Two to 4 days
   b. Five to 10 days
   c. Two to 10 weeks
   d. One year

5. Lymphogranuloma venereum is an infection caused by:
   a. *Neisseria gonorrhoeae*
   b. *Treponema pallidum*
   c. *Chlamydia trachomatis*
   d. *Ureaplasma urealyticum*

6. The causative agent for chancroid is:
   a. *Neisseria gonorrhoeae*
   b. *Treponema pallidum*
   c. *Haemophilus ducreyi*
   d. *Ureaplasma urealyticum*

7. The STI caused by *Klebsiella granulomatis* is:
   a. Syphilis
   b. Donovanosis
   c. Chancroid
   d. Chlamydia

8. A red-brown rash on the palms of the hands and soles of the feet is typical for:
   a. Syphilis
   b. Donovanosis
   c. Chancroid
   d. Chlamydia

9. Which of the following agents can be used in the treatment of balanitis?
   a. Tetracycline
   b. Tolnaftate
   c. Cefixime
   d. Ampicillin

10. Which of the following organisms can cause sexually transmitted toxic shock syndrome?
    a. *Staphylococcus aureus*
    b. *Neisseria gonorrhoeae*
    c. *Treponema pallidum*
    d. *Haemophilus ducreyi*

11. NGU is the abbreviation for _____.

12. Granuloma inguinale is also called _____.

13. HIV is the abbreviation for _____.

14. Vaccination is available for the sexually transmitted hepatitis _____ virus.

15. The only STI transmitted by a protozoan is _____.

16. Discuss and differentiate between the prevalence and incidence of STIs in the United States.

17. Describe the different symptoms of gonorrhea in males and females.

18. Explain the different stages of syphilis.

19. Describe the different stages of HIV infections and AIDS.

20. Discuss the most common fungal STIs.

Bibliography

Damjanov I: *Pathology for the health professions*, ed 3, St. Louis, 2006, Saunders.

Mims C, Dockrell HM, Goering RV, et al: *Medical microbiology*, ed 3, St. Louis, 2004, Mosby.

Murray PR, Rosenthal KS, Pfaller MA: *Medical microbiology*, ed 5, St. Louis, 2005, Mosby.

Internet Resources

CDC, Sexually Transmitted Diseases, http://www.cdc.gov/STD/

CDC, Sexually Transmitted Diseases, General Information, http://www.cdc.gov/nchstp/dstd/disease_info.htm

CDC, Sexually Transmitted Diseases, Division of STD Prevention, http://www.cdc.gov/nchstp/dstd/aboutdiv.htm

Gonorrhea—CDC Fact Sheet, http://www.cdc.gov/std/gonorrhea/STDFact-gonorrhea.htm

CDC, Sexually Transmitted Diseases, Chlamydia, http://www.cdc.gov/STD/chlamydia/default.htm

Bernstein A: AIDS and the next 25 years, *Science* 320:717, 2008 (downloaded from www.sciencemag.org), http://www.hvtn.org/media/Bernstein_editorial.pdf

CDC, Viral Hepatitis, http://www.cdc.gov/ncidod/diseases/Hepatitis/b/fact.htm

Genital Herpes—CDC Fact Sheet, http://www.cdc.gov/std/herpes/STDFact-herpes.htm

CDC, Sexually Transmitted Diseases, Human Papillomavirus Infection (HPV), http://www.cdc.gov/std/hpv/default.htm#fact

CDC, Vaccines and Preventable Diseases: HPV Vaccination, http://www.cdc.gov/vaccines/vpd-vac/hpv/default.htm

MayoClinic.com, Genital Herpes, http://www.mayoclinic.com/print/genital-herpes/DS00179/METHOD=print&DSECTION=all

CDC, Trichomoniasis—CDC Fact Sheet, http://www.cdc.gov/STD/Trichomonas/STDFact-Trichomoniasis.htm

Hill CS: How full automation of molecular diagnostic testing can increase accuracy, lab efficiency, cost savings, *Clinical Lab Products Magazine*, July, 2004. http://www.clpmag.com/issues/articles/2004-07_02.asp?mode=print

18

Emerging Infectious Diseases

OUTLINE

Introduction

Emerging/Reemerging Infectious Diseases
Factors of Emergence/Reemergence
Types of Emerging and Reemerging Diseases
Addressing and Preventing Emerging and Reemerging Diseases

Global Concerns
U.S. Global Public Health
Global Surveillance

LEARNING OBJECTIVES

After reading this chapter, the student will be able to:

- Explain the difference between newly emerging and reemerging infectious diseases in the United States and worldwide
- Describe the main factors responsible for the emergence of new infectious diseases
- Discuss the factors involved in the reemerging of infectious diseases that have previously been under control
- Describe how emerging infectious diseases can be divided into four groups based on the process of emergence
- Name and briefly describe the classification of emerging and reemerging infectious diseases set by the National Institute of Allergy and Infectious Diseases
- Explain how to address and prevent emerging infectious diseases
- Discuss the global concerns relating to emerging and reemerging infectious diseases
- Describe the role of the United States Centers for Disease Control and Prevention in protecting U.S. citizens from emerging infectious diseases
- Discuss the importance of global surveillance of infectious diseases
- Name and describe five infectious diseases that have emerged or reemerged between 1980 and the present

adoption
antigenic drift
antigenic shift
Centers for Disease
    Control and
    Prevention (CDC)
emerging infectious
    diseases
Food and Drug
    Administration (FDA)

International Emerging
    Infections Program
    (IEIP)
International Health
    Regulations (IHR)
National Center for
    Preparedness,
    Detection, and
    Control of Infectious
    Diseases (NCPDCID)

National Institute of
    Allergy and Infectious
    Diseases (NIAID)
reemerging infectious
    diseases
United Nations
urbanization

WHY YOU NEED TO KNOW

HISTORY

Microorganisms existed long before humans, and infectious diseases probably evolved with each developing species. Emerging infectious diseases have been feared throughout history and they are still emerging today. The devastating effects of infectious diseases have long been observed and most ancient peoples recognized that some diseases were communicable and, to prevent the spread, isolated individuals with infections. Entire villages were abandoned when the Black Death struck Europe, all in order to escape the highly infectious plague. In the Middle Ages the rich people of Europe fled to their country homes when smallpox struck. It was also recognized by many that people who recovered from a particular disease became immune to that disease, and survivors were often expected to nurse the ill. At the time, this knowledge did not help significantly and infectious diseases drastically cut the average human life span.

With the invention of the microscope it was finally possible to see the microorganisms and scientists started understanding the link between microorganisms and disease (see Germ Theory of Disease in Chapter 1, Scope of Microbiology). Soon thereafter hand washing (Semmelweis) and antiseptic methods (Lister) were used in many hospitals, to control the spread of disease. The breakthrough of vaccination against smallpox (Jenner) and the discovery of penicillin (Fleming) further helped the battle against infectious diseases.

IMPACT

After the discovery of penicillin, production methods were further developed, allowing large quantities of penicillin to be produced. By the end of World War II, enough penicillin was produced to treat 7 million patients a year. The golden age of antibiotics dawned with considerable achievements in the discovery and development of many different types of antibacterial drugs (see Chapter 22, Antimicrobial Drugs). Because of the success of these drugs the fight against bacteria seemed to have been won. It was reported that in 1967 and 1969, the U.S. Surgeon General, William H. Stewart, commented that we had essentially defeated infectious diseases and "we could close the book on infectious disease." During the same time frame, many pharmaceutical companies shifted their main priorities to drug development for chronic disease therapy and less to the development of new antibacterials. Unfortunately, microbial evolution has not stopped and many microbes, not only bacteria, have developed resistance to the currently available drug treatments. The incidence of multidrug-resistant pathogenic bacteria is on the rise.

FUTURE

Emerging and reemerging infectious diseases are on the rise because of globalization, urbanization, multidrug resistance, and many other factors. This is a global problem and new and advanced international surveillance methods have been developed. The World Health Organization is constantly striving to improve prevention and control methods. Furthermore, pharmaceutical companies, especially biotechnology-oriented ones, are actively pursuing the development of new antimicrobial drugs. Infectious diseases have emerged throughout history and new infections continue to emerge today, and most likely will continue to do so in the future.

Introduction

Emerging infectious diseases are diseases that are newly identified in a population, or that have existed but have changed. They show an increase in incidence, currently or in the recent past, or have a potential to increase in the near future. Emerging diseases can be caused by viruses, bacteria, fungi, protozoans, or helminths. Older diseases that have been known for a long time and were previously under control, but are recurring, are called **reemerging infectious diseases.**

Emerging/Reemerging Infectious Diseases

The increasing international threat of infectious diseases has received special attention in the past few decades. The emergence of infectious diseases generally involves two steps:

1. The introduction of the pathogen into a new host population, and
2. The establishment and further spreading of the pathogen within the new host population, a process referred to as **adoption.**

The occurrence of a new infectious disease often seems strange; however, there are specific factors that are generally responsible for such emergence. Although some infectious diseases have been successfully controlled by modern technology, new emerging infectious diseases such as HIV/AIDS, severe acute respiratory syndrome (SARS), and West Nile virus and Ebola infections are continually appearing and are on the rise. In addition, other infectious diseases including malaria, tuberculosis, and bacterial pneumonias are reappearing in strains that are resistant to antimicrobial drug treatments.

Factors of Emergence/Reemergence

Factors responsible for the emergence of new infectious diseases include human demographics and behavior, ecological changes and agricultural development, international travel and commerce, technology and industry, microbial adaptation and change, breakdown of public health measures, human susceptibility to infection, climate and weather, economic development and land use, war and starvation, and intent to harm.

Human Demographics and Behavior

Changes in human demographics due to migration or war are often significant factors in the emergence of infectious diseases. Population movements are often due to economic conditions, which encourage workers to move from rural areas into cities. Beginning in the twentieth century a rapid **urbanization** of the world's population occurred: whereas in 1950, 29% of the population lived in urban areas, the **United Nations** estimates that in 2030 approximately 60% will live in urban areas, increasing to more than 69% by the year 2050 (Figure 18.1 and Table 18.1). The population density in urban areas makes disease transmission easier as it allows infections that arise in isolated rural areas that previously remained vague and localized, to reach the larger urban population. Once in the city, the disease not only spreads locally, but can also spread farther by intraurban transport routes, along highways, and by airplane.

Human behavior, especially in large population centers, can have important effects on disease dissemination. Well-known examples include sexually transmitted infections, and intravenous drug use, which have contributed to the emergence and spread of HIV/AIDS and hepatitis.

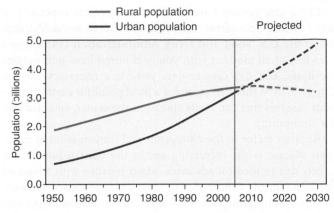

FIGURE 18.1 Urban and rural world population from 1950 to 2030.

TABLE 18.1 Urban and Rural Population Percentages from 1950 to 2050

Year	Percent Urban
Percent Urban Population from 1950 to 2050	
1950	29.1
1960	32.9
1970	36.0
1980	39.1
1990	43.0
2000	46.6
2010	50.6
2020	54.9
2030	59.7
2040	64.7
2050	69.6

Year	Percent Rural
Percent Rural Population from 1950 to 2050	
1950	70.9
1960	67.1
1970	64.0
1980	60.9
1990	57.0
2000	53.4
2010	49.4
2020	45.1
2030	40.3
2040	35.3
2050	30.4

Child care centers have become a way of life especially in many civilized countries, including the United States. According to the **U.S. Food and Drug Administration (FDA)** more than half of all mothers with young children have jobs outside the home and day care centers provide a necessary service. Unfortunately, this also provides a focal point for certain infectious diseases that can easily spread in the center, and also into the community.

Another factor in the emergence and transmission of infectious disease is the increasing age of the human population, largely due to medical advances. Many persons with advanced age or a chronic condition will have a compromised immune system, resulting in greater susceptibility to disease. Opportunistic organisms will then have the chance to develop an infection that normally would be prevented by an intact immune system. Once the disease has developed in an immunocompromised host, it can spread further into the community.

Ecological Changes and Agricultural Development

Changes in the ecosystem are frequently identified as factors increasing the occurrence of emerging infectious diseases. These ecological changes include changes in agricultural practices, economic development, and changes in land uses. Once the ecosystem is disturbed, outbreaks of previously unrecognized diseases occur and these often turn out to be of a zoonotic nature. Ecological changes often place people in contact with a natural reservoir or host that is unfamiliar to the population moving into the changed habitat. The building of dams and deforestation or reforestation are changes in the ecological makeup that will influence waterborne and vector-borne disease transmission. The movement of people into these areas will expose a larger population to wild animals and potential disease vectors. Agricultural development and urban development are the most common ways by which society alters the environment and introduces the population to previously unknown microbial challenges.

International Travel and Commerce

Persons infected with an exotic disease anywhere in the world can readily travel to any major city, including those in the United States. Even in the sixteenth and seventeenth centuries ships bringing slaves from West Africa to the New World also brought along infectious diseases, such as yellow fever and its mosquito vector. Other examples include the import of a filovirus into Marburg, Germany in 1967, with a shipment of African green monkeys used for laboratory purposes. The virus spread from the primate host to some of the human handlers, and subsequently to staff taking care of the infected people. This virus is now called the *Marburg virus,* which was responsible for seven deaths during that first outbreak. More outbreaks due to this virus occurred in many countries, including Angola in 2005. The mosquito-borne disease malaria is one of the most frequently imported diseases into nonendemic areas. The sporadic Ebola outbreaks in Central Africa could potentially be spread via air travel throughout the world within a matter of days.

Foods from other countries that are routinely imported, and vectors hitchhiking on imported products, also represent a potential for emerging infectious diseases all around the world.

Cruise ships are also a great environment for emerging diseases, because the passengers are frequently exposed to new environments, and live in a high population density.

Technology and Industry

Technical and industrial advancements in both the food and healthcare industries generally have a positive impact on the quality of life; however, they can also bring about the spread of infectious disease. Modern production methods tend to increase efficiency and reduce costs, but unfortunately also increase the chances of accidental contamination. This particular problem is amplified by globalization, because of the opportunity to intro-

LIFE APPLICATION

Pathogenic Hitchhikers: It's a Small World After All

In the 1960s the Surgeon General of the United States acknowledged that the time was at hand when we could "close the book on infectious disease". As a result of improvements of public health programs, hygiene, and advances in the development of new drugs and vaccines to combat infectious diseases, many public health officials stated that, at least in the Western world, death due to infectious diseases had been virtually eliminated. Unfortunately, this has not been the case as recent worldwide problems exist, with diseases such as malaria, West Nile virus, dengue fever, and SARS still spreading and claiming victims. There are a number of factors that contribute to the successful spread of pathogens to new host populations, but one that has changed considerably over the past century is the spread of disease through international travel and commerce. For instance, increases in cases of yellow fever in Africa have raised some serious concern in the international community regarding the potential epidemic should the virus and insect vector come together on a wide scale. There is fear that the virus, which is now confined mostly to the savannah and forest areas, may be transported to more urban areas as a result of migration due to economic development policies. If the virus is introduced to the mosquito vector in the urban environment, officials fear it could give rise to an urban epidemic. Air travel and transport shipping could then bring the virus to the United States, where the mosquito insect vector is already well established in the southern states. Once again, when the virus and vector are brought together, the potential for a devastating epidemic could arise. Although virtually any form of international transportation has the potential to transport a disease vector, the form that has historically proven to be most effective at spreading pathogens worldwide has been ship transport. The shipboard environment and the equipment and containers being transported favor the survival of animal vectors, with the bacterial/viral pathogens safely hitchhiking on or in their bodies.

duce microbes from different parts of the world. In bulk processing, a microbe present in raw material may end up in a large batch of the final product.

At present animal feed ingredients include rendered animal products, animal wastes, antibiotics, metals, and fats, all of which increase the potential for higher levels of bacteria, antibiotic-resistant bacteria, prions, and dioxin-like compounds in animals. Animal food products are then intended for human consumption. Although the FDA does closely monitor these practices, accidental outbreaks of old or emerging infections do occur.

Many technological advances have been made in healthcare during the twentieth century, yet there has been a dramatic increase in nosocomial infections (see Chapter 9, Infection and Disease), often due to the development of antibiotic resistance in microbes.

Microbial Adaptation and Change

Like other organisms microbes are constantly evolving, but at a much faster rate because of their rapid reproduction/generation cycles. Microbes, especially bacteria and viruses, can also adapt quickly to adverse environments and this change is a major contributing factor to the emergence of "new" pathogens. Almost all RNA viruses, such as influenza, HIV, and hemorrhagic fever viruses, undergo frequent and unpredictable genetic mutations. Microbes have enormous evolutionary potential as they are able to undergo changes in pathogenicity, as well as often being able to avoid the immune system of the host. Their capacity to adapt to new environments is often enhanced by human activities.

Antimicrobial resistance (see Chapter 22, Antimicrobial Drugs) due to the overuse of antimicrobial drugs and the failure to ensure proper diagnosis and adherence to treatment has become a significant public health problem. This widespread use of antibiotics and other antimicrobials has resulted in evolutionary adaptations in microbes, enabling them to survive many powerful drugs. Antimicrobial drug–resistant strains are a continuing source of emerging infections and diseases.

Breakdown of Public Health Measures

Public health and sanitation measures have proven their effectiveness at minimizing the distribution of infectious disease. Any breakdown of public health measures can potentially be responsible for the emergence or reemergence of disease. Human exposure to pathogens that are spread by traditional routes, such as water and food supply, can be largely controlled by appropriate health measures. Proper immunization and vector control are also tools to inhibit the emergence/reemergence of infectious disease.

It is clear that many infectious diseases can be adequately controlled with appropriate measures, even in areas that are endemic for a particular microbe. For example, cholera can be controlled by providing sufficient sewage disposal and water treatment. Although understood and recognized as a public health threat, lapses in public health measures in both developing countries and in some inner cities of the industrialized world have caused the reemergence of many previously controlled diseases. Inadequate vaccination programs can lead to

the reemergence of previously controlled diseases such as outbreaks of diphtheria in the former Soviet Union, and the increased number of pertussis cases in Eastern Europe and the United States.

Other Factors in Disease Emergence and Reemergence

Several other factors influence the emergence and reemergence of infectious disease. They include, but are not limited to:

- *Human susceptibility to infection:* A compromised immune system due to HIV infection, transplants, cancer treatment, chronic diseases, as well as aging increases the susceptibility to emerging and reemerging disease in individuals.
- *Poverty:* Malnutrition and poor living conditions also increase susceptibility to all infectious diseases.
- *War and famine:* Most casualties in modern wars are not soldiers but civilians as a result of the destruction of water supplies, malnutrition, and a collapse of the public healthcare system. All these will help contribute to the emergence and reemergence of infectious disease.
- *Climate, weather, and natural disasters:* Tsunamis, hurricanes, earthquakes, volcanic eruptions, and simple changes in weather pattern will force microbes to adapt to the new environment for survival—possibly creating new strains of organisms that are capable of causing a new disease, or the reemergence of old, disease-causing strains.
- *Intent to do harm:* Bioterrorism and biowarfare agents are covered in Chapter 24 (Microorganisms in the Environment and Environmental Safety)

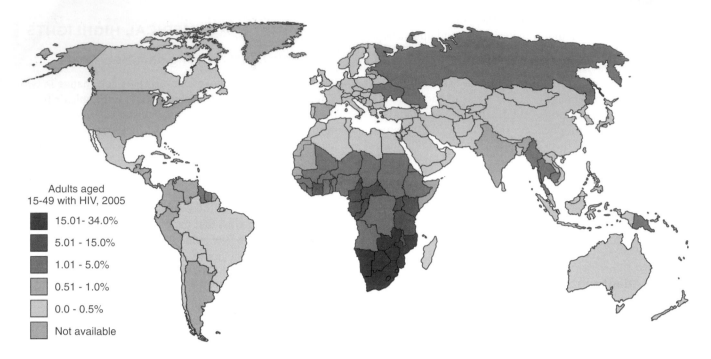

FIGURE 18.2 Global spread of HIV.

Adults aged
15-49 with HIV, 2005

- 15.01- 34.0%
- 5.01 - 15.0%
- 1.01 - 5.0%
- 0.51 - 1.0%
- 0.0 - 0.5%
- Not available

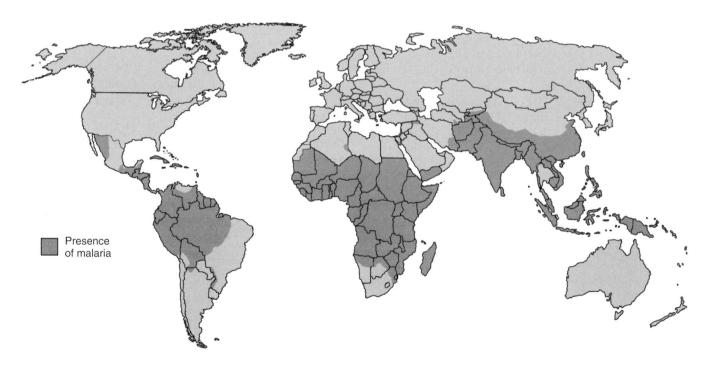

Presence
of malaria

FIGURE 18.3 Geographic distribution of malaria (2001–2002). (Data from the Centers for Disease Control and Prevention.)

Types of Emerging and Reemerging Diseases

Depending on the process of emergence, emerging infectious diseases can be divided into four major groups:

1. Newly emerging diseases that previously have not been known, such as hantavirus, Ebola, and AIDS (Figure 18.2)

2. Reemerging diseases such as tuberculosis and malaria (Figure 18.3)

3. New manifestations of known disease agents, for example, genital, respiratory, and cardiac manifestations of chlamydia

4. Introduction of known agents into new geographical territories such as the rapid spread of the West Nile virus in the United States

Mosquito Bites: "Fight the Bite" (CDC)

The West Nile virus is an infectious disease that first appeared in the United States in 1999. It is a known virus that has been introduced into a new geographical territory, and as of 2007 human cases have been reported in almost all states of the United States. The virus is spread by infected mosquitoes. People infected with the virus generally show mild or no symptoms at all; however, if the virus enters the brain it can be deadly. The "fight the bite" call by the CDC emphasizes the following (http://www.cdc.gov/ncidod/dvbid/westnile/index.htm):

- Avoid mosquito bites
- Use insect repellent
- Be aware of peak mosquito hours
- Drain all standing water
- Install or repair screens

Furthermore, report dead birds to local authorities, as this may be a sign that the virus is circulating between birds and mosquitoes in an area. More than 130 species of birds are known to have been infected with the West Nile virus. It is important to note that all infected birds die from the virus; however, one should not assume that every dead bird is a victim of this virus.

H1N1: Return of a Killer

In 1918, Influenza A virus subtype H1N1 swept across the world and killed 50–100 million people worldwide. The particular strain of H1N1 that caused this pandemic is often referred to as *avian flu*, as this specific strain is endemic in birds. In 1976, 1988, 1998, and in 2007 there were minor outbreaks of a flu caused by another strain of H1N1 endemic to pigs, and it was thus referred to as *swine flu*. In 2009 a new strain of the H1N1 subtype returned, but this time it has a very different genetic makeup. Six genes isolated from cases of the flu in America have been found to be mixtures of swine, avian, and human influenza viruses. Due to this unique mix of genes, there is a serious concern among many health agencies that the existing stocks of vaccines for the "old" strains of H1N1 will not be very effective against this new strain. Recently identified as a full-scale pandemic, the spread of the new H1N1 subtype is being carefully tracked by the WHO. As of June 2009, 74 countries have reported cases of influenza A(H1N1), with more than 27,000 infected and over 150 deaths. It is apparent that this new strain will present a challenge to health organizations everywhere, and its future effects on the world health situation are at this time unknown.

The **National Institute of Allergy and Infectious Diseases (NIAID)** has classified emerging and reemerging infectious diseases into only three groups:

- Group I: Pathogens that have been newly recognized in the past two decades
- Group II: Reemerging pathogens
- Group III: Agents with bioterrorism potential, subdivided into categories A, B, and C (see Chapter 24, Microorganisms in the Environment and Environmental Safety). Only NIAID category A organisms are included in the tables of this chapter

Bacterial, viral, fungal, protozoan, as well as prion-related emerging diseases are included in these groups (Tables 18.2 through 18.5). According to the **Centers for Disease Control and Prevention** (CDC, Atlanta, GA), almost 70% of emerging infectious disease episodes in the last decade or more have been zoonotic diseases. The recurrent examples of infections originating as zoonoses suggest that this reservoir of infections is a potentially rich source of emerging diseases and the periodic appearance of new zoonoses indicates that this pool is not exhausted. Although zoonotic agents generally do not spread easily from person to person, other factors, as discussed previously, might help to transmit the infection.

Addressing and Preventing Emerging and Reemerging Diseases

Many infectious diseases that occur in the United States are in the category of Nationally Notifiable Diseases (see Box 9-1 in Chapter 9, Infection and Disease). In other words, they need to be reported to the public health system. Numerous other emerging diseases are not yet in this reportable category because of continuous changes and the need for constant updates. General provisions for fighting infectious diseases in the United States include the responsibilities for monitoring, preventing, and controlling infectious disease. These responsibilities are carried out by hospitals, clinical laboratories, pharmaceutical companies, healthcare providers, universities, and various other research groups. Although these are part of a large system working to reduce the impact of pathogenic organisms, it is the CDC that acts as the lead U.S. federal agency responsible for providing information, recommendations, and technical assistance to support state and local public health departments (see Epidemiology and Public Health in Chapter 9, Infection and Disease).

Surveillance

In the United States, surveillance of infectious diseases, including new and reemerging ones, includes efforts at the state and federal levels. State departments collect and analyze data on infectious disease cases that were reported to the departments by healthcare providers. The reported cases are then verified by the state public health departments, which in turn report the information to the CDC. At the federal level, agencies and departments collect and analyze disease surveillance data and maintain the disease surveillance systems.

TABLE 18.2 Bacterial Emerging and Reemerging Infectious Diseases

Disease	Organism	Category	Transmission
Anthrax (Chapters 9, 11, and 24)	*Bacillus anthracis*	Group III	Cutaneous, inhalation, gastrointestinal
Cat scratch disease	*Bartonella henselae*	Group I	Cat bite or scratch, but recently tick-borne and transmitted
Lyme borreliosis (Chapter 9)	*Borrelia burgdorferi*	Group I	Tick
Botulism (Chapters 9, 12, and 13)	*Clostridium botulinum*	Group III	Four types: foodborne, infant, wound, undetermined
Pseudomembranous colitis	*Clostridium difficile*	Group II	Fecal–oral route
Ehrlichiosis (Chapter 9)	*Ehrlichia* spp.	Group I	Lone star tick *(Amblyomma americanum)*
Tularemia	*Francisella tularensis*	Group III	Tick, deerfly, other insect; handling infected animal carcasses; contaminated food or water; inhalation
Peptic ulcer (Chapter 12)	*Helicobacter pylori*	Group I	Fecal–oral; kissing
MRSA infections (Chapter 22)	*Staphylococcus aureus*	Group II	Usually nosocomial, but also community acquired
Group A streptococcal disease (GAS) (Chapter 11)	*Streptococcus*, group A	Group II	Direct contact with nasal or pharyngeal mucus from infected persons; contact with infected wounds or sores of the skin
Plague (Chapter 24)	*Yersinia pestis*	Group III	Flea bites

MRSA, Methicillin-resistant *Staphylococcus aureus*.

TABLE 18.3 Viral Emerging and Reemerging Infectious Diseases

Disease	Organism	Category	Transmission
ABL infection (Chapters 7 and 9)	Australian bat lyssavirus	Group I	Scratch or bite from infected bat
Neurological disease, hand, foot and mouth disease	Enterovirus 71	Group II	Fecal-oral, some indications of respiratory transmission
Respiratory illness (Chapter 7)	Hendra virus (equine morbillivirus)	Group I	Flying foxes (Australia)
Hepatitis (Chapters 9 and 12)	Hepatitis C virus	Group I	Blood-borne
Hepatitis (Chapters 9 and 12)	Hepatitis E virus	Group I	Contaminated food or water
Discovered in Kaposi's sarcoma (Chapter 7)	Human herpesvirus 8	Group I	Not established
Associated with roseola (Chapters 7 and 10)	Human herpesvirus 6	Group I	Opportunistic
"Fifth disease" (Chapters 7 and 9)	Human parvovirus B19	Group I	Person-to-person contact, or direct contact with saliva, sputum, or nasal secretion of infected person
Mumps (Chapters 7, 9, and 11)	Mumps virus	Group II	Person to person by saliva droplets or direct contact with contaminated articles
Smallpox (Chapters 10 and 24)	Variola virus	Group III	Person to person, infected aerosols, face-to-face contact with infected person after fever has begun
Viral hemorrhagic fevers (Chapter 24)	Arenaviruses Bunyaviruses Flaviviruses Filoviruses	Group III	Zoonotic with exception of the filovirus (can also be transmitted from person to person)

ABL, Australian bat lyssavirus.

TABLE 18.4 Fungal Emerging and Reemerging Infectious Diseases

Disease	Organism	Category	Transmission
Coccidioidomycosis	*Coccidioides immitis*	Group II	Inhalation of the conidia
Human microsporidiosis	*Encephalitozoon cuniculi* *Encephalitozoon hellem* *Encephalitozoon intestinalis*	Group I	Zoonotic and environmental (spores on water surface)

TABLE 18.5 Protozoan Emerging and Reemerging Infectious Diseases

Disease	Organism	Category	Transmission
Acanthamebiasis	*Acanthamoeba*	Group I	Contact lenses; through skin
Babesiosis (Chapter 8)	*Babesia* spp.	Group I	Bite of *Ixodes* tick

The first step in disease detection involves surveillance to determine whether clinical symptoms associated with a particular incident warrant intensive public health attention. These may include the following:

- Acute respiratory disease
- Acute diarrhea
- Encephalitis
- Meningitis
- Hemorrhagic fever
- Unusual clustering of disease or deaths
- Resistance to common drug treatments

An epidemic is often detected through routine surveillance or through an unusual cluster of cases recognized by a healthcare provider. Examples of such cases are the hantavirus outbreak in 1993 in the American Southwest, or the presence of the West Nile virus in the western hemisphere. Consequently, new infectious diseases are recognized mainly because of incidences of an actual epidemic.

Investigation

One of the most important reasons to investigate an outbreak of infectious disease, regardless of whether it is a newly emerging or reemerging disease, is that exposure to the source of infection may be continuing. Quick and precise identification of the pathogen, its transmission, and an appropriate response may be necessary to prevent additional cases of a potentially dangerous disease. In general, once a decision has been made to investigate an outbreak the following activities are involved:

- Epidemiologic investigation (see Chapter 9, Infection and Disease)
- Environmental investigation
- Interaction with the public

Even if an investigation is done after an outbreak it may still be important in order to prevent other outbreaks, describe new

disease, evaluate existing prevention strategies, and address public concerns about the outbreak. Again, the CDC supports state and local health officials in this effort and the CDC's **National Center for Preparedness, Detection, and Control of Infectious Diseases (NCPDCID)** provides public health laboratories with reliable microbiological references and reagents that may not be available commercially.

Response

The intervention/prevention/response to emerging diseases will depend on the disease and should be a public health response utilizing a variety of methods. One of the most successful tools in preventing infectious diseases is appropriate immunization programs. The National Immunization Program supports local health departments in planning, developing, and implementing immunization programs (http://www.cdc.gov/vaccines/). Other measures to prevent or interrupt the transmission process of infectious agents include rodent or insect vector control, food recall, isolation, and quarantine. Because human behavior is an important factor in infectious disease transmission, education and information campaigns are also an essential feature of most disease response activities.

Global Concerns

One of the roles of the Centers for Disease Control and Prevention (CDC) is to protect people in the United States from infectious disease. Yet, the health of a nation cannot be sufficiently protected without addressing infectious disease problems that occur elsewhere in the world. Because of expanding air travel and international trade, infectious microbes can be easily transported across borders on a daily basis. Microbes can be carried by infected people, animals, and insects. In addition, commercial shipments can contain contaminated materials, such as food.

The National Center for Infectious Diseases (NCID), a branch of the CDC, has now been officially reorganized. The former divisions and programs of the NCID have been reorganized into multiple national centers. The National Center for Preparedness, Detection, and Control of Infectious Diseases (NCPDCID) is now the agency responsible for the protection of domestic and international populations. Through their leadership, partnership, epidemiologic and laboratory studies, and the use of quality systems, this agency establishes standards and practices for response to infectious diseases (http://www.cdc.gov/ncpdcid/).

The **International Emerging Infections Program (IEIP)** is an integral component of the CDC's Global Disease Detection Program. This is the agency's principal program to reinforce the identification of emerging infections around the world, and to effectively respond to them (http://www.cdc.gov/ieip/).

U.S. Global Public Health

According to the CDC the United States should continue to increase its participation in combating all infectious disease threats around the world. These include the following:

- Protecting the health of U.S. citizens at home and abroad by controlling disease outbreaks and also dangerous endemic diseases. Wherever endemic diseases occur, the disease must be prevented from spreading internationally.
- Furthering U.S. humanitarian efforts potentially saves many human lives by preventing infectious diseases overseas. The prevention of many infectious diseases can be achieved by vaccination.
- Providing diplomatic and economic benefits for international projects that address infectious diseases. Improvements in global health will not only enhance the economy but also reduce U.S. healthcare costs by decreasing the number of imported diseases.
- Enhancing security to prevent the intentional release of biological agents by terrorist organizations (see Bioterrorism in Chapter 24, Microorganisms in the Environment and Environmental Safety).

Furthermore, in consultation with global public health partners the CDC defines global infectious disease priorities in six areas:

1. International outbreak assistance is considered to be an integral function of the CDC. This needs to include follow-up assistance after each acute emergency response to maintain control of new pathogens after the outbreak.
2. A global approach to disease surveillance needs to evolve into a global "network of networks" to provide early warning of emerging health threats. Such a network also increases the capacity to monitor the effectiveness of public health control measures.
3. Applied research on diseases of global importance, including those that are uncommon in the United States, is a valuable resource because of the dangers represented by certain imported diseases.
4. Applications of proven public health tools need to be identified and shared with the international community.

5. Global initiatives for disease control are needed to reduce the prevalence of HIV/AIDS in young people by 25% and to reduce deaths from tuberculosis and malaria by 50% by the year 2010. To reduce infant mortality the CDC shall work with the Global Alliance for Vaccines and Immunization to enhance delivery and use of new vaccines against respiratory illnesses and other childhood diseases.
6. Public health training through the encouragement and support of the CDC should result in the establishment of International Emerging Infections Programs (IEIPs) in developing countries. These centers of excellence will integrate disease surveillance, applied research, prevention, and control activities.

Global Surveillance

In industrialized countries communicable disease mortality has significantly decreased over the past century. Health agencies in these countries are concerned mostly with preventing diseases from entering the country and causing an outbreak or reemergence. Developing countries are concerned with the early detection of communicable disease outbreaks; and stopping their mortality, spread, and potential impact on trade and tourism.

To rapidly identify and contain public health emergencies the world requires a reliable global system. The **International Health Regulations (IHR),** revised in 2005, provide such a global framework to address these needs through a collective approach for prevention, detection, and timely response to any public health emergency of international concern. Once a communicable disease outbreak has been confirmed, the information is posted on the World Wide Web, and is accessible by healthcare professionals and the general public (http://www.who.int/csr/don/en/). The international response to an outbreak involves a World Health Organization (WHO) team that arrives on site within 24 hours of the information release, for initial assessment and the beginning of immediate control measures. The international response linked to the global surveillance presents a worldwide "network of networks," available for technical or humanitarian support, ensuring that no one country has to bear the entire burden.

Summary

- Emerging infectious diseases are diseases newly identified in a population; reemerging infectious diseases are known diseases that have previously been under control but are recurring.
- The emergence of infectious diseases generally involves two steps: the introduction of a pathogen into a new host population, and the establishment and further spreading within the new host population, which is referred to as *adoption.*
- Factors responsible for the emergence of new infectious diseases include human demographics and behavior, ecological changes and agricultural development, international travel and commerce, technology and industry, microbial adaptation and change, breakdown of public

Examples of Epidemic and Pandemic Alert and Response*

Date	Disease	Location	Comments
April 30, 2008	Avian influenza	Situation in Indonesia	New case of human infection of H5N1 avian influenza: 3-yr-old male
April 25, 2008	Yellow fever	Liberia	30-yr-old male, same community as index case; two confirmed cases, one death
April 22, 2008	Severe acute watery diarrhea with *Vibrio cholerae*–positive cases	Vietnam	2490 cases between March 5 and April 22, 377 cases positive for *V. cholerae*
April 18, 2008	Rift Valley fever	Madagascar	418 suspected cases, including 17 deaths
April 17, 2008	Avian influenza	Egypt	Update 10: New case, 2-yr-old male

*Examples of the cases are reported as soon as information is available. Current updates can be found at http://www.who.int/csr/don/archive/year/2008/en/index.html.

health measures, human susceptibility to infection, climate and weather, economic development and land use, war and starvation, and intent to harm.

- Emerging infectious diseases can be divided into four major groups: newly emerging diseases, reemerging diseases, new manifestations of known disease agents, and the introduction of known agents into new geographical territories.
- The NIAID has classified emerging and reemerging infectious diseases as being caused by group I, II, and III pathogens.
- Provisions for fighting infectious diseases in the United States include monitoring, preventing, and controlling infectious disease. The CDC acts as the lead U.S. federal agency responsible for providing information, recommen-

dations, and technical assistance to state and local public health departments.

- Steps in addressing and preventing emerging diseases include surveillance, investigation, and response measures.
- To protect U.S. citizens from infectious disease at home and abroad the United States must participate in combating infectious disease threats around the world.
- The International Emerging Infections Program (IEIP) is an integral component of the CDC's Global Disease Detection Program.
- The International Health Regulations (IHR) provide a global framework to address prevention, detection, and timely response to any public health emergency of international concern.

Review Questions

1. The establishment and further spreading of an infectious disease within a new population is a process called:
   a. Emergence
   b. Adoption
   c. Inclusion
   d. Appearance

2. The United Nations estimates that by the year 2050 more than _____ of the world's population will live in urban areas.
   a. 35%
   b. 56%
   c. 60%
   d. 69%

3. The Marburg virus was originally spread by:
   a. Laboratory rats
   b. Birds
   c. Green monkeys
   d. Wild turkeys

4. Which of the following infectious diseases is considered a newly emerging disease?
   a. Hantavirus
   b. Malaria
   c. Tuberculosis
   d. Chlamydia

5. Which of the following infectious diseases is considered to be a reemerging disease?
   a. AIDS
   b. Ebola
   c. West Nile virus
   d. Tuberculosis

6. Which of the following organisms belongs in the group I category?
   a. *Francisella tularensis*
   b. *Clostridium difficile*
   c. *Helicobacter pylori*
   d. *Bacillus anthracis*

7. Which of the following diseases is considered to fall in the group II category?
   a. Anthrax
   b. Lyme disease
   c. Mumps
   d. Smallpox

8. Protozoan emerging and reemerging diseases generally belong to category:
   a. I
   b. II
   c. III
   d. IV

9. Which of the following diseases is transmitted by the fecal–oral route?
   a. Ehrlichiosis
   b. Peptic ulcer
   c. Lyme disease
   d. Tularemia

10. Which of the following diseases can be transmitted by a tick?
    a. Botulism
    b. Anthrax
    c. Tularemia
    d. MRSA

11. Small changes in the viral coat that happen over time are referred to as an antigenic _____.

12. The lead federal agency whose primary responsibility is to protect the people of the United States from infectious diseases is the _____.

13. The Hendra virus is transmitted by _____.

14. "Fifth disease" is caused by _____.

15. Acanthamebiasis is a group _____ emerging/reemerging infectious disease.

16. Define emerging and reemerging infectious diseases.

17. Describe five factors that play a role in the emerging of infectious disease.

18. Describe what type of agent would be placed in group I of emerging and reemerging infectious diseases.

19. Name and briefly describe the six priority areas dealing with global infectious disease.

20. Discuss the role of continuing urbanization in the emerging/reemerging of infectious diseases.

Bibliography

Madigan MT, Martinko JM, Dunlap PV, et al: Biology of microorganisms, ed 12, San Francisco, 2009, Benjamin Cummings/Pearson Education.

Bower J, Chalk P: The Global Threat of New and Reemerging Infectious Diseases, Santa Monica, 2003, RAND.

Internet Resources

Oshitani H, Kamagaki T, Suzuki A: Major issues and challenges of influenza pandemic preparedness in developing countries, *Emerg Infect Dis* 2008;14:875–880. http://www.cdc.gov/eid/content/14/6/pdfs/07-0839.pdf

CDC, National Center for Infectious Diseases, Emerging Infectious Diseases, http://www.cdc.gov/ncidod/diseases/eid/#overviews

National Institute of Allergy and Infectious Diseases, Emerging and Re-emerging Infectious Diseases, http://www3.niaid.nih.gov/research/topics/emerging/

Morse SS: Factors in the emergence of infectious diseases, *Emerging Infectious Diseases* 1995;1:7–15. http://www.cdc.gov/ncidod/eid/vol1no1/morse.htm

Institute of Medicine (PowerPoint presentation): New Perspectives on Emerging Diseases, Biocomplexity and Teaching for Context, http://www.bioquest.org/summer2004/newEIDBQ.ppt

United Nations, World Urbanization Prospects: The 2007 Revision Population Database, http://esa.un.org/unup/

ScienceDirect, http://www.sciencedirect.com/science

Health Talk With Dr. Frank Young: In Day-Care Centers, Cleanliness Is a Must, FDA Consumer, August 1989 (Updated June 2002 and January 2003), U.S. Food and Drug Administration, http://www.cfsan.fda.gov/~dms/wh-dcare.html

CDC, Division of Foodborne, Bacterial and Mycotic Diseases (DFBMD), Disease Listing, http://www.cdc.gov/nczved/dfbmd/disease_listing.html

CDC, Tickborne Rickettsial Diseases, Ehrlichiosis, http://www.cdc.gov/ticks/diseases/ehrlichiosis/

CDC, Information about a new strain of *Clostridium difficile*, http://www.cdc.gov/ncidod/dhqp/id_CdiffFAQ_newstrain.html#1

Sunenshine RH, McDonald LC: Clostridium difficile–associated disease: New challenges from an established pathogen, Cleveland Clinic Journal of Medicine, 73(2): 187–197, 2006. http://www.cdc.gov/ncidod/dhqp/pdf/infDis/Cdiff_CCJM02_06.pdf

Campadelli-Fiume G, Mirandola P, Menotti L: Human herpesvirus 6: An emerging pathogen, *Emerging Infectious Diseases* 5(3): 353–367, 1999. http://www.cdc.gov/Ncidod/eid/vol5no3/pdf/campadelli.pdf

Slodkowicz-Kowalska A, Graczyk TK, Tamang L, et al: Microsporidian species known to infect humans are present in aquatic birds: Implications for transmission via water? *Appl Environ Microbiol* 72(7):4540–4544, 2006. Copyright © 2006, American Society for Microbiology. http://www.pubmedcentral.nih.gov/articlerender.fcgi?artid=1489349

emedicine by WebMD, Coccidioidomycosis (Infectious Diseases), http://www.emedicine.com/MED/topic539.htm

emedicine by WebMD, Babesiosis, http://www.emedicine.com/EMERG/topic49.htm

World Health Organization, Disease Outbreak News, http://www.who.int/csr/don/en/

CDC, Division of Vector-borne Infectious Diseases, West Nile Virus, Fight the Bite! http://www.cdc.gov/ncidod/dvbid/westnile/index.htm

19

Physical and Chemical Methods of Control

OUTLINE

Introduction

Microbial Control
General Considerations in Microbial Control
Resistance of Microbes
Terminology for Microbial Control
Microbial Death

Physical Control
Temperature
Osmotic Pressure
Radiation
Filtration

Chemical Control
Disinfectants and Antiseptics
Factors Influencing Antimicrobial Effectiveness
Evaluating Disinfectants
Antimicrobial Agents

Food Preservation
Pasteurization
Pressure Canning
Food Irradiation
Other Methods

LEARNING OBJECTIVES

After reading this chapter, the student should be able to:
- Describe the factors that need to be considered before deciding on the most appropriate method to be used for microbial control
- Differentiate between sterilization, disinfection, antisepsis, degermination, sanitization, and pasteurization and explain their practical uses
- Define microbial death and describe its significance in microbial control
- Describe the different physical methods that can be used in the control of microbial growth
- Define the terms microbicidal and microbiostatic
- Describe the factors influencing antimicrobial effectiveness
- Compare and contrast the methods used to measure the effectiveness of disinfectants and antiseptics
- Compare and contrast the different types of antimicrobial chemicals, and discuss the advantages and disadvantages of each
- Describe the different methods used in food preservation and explain their effectiveness in the control of microbial growth

KEY TERMS	aldehydes	disinfectants	sanitization
	algicides	disinfection	sterilization
	antisepsis	disk-diffusion method	thermal death point
	antiseptics	fungicides	(TDP)
	bactericides	ionizing radiation	thermal death time
	decimal reduction	lyophilization	(TDT)
	time (DRT)	microbicidal	use-dilution test
	decontamination	microbiostatic	virucides
	degermination	nonionizing radiation	
	desiccation	pasteurization	

WHY YOU NEED TO KNOW

HISTORY

Millennia before "animalcules" were viewed by van Leuwenhoek (see Chapter 1, Scope of Microbiology), and before the germ theory of disease and Koch's postulates had been accepted, references to germicidal agents had been made in the ancient writings of the Egyptians. Their embalmers applied spices, vegetable oils, and gums to their dead, using techniques that have kept them in a superior state of preservation even today. Persians, Greeks, and Romans had legal documents requesting the use of bright copper and silver vessels for the storage of public drinking water. The armies of Alexander the Great boiled their drinking water and buried their wastes. Very early on, salting, spicing, and smoking of foods were practiced as means of preservation. Moreover, the use of wine and vinegar in wound dressings dates back to the time of Hippocrates. Iodine was used to treat wounds before pus formation was understood because putrefaction and disease were believed to be associated.

Food preservation techniques have evolved along with culture and technology, with drying and freezing markedly influenced by the climates in which we live. Although humankind invented many methods of food preservation, fermentation was more or less discovered, not invented. Not to be upstaged by past authors who emphasized the impact of religion on science, Benjamin Franklin wrote that "...wine [is] constant proof that God loves us, and loves to see us happy." Pickling, curing (actually dehydration), the use of honey and sugars to make jams and jellies, and canning have historically impacted food-processing technologies as well.

IMPACT

Ignaz Semmelweis (see Chapter 1), in 1847 at the maternity clinic of Vienna's General Hospital, requested that interns who had performed autopsies wash their hands with chlorinated lime before examining expectant mothers. After hand-washing procedures had been instituted the incidence of death due to post delivery infection fell to about 1%.

Joseph Lister (see Chapter 1) instituted aseptic surgical techniques by the use of carbolic acid on surgeons' hands, the operating field, the surgical instruments used, and the hospital environment in general. Protective surgical gloves were developed to protect both patients and surgeons, which greatly reduced infection during and after surgical procedures.

Food preservation by canning procedures was pioneered in the late 1700s by the French and later perfected by the British, who instituted the use of tin cans in 1810. Coupled with Pasteur's work on the relationship between microbes and food spoilage/sickness, pressure canners led to canning at temperatures in excess of 100° C (212° F) and in the 1920s this canning procedure showed a significant reduction in the survival of the spores of *Clostridium botulinum*.

FUTURE

Improvements in disinfection techniques along with food preservation processes are essential to the future of physical and chemical methods of control of microorganisms in our environments. For example, better control of biofilms and of new and/or emerging resistant strains of microbes such as methicillin-resistant *Staphylococcus aureus* (MRSA) will all benefit from renewed attention.

The use of minimal food-processing techniques results in increased susceptibilities to resistant microbial strains. Therefore, in addition to developing better technologies for the improvement of disinfection and antisepsis, much greater shelf life of food is being emphasized because of the movement of population centers from the countryside to the city and the coming of the space age. Current conventional, thermal, and nonthermal methods are being investigated as potential preservation technologies for future space mission products, where minimization of mass and volume, water use, power requirements, crew size, time, and resistance to breakthrough contaminants are only some of the factors essential to the success of mission products and products having greater shelf lives.

Introduction

Under natural conditions humans and a large number of different microorganisms share the environment. Although the majority of microorganisms are harmless others can cause infection and disease, food spoilage, and water contamination. It is neither possible nor desirable to remove all microorganisms from the environment, but the control of microbial growth is necessary under many circumstances.

Microbial Control

General Considerations in Microbial Control

The control of microorganisms in the environment is a never-ending concern in healthcare, in the laboratory environment (see Chapter 4, Microbiological Laboratory Techniques), as well as in various industries, especially the food industry. Microbial control can be achieved by physical methods, chemical agents, or a combination of both. Under ideal circumstances the methods used for microbial control should be inexpensive and fast-acting. Several factors need to be considered before deciding which method is most appropriate in a given circumstance. These factors include the following:

- *Site to be treated:* The nature of the site or item to be treated will determine the method of treatment. It needs to be determined whether or not the item is treatable with harsh chemicals, heat, or radiation, or a combination thereof, without undue damage to the item.
- *Environmental conditions:* Environmental conditions have an impact on the effectiveness (efficacy) of the antimicrobial method. For example, warm disinfectants generally work better than cold ones, because chemical reactions usually occur faster at warm temperatures, therefore reducing the time of exposure. Furthermore, certain chemical agents will perform better under acidic or alkaline conditions. Items contaminated with organic substances such as feces, vomit, blood, and so on need to be cleaned before disinfection or sterilization is performed for optimal results. Biofilms notoriously prevent the penetration of chemicals into all layers of the biofilms, and physical methods may have to be used before chemical methods can be effective.
- *Susceptibility:* Susceptibility of the microorganisms needs to be considered for any of the treatments (see later).

The methods used in the control of microbes belong to the general measures of **decontamination.** In the world of microbiology, contaminants are microorganisms present at a place and a time when they're undesirable for human health. Decontamination is defined as the reduction or removal of chemical or biological agents so that they no longer present a hazard. The prerequisite for any decontamination procedure is adequate precleaning of the item to be decontaminated. Organic material such as feces, blood, and soil may inactivate disinfectants and protect microorganisms from the decontamination process; therefore, the actual physical removal of microorganisms by scrubbing is as important as the antimicrobial effect of disinfectants.

In addition to everyday management of microbial control, emergency departments and emergency medical services are responsible for the management of potential biological and chemical disasters caused by accident or by terrorist activities. Details on this topic are provided in the section First Responders to Natural Disasters and Bioterrorism in Chapter 24 (Microorganisms in the Environment and Environmental Safety).

Resistance of Microbes

Contamination with microbes is a concern in many environments; industrial, home, and healthcare, to name a few. The adequate control of these contaminants is necessary to avoid infections and disease. Although physical and chemical methods of control are available, the resistance of microbes to these methods of control varies greatly, depending on the type of microbe as well as the life stage the microorganism is in. Resistance ranges from the least resistant organisms to those with highest resistance (Box 19.1).

- Least resistant organisms include most bacterial vegetative cells, most fungal spores and hyphae, yeasts, enveloped viruses, and protozoan trophozoites.
- Moderate resistance is shown by some fungal sexual spores, protozoan cysts, and some viruses—mostly naked ones. Some of the most resistant viruses include hepatitis B virus and poliovirus. The bacteria *Pseudomonas* spp., *Mycobacterium tuberculosis,* and *Staphylococcus aureus* also are moderately resistant organisms.
- Highest resistance is demonstrated by bacterial endospores and prions. Endospores are considered the most resistant microbial form and when killed other nonpathogenic organisms are killed as well.

Endospores

Bacterial endospores are dormant, highly resistant structures formed by vegetative bacterial cells when unfavorable environments are present. Endospore-forming bacteria have a two-phase life cycle—a vegetative state and an endospores state. In the vegetative state, the cell is metabolically active, replicates, and grows. As endospores, they are a dormant alternate life form that allows the organism to withstand extremely hostile conditions and increase the chances of survival. Endospores are rather resistant to high temperatures (including boiling), most disinfectants, antibiotics, and even some radiation. It is possible for endospores to survive thousands of years until environmental stimuli trigger germination. *Bacillus, Clostridium, Desulfotomaculum, Sporosarcina, Sporolactobacillus, Oscillospira,* and *Thermoactinomyces* are some of the genera that are capable of endospore formation.

Endospores can threaten human health by causing infections such as tetanus, anthrax, and botulism. Bacterial endospores can enter the body by a break in the skin, inhalation, and/or

TABLE 19.1 Terminology in the Control of Microbial Growth

Term	Definition
Asepsis	Technique to prevent the entry of microorganisms into sterile tissues
Antisepsis	Destruction of pathogens on living tissue
Commercial sterilization	Sufficient treatment with heat to kill *Clostridium botulinum* endospores; used in the food industry
Decontamination	Destruction, removal, or reduction of the number of undesirable microbes
Degermination	Removal of microbes from a limited area (i.e., area of skin being prepared for injection)
Disinfection	Destruction of vegetative pathogens
Sanitization	Treatment to reduce microbial counts on eating and drinking utensils to achieve safe public health levels
Sterilization	The complete destruction of all forms of microbial life to include endospores and prions

ingestion. Once the bacterial spores are in the human body and they find favorable conditions, the bacteria may germinate and cause infection and disease.

Terminology for Microbial Control

All healthcare professionals, scientists, and government workers need to be familiar with, and use the precise terminology pertaining to, the control of microbial growth (Table 19.1). Some of this terminology is also explained in Chapter 4 (Microbiological Laboratory Techniques).

Sterilization

Sterilization occurs when all forms of microbial life including the most resistant forms, the bacterial endospores and prions, are eliminated. Items to be sterilized can be surfaces, equipment, foods, medications, as well as biological culture media. Sterilization can be achieved by application of heat, pressure, chemicals (liquid and gas), irradiation, or filtration. Extreme heat is the most common method used to kill microorganisms. Filtration is also an effective method to use for the removal of microbes from liquids or air. In the case of prions, the sterilization procedure typically utilizes both chemical and physical approaches, as prions are destroyed by autoclaving the contaminated items in a broth of 1 *N* NaOH.

Commercial Sterilization

Unfortunately for the food industry, temperatures used to kill all living microbes will also result in degrading the quality of food during the canning process. Instead, commercial sterilization is used, which applies just enough heat to destroy the endospores of *Clostridium botulinum,* an organism capable of producing a toxin deadly to humans.

Disinfection

Disinfection is the destruction of vegetative microorganisms via chemical or physical methods. Disinfection does not destroy bacterial endospores and can be achieved by chemicals, ultraviolet radiation, boiling water, or steam. Usually the term dis-

infection is used when inert substances or surfaces are treated chemically, and any disinfection of living tissue is called **antisepsis** and the chemical used is an antiseptic.

Degermination

Degermination is the mechanical removing of most of the microbes in a limited area. An example of degerming is the cleaning of skin with alcohol before receiving an injection.

Sanitization

Medical instruments require sterilization, but in other areas of life, microbes do not have to be completely eliminated, just reduced in sufficient numbers to prevent infection, disease, and the transmission of infection and disease. **Sanitization** is a process that intends to lower microbial counts to safe public health levels and therefore minimize the chances of disease transmission between users. For example, sanitization is used for glassware and other tableware in restaurants, institutions, as well as in the home environment.

Pasteurization

Pasteurization was introduced by Louis Pasteur in 1857 (see Chapter 1, Scope of Microbiology), using heat to kill vegetative bacteria and therefore reducing the number of microorganisms that have the potential to spoil food. To this day, pasteurization is used in the food industry in the preparation of milk, fruit juices, wine, and beer. Pasteurization does not kill all the microorganisms but reduces their numbers, or eliminates dangerous pathogens enough to prevent foodborne diseases and food spoilage.

Microbicidal Agents

The term **microbicidal** agent describes an agent that is designed to destroy microbes. They can be further subgrouped into bactericidal agents that kill bacteria, fungicidal agents that lead to fungal death, and virucides that inactivate viruses.

Microbiostatic Agents

The term **microbiostatic** indicates that microbial growth is at a standstill. Therefore a bacteriostatic agent prevents further bacterial growth, and fungistatic agents inhibit fungal growth.

Microbial Death

Microbial death is the permanent loss of the reproductive ability of microbes, as well as the permanent loss of all other vital activities. Lethal agents do not always alter the appearance of a microbial cell, even if the motility of the organism is gone. Therefore, the term microbial death can be used only if reproduction cannot occur even if the organism is given the optimal growth conditions.

The destructive forces of chemical or physical agents act on the individual cells and if exposed intensively and long enough, the cell structures become dysfunctional and the cells show irreversible damage. In general, cells in a given culture/environment vary in their susceptibility to antimicrobial agents depending on their level of metabolic activity. Young, rapidly dividing cells have the tendency to die more rapidly than older, less active cells. When microorganisms are killed by any method of control, they have the tendency to display exponential death curves. In other words, they die at some fractional rate per unit time. If 50% of microorganisms in a population die every minute, after 2 minutes 25% will still be alive, after 3 minutes 12.5% are still alive, and so on (Figure 19.1). It is therefore safe to say that the total number of organisms present when the disinfection process began determines the time required to eliminate all microbes. The effectiveness of an agent is influenced by other factors besides time, such as:

- The number of microorganisms, which dictates the amount of time required for the destruction of all contaminants.
- The nature of the organism(s) to be destroyed. Biofilms, for example, include a number of different organisms and species. Other contaminants can include vegetative organisms as well as spores. Any target population that contains more than one organism can present a broad spectrum of resistance.
- The temperature and pH of the environment have an influence on the effectiveness of the antimicrobial agent.
- The overall concentration of the microbial control agent: Most are more active at higher concentrations.
- The presence of other materials, such as organic matter, solvents, and other substances, can inhibit or interfere with the actions of antimicrobial agents.

Microbial control requires many considerations to find the most appropriate method to achieve the desired control in a

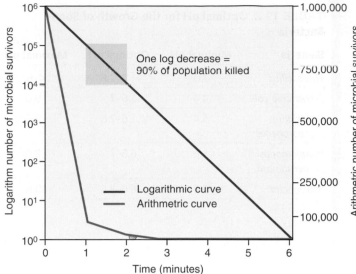

FIGURE 19.1 Exponential death of microbes. As this graph demonstrates, the microbial population shows an exponential death curve as the method of microbial control is applied.

given environment. Several questions need to be answered before a given method and/or agent is selected for microbial control. Some of these questions are as follows:

- Is the goal disinfection or sterilization?
- Will the item be discarded or is it reused?
- If dealing with a reusable item, which temperatures, pressures, chemicals, or types of radiation are acceptable?
- Will the treatment leave an undesirable residue?
- Is the agent able to penetrate to the necessary extent, that is, removal of biofilms?
- Is the process cost and labor efficient, in addition to being safe?

Physical Control

The optimal growth of most microorganisms depends on the most favorable environmental conditions for each species; most grow best in a narrow range of temperature, pH, osmotic pressure, and atmospheric conditions (Table 19.2). For example, obligate anaerobic bacteria will be killed instantly by exposure to oxygen. If the nature of the contaminant is known, the best agent of control can be determined rather easily and selectively. However, under most circumstances the exact nature of the microbe is unknown and rather stringent methods of decontamination will have to be employed.

The nature of the contaminated item(s) or areas needs to be considered to efficiently and effectively remove the unwanted organisms without destroying the item. In the case of the food industry, nutrients might be inactivated by improper treatment (see Food Preservation, later in this chapter). A summary of physical methods for the control of microbial growth is provided in Table 19.3.

TABLE 19.2 Optimal pH for the Growth of Some Bacteria

Bacteria	Minimal pH	Optimal pH	Maximal pH
Thiobacillus	1.0	2–2.8	4–6
Escherichia coli	4.4	6–7	9.0
Clostridium sporogenes	5.4	6–7.6	9.0
Pseudomonas aeruginosa	5.6	6.6–7	8.0
Nitrobacter	6.6	6.6–8.6	10.0

Temperature

Each species of microorganism has an optimal temperature range for growth, and any deviation from this will either slow down growth or stop growth altogether (Figure 19.2). For example, human pathogens prefer normal body temperature for optimal growth. In response to an infection, the human immune system (see Chapter 20, The Immune System) will increase the body temperature in an attempt to kill the invading microorganism. Microorganisms involved in the spoilage of food also generally prefer a moderate temperature for growth. Refrigeration commonly slows their growth, and appropriate cooking will kill the vegetative organisms. In other words, the majority of microbes that humans are most interested in controlling will be sensitive to abrupt changes in their environmental temperature.

TABLE 19.3 Summary of Physical Methods Available for the Control of Microbial Growth

Method	Mechanism	Comments	Use
Dry Heat			
Flaming	Burning to ashes	Sterilization	Inoculating loops
Incineration	Burning to ashes	Sterilization	Dressings, wipes, animal carcasses
Hot air sterilization	Oxidation	170° C/2 h	Glassware, needles, glass syringes
Moist Heat			
Boiling	Denaturation	Kills vegetative cells but not spores and prions	Equipment, dishes
Autoclaving	Denaturation	Sterilization	Media, linens, equipment
Tyndallization	Denaturation	Intermittent sterilization; free-flowing steam (30–60 min) for 3 d in a row	Substances that cannot withhold the high temperature of an autoclave
Pasteurization			
LTLT (low temperature, long time)	Denaturation	63° C for 30 min	Milk, milk products
UHT (ultrahigh temperature)	Denaturation	138° C for a fraction of a second	Milk, juices
Low Temperatures			
Refrigeration	Slows down microbial growth	Bacteriostatic for most bacteria	Foods, drugs
Deep freezing	Stops most microbial growth	Preservation	Foods, drugs, cultures
Desiccation, Lyophilization, Osmotic Pressure			
Desiccation	Inhibits microbial growth	Loss of water; preservation	Foods
Lyophilization	Inhibits growth	Loss of water; preservation; combination of drying and freezing	Storage of cultures, vaccines, cells
Osmotic pressure	Plasmolysis	Loss of water	Food preservation
Ionizing Radiation			
	DNA destruction	Electron beams, gamma rays, x-rays	Sterilizing medical and dental supplies
Nonionizing	DNA damage	Ultraviolet light, visible light, infrared radiation, microwaves, radio waves	Disinfecting air; transparent fluids; germicidal lamps

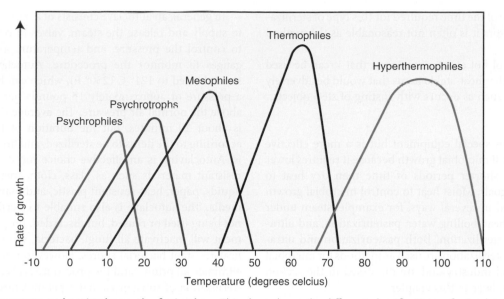

FIGURE 19.2 **Temperature and optimal growth of microbes.** This chart shows the different classifications of microbes based on optimal growth characteristics. Note that although the classifications show definite differences in the temperature optimums for groups of organisms there is some overlap in the upper and lower limits of each classification.

The most common physical method of microbial control is heat, either dry or moist. Enough heat denatures proteins, and therefore enzymes necessary for microbial growth will be inactivated and the microbe will cease to exist in its vegetative form.

Heat resistance among different microbes exists, is variable, and is expressed as the **thermal death point (TDP).** This point is the lowest temperature at which all the microorganisms in a particular liquid will be killed within 10 minutes. Another factor to be considered is the length of time required to kill the microorganisms in a particular liquid at a given temperature. This period of time is referred to as the **thermal death time (TDT).** TDP and TDT are valuable guidelines used to determine the level of treatment required to kill a given population of microorganisms, especially bacteria. Another concept, the **decimal reduction time (DRT),** is related to bacterial resistance and indicates time in minutes in which 90% of the bacterial population in question will be killed at a given temperature.

Dry Heat

One of the simplest methods of dry heat sterilization is to expose the object to direct flaming or electric heating. If contaminated objects, such as wound dressings, are expendable, incineration is usually recommended, because it is the most rigorous of all heat treatments. Direct exposure to intense heat ignites substances and reduces them to ashes and gas. Incineration of microbial samples on inoculating loops or needles is a common practice in microbiology laboratories, but although it is fast and effective it is also limited to metals and heat-resistant glass materials. The method of flaming inoculating loops and needles also produces a potential hazard to the operator through the possible splattering of contaminants when the loop is placed into the flame. For this reason tabletop infrared incinerators (Figure 19.3) have replaced the traditionally used Bunsen burners in many laboratories. However, many clinical laborato-

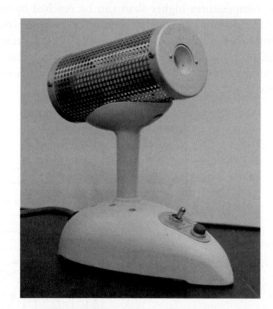

FIGURE 19.3 **Tabletop infrared incinerator.** These are sometimes used instead of Bunsen burners, when there may be a risk of dangerous aerosols being produced if a loop is sterilized in the open flame of the burner.

ries and also educational facilities are now using sterile, disposable, plastic inoculation loops and needles.

Other than incineration, dry heat is less efficient than moist/wet heat sterilization because it requires longer times and/or higher temperatures. Furthermore, not all objects that require sterilization can withstand direct flaming, and the specific times and temperatures must be determined for each type of material to be sterilized. Higher temperatures and shorter times can be used for heat-resistant materials. To accomplish sterilization with dry heat in an oven, the objects must be exposed to temperatures of 160° C to 170° C (320° F–338° F) for a period of 2 to 4 hours. Because of the time required for this type of sterilization and other factors it is often not reasonable as the method of choice.

The advantage of hot air sterilization is that it can be used on powders and other heat-stable items that would be adversely affected by steam, such as occurs with rusting of steel objects.

Moist Heat

Moist heat requires special equipment but is a more effective way to control or kill microbial growth because it requires lower temperatures and shorter periods of time than dry heat to achieve the same goals. Moist heat to control microbial growth is applied and used in several ways, for example, steam under pressure, flowing heat, boiling water, pasteurization, and ultra-high-temperature sterilization. Both pasteurization and ultra-high-temperature sterilization are used as methods for microbial control in the food industry and are discussed in the section Food Preservation, later in this chapter.

Steam Under Pressure The most dependable procedure to destroy all forms of microbial life with moist heat is steam sterilization under pressure. True sterilization using moist/wet heat requires temperatures higher than can be reached by boiling water. To achieve these higher temperatures pressure is applied to boiling water to increase the boiling point, and the temperature will proportionally increase with increasing pressure. A widely used instrument for pressurized steam sterilization is the autoclave (Figure 19.4).

In general, an autoclave consists of a pressure chamber, pipes to supply and release the steam, valves to remove air in order to control the pressure, and temperature as well as pressure gauges to monitor the procedure. Autoclaves generally use steam heated to 121° C (250° F), which can be achieved under a pressure of approximately 15 pounds per square inch (psi) above the normal air pressure. The average time of autoclaving is about 20 minutes, but the duration of the process varies according to the items to be sterilized, and how full the chamber is. Autoclaving is an effective choice for sterilization of heat-resistant materials such as glass, cloth, metallic instruments, liquids, paper, heat-resistant plastic, and many types of culture media. The autoclave is also suitable to sterilize items that are not being used or reused, but discarded. Proper autoclave treatment will inactivate all fungi, bacteria, viruses and even most heat-resistant bacterial spores. However, it will not necessarily eliminate all prions, and the procedure is also ineffective for the sterilization of substances that repel moisture, such as oils and waxes; or for powders, which will absorb the moisture and cause the particles to cake together.

Other than instrumentation to ensure that the autoclaving process displays the pertinent information abut the process, heat-sensitive indicator tape is often placed on packages of products to be sterilized before autoclaving. The chemical in the tape will change color when the desired heating conditions have been met. In addition, biological indicators distributed throughout the autoclave can be used to verify the performance of the autoclave.

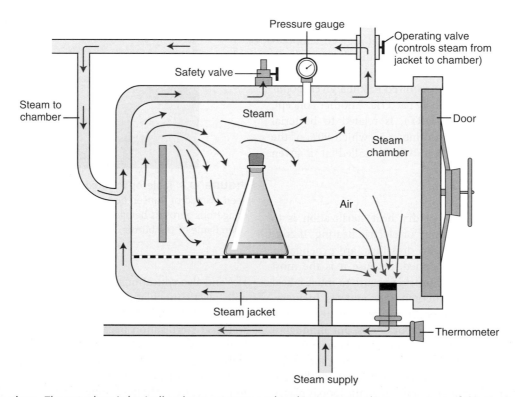

FIGURE 19.4 Autoclave. The autoclave is basically a large pressure cooker that increases the temperature of the steam in the chamber above the normal boiling point of water. It accomplishes this by raising the boiling point of the water through an increase in the pressure in the chamber.

Flowing Steam Certain substances cannot withstand the high temperature of the autoclave, but can be subjected to intermittent sterilization, a process called *tyndallization,* named after John Tyndall, the inventor of this process. This procedure is designed to reduce the level of sporulating bacteria. The technique requires a chamber to hold the materials and a reservoir for boiling water. The items are exposed to free-flowing steam for 30 to 60 minutes. The procedure is based on the assumption that some spores will survive the procedure and germinate given the appropriate environment. Furthermore, it is assumed that this germination will result in less resistant vegetative cells and, after incubation and subsequent additional exposure to steam, more of the resistant cells will be eliminated. . The procedure is repeated for 3 days in a row. Although many resistant spores will no longer germinate, the most resistant ones still may survive. Intermittent sterilization is often used to process heat-sensitive culture media containing sera, egg, other sensitive proteins, or carbohydrates.

Boiling Water Boiling items in water for 10 to 15 minutes will kill most vegetative bacteria and viruses, but it is ineffective against bacterial and fungal spores, as well as prions. On the other hand, although boiling water cannot sterilize, it is an effective, simple way to quickly decontaminate and disinfect items in the home and even in clinical environments. Boiling in water for 30 minutes will kill most nonsporing pathogens including some resistant species such as tuberculosis bacilli and staphylococci. Boiling is a recommended method for disinfecting unsafe drinking water and it is also a useful method to sanitize and disinfect materials needed for food preparation, utensils, bedding for humans, as well as materials used in the care of infants.

Refrigeration and Freezing

Another method used in the control of microbial growth is the use of cold temperatures. This method is only bacteriostatic for many microbes, and certainly cannot be applied to disinfect or sterilize items. It is, however, a convenient method to control microbial growth for limited times during food preparation and storage:

- Refrigeration halts the growth of many pathogens because they are predominantly mesophiles, yet some pathogens are perfectly capable of reproduction in a refrigerated environment.
- Slow freezing forms ice crystals that can puncture cell membranes and therefore is generally more effective in inhibiting microbial metabolism than quick freezing; however, many bacterial cells, endospores, and viruses can survive ultralow temperature for years. Because they are able to become viable microbes given the appropriate temperature and medium, many bacteria and viruses can be stored in ultralow-temperature freezers for later use in the laboratory environment. Bacteria, viruses, and tapeworms can survive in frozen food for days and months, which needs to be considered when thawing and using frozen foods (later in this chapter).

Desiccation and Lyophilization

Microbial metabolism requires water; therefore **desiccation** (drying) inhibits microbial growth. This method has been used over the years by many cultures for the preservation of a variety of foods.

Lyophilization is a technique that combines (1) freezing and (2) drying to preserve microbes, other cells, and materials for many years. It is successfully used by scientists to preserve organisms for later use. For the preservation of microbes the culture is instantly frozen in liquid nitrogen or dry ice and then subjected to a vacuum treatment that removes the water by transforming water instantly from the solid state into a gas. Therefore, lyophilization prevents the formation of ice crystals that otherwise would damage the cells. Although not all cells will survive this treatment, enough will be viable to restart the cultures many years later.

Osmotic Pressure

Subjecting microorganisms to hypertonic environments will lead to the loss of water within the cell, which interrupts the cell's metabolism. The use of osmotic pressure by high salt or sugar concentrations has long been used for food preservation. However, this method of microbial growth control is not always effective against molds which have a greater ability to grow in hypertonic environments than do bacteria.

Radiation

Radiation is also a method used in the control of microbial growth and one of the most controversial ones. By definition, radiation is the propagation of energy through space in the form of electromagnetic waves. Radiation has a variety of effects on cells, depending on the type of radiation used. These types include **ionizing radiation,** and **nonionizing radiation.** The effects of the different kinds of radiation greatly depend on the following factors:

- Time of exposure
- Distance from the source
- Shielding

Ionizing Radiation

Gamma rays, electron beams, and x-rays have wavelengths of about 1 nanometer (nm) and cause ionization. This energy has the potential to ionize atoms or molecules through atomic interactions. Ionizing radiation has enough energy to disrupt hydrogen bonding, for oxidation of double covalent bonds, and so create highly reactive hydroxide ions. These ionized molecules can denature other molecules including DNA molecules in biological organisms. The DNA damage can cause mutations and cell death.

- Electron beams are highly energetic and very effective at killing microbes within just a few seconds. However, because they do not penetrate deep into matter they cannot be used to sterilize thick objects, or objects that are covered with a large amount of organic matter. They can be used for the sterilization of microbiology plastic ware, and medical supplies including gloves, syringes, and suturing material.

- Gamma rays penetrate deep into material but may require more time to sterilize large masses. Irradiation with gamma rays not only kills microbes, but also the larvae and eggs of insects. Gamma rays are often used for sterilization of disposable medical equipment, such as needles, syringes, cannulas, and intravenous sets. This type of radiation requires bulky shielding for the safety of the operators. Irradiation with x-rays or gamma rays does not make the materials radioactive. Irradiation is used by the United States Postal Service to sterilize mail in the Washington, DC area.
- X-rays penetrate the deepest but they have less energy than gamma rays and require too much time to be useful for the control of microbial growth.

Nonionizing Radiation

Unlike ionizing radiation, nonionizing radiation, a type of electromagnetic radiation with a wavelength greater than 1 nm, does not have enough energy to remove an electron from an atom. But nonionizing radiation has enough energy to cause the formation of new covalent bonds, which affects the three-dimensional structure of proteins and nucleic acids. Nonionizing radiation includes the spectrum of ultraviolet (UV) light, visible light, infrared radiation, microwaves, and radio waves. UV light, with a wavelength of about 260 nm, is the only form of nonionizing radiation with enough energy to kill microbes in a practical setting. UV light damages DNA by causing bonds to form between adjacent pyrimidine bases, resulting in the inhibition of DNA reproduction in cells.

A disadvantage of the use of UV light as a means of disinfection is the poor penetration capacity of UV light, and organisms must be directly exposed to the rays to cause their destruction. Therefore, UV radiation is used primarily to disinfect air, transparent fluids, and the surfaces of objects. UV or "germicidal" lamps are commonly found in hospital rooms, nurseries, operating rooms, and cafeterias. UV light is also used to disinfect vaccines and other medical products. In addition, some cities use UV irradiation in sewer treatment plants by passing wastewater past UV light sources in order to reduce the number of bacteria without the use of chlorine.

Microwaves do not affect microbes directly; however, moisture-containing foods are heated by microwave action and this heat will kill most vegetative pathogens. The uneven distribution of moisture in solid foods reduces the ability of microwaves to kill the microorganisms.

Filtration

Filtration is the mechanical separation of solids from fluid or gas by means of filters, which have various pore sizes. The separation of solids from liquid is based on the molecular size of the solutes. In microbiology filters must have pores small enough to retain microorganisms. Filtration traps only particles that are larger than the pores of the filter, and in the early years of

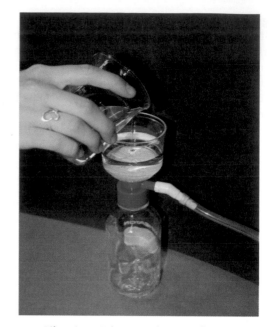

FIGURE 19.5 Filtration. When supplements for media are not heat stable, the supplements may be sterilized by filtration through a membrane. This photograph shows a simple vacuum flask setup in which the liquid to be sterilized is pulled down through a funnel with a filter by a vacuum created in the lower collection flask. Filter pore size may vary, but the two sizes used frequently when filtering for bacteria/fungus and spores are 0.22 and 0.45 μm.

microbiological studies filters were able to trap bacteria, but the pores were too large to trap the pathogens causing diseases such as rabies and measles. These pathogens were then named *"filterable viruses"* (an example being the 1918 influenza virus) and are now known simply as *viruses.* Today, filters are produced with pores small enough to sterilize—that is, eliminate all microbes, both bacteria and viruses—heat-sensitive materials such as ophthalmic solutions, antibiotics, vaccines, liquid vitamins, enzymes, sera, and culture media.

Liquids usually flow through filters by gravity, such as in coffeemakers, but in the laboratory environment a vacuum is often used to assist the movement of fluid through the filter (Figure 19.5). Filters originally were constructed from porcelain, glass, cotton, asbestos, and other special materials. Today's scientists use membrane filters manufactured from nitrocellulose or plastic with specific pore and filter sizes. The pore sizes of these membrane filters range from 25 μm to less than 0.01 μm in diameter; these pore sizes are small enough to trap small viruses and even some of the larger protein molecules (Table 19.4).

Chemical Control

In addition to the physical factors used to control microbial growth, chemical factors can also be employed both to kill microbes (bactericidal) and/or to inhibit growth (bacteriostatic). Different types of chemical agents are used to control

TABLE 19.4 Membrane Filters

Pore Size (μm)	Microbes Retained
5	Multicellular algae and fungi
3	Yeasts and large unicellular algae
1.2	Protozoa and small unicellular algae
0.45	Largest bacteria
0.22	Largest viruses and most bacteria
0.025	Larger viruses, mycoplasmas, rickettsias, chlamydias, and some spirochetes
0.01	Smallest viruses

microbial growth on both nonliving objects and living tissues. They are used to control microbes on surgical instruments and kitchen countertops, to clean toilets, and to prevent microbial growth in food and pharmaceutical products, just to name a few.

Disinfectants and Antiseptics

Antimicrobial chemicals are available in the form of liquids, gases, or solids. Few chemicals accomplish sterility; therefore most of the chemical methods of microbial control are aimed at disinfection and antisepsis. Chemicals specifically designed to be used on nonliving surfaces are referred to as **disinfectants** and those to be used on living tissues are referred to as **antiseptics.** Each category is designed for a specific task, and because no single chemical control agent is suitable for all circumstances, the selection of the appropriate agent is crucial for safety and quality control purposes. Chemical disinfectants and antiseptics have various characteristics that must be considered before any of them is used for a particular purpose.

Not all chemical agents are used to kill all microbes, because there may be circumstances in which the complete elimination of all microbes may not be desirable; instead, the inhibition of growth may be the desired effect. For example, the complete elimination of microorganisms might include the destruction of a population of normal flora, thus opening the potential for repopulation by a pathogenic microbe.

Although many antimicrobial agents have similar mechanisms of action they often vary in their effectiveness against different types of microbes. In these cases the groups of disinfectants/antiseptics may be further classified as **bactericides, fungicides, algicides,** or **virucides.** No matter what the chemical agent of choice, unless an aggressive protocol is used, a disinfectant/antiseptic typically does not sterilize an object because some resistant organisms or spores survive the treatment.

Factors Influencing Antimicrobial Effectiveness

Chemical disinfectants are commonly used in laboratory and healthcare settings for the decontamination and disinfection of benches, furniture, equipment, floors, and bathrooms, to

mention a few. In addition to the nature of the chemical agent itself, other conditions influence the effectiveness of antimicrobial chemical agents as well. These factors include the following:

- *Population size:* Most agents kill organisms at a constant rate, and therefore require a longer period of time to kill or reduce a larger population.
- *Population composition:* As previously mentioned, the effectiveness of a chemical agent can vary greatly depending on the nature of the organisms being targeted. Because of differences in susceptibility, conditions in which there are a number of populations of different organisms may significantly decrease the overall effectiveness of the agent being used.
- *Duration of exposure:* As most agents kill at a constant rate, the longer the population of microbes is exposed to an agent, the more microbes are killed. Typically an exposure time long enough to reduce the probability of survival to 10^{-6} is required to achieve sterilization.
- *Local environment:* A bacterial population is surrounded and affected by various environmental factors that may alter the effectiveness of chemical agents. The formation of a biofilm is a good example of a population condition that could dramatically decrease the activity of a chemical agent.
- *Concentration of the chemical agent:* During the initial period of exposure, an increase in the concentration of a chemical agent will typically lead to a rise in the killing rate against the target organisms. Beyond a certain point, however, a concentration increase will not alter the killing rate. Sometimes a chemical agent is actually more effective at lower concentrations. For example, ethyl alcohol is more effective at 70% concentration than at 95% concentration because of the fact that as the alcohol denatures proteins, the higher concentration will cause the proteins to coagulate rapidly throughout the entire cell wall/membrane thus preventing a more complete penetration of the alcohol deeper into the cell. A lower concentration allows the denaturing process to proceed more slowly thus allowing a deeper penetration into the cell.
- *Temperature:* An increase in temperature often increases the effectiveness of a chemical agent, provided the chemical stability of the compound is not exceeded. It is frequently possible to use lower concentrations of a chemical agent if it is used at higher temperatures.
- *Organic matter:* The presence of organic matter such as feces, vomit, or sputum can decrease the effectiveness of chemical disinfectants.

In addition, microorganisms have a range of resistances to chemical disinfectants, and the following points should be considered before choosing a particular one:

- Type of microorganisms, numbers, possible presence of spores
- Physical situation, such as surface type and suspension
- Noncorrosive or nonstaining properties with regards to the surface being treated

- Available contact between disinfectant and microorganism
- Possible interaction between disinfectant and materials
- Allowable contact time
- Concentration of the chemical: Remember, it is essential to follow the manufacturer's recommendations for dilution of a concentrate

Evaluating Disinfectants

Formal testing of the effectiveness of chemical agents is a somewhat complicated process regulated by the U.S. Environmental Protection Agency (EPA) and the U.S. Food and Drug Administration (FDA). The EPA is concerned primarily with the testing and regulation of disinfectants, whereas the FDA oversees the regulation of chemical agents that are used on humans or animals. As stated previously, antiseptics and disinfectants are used in different ways to control microbial growth. The efficiency of a particular disinfectant or antiseptic can be determined by the **use-dilution test** and/or the **disk-diffusion method.**

Use-dilution Test

The use-dilution test is a bioassay method for testing the effectiveness of disinfectants and antiseptics on microorganisms. In the past, disinfectants and antiseptics were tested by the so-called *phenol coefficient test,* a procedure that compared the activity of a disinfectant with that of phenol, and has been replaced by the use-dilution test (Association of Analytical Communities). The test organisms used for this testing procedure are *Salmonella enterica, Staphylococcus aureus,* and *Pseudomonas aeruginosa.*

Disk-diffusion Method

In the disk-diffusion method a filter paper disk impregnated with a chemical disinfectant or antiseptic is placed on an agar plate on which a bacterial culture has been spread-plated. The chemical will diffuse from the disk into the agar around the disk. The size of the area of chemical infiltration around the disk is a function of the solubility of the chemical in agar, and of its molecular size. Microbes on the agar will not grow in the area around the disk if the organism is susceptible to the chemical. The area of no growth around the disk is called the *"zone of inhibition"* (Figure 19.6).

Because several conditions may affect the disk-diffusion susceptibility test, conditions must be constant from test to test, so that only the size of the zone of inhibition is variable. These conditions include the following:

- Agar used
- Amount of organism used
- Concentration of chemical used
- The incubation conditions, such as time, temperature, and atmosphere

The amount of organism needs to be standardized according to a turbidity standard, either a visual approximation or by means of a spectrophotometer.

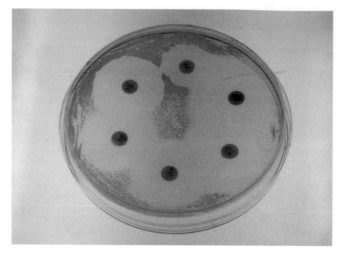

FIGURE 19.6 Disk-diffusion method. The Kirby-Bauer method for testing the effectiveness of antimicrobial agents uses a plate of Mueller Hinton agar on which a lawn of bacteria is spread. Disks impregnated with antimicrobial compounds are then placed on the surface of the plate, which is incubated for about 24 hours. The clear zones around the disks seen in this photograph are called *zones of inhibition* and are a relative measure of the effectiveness of the compound when used against a particular organism.

Antimicrobial Agents

A wide variety of chemical compounds is available to meet the varied requirements for control of microbial growth. The main groups of compounds include phenols and phenolics, halogens, alcohols, surfactants, quaternary ammonium compounds, heavy metals, and aldehydes (Table 19.5).

Phenols and Phenolics

Phenol, also known as *carbolic acid,* and phenolics (substances chemically related to phenol) are disinfectants that denature proteins and therefore disrupt the cell membranes of a wide variety of pathogens. Joseph Lister introduced and started the use of phenol in 1867 to reduce infection during surgeries. Although often replaced by the use-dilution test, the efficacy of phenol remains a standard against which the actions of other antimicrobial agents can be compared.

Phenol and phenolics have been shown to be effective even in the presence of organic contaminants such as vomit, feces, saliva, and pus. Furthermore, these chemicals remain active on surfaces for prolonged periods of time. Although they are effective agents for microbial control, phenolics do have an intense odor and can irritate the skin and mucous membranes of some individuals. Phenol itself is still used for general disinfection of drains, cesspools, and animal quarters, but rarely as a medical germicide. Phenol derivatives such as cresols, combined with soap, are used for low-level disinfection in the hospital environment. One percent to 3% emulsions of lysol and creolin are commonly used household disinfectants. Several phenolics are major ingredients in disinfectant aerosol sprays used in hospitals and as laboratory disinfectants. One of the most widely used phenolics is 5 chloro-2-(2,4-dichlorophenoxy)phenol (triclo-

TABLE 19.5 Chemicals Used in the Control of Microbes

Chemical Compound	Effectiveness	Advantages	Disadvantages	Preferred Use
Halogens				
Chlorine	Kills most vegetative cells, some viruses and fungi	Good deodorant, inexpensive	Reduced by organic material; irritating odor and residue; solutions somewhat unstable	Purification of drinking water; disinfectant in food industry and hospitals
Iodine	Kills vegetative cells, some spores and viruses, if used in high concentrations	Useful as skin disinfectant; can be used over a wide pH range	Irritating odor and residue, except with iodophors; toxic if ingested	Wound dressing, preoperative preparation, sterilization of dairy equipment
Alcohols	Kill vegetative cells and many viruses and fungi	Unaffected by organic compounds; no residue; stable and easily handled; rapid effect	Flammable	Skin and surfaces
Phenols and phenolics	Kill vegetative cells and some fungi; only moderately effective against spores	Stable to heating and drying; unaffected by organic compounds	Pure phenol is harmful to tissues; disagreeable odor; expensive; corrosive	In combination with halogens and detergents, make excellent disinfectants
Surfactants	Disrupt bacterial attachment to surfaces	Inexpensive, usually nontoxic	Usually dislodge, not kill, bacteria	Surfaces including skin and counters
Quaternary ammonium compounds	Kill bacteria (including staphylococci; *Mycobacterium tuberculosis*) and enveloped viruses	Stable in presence of organic compounds; easy to handle; no irritation residue	Hard water, detergents, and fibrous material can interfere with activity; can rust metals; low concentrations can support some bacterial growth	Small metal instruments
Heavy metals	Kill some vegetative cells and viruses	Fast and inexpensive; no special equipment required	Inactivated by organic compounds and chemical antagonists	Rarely used except as preservatives and in fungal and protozoan infections
Alkylating agents				
Aldehydes	Readily kill staphylococci, TB, and viruses; spores killed on prolonged exposure	Wide range of activity; noncorrosive	Prolonged exposure may be required; irritating to tissue, can be toxic	Instrument disinfection
Ethylene oxide (ETO)	Kills all microorganisms, including spores	Rapidly penetrates packing material	Extremely toxic, must be aerated; absorbed by porous materials, pure ETO is explosive	Sterilization of heat-sensitive materials and unwieldy objects in hospitals

san), an antibacterial compound that is added to many household products.

Halogens

Halogens are reactive nonmetallic elements: iodine, chlorine, bromine, and fluorine. The mechanism of action of the halogens in controlling microbes is the oxidation of various cellular materials, including enzymes. This denaturation of enzymes is permanent and stops all metabolic activities of the microbes. Fluorine and bromine are hazardous to handle and are no more effective than iodine and chloride, and therefore the choices for germicidal preparations are iodine and chlorine. In fact, a common example of a microbicidal halogen compound is bleach. Both chlorine and iodine are routinely used in germicidal preparations, because they are not only microbiostatic, they are microbicidal and even sporicidal given longer exposure times.

Chlorine Chlorine and its compounds have been used as disinfectants for more than 200 years. Chlorine not only kills bacteria and their endospores, but also fungi and viruses. Gaseous and liquid chlorine are used for large-scale disinfection of drinking water, swimming pools, sewage, and industrial and agricultural wastewaters. Furthermore, hypochlorite, a chlorine compound, is used to disinfect food equipment in dairies, restaurants, canneries, and more. Common household bleach is an effective all-around disinfectant, deodorizer, and even stain remover.

Iodine Iodine, when dissolved in water, forms a brown-colored solution that rapidly penetrates microorganisms and interferes with their metabolism. With proper exposure times and concentration, iodine kills all classes of microorganisms. Weak iodine solutions (1% to 5%) are used as a topical antiseptic before surgery and also in the treatment of burned or infected skin. Disinfection of nonliving objects is done with stronger solutions, up to 10%.

Alcohols

Alcohols are bactericidal, fungicidal, and virucidal, but are ineffective against fungal spores and bacterial endospores. Commonly used alcohols include rubbing alcohol (isopropanol) and drinking alcohol (ethanol). The common antiseptic isopropyl alcohol (isopropanol) is slightly superior to ethanol as a disinfectant and antiseptic. The mechanism of action of alcohols in controlling microbes is the denaturing of cellular proteins and the dissolving of lipid membranes. Because the denaturation of proteins requires water, pure alcohol is not as effective an antimicrobial agent as the 70% or 90% alcohols that are commonly used to control microbial growth.

Surfactants

Surfactants are surface-active chemicals that reduce the surface tension of solvents so that the solvent becomes more effective at dissolving solute molecules. Two common surfactants in the control of microbes are soaps and detergents. These compounds do not directly affect microbial cells but instead reduce or prevent their attachment to surfaces. For these reasons, soaps and detergents are good degerming agents, but poor antimicrobial agents. Surgical and household soaps that are antiseptic contain antimicrobial chemicals.

Quaternary Compounds

Quaternary compounds or "quats" are the most popular detergents for microbial control. They are cationic detergents that not only act as emulsifiers and wetting agents but are also microbicidal. These compounds contain positively charged quaternary nitrogen and a long hydrophobic chain that can disrupt microbial membranes and may denature some proteins. In addition, quats are colorless, tasteless, and harmless to humans, except in high concentrations.

Quats are bactericidal, fungicidal, and virucidal against enveloped viruses, but are ineffective against naked viruses, mycobacteria, or endospores. Organic compounds and soaps eliminate the action of quaternary ammonium compounds. Some pathogens such as *P. aeruginosa* will thrive in the presence of these compounds; therefore, surfactants are classified as low-level disinfectants.

Heavy Metals

Heavy metal compounds (so called because of their relatively high atomic weight), such as the elements mercury, silver, gold, copper, arsenic, and zinc, have been used in microbial control for centuries. Their mechanism of action involves altering the three-dimensional shape of proteins, thereby interfering with or eliminating the appropriate function of cellular proteins.

For many decades, a large number of states in the United States required that the eyes of newborns be treated with cream containing 1% silver nitrate to prevent possible blindness caused by *Neisseria gonorrhoeae*, which newborns could acquire during passage through the birth canal. Although silver is still used in some surgical dressings, burn creams, as well as catheters, it has largely been replaced by other antimicrobial treatments that have been proven to be less irritating but still effective against pathogens.

Copper is used to control algal growth in fish tanks, swimming pools, reservoirs, and water storage tanks. Copper interferes with chlorophyll and is an effective algicide in the absence of organic contaminants.

Alkylating Agents

Alkylating agents constitute a diverse group of chemicals, often toxic because of their ability to inactivate nucleic acids and proteins. Agents used in the control of microorganisms include aldehydes and ethylene oxide.

- The **aldehydes** most often used in microbial control are glutaraldehyde, a liquid, and formaldehyde, a gas.

MEDICAL HIGHLIGHTS

Thimerosal in Vaccines

Pharmaceutical companies have used thimerosal, a mercury-containing compound (an organomercurial), for decades to preserve some vaccines and other products, beginning in the 1930s. Mercury is a metabolic poison; however, no harmful effects have been reported from thimerosal at doses used in vaccines. However, concern about the theoretical potential for neurotoxicity of even low levels of organomercurials has grown over the years. Furthermore, an increased number of thimerosal-containing vaccines have been added to the infant immunization schedule. As a result, concerns about the use of thimerosal in vaccines and other products have been raised. Because of public pressure, in July 1999 agencies of the U.S. Public Health Service, the American Academy of Pediatrics, and vaccine manufacturers agreed that as a precautionary measure thimerosal should be reduced or eliminated in vaccine preparation and storage. With the exception of some influenza vaccines, none of the vaccines in the United States used for the protection of preschool children against 12 infectious diseases contain thimerosal.

Glutaraldehyde is a yellow acidic liquid and is one of the few chemicals that are accepted as a sterilant and high-level disinfectant. A 2% solution of glutaraldehyde will kill bacteria, viruses, and fungi within a 10-minute period of time for most objects. Spores and fungi can be killed within 3 hours, and an exposure time of 10 hours will achieve sterilization. Glutaraldehyde is less irritating and more effective than formaldehyde, but also more expensive. Formaldehyde is an irritating, strong-smelling gas that readily dissolves in water to form a solution called *formalin*. Although formalin is an intermediate to high-level disinfectant, it is extremely toxic (carcinogen), which limits its clinical usefulness.

- **Ethylene oxide** (ETO) is colorless, exists as a gas at room temperature, and is used as a sterilizing agent in hospitals and dental offices. It provides an effective method to sterilize and disinfect plastic materials and delicate, heat-sensitive instruments in hospitals and industries. Because of their toxicity and explosive properties, gaseous agents can be extremely hazardous to the people using them. Specially designed ETO sterilizers with safety features should be used by trained personnel only.

Food Preservation

Food preservation refers to a variety of techniques used in handling/preparing and treating food to avoid or slow down food spoilage, and to prevent foodborne illnesses. At the same time, food preservation processes should result in the maintenance of nutritional value, density, texture, and flavor.

Food poisoning is a common and usually mild illness; however, at times it can turn deadly. Symptoms include nausea, vomiting, abdominal cramps, and diarrhea, which occur within 48 hours of consuming a contaminated food or drink. Foodborne diseases (also see the Healthcare Application tables in Chapter 1, Scope of Microbiology) are caused by either the contaminating microbe itself or by its toxins. Infectious diseases can be spread through food or beverages and are a problem for millions of people in the United States and around the world. The Centers for Disease Control and Prevention (CDC) estimates that 76 million people annually suffer from foodborne illnesses in the United States alone, causing approximately 325,000 hospitalizations and more than 5000 deaths. According to the National Institutes of Health (NIH) the annual cost of all foodborne diseases in the United States is 5 to 6 billion dollars in direct medical costs and lost productivity. An increase in reported food poisoning cases has been noted by the CDC, and it is estimated that nearly 25% of the U.S. population suffers from some sort of food poisoning each year. It has been suggested that this increase is due to the mass production and distribution of processed foods, including raw vegetables, fruits, and meats. Any type of safety shortcuts and improper handling will lead to contamination of large masses of food with dirt, water, or animal wastes.

Safe food preservation involves preventing the growth of bacteria, fungi, and other microorganisms. It also involves stop-

ping fat oxidation, which results in spoilage (rancidity), as well as processes that will inhibit the natural aging and discoloration that occur during food processing. Methods to prevent these processes include canning, pickling, drying, freeze-drying, pasteurization, smoking, addition of chemical additives, and irradiation.

Pasteurization

Pasteurization (also see Chapter 1, Scope of Microbiology) is a method by which heat is applied to liquids to kill potential pathogens, as well as microbes that could lead to food spoilage, without changing the flavor and food value of the material. Pasteurization is designed to achieve a mathematical "log reduction" in the number of viable organisms to such a point that they are unlikely to cause disease. Although pasteurization does eliminate most pathogens, it does not sterilize, and heat-loving and heat-tolerant bacteria survive the procedure. These swimming organisms do not cause food spoilage over a relatively short time period, if appropriately refrigerated, and they are generally not pathogenic.

Effective pasteurization varies with the product and the time and temperature required for effectiveness, all of which must be adjusted accordingly. Pasteurization uses temperatures below the boiling point to avoid damage to the food. Today, two types of pasteurization are typically used: high temperature short time (HTST) and ultrahigh temperature (UHT).

- HTST pasteurization can be achieved in two ways: by batch or continuous flow. In the batch process the fluid is held at 63° C for 30 minutes and then quickly cooled to about 4° C. In the continuous flow process, liquid is guided between metal plates or pipes that are heated from the outside by hot water.
- UHT pasteurization is done by holding the liquid at a temperature of 138° C for a fraction of second; products are accordingly labeled and can be stored at room tem-

Milk: Pasteurized or Raw?

Since its adoption in the early 1900s, pasteurization has resulted in the reduction of foodborne illnesses due to contaminated milk. By carefully processing milk and milk products many illnesses can be prevented. However, some groups of people firmly believe that the processed milk destroys the natural nutritive properties of milk and may make it harmful for human consumption. Although pasteurization will change some proteins within milk through denaturation, it also will prevent disease from organisms that contaminate raw milk—milk cannot be harvested without some contamination by pathogens, because our environment is not sterile. According to the U.S. Department of Agriculture, drinking untreated (raw) milk or eating raw milk products is equivalent to playing "Russian roulette" with your health. Annually the Centers for Disease Control and Prevention reports contain many cases of foodborne diseases due to consumption of raw milk or raw milk products.

perature without microbial spoilage. After months the food prepared by this method may lose some of its flavor.

In the United States, pasteurization methods are standardized and controlled by the U.S. Department of Agriculture (USDA). Different standards are applied for different products, usually depending on the content and intended use.

Pressure Canning

All foods contain microbes, which are the major cause of food spoilage. Using heat in canning is at least a century-old technique. Boiling forces the air out of the jar, a vacuum is formed as the jar cools and, with the proper type of lid, it seals, thereby preventing microorganisms from reentering and contaminating the food. This process also creates an anaerobic environment in the food, which limits the growth of many organisms. Although a specific amount of heat applied for a specific amount of time kills certain bacteria, not all bacteria are necessarily killed.

Acid in pickled products, or sugar in jams and jellies, prevents the growth of some microorganisms, but does not protect low-acid foods from some microorganisms. Foods low in acid such as vegetables, meat, poultry, and fish must be pressure canned at higher temperatures than the normal boiling point in order to destroy the obligate anaerobe *Clostridium botulinum,* the organism that causes botulism, a deadly form of food poisoning. These high temperatures can be reached under pressure and are necessary to ensure the safety of these food products. Canned foods in which the pressure seal is broken generally require refrigeration. If the seal is not effective after the pressurized boiling it becomes a "high-risk" consumable food item.

Food Irradiation

Food irradiation is a fairly new food safety technology for preventing food spoilage and eliminating foodborne pathogens. This technology is similar to the technology used to sterilize medical devices. Food for space travel is sterilized by irradiation to avoid foodborne illness. Extensive studies on irradiated food products have shown that irradiated food does not have an adverse effect on humans or animals. Furthermore, studies have indicated the following about irradiated food:

- Disease-causing organisms are reduced or eliminated.
- The food does not become radioactive.
- No dangerous substances are produced as a result of the process.
- The nutritional value is essentially unchanged.

When ionizing radiation strikes microorganisms, its high-energy wavelengths create transient reactive chemicals that change the DNA of the microbes, killing the organisms. The sensitivity of the various microorganisms varies depending on the size of their DNA, the rate at which they can repair DNA, and other issues. The size of the DNA is the major factor for elimination of an organism by irradiation. Parasites and insects, which have large amounts of DNA, are killed rapidly even with low doses of irradiation. More radiation is necessary to kill bacteria because of their smaller DNA, and it takes additional radiation to kill bacterial endospores. Viruses, which have even smaller DNA, are generally resistant to irradiation at doses approved for foods. Prion particles such as those associated with bovine spongiform encephalopathy (mad cow disease) lack DNA and are not inactivated by irradiation, except at extremely high doses. In other words, irradiation is effective in eliminating parasites and bacteria from food, but will not be effective in eliminating viruses or prions.

Other Methods

Many other methods of food preservation have been used by various cultures under various environmental conditions. Food begins to spoil from the moment it is harvested and previously each culture preserved their local food sources by using the same basic methods of food preservation. These include drying, freezing, pickling, curing, fermenting, and the preparation of jams and jellies:

- Drying is probably the oldest method of preserving foods. The food will keep well because the water available for metabolism is so low that spoilage organisms cannot grow. Various methods of drying can be used, including sun drying, oven drying, and food dryers.
- Freezing does preserve foods and inactivate many microbes; however, once thawed these microbes can again become active and multiply under the right conditions, which then can lead to foodborne illnesses.
- Pickling is the process of preserving food by anaerobic fermentation in a salt solution to produce lactic acid. It

also includes marinating and storing food in an acid solution, usually vinegar.

- Curing is the addition of some combination of salt, sugar, nitrite, and/or nitrate to meats for the purposes of preservation, flavor, and color. Salts inhibit microbial growth by plasmolysis. The concentration of salt needed to inhibit the growth of microorganisms is genus and species dependent.
- Fermentation typically refers to the conversion of sugar to alcohol by yeast under anaerobic conditions. Furthermore, fermentation implies that the action of microorganisms is desirable, and the process is used to produce products such as wine, beer, cider, and vinegar.
- Jams, jellies, and marmalades are thickened or gelled fruit products. Most of them are cooked and preserved with sugar, which creates an osmotic gradient inhibiting microbial growth.

Summary

- Most microorganisms are harmless, but many can cause infection and disease, water contamination, food spoilage, and other undesirable effects. Controlling them is a constant, never-ending concern in the healthcare environment, in laboratories, and in industry, especially in the food industry.
- Microbial control can be achieved by physical methods, chemical agents, or a combination of both in order to destroy, remove, or reduce microbes within a given area.
- Several factors need to be taken into consideration before a method of control is decided on, including the site or material to be treated, the type and number of microbes involved, the environmental conditions, the time available for management, as well as the effect desired.

- Sterilization is the elimination of all forms of microorganisms. Disinfection is the destruction of all vegetative microorganisms. The term disinfection when applied to living tissue is antisepsis. Degermination means the mechanical removal of most microbes within a given area, whereas sanitation provides a significant reduction of microbial numbers, and pasteurization kills enough microbes to prevent foodborne disease and food spoilage.
- Physical control of microbial growth involves different types of treatments such as temperature, osmotic pressure, radiation, and/filtration.
- Various types of chemical agents are used to control microbial growth on nonliving objects such as surgical instruments, laboratory and kitchen countertops, and toilets, as well as on living tissues, to mention a few.
- Antimicrobial chemicals are available in the form of liquids, gases, or solids, but few can achieve sterility; therefore chemical methods of control are aimed mainly at disinfecting nonliving items, and antisepsis of living tissues.
- Conditions such as the size of the microbial population and its composition, as well as the duration of chemical exposure, its concentration, the ambient environment, and temperature influence the effectiveness of antimicrobial agents.
- Formal testing of the effectiveness of antimicrobial agents is regulated by the Environmental Protection Agency (EPA) and Food and Drug Administration (FDA), and the efficacy of a disinfectant or antiseptic can be determined by the use-dilution test or the disk-diffusion method.
- Food preservation is achieved by a variety of techniques in handling, preparing, and treating food to prevent foodborne illnesses and to avoid or slow down food spoilage.

Review Questions

1. Decontamination is defined as the:
   a. Killing of all microorganisms in a given area.
   b. Reduction or removal of unwanted chemical or biological agents.
   c. Stopping of growth of microorganisms in a given area.
   d. Removal of all vegetative organisms.

2. Which of the following organisms has higher resistance to most physical control methods than the others?
   a. Protozoan cysts
   b. Fungal spores
   c. Enveloped viruses
   d. Vegetative bacterial cells

3. The cleaning of glassware and tableware in restaurants falls in the category of
   a. Degermination
   b. Sterilization
   c. Disinfection
   d. Sanitation

4. Which of the following methods is the simplest heat-related method to sterilize metal?
   a. Boiling
   b. Autoclaving
   c. Direct flaming
   d. Indirect heating

5. Boiling items in water for _____ minutes will kill most vegetative bacteria and viruses.
   a. 3–5
   b. 5–6
   c. 6–8
   d. 10–15

6. The technique that combines freezing and drying to preserve microbes and other cells is:
   a. Desiccation
   b. Lyophilization
   c. Pasteurization
   d. Radiation

7. Ionizing radiation involves all of the following *except*:
   a. UV light
   b. Gamma rays
   c. Electron beams
   d. X-rays

8. The term "zone of inhibition" is used in which of the following procedures?
   a. Use-dilution test
   b. Growth inhibition test
   c. Disk-diffusion test
   d. Multiple inhibition test

9. Chlorine belongs to which of the following chemical groups?
   a. Halogens
   c. Phenols
   b. Heavy metals
   d. Alcohols

10. All of the following are methods for food preservation *except*:
    a. Pasteurization
    b. Sterilization
    c. Irradiation
    d. Ultrahigh-temperature pasteurization

11. The destruction of vegetative organisms by chemical or physical methods is called _____.

12. The term used to describe an agent that causes microbial growth to come to a standstill is _____.

13. The lowest temperature by which all microorganisms in a particular liquid will be killed within 10 minutes is the _____.

14. Antimicrobial agents that are specifically designed to be used on living tissues are referred to as _____.

15. Agents that kill microbes are classified as _____.

16. Explain and differentiate between sterilization and commercial sterilization.

17. Define decontamination.

18. Name two organisms that are moderately resistant to antibiotics.

19. Describe the factors influencing the antimicrobial effectiveness of chemical agents.

20. Describe the two different types of pasteurization.

Bibliography

Bauman R: *Microbiology: with diseases by taxonomy*, ed 2, San Francisco, 2007, Benjamin Cummings/Pearson Education.

Mims C, Dockrell HM, Goering RV, et al: *Medical microbiology*, ed 3, St. Louis, 2004, Mosby/Elsevier.

Murray PR, Rosenthal KS, Pfaller MA: *Medical microbiology*, ed 5, St. Louis, 2005, Mosby/Elsevier.

Talaro KP: *Foundations in microbiology*, ed 6, New York, 2005, McGraw-Hill.

Totora GJ, Funke BR, Case CL: *Microbiology: an introduction*, ed 9, San Francisco, 2007, Benjamin Cummings/Pearson Education.

Internet Resources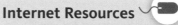

CDC, *Vaccine Safety*, http://www.cdc.gov/vaccinesafety/?

Real Milk Articles, Why Milk Pasteurization? Sowing the Seeds of Fear, http://www.realmilk.com/propaganda.html

CDC, Outbreak Surveillance Data, http://www.cdc.gov/foodborne-outbreaks/outbreak_data.htm

Suite101.com, The Raw Milk Debate: Controversy Surrounding Raw, Unprocessed Milk, http://beverages.suite101.com/article.cfm/the_raw_milk_debate

FDA Consumer Magazine (Sept-Oct, 2004), Got Milk? Make Sure It's Pasteurized, http://www.fda.gov/fdac/features/2004/504_milk.html

CDC, Food Irradiation, http://www.cdc.gov/ncidod/dbmd/diseaseinfo/foodirradiation.htm

The Immune System

20

OUTLINE

Fundamentals of the Immune System
Immunology
Immunity
Antigens
Antibodies

Components of the Immune System
Tissues and Organs of the Immune System
Cells of the Immune System

Host Defense
First Line of Defense
Second Line of Defense
Third Line of Defense

Diseases Caused by the Immune System
Allergy–Hypersensitivity Reactions
Autoimmune Diseases
Immune Deficiency Diseases

Aging and the Immune System

LEARNING OBJECTIVES

After reading this chapter, the student will be able to:
- Describe the chemical composition and function of antigens and antibodies
- Name and explain the functions of the different classes of antibodies
- Describe the components and functions of the lymphatic and immune systems
- Discuss the lines of defense against microbes
- Describe the processes and steps of phagocytosis and inflammation
- Differentiate between innate (nonspecific) and acquired (specific) immunity
- Discuss active and passive immunity—both naturally and artificially acquired
- Identify and discuss autoimmune diseases
- Describe the four types of hypersensitivity reactions
- Explain how the aging process influences the immune system

adaptive immune system
allergens
allografts
alternative complement
  pathway
antibody
antibody titer
antigen
antigen-presenting cell
autoantigens
autografts
autoimmune diseases
B cells
basophils
chemotaxis
classical complement
  pathway
clonal selection
cytokines
dendritic cells (DCs)
eosinophils

epitope
erythropoiesis
hapten
hemocytoblasts
hemopoiesis
immunity
immunocompetent
immunogens
immunoglobulins (Igs)
immunology
immunosuppressed
inflammation
innate
interferons
isografts
lectin pathway
leukopoiesis
lymphocytes
lymphopoiesis
lysozymes

macrophages
major histocompatibility
  complex (MHC)
monocytes
myelopoiesis
neutrophils
nonself-antigens
phagocytosis
phagosome
primary response
pyrexia
pyrogens
secondary immune
  response
self-antigens
T cells
tolerogens
tumor antigens
vaccine
xenografts

WHY YOU NEED TO KNOW

HISTORY

Outbreaks of infectious pathogenic diseases, pestilences, epidemics, pandemics, and plagues have and continue to threaten annihilation of the human race. One of the earliest, chronicled by Thucydides in 431 bce, was a plague in Athens that lasted for more than a year. Later, in the 1300s ce, the Black Death from *Yersinia pestis* and opportunistic microbes killed an estimated one third of the known population of Asia and Europe. In the twentieth century, the Spanish Influenza virus of 1917–1918 killed an estimated 100 million worldwide in just over 9 months!

Can the "fittest" survive without an immune system? No. Immediately after exposure and later survival ultimately becomes a game of numbers. How many invaders (antigens) against how many antibodies? How virulent are the microbes versus how specific are the antibodies or the T cell response? How able is our own immune system to effectively challenge and control the antigens?

IMPACT

Today we are threatened by Ebola virus, bird flu viruses, HIV, the reemergence of smallpox virus, and, most recently in 2004, the severe acute respiratory syndrome (SARS) virus. The SARS virus is a coronavirus and coronaviruses are generally weak, causing diarrhea or other mild symptoms. But the SARS virus is extremely virulent and can be lethal, particularly among those over 40 years of age. Although a measure of protection against the flu viruses in general is afforded by annual flu shots with vaccines grown in egg culture that is purified and chemically killed, the best protection against the SARS virus is a healthy immune system. Although vaccines are effective, many of these viruses mutate and spread rapidly. For vaccines to be useful, they must be produced in quantity, and delivered in time to meet the viral challenge *du jour*.

Immunity first comes from the mother, through the umbilical cord before birth, but this is only temporary and helps us survive exposure to pathogens until our own immune system has matured and is functional. The effectiveness of the immediate response of our immune system to pathogens initially depends on our general state of health. This response is enhanced by the presence of antibodies from previous exposure to the same or similar pathogens. Further strengthening is obtained by timely vaccinations. Compliance with all these factors shifts the balance toward a more successful response to and survival after exposure to pathogens.

THE FUTURE

Egg culture vaccines are effective but are produced slowly. New methods being explored that more rapidly produce better vaccines include growing virus in human cell cultures and the development of genetically engineered vaccines. Yet any of these deadly flu viruses, as well as HIV, Ebola, and smallpox viruses, left unchecked, could either decimate or wipe out civilization.

Although our current armory of drugs is generally effective, the occurrence of microbial mutations is eliciting a rising resistance of pathogens to successful, well-established antibiotic therapies. The tried-and-true drugs of the past are becoming ineffective. New and improved therapies, based on better understanding of what assists the immune system, are needed to confront "new and improved" pathogens.

In other words, serendipitous trial and error can only take us so far. It is essential to understand how our immune system works and responds to the presence of any antigens or foreign substances so that we can strengthen our response to them and rationally tip the numbers in favor of survival.

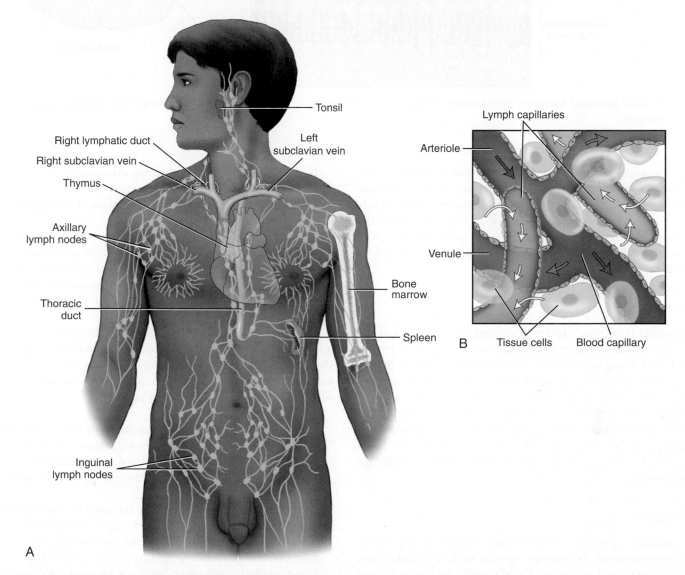

FIGURE 20.1 Overview of the lymphatic system. The lymphatic system consists of lymphatic vessels, lymphoid tissue and cells, and lymphatic organs.

Fundamentals of the Immune System

Immunology

Immunology is the study of the genetic, biological, chemical, and physical characteristics of the immune system. It describes the actions of cells, tissues, and organs that are specialized to protect the body from microorganisms and other foreign substances (Figure 20.1). In essence, immunology is concerned with how the body uses protective mechanisms to recognize self from nonself-molecules. Self and nonself are determined by specific receptors on the surface of cell membranes that recognize and differentiate among antigens. These receptors, specific to a cell or particle, are called *self-antigens* or *cell surface markers*. In response to foreign antigens, cells of the immune system produce specific antibodies that bind to spe-

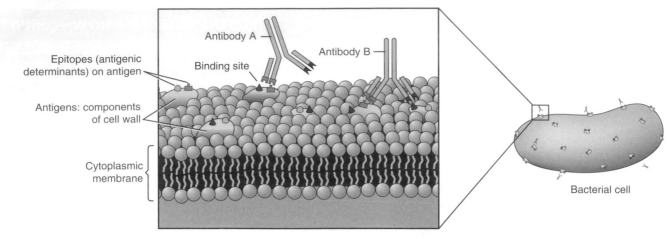

FIGURE 20.2 Epitopes: Antigenic determinants. Antigens are a component of cell walls and/or plasma membranes and have one or more epitopes.

cific antigens. An antigen–antibody complex is formed, which is then destroyed by the immune system. Another immune reaction to protect the body is *cell-mediated immunity*. This is an immune response that does not include antibodies but involves the activation of macrophages, natural killer (NK) cells, and cytotoxic T lymphocytes, and the release of various cytokines.

Immunity

Immunity is the body's ability to respond to the presence of any foreign substance. The immune response that begins after exposure to invading organisms or substances is controlled by two immune system response mechanisms: (1) the innate (nonspecific) immune response and (2) the adaptive (specific) immune response. The immune system of a person is considered to be **immunocompetent** when it functions properly, and **immunosuppressed** (immunodepressed, immunocompromised) if part or all of the system cannot respond appropriately to a challenge by antigens.

Antigens

An **antigen** is any agent that is capable of binding specifically to components of the immune system such as lymphocytes, macrophages, and antibodies. Usually, only a part of an antigen triggers the immune response. The smallest part of an antigen molecule that can bind with an **antibody** is called an **epitope** or antigenic determinant. All antigens have one or more epitopes (Figure 20.2). Proteins, carbohydrates, lipids, and nucleic acids can all be antigens under certain circumstances.

- Proteins are the most immunogenic molecules and often have several epitopes for antibody recognition.
- Carbohydrates are potentially immunogenic when bound to a protein, forming complex glycoprotein molecules. These are located in the cell membrane and can cause an immune response. Examples of the antigenicity of carbohydrates are the polysaccharides on the surface of red

blood cells (see ABO blood typing discussed in the Antigens section, later in this chapter).
- Lipids also can cause an immune response if conjugated with a protein carrier.
- Nucleic acids are poor immunogens themselves, but when bound to a carrier protein they can become immunogenic. A clinical example is the presence of anti-DNA antibodies in patients with systemic lupus erythematosus (see the section Autoimmune Diseases later in this chapter).

Moreover, a distinction between antigens is required because many of them are incapable of inducing an immune response. On the basis of the reaction of the immune system to a given antigen, antigens can be classified as immunogens, tolerogens, allergens, autoantigens, and tumor antigens.

- **Immunogens** are substances that stimulate the production of specific antibodies by the immune system. All immunogens are antigens but not all antigens are necessarily immunogens. Pathogenic organisms such as bacteria and viruses are immunogens.
- **Tolerogens,** like self-antigens, are tolerated by the immune system. However, if the molecular weight or form of a tolerogen changes, it can become an immunogen. For example, low molecular weight compounds, including some antibiotics and other drugs, are incapable of eliciting an immune response themselves, but become immunogens when conjugated with a high molecular weight molecule. The low molecular weight compound is called a **hapten** (Figure 20.3) and the high molecular weight compound is referred to as a carrier.
- **Allergens** are substances causing allergic reactions. They can be ingested, inhaled, injected, or come into contact with the skin to evoke an allergic response. Substances such as pollen, egg white, honey, and many others can cause such reactions in some individuals and therefore are referred to as allergens.
- **Autoantigens** are molecules, usually proteins, that are interpreted by the immune system as nonself-antigens,

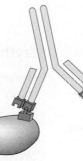

| Hapten molecule | Carrier molecule | Hapten-carrier conjugate | Conjugate with antibody |

such as in the case of **autoimmune diseases.** Autoantigens are frequently components of multimolecular, subcellular particles that are involved in a variety of cell functions. Under normal circumstances these antigens would be accepted (tolerated) as self-antigens and not targeted by the immune system.

- **Tumor antigens** are always presented by tumor cells and never by normal cells of the body. In this case the antigens are tumor specific and typically result from tumor-specific mutations. Lymphocytes that recognize these antigens as nonself destroy these tumor cells before they can proliferate and metastasize. Examples of the origin of these tumor antigens include new genetic information introduced by a virus such as the human papillomavirus of cervical cancer, or the alteration of oncogenes by carcinogens.

A microbe or parts of a microbe such as flagella, capsules, portions of the bacterial cell wall, bacterial and viral toxins, spike proteins in the coat of viruses, and external structures of fungi and protozoans all can be antigenic. Nonmicrobial antigens include components of pollen, egg white, beeswax, cat dandruff, dog hair, foreign blood cells, as well as tissue and organ transplants (see Allergy–Hypersensitivity Reactions later in this chapter).

An organism's self-antigens are located on the cell membrane and are unique for each individual, with the exception of identical twins, who carry the same genetic code. These antigen molecules are coded by a group of genes located on chromosome 6 and form the **major histocompatibility complex (MHC).** Antigens resulting from the MHC are glycoproteins and are found on all cells except red blood cells (see later in this section). These antigens were originally identified on the surface of white blood cells and therefore the MHC is sometimes referred to as the human leukocyte antigen (HLA) system. The MHC plays a major role in an individual's immune system by recognizing and tolerating self-antigens and rejecting foreign antigens. This phenomenon of self-recognition is referred to as immunological tolerance. A healthy immune system can distinguish between the body's self-antigens and nonself-antigens. However, in the case of an autoimmune disease, the immune system has lost its tolerance to the self-antigens and attacks the body's own cells or cell structures.

Moreover, the MHC genes are clustered to form a multigene complex made of three subgroups called *class I, class II,* and *class*

III. The class I genes encode the unique self-antigen characteristics and aid in the recognition of self-antigen molecules, and the class II genes encode receptors that recognize foreign antigens. These regulatory receptors are located mainly on macrophages and B cells and are involved in presenting antigens to the T cells during the immune response. Class III genes, in contrast to class I and class II MHC genes, which encode cell surface molecules, encode secreted complement components such as C2 and C4 (see Complement System later in this chapter).

Transplantation is a solution for replacement of damaged tissues or organs. However, for a transplant to be successful, matching as many MHC molecules (self-antigens) as possible is essential to avoid a serious immune reaction called *rejection*. Transplants are classified according to donor characteristics as autografts, isografts, allografts, and xenografts.

- **Autografts** are tissues transplanted from one site in an individual to another site. An example is the removal of a portion of a blood vessel from one site and transplanted to another, in order to provide a healthy blood vessel for a dialysis stent.
- **Isografts** are tissues or organs transplanted between genetically identical entities such as identical twins, for whom tissue or organ rejection is not an issue. For example, a kidney or part of the liver can be transplanted from one identical twin to the other without resulting in major transplant rejection.
- **Allografts** are transplants between genetically different individuals from the same species (e.g., humans) but with different genomes (genetic information). In other words, the MHC molecules are different and rejection of the transplant can occur.
- **Xenografts** are transplants between individuals of different species such as pigs and humans. Although xenografts are often less successful than same-species grafts, pig heart valves have been used extensively and with great success for human cardiac valve replacement.

Normally the most successful transplants are ranked in order as autografts followed by isografts, allografts, and xenografts. Rejections may occur immediately after transplantation, or after several weeks, months, or years. To reduce the immune response and prevent transplant rejection, immunosuppressive drugs such as cyclosporine and prednisone are used. However, the

TABLE 20.1 ABO Blood Typing

Blood Type	Antigen	Antibody
A	A	Anti-B
B	B	Anti-A
AB	A, B	None
O	None	Anti-A, anti-B

Erythroblastosis Fetalis

Hemolytic disease of the newborn (erythroblastosis fetalis) occurs if an Rh-negative (Rh⁻) mother carries an Rh-positive (Rh⁺) fetus. The mother's immune system develops antibodies against Rh⁺ blood when red blood cells (RBCs) of the fetus cross the placenta and enter the mother's circulation. This can occur during childbirth. The mother's immune system maintains the antibodies in case foreign blood cells enter her system again, such as in a future pregnancy. The mother's body is now considered to be Rh sensitized. During the first pregnancy, Rh sensitization is not likely but does become a problem in subsequent pregnancies with another Rh⁺ fetus. In this instance, the mother's antibodies cross the placenta and attack the fetus's RBCs. The destruction of the fetus's RBCs can result in a worst-case scenario in which the fetus is at great risk of erythroblastosis fetalis and can be stillborn. Prevention of this condition can be achieved by injecting the mother with anti-Rh immune globulin to prevent the sensitization of her immune system during the first pregnancy with an Rh⁺ fetus.

A fetus born with erythroblastosis fetalis is said to have hemolytic disease of the newborn and its treatment will be determined by the physician, based on the severity of the disease and the overall health of the infant.

---

resulting compromised immune system puts the recipient of the transplant at a higher risk of infection and is a major concern when immunosuppressive drugs are used.

Blood typing, for compatibility before blood transfusion, is also based on genetically determined surface antigens on red blood cells (RBCs). Although more than 20 blood group systems are known today the ABO and Rh systems are used most often. The ABO system is based on the presence of type A or B antigens on the surface of RBCs. The RBCs of blood type A have A antigens, blood type B cells have B antigens, blood type AB cells have both antigens, and blood type O cells have neither A nor B antigens. The immune system does not normally produce antibodies against its own RBC antigens, but antibodies against another blood type are present in the blood plasma (Table 20.1). Type A blood contains antibodies against type B blood (anti-B) and type B blood contains antibodies against type A blood (anti-A). Type O blood contains both anti-A and anti-B, whereas type AB blood does not contain either.

Because of the presence or absence of antigens and antibodies, people with type AB blood can donate only to persons with type AB blood, but can receive blood from all other ABO groups, thus they are often referred to as universal recipients. A person with blood type O does not have any antigens and therefore can donate to anyone. This group is often referred to as the universal donor group.

Because of the different antigens, not all blood groups are compatible with each other and mixing incompatible blood groups leads to agglutination [see Cytotoxic Hypersensitivity Reactions (Type II) later in this chapter].

In addition, many people have an additional antigen, the Rh factor (or D antigen), on the surface of their RBCs. This antigen was first discovered during experiments in rhesus monkeys and is therefore called the *Rh factor*. A person with the D antigen is called *Rh positive* (Rh⁺) and someone without D antigen is referred to as *Rh negative* (Rh⁻). Although a person with Rh⁻ blood does not normally contain Rh antibodies in the serum, exposure to Rh⁺ blood will trigger the production of Rh antibodies. An example of this is erythroblastosis fetalis, or hemolytic disease, which occurs when an Rh⁻ mother begins to develop antibodies because she is carrying an Rh⁺ fetus (for more information, please refer to the Medical Highlights box).

Antibodies

One of the major functions of the immune system is to produce freely circulating soluble proteins that contribute specifically to the protection against foreign substances. These proteins are called *antibodies* and due to their globular structure are also known as **immunoglobulins (Igs)** or gamma (γ) globulins. In addition to acting as antibodies in the circulation, immunoglobulins serve as specific receptors on B cells. Produced by B lymphocytes, they recognize and bind to foreign antigens, forming an antigen–antibody complex, marking the antigen for destruction.

Structurally, antibodies are fork- or Y-shaped molecules composed of a pair of two identical long polypeptide chains (heavy chains) and a pair of identical short (light) polypeptide chains (Figure 20.4). At the end of the Y shape, formed by the heavy and light chains, are specific antigen-binding sites that differ from antibody to antibody. Because of the high variability of this region, it is referred to as the variable (V) region of the antibody. This variable region is composed of 110 to 130 amino acids, which gives the antibody its specificity for the antigen through its antigen-binding site. The remainder of the molecule is the constant (C) region that does not vary significantly from antibody to antibody. It is the variable region of antibodies that meets the enormous variety of antigenic challenges. The tips of the Y-shaped molecule consisting of the V and C regions are referred to as the *Fab* (fragment, antigen-binding) region, and the stem of the molecule is called the *crystallized fragment* or *Fc fragment* and plays a role in modulating immune cell activity. The Fc region can bind to various cell receptors including Fc receptors and complement proteins. This binding mediates different physiological effects, including opsonization (the

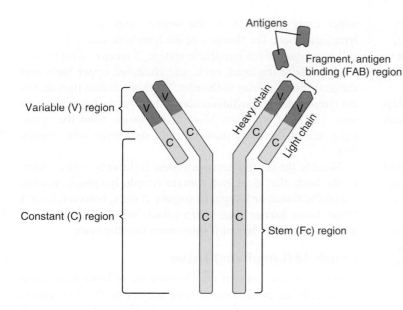

Antigens

Fragment, antigen
binding (FAB) region

Variable (V) region

Heavy chain

Light chain

Constant (C) region

Stem (Fc) region

FIGURE 20.4 Basic antibody (immunoglobulin) structure.
Antibodies are Y-shaped structures with two heavy chains
and two light chains with specific antigen-binding sites.

TABLE 20.2 Summary of Immunoglobulin Classes

Characteristic	IgG	IgD	IgE	IgA	IgM
Structure	Monomer	Monomer	Monomer	Monomer, dimer	Pentamer
Number of antigen-binding sites	2	2	2	2 (monomer), 4 (dimer)	10
Percentage of total serum antibody	80%	0.2%	0.002%	10–15%	5–10%
Average life span in serum	23 d	3 d	2–2.5 d	6 d	5 d
Function	Major antibody in circulation; long-term immunity	Receptor on B cells	Antibody in allergies and worm infections	Secretory antibody	First response to antigen; can serve as B-cell receptor

action of making bacteric and other cells easier to phagocytize
by marking or "tagging" them chemically), cell lysis, and
degranulation of mast cells, basophils, and eosinophils.

Although all immunoglobulins share common features, different classes of antibodies trigger different responses when
combining with the same epitope (antigenic determinant). Five
classes of immunoglobulins have been identified (Table 20.2).

1. *IgG,* a monomer produced by B cells, is the major antibody
   in the blood and lymphatic circulation. This class of

antibody can cross the placenta and provide passive
immunity to the newborn.

2. *IgA,* a monomer in blood and a dimer in secretions
   such as tears, saliva, and secretions of the respiratory
   and digestive tracts, provides local protection against
   bacteria and viruses. IgA is also found in colostrum and
   mother's milk, providing additional passive immunity to
   the newborn.

3. *IgM* is a pentamer and the largest of the immunoglobulins.
   Because of its large molecular size, it does not diffuse

readily from the bloodstream, where it remains and is efficient in reacting with bacteria and foreign cells. IgMs provide the first immunoglobulin activity in an immune response. These antibodies are also mainly responsible for the clumping of red blood cells in transfusion reactions.

4. *IgD* is a monomer bound to the surface of B cells and plays a role in B-cell activation. Although IgD is present in small amounts in serum its function in the circulation is unknown.

5. *IgE* is a monomer that binds to receptors on mast cells and basophils. It is the least abundant antibody type in serum. Functionally, it is implicated in allergic reactions and stimulates basophils to release histamines. Research indicates that IgE production can occur locally in the nasal mucosa of patients with allergic rhinitis. IgEs also provide protection against parasites and a 10- to 100-fold increase in serum IgE levels has been detected in patients with parasitic infections.

Components of the Immune System

Tissues and Organs of the Immune System

Lymphatic Vessels

Lymphatic vessels anatomically communicate with the vessels of the cardiovascular system. They originate as microscopic blind-ended vessels in the capillary beds of tissues (Figure 20.5). The function of lymph capillaries is to absorb excess extracellular (interstitial) fluid generated by the hydrostatic pressure of blood capillaries in these areas. As soon as the interstitial fluid enters the lymph capillaries it is called *lymph*. The plasma-like, watery lymph contains white blood cells, which are important in the immune response, and also transports dietary lipids from the small intestine to the liver.

The lymph capillaries drain the lymph into larger lymphatic vessels, which resemble veins of the cardiovascular system in their structure but have thinner walls and more valves. At various intervals throughout the body's lymph vessels, lymph passes through lymph nodes (where lymphocytes first interact with a specific antigen) and then is collected by lymphatic trunks, which carry the lymph to the largest lymphatic vessels, the lymphatic ducts. The thoracic or left lymphatic duct is the main collecting duct of the lymphatic system. It receives lymph from the left side of the head, neck, and chest, left upper limb, and the entire body inferior to the ribs. The thoracic duct then drains the lymph into the cardiovascular system via the left subclavian vein. The right lymphatic duct drains lymph from the upper right side of the body into the right subclavian vein (Figure 20.6).

Notably, the central nervous system is the only organ system in the body that does not contain lymph, lymphatic vessels, lymphatic tissue, or lymphatic organs. It does, however, have a blood–brain barrier that, when intact, impedes the entry of proteins and other harmful substances into the brain.

Lymphoid (Lymphatic) Tissue

Lymphoid tissue consists of a framework of loose connective tissue with accumulations of lymphocytes in the interspaces. Lymphoid tissues are the secondary lymphoid organs and can be divided into two basic types: diffuse and nodular lymphatic tissue. Diffuse lymphatic tissue consists of any unorganized collections of lymphocytes, whereas nodular lymphatic tissue is much more organized (see the next section, Lymphatic Nodules). Lymphoid tissue is widely distributed in the body and is typically found at sites that provide possible routes of entry for pathogens. This type of tissue therefore plays a major role in the defense against microorganisms and is found in the connective tissues of mucous membranes in the gastrointestinal, respiratory, urinary, and reproductive tracts (Figure 20.7).

Lymphatic Nodules

Lymphatic nodules are oval-shaped concentrations of lymphoid tissue (nodular lymphatic tissue) not surrounded by a connective tissue capsule. The lymphocytes are densely packed within loose connective tissue in the mucous membranes of the gastrointestinal tract, the respiratory tract, the urinary tract, and the reproductive tract. Collectively this type of tissue is referred to as mucosa-associated lymphoid tissue (MALT). The extensive collections of lymphoid nodules in the digestive tract are specifically called *gut-associated lymphoid tissue* (GALT). Examples of GALT are the Peyer's patches, which are concentrated in the ileum. Lymphatic nodules should not be confused with lymph nodes, which are specific anatomical organs surrounded by a distinct connective tissue capsule (see the section Lymph Nodes, later in this chapter).

Tonsils

Tonsils are large lymphatic nodules that are essential components of early defense mechanisms. Located strategically in the wall of the pharynx, they can remove foreign substances entering the body by ingestion or inhalation. The five tonsils are as follows:

- A single pharyngeal tonsil, also called the *adenoid,* that is embedded in the posterior wall of the nasopharynx
- A pair of palatine tonsils located in the posterior region of the oral cavity
- A pair of lingual tonsils, located at the base of the tongue

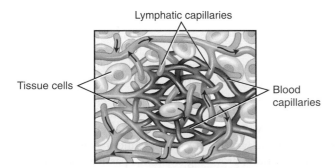

Lymphatic capillaries

Tissue cells

Blood capillaries

FIGURE 20.5 Origin of lymph capillaries. Lymph capillaries are microscopic blind-ended vessels originating in the capillary beds of tissues.

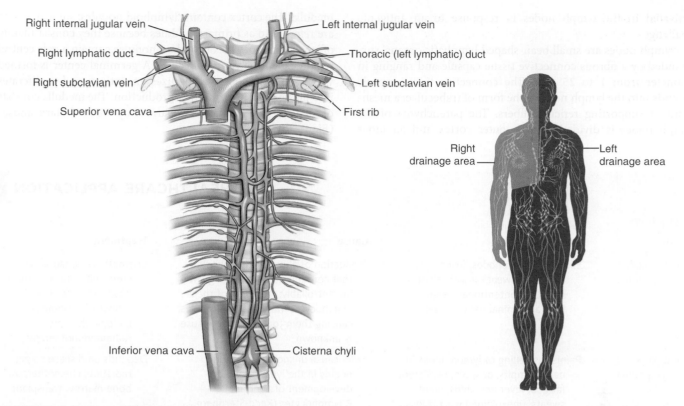

Right internal jugular vein

Right lymphatic duct

Right subclavian vein

Superior vena cava

Left internal jugular vein

Thoracic (left lymphatic) duct

Left subclavian vein

First rib

Right drainage area

Left drainage area

Inferior vena cava

Cisterna chyli

FIGURE 20.6 Drainage of lymph capillaries. Lymph capillaries drain into larger lymphatic vessels that drain into lymphatic trunks and then into the thoracic and right lymphatic ducts. The thoracic and right lymphatic ducts deliver the lymph into the left and right subclavian veins.

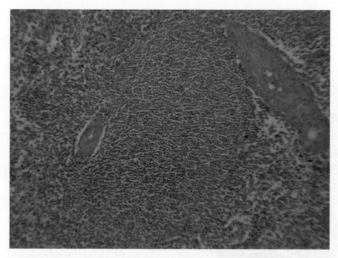

FIGURE 20.7 Lymphoid tissue in the submucosa of the large intestine.

Tonsils are comparatively larger in children than in adults, and can obstruct the air passageways if enlarged, such as can occur in tonsillitis. The palatine tonsils are the ones commonly removed in a tonsillectomy. However, lingual tonsils may require removal such as in chronic tonsillitis, sleep apnea, difficulty swallowing, or cancer.

Lymph Nodes

Approximately 600 lymph nodes are located along the lymphatic vessels, with clusters in various areas of the body. Lymph enters the lymph nodes via afferent lymphatic vessels and exits through efferent lymphatic vessels. Before the lymph is returned to the cardiovascular system, it is filtered through the lymph nodes. In addition to phagocytosis to remove pathogens and other foreign substances, B lymphocytes and T lymphocytes are activated in the lymph nodes in response to an antigenic challenge.

Lymph nodes are small bean-shaped lymphatic organs, surrounded by a fibrous connective tissue capsule and ranging in diameter from 1 to 25 mm. The connective tissue capsule extends into the lymph node in the form of trabeculae, a meshwork of supporting reticular fibers. The parenchyma of the lymph nodes is divided into an outer cortex and an inner medulla. The cortex contains lymphoid nodules, some of which are referred to as primary nodules because they consist mainly of small lymphocytes. Secondary nodules contain a pale central region called the *germinal center*. A germinal center is formed when a B lymphocyte recognizes an antigen and proliferates into plasma cells for antibody production. The medulla consists of medullary cords that are separated by the medullary sinuses (Figure 20.8).

HEALTHCARE APPLICATION

Lymphoma

Term	Symptoms	Cause	Treatment
Non-Hodgkin's lymphoma	Enlarged lymph nodes, fever, excessive sweating with night sweats, unintentional weight loss, abdominal pain or swelling	Production of abnormal lymphocytes that continue to divide and grow uncontrollably; crowding of these lymphocytes into the lymph nodes, causing them to swell; exact cause is unknown	Chemotherapy, radiation, stem cell transplantation, observation for slow-growing lymphomas, biologic therapy, radioimmunotherapy
Hodgkin's lymphoma	Painless swelling of lymph nodes in neck, armpits, or groin; persistent fatigue; fever and chills; night sweats; unexplained weight loss; loss of appetite; itching	Exact cause unknown, commonly begins in the lymph nodes; development of abnormal B lymphocytes (Reed-Sternberg cells)	Depends on disease stage; radiation, chemotherapy, bone marrow transplant

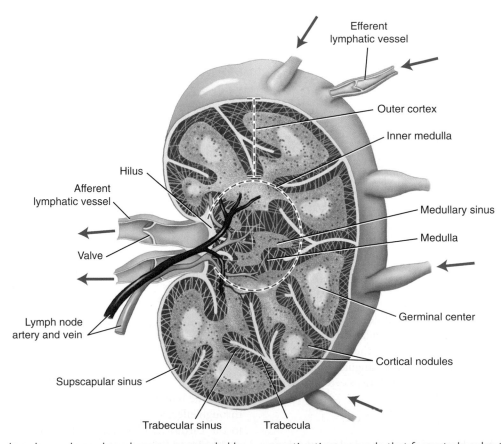

FIGURE 20.8 Lymph nodes are bean-shaped organs surrounded by a connective tissue capsule that forms trabeculae to provide the framework for the node. Afferent lymphatic vessels enter the node and efferent lymphatic vessels leave the node.

Spleen

The spleen is the largest lymphatic organ of the body and is located in the upper left abdominal cavity between the stomach and diaphragm (Figure 20.9). The cellular components of the spleen consist of the red pulp, containing large quantities of blood, and the white pulp, which contains lymphoid tissue resembling lymphoid nodules. Approximately 25% of the body's lymphocytes are located in the spleen. The spleen filters the blood, removing damaged blood cells and other cells with non-self-antigens. In response to circulating antigens, B cells, T cells, and macrophages are activated to eliminate any pathogens.

Thymus Gland

The thymus gland is a bilobate organ located in the mediastinum (Figure 20.10). The cells of the thymus produce thymosins, which are hormones essential for the maturation of the T lymphocytes. The thymus is large after birth and is essential in the development of the immune system in newborns. Although large in childhood, it gradually atrophies throughout adulthood. Functionally, after being active during the first years of life, its capacity slows down during puberty. By age 60 years the thymus gland is small and many of its cells have been replaced by adipose (fat) cells. As a result, the production of thymosin

HEALTHCARE APPLICATION

Spleen Disorders

Term	Symptoms	Cause	Treatment
Trauma (damage or rupture)	Painful and tender abdomen, abdominal muscles contract and feel rigid, low blood pressure, light-headedness, blurred vision, confusion, loss of consciousness	Severe blow to the stomach, abdominal injury (e.g., car accidents), athletic mishaps	Immediate blood transfusions, followed by removal of the spleen (splenectomy), if required by the severity of tissue damage
Splenomegaly	Abdominal pain, early satiety (fullness) due to splenic encroachment, anemia	Mononucleosis caused by the Epstein-Barr virus, other viral infections, bacterial infections, parasitic infections; diseases involving the liver, hemolytic anemias, cancer, sarcoidosis	No treatment for the disease; treatment of the underlying conditions; treatment of symptoms

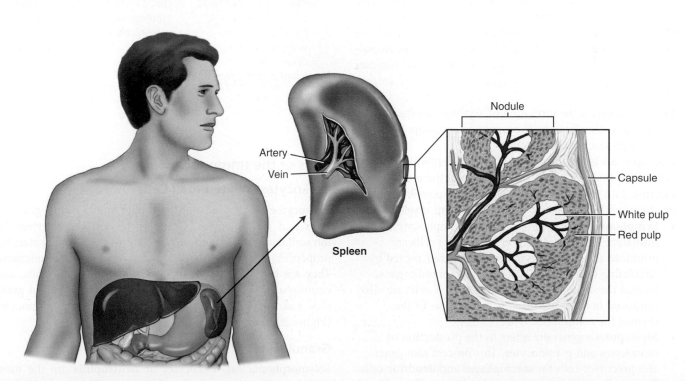

FIGURE 20.9 Spleen. The spleen is the largest lymphatic organ, and is located in the upper left abdominal cavity. The spleen consists of red pulp, which contains a large quantity of blood, and white pulp, composed of lymphoid tissue.

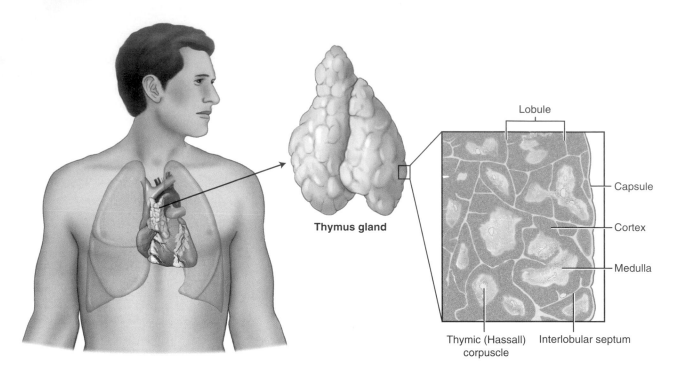

FIGURE 20.10 Thymus. The thymus gland is located superior to the heart; it is a bilobate organ, with the two lobes connected by an isthmus.

may have stopped, which negatively influences the maturation of T lymphocytes.

Red Bone Marrow (Myeloid Tissue)

Red bone marrow is found in flat and irregularly shaped bones and is considered the primary lymphoid organ. All blood cells, including the cells of the immune system, originate from hematopoietic stem cells, the **hemocytoblasts** located in the red bone marrow. The process of blood cell formation is called **hemopoiesis** or hematopoiesis and includes the following processes (Figure 20.11):

- **Erythropoiesis** is the formation of erythrocytes (red blood cells) and is stimulated by the hormone erythropoietin, which is produced in the kidneys.
- **Leukopoiesis** is the formation of leukocytes (white blood cells) from the hematopoietic stem cells of the red bone marrow. Two pathways or processes are responsible for the production of leukocytes: lymphopoiesis and myelopoiesis.
  - **Lymphopoiesis** is the production of lymphocytes. Immature B cells and natural killer (NK) cells are produced in red bone marrow and are transported by circulating blood to the secondary lymphoid organs, located throughout the body. Immature T cells are also produced in red bone marrow but migrate to the thymus for maturation.
  - **Myelopoiesis** generally refers to the production of monocytes and granulocytes. This process also generates precursor cells for macrophages and dendritic cells. These cells are also transported by the circulating blood to the secondary lymphoid organs.

Cells of the Immune System

Leukocytes: White Blood Cells

Leukocytes are divided into two main subdivisions: granulocytes and agranulocytes. Granulocytes are characterized by intracellular granules and on the basis of their special staining properties, differently shaped nuclei, and specific functions. They are further subdivided into basophils, eosinophils, and neutrophils (Figure 20.12). Agranulocytes are devoid of granules and are subdivided into lymphocytes and monocytes (Figure 20.13).

Granulocytes

Polymorphonuclear leukocytes or **neutrophils** are the most abundant of actively motile phagocytes. They contain large numbers of small lysosomes and migrate to the site of infection

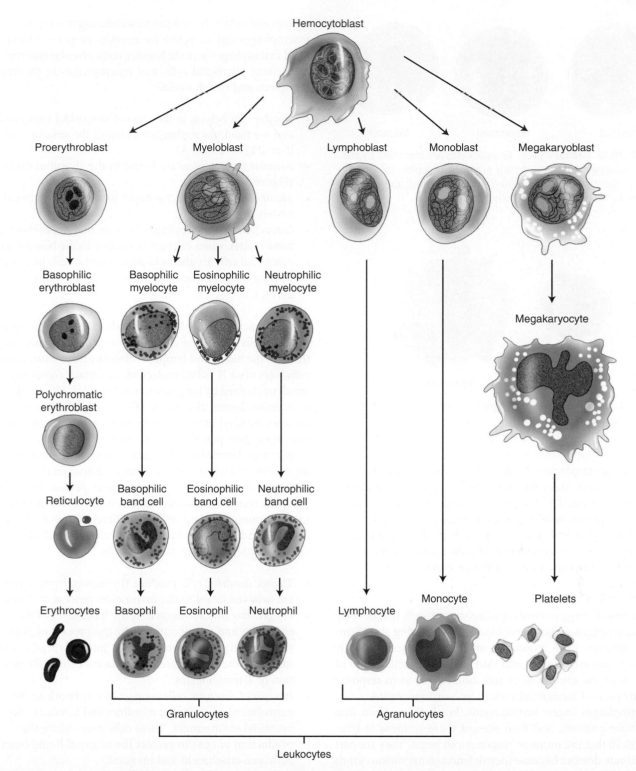

Hemocytoblast

Proerythroblast Myeloblast Lymphoblast Monoblast Megakaryoblast

Basophilic erythroblast

Basophilic myelocyte Eosinophilic myelocyte Neutrophilic myelocyte

Megakaryocyte

Polychromatic erythroblast

Reticulocyte

Basophilic band cell Eosinophilic band cell Neutrophilic band cell

Monocyte Platelets

Erythrocytes Basophil Eosinophil Neutrophil Lymphocyte

Granulocytes Agranulocytes

Leukocytes

FIGURE 20.11 Development of blood cells. Blood cell production is called *hemopoiesis* and occurs in the red bone marrow. The stem cell of all blood cells is the hemocytoblast, which undergoes differentiation to form the cell lines for all blood cells.

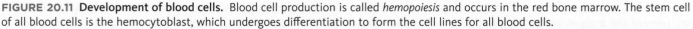

to phagocytose invading organisms, after which they die. The death of neutrophils releases the digestive enzymes from their lysosomes, dissolves cellular debris, and prepares the site for healing.

Eosinophils are distinguished from other granulocytes by their large reddish-staining granules. They have phagocytotic capability but are less effective in this action than are neutro-

phils. Eosinophils increase in numbers during hypersensitivity (allergic) reactions and stimulate the release of histamines by basophils and macrophages. They also provide defense against parasitic infestation by increasing their numbers.

Basophils are the least common of the five leukocyte types. They have dark, bluish purple granules that contain chemical mediators promoting **inflammation.** These chemicals include

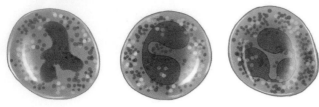

Basophil   Eosinophil   Neutrophil

FIGURE 20.12 Granulocytes. Granulocytes are identified by the specific staining properties of their granules: basophils (blue/purple granules), eosinophils (pink/reddish granules), and neutrophils, in which granules do not stain.

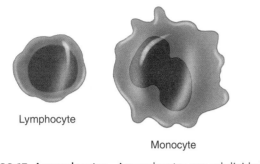

Lymphocyte

Monocyte

FIGURE 20.13 Agranulocytes. Agranulocytes are subdivided into lymphocytes and monocytes.

histamine, proteoglycans, bradykinin, serotonin, and the anticoagulant heparin. Basophils leave the blood and accumulate at the site of infection. Discharge of the granular contents releases chemical mediators resulting in an increase in blood flow to the affected area. Basophils play a major role in allergic responses, particularly in type I hypersensitivity reactions, and also in the inflammatory response (see later in this chapter).

Agranulocytes

Monocytes are large circulating phagocytotic cells that develop into macrophages as they leave blood vessels during an inflammatory reaction. Both monocytes and macrophages are highly efficient in the engulfment and destruction of bacteria and of cellular debris at the site of an infection as well as in response to an invasion of foreign substances into various organs.

Macrophages ingest immunogens, break them down into smaller components, and then present these antigens to lymphocytes so that the immune response can begin. They are part of the innate defense because they defend against various kinds of agents, but they also play a role in the adaptive defense as they present the antigen to the lymphocytes. Cells presenting antigens to lymphocytes are called *antigen-presenting cells*. They are classified as wandering macrophages or fixed macrophages depending on their location and function.

Wandering macrophages develop from circulating monocytes that leave the bloodstream during the inflammatory response and act at the infected site. These macrophages usually have a short life span.

Fixed macrophages migrate to specific areas and remain in the specific organs and tissues, where they trap foreign sub-

stances and debris. In contrast to wandering macrophages, fixed macrophages can be active for months or years. Examples of fixed macrophages include Kupffer cells, alveolar macrophages, osteoclasts, microglial cells, and macrophages in the lining of the spleen and lymph nodes:

- *Kupffer cells* belong to the class of sinusoidal lining cells and are fixed macrophages located in the sinusoids of the liver (Figure 20.14, *A*).
- *Alveolar macrophages* are found in the alveoli of the lungs (Figure 20.14, *B*).
- *Mesangial cells* are macrophages located around blood vessels in the kidneys.
- *Osteoclasts* are macrophages in bone that break down the bone matrix when calcium is needed in the bloodstream.
- *Microglial cells* are the only phagocytotic cells in the brain, moving to areas where cell debris must be removed (Figure 20.14, *C*).

Like macrophages, **dendritic cells (DCs)** are antigen-presenting cells that arise from monocytes and then migrate through the blood and lymph to almost every tissue. Dendritic cells have class II MHC molecules as surface components and are characterized by long extensions that look like the dendrites of neurons, hence their name (Figure 20.15). In general, they are concentrated at sites where antigen-bearing microorganisms seek their portal of entry, such as the skin and mucous membranes. Dendritic cells check their environment for microorganisms, and when they encounter a pathogen they ingest the organism, break it down, and transport protein fragments to their cell membrane, where these cell fragments are presented to other immune system cells. The different types of DCs include thymic dendritic cells, Langerhans cells, interstitial dendritic cells, and interdigitating dendritic cells.

- *Thymic dendritic cells* produce thymosins, hormones that are believed to aid in the maturation process of T cells.
- *Langerhans cells* are located in the basal layer of the epidermis and engulf antigens by the process of pinocytosis. The antigens are broken down into polypeptides and moved to the cell surface. This process evokes the activation of T lymphocytes.
- *Interstitial dendritic cells* are part of a network in the gastrointestinal tract that monitors and interacts with the intestinal environment. These cells may induce the production of IgAs to protect the mucosal lining from pathogen attachment and invasion.
- *Interdigitating dendritic cells* are found in lymph nodes and play a major role in antigen presentation to the lymphocytes in these lymphatic organs.

Lymphocytes (mononuclear leukocytes) make up 30% to 40% of the white blood cells and they are the primary cells of the immune response. B lymphocytes (B cells) complete the first stage of development in the bone marrow before they enter the blood circulation and migrate to the secondary lymphoid organs. They are ultimately responsible for antigen interaction, the production of antibodies, and immune memory. The naive

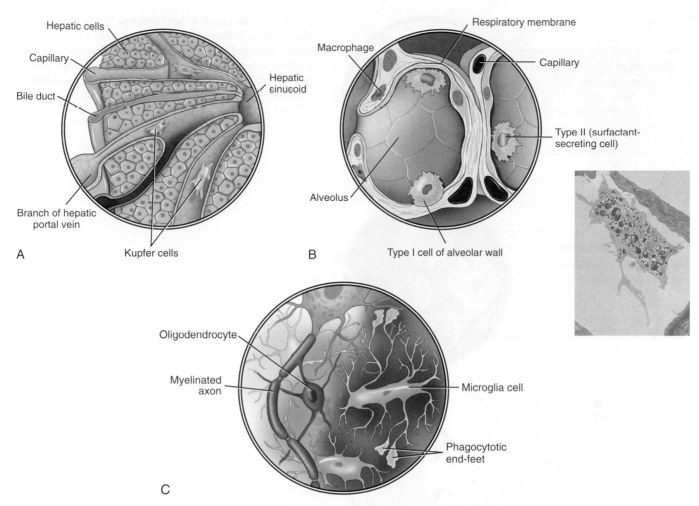

FIGURE 20.14 **A,** Kupffer cells in the sinusoids of the liver; **B,** alveolar macrophage, drawing and electron micrograph; **C,** microglia.

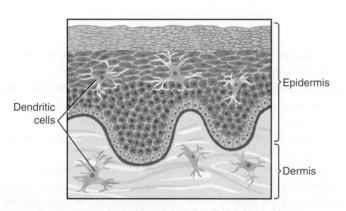

FIGURE 20.15 Dendritic (Langerhans) cells in the epidermis.

(inactive) B cells are small lymphocytes with antibodies located in the cell membrane. These surface antibody molecules serve as receptors for specific antigens (antigen-binding sites). One set of these surface immunoglobulins is responsible for antigen recognition and another molecule, a class II MHC molecule, is responsible for antigen presentation. Once an antigen binds to the antibody on the B cell, the B cell rapidly divides and forms plasma cells and memory B cells (see Antibody-mediated Immunity, later in this chapter).

T lymphocytes (T cells) mature in the thymus gland and are necessary for B-cell proliferation as well as cell-mediated immunity (discussed later in this chapter). B cells and T cells have unique surface antigens that distinguish them from each other and subdivide each group into subsets. The international naming system of surface antigens in blood cells is the CD system, which is of clinical importance (i.e., in the diagnosis of AIDS involving the CD4 and CD8 T-cell subsets).

Host Defense

Host defense mechanisms protect against foreign substances and microbes. Certain defense mechanisms are always present **(innate)** and often are sufficient to impede the replication and spreading of infectious agents. The function of the innate immune defense is to prevent the development of disease by mechanisms of the first and second lines of defense. Innate defense mechanisms are nonspecific because they challenge all invaders via general defense mechanisms. If the innate immune defense is insufficient to stop the invasion of the infectious agent, the **adaptive immune system** is activated. This process takes time to attain maximal strength. The adaptive immune

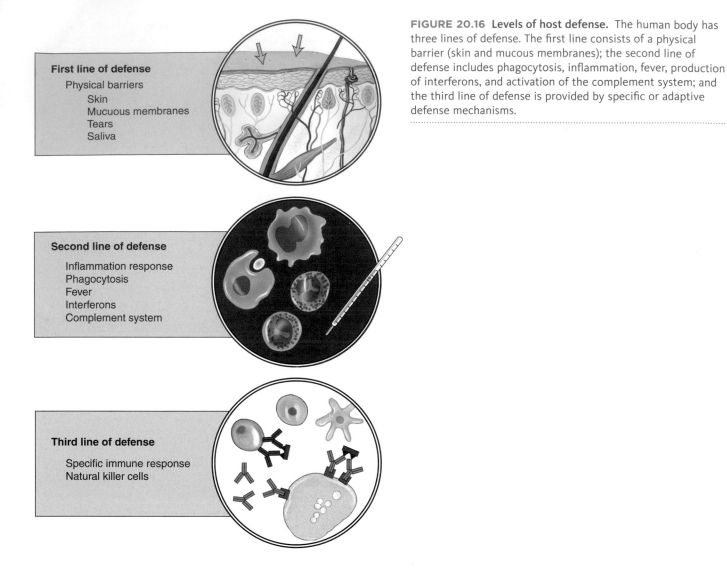

First line of defense

Physical barriers
    Skin
    Mucuous membranes
    Tears
    Saliva

Second line of defense

Inflammation response
Phagocytosis
Fever
Interferons
Complement system

Third line of defense

Specific immune response
Natural killer cells

FIGURE 20.16 Levels of host defense. The human body has three lines of defense. The first line consists of a physical barrier (skin and mucous membranes); the second line of defense includes phagocytosis, inflammation, fever, production of interferons, and activation of the complement system; and the third line of defense is provided by specific or adaptive defense mechanisms.

system response is specific to a specific antigen and is therefore also referred to as specific defense. It represents the third line of defense (Figure 20.16).

First Line of Defense

The first line of defense includes physical and chemical barriers to prevent microbes from entering the body.

Physical Barriers

The intact skin and mucous membranes lining the respiratory, digestive, gastrointestinal, urinary, and reproductive systems provide physical protection against microbial invasion. The smallest of injuries to these physical barriers can provide a portal of entry for pathogens. The mucus of mucous membranes traps particles, which are then removed by the mechanical actions of cilia, called the *ciliary escalator* (Figure 20.17). The term ciliary escalator describes the process by which the ciliary action moves the mucus from the apical surface of the mucous membrane of the trachea to the oral cavity. The mucus, together with the trapped particles, is then swallowed together with the trapped particles and moved to the stomach, where the particles

and microbes are destroyed by the acidity (pH 2) of the stomach's environment. Sneezing and coughing assist in the removal of mucus from the upper respiratory tract. In smokers, the cilia of the respiratory tract are damaged and the ciliary action is impaired or absent; therefore the mucus is not easily transported to the oral cavity and must be removed by coughing actions (smoker's cough).

Perspiration mechanically flushes organisms from pores of the sweat glands and also washes the surface of the skin. Tears, saliva, and the flow of urine produce flushing actions against invaders. Infrequent urination, for example, promotes urinary tract infection due to bacterial invasion.

Chemical Barriers

The pH 4.5 to 6 of the skin inhibits the colonization of many pathogens. Sebum produced by sebaceous (oil) glands contains fatty acids and lactic acids that are toxic to many pathogens. Sweat glands also produce fatty acids and lactic acids, which prevent undesirable bacterial colonization on the skin. Mucus produced by the mucous membranes of epithelial tissue contains lysozyme, lactoferrin, and lactoperoxidase, all of which are either bacteriostatic or bactericidal.

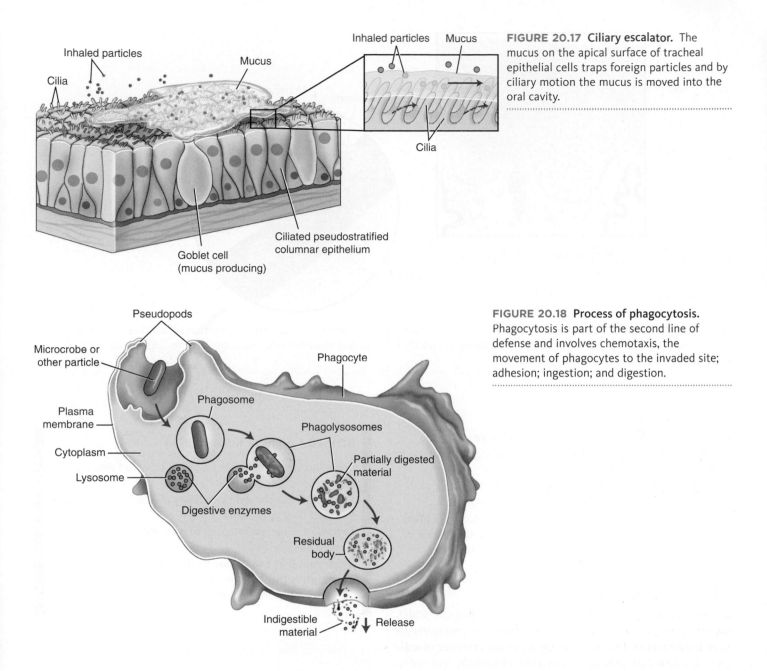

Inhaled particles
Cilia
Mucus
Inhaled particles
Mucus

FIGURE 20.17 Ciliary escalator. The mucus on the apical surface of tracheal epithelial cells traps foreign particles and by ciliary motion the mucus is moved into the oral cavity.

Cilia

Goblet cell
(mucus producing)
Ciliated pseudostratified columnar epithelium

Pseudopods
Microcrobe or other particle
Phagocyte
Plasma membrane
Phagosome
Phagolysosomes
Cytoplasm
Lysosome
Partially digested material
Digestive enzymes
Residual body
Indigestible material
Release

FIGURE 20.18 Process of phagocytosis. Phagocytosis is part of the second line of defense and involves chemotaxis, the movement of phagocytes to the invaded site; adhesion; ingestion; and digestion.

Lysozymes, enzymes that attack the peptidoglycan layer of the bacterial cell wall, are present in perspiration, nasal secretions, saliva, and tears. In addition, the acidity of the stomach, the alkalinity of the intestines, and the digestive enzymes all help to protect the digestive tract from unwanted, pathogenic bacterial colonization.

Second Line of Defense

Pathogens that penetrate the first line of defense usually are eliminated by a combination of nonspecific cellular and chemical responses provided by the second line of defense. These responses include phagocytosis, inflammation, fever, production of interferons, and activation of the complement system.

Phagocytosis and Phagocytes

Phagocytosis is a process by which invading foreign substances are destroyed by phagocytes. There are many cells of the immune system that are capable of phagocytosis. Phagocytes approach a microorganism or other particle and extend pseudopods (footlike projections) to engulf the organism. The complete encircling of the organism forms a sac called the **phagosome,** which fuses with lysosomes containing bactericidal chemicals. After destroying the invader, the phagocyte processes the proteins and presents parts of the antigen protein at the cell surface for lymphocyte recognition.

Steps in phagocytosis (Figure 20.18):

- **Chemotaxis** is the guided movement of phagocytes to the invaded site. It is the result of a chemical attraction caused by chemotactic agents. In general, this is achieved through the action of chemokines produced during the complement cascade (see Complement System later in this chapter).
- Adhesion is the process by which phagocytes attach to foreign substances before their ingestion.

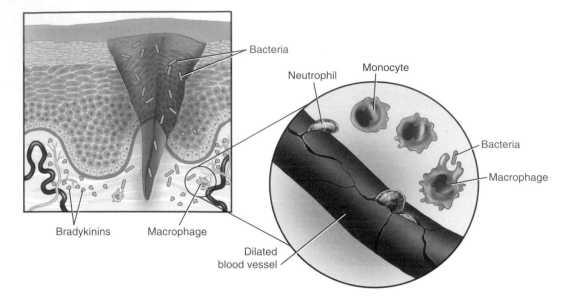

FIGURE 20.19 Steps of inflammation. Inflammation occurs when microbes enter damaged tissue. In response to tissue damage blood vessels also dilate, bradykinin is released by the damaged endothelial cells, and monocytes/macrophages and neutrophils leave the blood vessels in an effort to destroy the invaders.

- Ingestion is the process by which the membrane of the phagocyte extends pseudopods, surrounding the particle to be ingested.
- Digestion occurs when the phagosome merges with lysosomes within the phagocytotic cell to produce a phagolysosome. The digestive enzymes of lysosomes break down and dissolve the invaders, followed by the release of these digested materials from the phagocyte into the extracellular fluid compartment.

Inflammatory Response

The inflammatory reaction is a protective mechanism, which under certain circumstances may be harmful. Initiating events of an inflammation can be either injury or the presence of antigens, but also extremes of temperature, chemicals, and radiation. If the inflammatory reaction begins when the skin is broken due to a minor injury, it is often strong enough to prevent disease by stopping pathogenic microbes from entering other tissues (Figure 20.19).

Steps of inflammation include the following:

1. An injury to capillaries and tissue cells is followed by the release of bradykinin from the injured cells.
2. Bradykinin activates sensory nerve impulses, which initiate pain.
3. The sensation of pain stimulates mast cells and basophils to release histamine.
4. Both bradykinin and histamine cause capillary dilation, increase blood flow, and increase capillary permeability in the infected area.
5. The break in the skin allows bacteria to enter the tissue, which results in the migration of neutrophils and monocytes to the site of injury.

> **BOX 20.1 Signs of Inflammation**
>
> *Calor:* Increased temperature of the inflamed area due to increased blood flow
> *Rubor:* Redness caused by capillary dilation and increased blood flow to the area
> *Tumor:* Swelling (edema) due to increased capillary permeability
> *Dolor:* Pain that can be due to stimulation of pain receptors (nociceptors) by prostaglandin release, microbial toxins, and edema

6. Neutrophils phagocytize bacteria and destroy them via the hydrolytic enzymes of their lysosomes.
7. Monocytes that matured into macrophages leave the bloodstream and quickly phagocytize microbes.

The symptoms of inflammation (Box 20.1) include redness (rubor), increased temperature (calor), swelling (tumor), and pain (dolor) in the inflamed area. The redness and increased temperature are caused by the dilation of capillaries and increased blood flow in the region. The increased temperature increases the metabolic rate of the cells to increase the speed of healing. Heat also increases the activities of phagocytotic and other defensive cells. The sensation of pain results from stimulation of nociceptors (sensory receptors) caused by edema (excessive tissue fluid), and the release of prostaglandins by injured cells or bacterial toxins. Swelling (edema) is due to increased permeability of the capillaries and results in seeping of blood plasma components into the tissues. This capillary leakage pro-

BOX 20.2 Benefits of Fever

- Inhibits multiplication of microorganisms sensitive to higher temperatures
- Reduces the availability of iron to bacteria, resulting in a decline in their nutrition
- Stimulates the immune reaction by increasing the metabolism of the cells responsible to fight infection
- Speeds up hematopoiesis, phagocytosis, and other specific immune reactions

TABLE 20.3 Selected Cytokines and Their Activities

Cytokine	Source	Function
IL-1	Macrophage, monocytes	T- and B-cell activation; fever; inflammation
IL-2	T cells	T-cell proliferation; activation of B cells
IL-3	T cells	Stimulates growth of stem cells and mast cells
IL-4	T cells	Stimulates growth of B cells and some T cells
IL-5	T cells	B cells; eosinophil differentiation
IL-6	Macrophages, B cells and T cells, other cells	Inflammation, hematopoiesis, differentiation of B cells
IL-7	Fibroblasts, endothelial cells	Early B- and T-cell differentiation
IL-8	Monocytes	Attracts granulocytes
IL-11	Bone marrow	Hematopoiesis
IL-14	Dendritic cells, T cells	B-cell memory

vides a path to the site of infection for rapid action of infection-fighting cells and clotting factors.

Fever

Fever or **pyrexia** is a systemic response to extensive inflammation or microbial invasion (Box 20.2). A body temperature above 37.8° C (100° F) is generally considered to be a slight (mild) fever and helps the body to eliminate pathogenic organisms. Although high fever is dangerous, within limits it can also be beneficial if it reduces or eliminates the growth and reproduction of the invading microorganisms. The increase in body temperature is regulated by the hypothalamus in response to **pyrogens,** which are fever-producing substances released from white blood cells in response to microbial invasion. Also, microbial toxins released into the bloodstream can act as pyrogens. Pyrogens are transported by the bloodstream to the hypothalamus, where they stimulate specific neurons that release prostaglandins. Prostaglandins raise the physiological set point of the body temperature, which results in shivering (chills), a physiological response that initiates a rise in body temperature. Shivering involves increased muscle contraction, generating the heat necessary to increase body temperature. When the pathogens are eliminated the set point of the body temperature is lowered to pre-fever levels by evoking the physiological response of perspiration to cool off the body (the fever breaks).

Interferons

Interferons are glycoproteins produced by cells infected with a virus. These proteins are considered antiviral because they interfere with the replication of a virus and impede the spread of the pathogen. The different types of interferons (alpha, α; beta, β; gamma, γ) are activated by different stimuli: bacteria, viruses, foreign cells, and tumors. Interferon-α proteins are produced by B cells, monocytes, and macrophages. Interferon-β proteins are produced by fibroblasts and other virus-infected cells, whereas interferon-γ proteins are released by T cells and natural killer (NK) cells. These interferons do not save the infected cell but bind to receptors on uninfected cells, where they stimulate the production of antiviral proteins. Interferons are species specific but not virus specific. In other words, interferons from a rabbit are ineffective in humans. Although interferons can prevent the spread of viruses they also can elicit nonspecific flulike symptoms that are associated with viral infections.

Cytokines

Cytokines are small proteins considered to be chemical mediators of the immune response and are secreted by cells of the immune system. They are chemical messengers that allow cells within the immune system to communicate with each other and organize the attack on an invader. The same cytokine may be produced by several different cells and the same cytokine might have a different effect in different circumstances. This phenomenon is called *pleiotropy.* In addition, different cytokines may mediate the same activity depending on the situation; this is called *redundancy.* Many cytokines are referred to as interleukins (ILs) and are numbered according to when they were discovered, similar to the numbering of blood-clotting factors. The term interleukin describes the chemicals that function as mediators between the white blood cells (inter + leukocytes). Three groups of cytokines have been described according to their functional properties: cytokines that play a role in the regulation of hematopoiesis, cytokines that affect the inflammatory response, and cytokines that regulate the adaptive immune response (Table 20.3).

Complement System

The complement system can be activated by the immune system for the recruitment of phagocytes to areas of microbial invasion. This system consists of more than 35 different soluble proteins found in extracellular fluid and influences both innate and acquired immunity. The complement proteins are synthesized primarily by hepatocytes but are also produced by monocytes, macrophages, and epithelial cells of the gastrointestinal and genitourinary tracts. The major complement proteins are named

C1 through *C9* according to their time of discovery and not the order of their activation in the immune response. Activation of the complement system is called the *complement cascade,* and it is activated through three biochemical pathways:

1. The **classical complement pathway,** triggered when an antigen–antibody complex (IgG or IgM) binds to the C1 component
2. The **alternative complement pathway,** activated by C3 component hydrolysis on the surface of a pathogen
3. The **lectin pathway,** activated when mannose-binding lectin bound to carbohydrate of a pathogen interacts with an enzyme similar to C1

The three pathways merge at the final stages into a common pathway, with similar end results, namely inflammation, phagocytosis, and/or direct lysis of the antigen.

Third Line of Defense

The third line of defense is provided by the specific or adaptive defense mechanisms. These mechanisms are triggered by a specific antigen. The two fundamental mechanisms in adaptive defense are cell-mediated immunity and humoral immunity. When challenged by an antigen, both B cells and T cells further differentiate, proliferate, and elicit the antigen-specific immune response.

Cell-mediated Immunity

The cell-mediated immune system is controlled by **T cells,** which are highly specialized lymphocytes circulating in the blood and lymph to fight bacteria, viruses, fungi, protozoans, and any other substances or cells that are foreign to the body. Neither cytotoxic T cells nor helper T cells can recognize an antigen floating in the blood or lymph and must be activated by an **antigen-presenting cell,** such as a macrophage (Figure 20.20).

The categories of T cells (T lymphocytes) are as follows:

- *Cytotoxic/killer T cells* (CD8) recognize antigens presented within class I MHC molecules and will attack and destroy antigen-bearing cells such as virus-infected cells and cancer cells by releasing perforin and granzymes. Perforin molecules form a hole in the infected cells, allowing entry of the granzymes, which initiate apoptosis.
- *Helper T cells* (CD4) recognize antigens presented within class II MHC molecules and will aid the immune response by releasing cytokines that stimulate growth and division of cytotoxic T cells and B cells. In addition, they attract macrophages and further enhance the capabilities of macrophages to phagocytose microbes.
- *Suppressor T cells* (a subpopulation of CD8 T cells) release chemicals to regulate the immune response by suppressing both the further development of helper T cells and the antibody production by plasma B cells.
- *Memory T cells* represent the population of T cells that persists after suppression of the immune response. These cells recognize and respond to pathogens that previously invaded the body. They secrete cytokines to stimulate macrophages and B cells in response to repeated invasions.

Antibody-mediated Immunity (Humoral Immunity)

B cells produce specific antibodies and regulate the antibody-mediated immune response to viral and bacterial antigens. Small, naive B cells are mature immunocompetent cells that are stimulated to proliferate and differentiate by antigens that bind to their surface receptors. Each B cell carries a specific surface antibody that recognizes a specific antigen. After an antigen has been recognized, B cells become activated (sensitized) and start dividing into plasma cells and memory cells. This process is called **clonal selection** (Figure 20.21) and is enhanced by helper T cells (CD4). The majority of the clones become short-lived plasma cells that produce the specific antibodies and the others

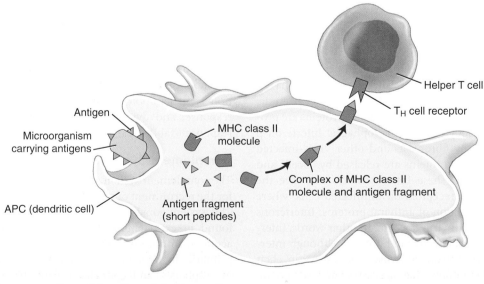

FIGURE 20.20 Antigen-presenting cell in cell-mediated immunity.

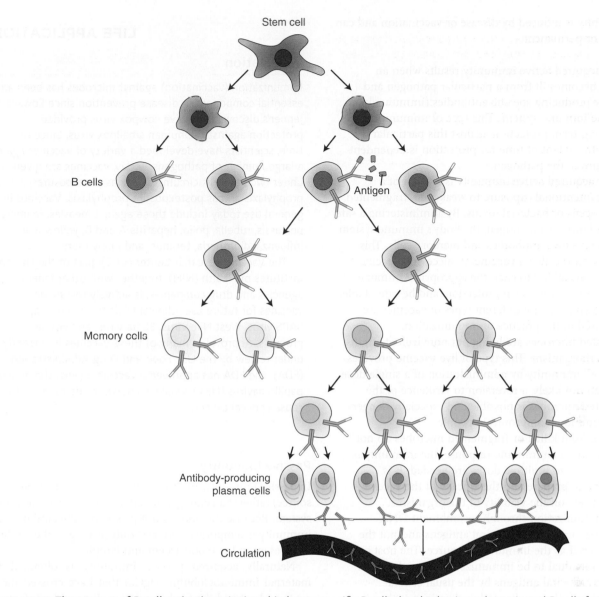

FIGURE 20.21 **The process of B-cell activation.** Antigen binds to a specific B cell, clonal selection—the activated B cells form one colony of plasma cells and one colony of memory cells; antibody synthesis—B cells produce specific antibodies to the invading antigen.

become long-lasting memory cells. Once enough antibodies have been produced by the B cells to eliminate the antigens, the development of plasma cells ceases under the direction of suppressor T cells. Memory B cells remain and they are responsible for long-term immunity. They will recognize the same antigen when it enters the system again and will divide quickly to produce new plasma and memory cells.

When the immune system is exposed to a specific antigen for the first time, it undergoes a **primary response.** The earliest part of the response is characterized by a latent period (lag period) during which no antibodies specific to the antigen are present. Recognition of foreign substances occurs when the epitope of an antigen fits into the antigen-binding site of the antibody. The antigen is concentrated in lymphoid tissue during this time period and processed by the appropriate B lymphocyte, which then undergoes clonal expansion. Early in the primary response the B cells produce primarily IgM-type antibodies, which are later switched to IgG or another class such as

IgE or IgA. The specificity of the antibody for this antigen does not change.

A **secondary immune response** occurs when the system is exposed to the same immunogen weeks, months, or years later. The rate of antibody synthesis is significantly higher during the secondary response compared with the primary response. The antibody concentration in serum is referred to as the **antibody titer.** The rapid amplification of antibodies is due to the presence of memory B cells in the secondary immune response. This occurrence is the basis for booster shots in vaccination to increase the antibody titer against dangerous pathogens (see next section). Humeral immunity can also be divided into two categories: active immunity and passive immunity.

Active Immunity

In active immunity, antigens enter the body, which then responds by making its own antibodies via B lymphocytes. This type of immunity is induced by disease or vaccination and can be long-lived or permanent.

- Naturally acquired active immunity results when an individual becomes ill from a particular pathogen and recovers by producing specific antibodies (immunoglobulins) via the immune system. This type of immunity provides long-term protection against this particular pathogen. The extent of time for protection is dependent on the nature of the pathogen.
- Artificially acquired active immunity is a result of a controlled, intentional exposure to weakened, fragmented, killed pathogens or bacterial toxins. By administering a safe amount and form of an antigen, the body's immune system will produce its own antibodies and memory cells. This type of antigen is called a **vaccine.** A successful vaccine should have the ability to elicit the appropriate immune response, provide long-term protection, and be safe, stable, and inexpensive. Several different types of vaccines are currently used in the practice of immunization.
    - Attenuated microbes are living but nonvirulent strains of a microorganism. This type of live vaccine provides long-lived immunity by administration of a single dose. Although not likely, a reversion to virulence of the attenuated microbes is possible and especially dangerous for immunocompromised people.
    - Vaccines from killed or fragmented microbes do not elicit as strong an immune response, the immunity is short-lived, and multiple doses are needed. It is expensive to prepare and the efficacy of the vaccine does not rely on the viability of the organisms.
    - DNA immunization through recombinant DNA technology uses genes for viral antigens and not the antigen itself as the immunogen source. The host cells in the individual to be immunized take up the DNA and produce viral antigens by the usual cellular mechanisms. The newly produced antigen is then presented on the cell surface with host MHC class I and class II molecules. Subsequent contact with immunocompetent cells evokes an immune response.
    - Toxoids are bacterial or viral toxins that have been altered to become nontoxic. Injections of toxoids provide protection against the toxin, but not against the pathogen itself.

The quantity of antibodies produced and ultimately found in serum after vaccination or an actual infection is the antibody titer. The initial vaccination triggers a rise in the antibody titer that gradually weakens, and booster shots (second injections) are often administered to keep the antibody titer high enough to prevent infection. The secondary response is more effective than the primary response. The memory B cells quickly divide to form more memory B cells and a large number of plasma cells produce a great number of antibodies at a moment's notice. When an immunized individual is later exposed to the particular pathogen, the immune response is even more intense, thus preventing the infection. For more information about vaccination, see the Life Application box.

LIFE APPLICATION

Vaccination

Immunization (vaccination) against microbes has been an essential component in disease prevention since Edward Jenner's discovery that live cowpox virus provided protection against the human smallpox virus. Since that time, scientists have developed a variety of vaccines against a large number of pathogens. Today, vaccines are given under two different circumstances: as preexposure prophylaxis and as postexposure prophylaxis. Vaccines in general use today include those against measles, mumps, pertussis, rubella, polio, hepatitis A and B, yellow fever, influenza, diphtheria, tetanus, and many more.

The Vaccine Research Center (VRC), part of the National Institutes of Health (NIH), together with other federal agencies and drug companies, is actively testing new vaccines for future use. Clinical trials for vaccines against SARS virus, West Nile virus, Ebola virus, and HIV are in progress. Approval of many of these vaccines is currently under review by the U.S. Food and Drug Administration (FDA). The FDA has approved a vaccine against the human papillomavirus (HPV), which is known for its capacity to cause cervical cancer.

Passive Immunity

In passive immunity, antibodies are exogenous (from an outside source) rather than endogenous after stimulation of the immune system. Because the body is not producing the antibodies, this immunity is temporary and lasts only as long as the antibodies are present in the bloodstream and lymph.

Naturally acquired passive immunity is obtained from maternal immunoglobulins (IgGs) that have crossed the placenta and entered the fetal circulation. It provides infants with antibodies from the mother for immunity against a specific pathogen. This type of immunity generally lasts for 6 to 12 months after birth, during which time the newborn's immune system is developing. IgA and IgG in colostrum and breast milk provide additional passive immunity for the newborn. In addition, colostrum and breast milk contain the following substances to help the infant fight infection:

- Oligosaccharides and mucins, which interfere with the adherence of microbes to host cells
- The iron-binding substance lactoferrin, which makes iron unavailable to most bacteria
- Fibronectin, which increases the activity of the infant's macrophages
- Cytokines, which enhance the activity of certain immune cells
- Lysozymes, which break down the peptidoglycan layer in bacterial cell walls

Artificially acquired passive immunity is achieved by the administration of exogenous protective antibodies from another person or animal. These antibodies may be serum immunoglobulins, or monoclonal antibodies produced in the laboratory. The injection of serum carries a risk of allergic responses to foreign antigens, resulting in serum sickness.

Diseases Caused by the Immune System

Immune system diseases and disorders occur when the immune response is faulty, excessive, or lacking. An altered immune response can occur when one or many of the components of the immune system are structurally or functionally impaired.

Allergy/Hypersensitivity Reactions

An allergy is a strong immune response to an **allergen,** a substance that usually is not harmful to the body but causes hypersensitivity reactions. Substances such as pollen, mold, dust (most likely dust mites), cat dander, foods, insect stings or bites, certain foods, and medicines can cause these reactions (Table 20.4). Allergies are caused by an overactive immune system producing antibodies against substances that are nonpathogenic and do not cause problems for the human body.

Immediate Hypersensitivity (Type I)

The type of allergy called *immediate hypersensitivity type I* is caused by an excessive response of B lymphocytes to an allergen. Symptoms occur within seconds or minutes of exposure in type I hypersensitivity reactions. These symptoms include the following:

- A runny or stuffy nose
- Watering eyes
- Conjunctivitis
- Asthma
- Hives
- Fever
- Dermatitis
- Gastrointestinal symptoms

The various types of reactions in this category are either local or systemic, involving airway obstruction and even circulatory collapse. A genetic predisposition to allergies is believed to play an important role in the development of this hypersensitivity reaction. However, other factors such as age, the type of allergen, portal of entry, geographic location, and general health of the patient have an impact on the development of hypersensitivity type I reactions.

The production of IgE antibodies instead of IgG antibodies is responsible for the allergic reactions. IgEs do not circulate in the blood but attach to mast cells and basophils within the tissues and bind to the surface receptors of these cells. Mast cells and basophils then release various substances including histamines. The symptoms of hay fever are caused primarily by histamines and are often treated effectively with antihistamines. On the other hand, food allergies are mediated primarily by prostaglandins and are often treated with aspirin, which inhibits prostaglandin synthesis. The difficulty with breathing that occurs in asthma is due to inflammation and smooth muscle contraction of the respiratory system, which can be treated with epinephrine. Probably the most commonly observed allergic symptoms are fever, asthma, hives, and gastrointestinal symptoms.

Cytotoxic Hypersensitivity Reactions (Type II)

In type II hypersensitivity (cytotoxic hypersensitivity) the antigens are located on the surface of specific cells or tissues and provide the binding site for circulating antibodies. All type II reactions involve IgG or IgM antibodies, resulting in destruction of the antigen-bearing cells by activating cytolytic enzymes of the complement system (C1 of the classical pathway) or by phagocytosis. Examples of such a reaction would be blood transfusion with an incompatible ABO blood group as well as Rh incompatibility reactions. Damage caused by type II reactions is localized to a particular tissue or cell type, in contrast with type III reactions, which affect organs where antigen–antibody complexes are deposited.

Immune Complex Hypersensitivity Reactions (Type III)

Type III hypersensitivity reactions form immune complexes found in certain autoimmune diseases. These reactions include

TABLE 20.4 Examples of Allergic Responses, Symptoms, and the Causative Allergens

Allergic Response	Symptoms	Allergen
Allergic rhinitis (hay fever), asthma	Sneezing, nasal congestion, difficulty breathing	Mold, pollen, animal dander, dust mites
Food allergy	Nausea, vomiting, abdominal cramps, diarrhea	Eggs (mostly egg white), fish (especially shellfish), chicken, milk and milk products, nuts, wheat, soybeans
Hives	Reddening and swelling of specific skin areas	Selected foods and food additives, insect bites, drugs (e.g., penicillin), cosmetics
Anaphylactic shock	Dilation of blood vessels, dizziness, nausea, diarrhea, unconsciousness, possibly death	Insect stings, medications, certain foods

Examples of Hypersensitivity Reactions

Allergy	Symptoms	Cause	Treatment
Type I Hypersensitivity Reactions: Immediate or Anaphylactic			
Dermatitis (eczema)	Itchy, inflamed skin caused by a variety of antigens with different ports of entry	Contact with an antigen found in gloves, new clothes, plants, foods; stress or neurological conditions	Frequent washing and shampooing with medicated soap; topical corticosteroids, and antibiotics
Allergic rhinitis (hay fever)	Nasal congestion, sneezing, coughing, extensive mucous secretion, itchy and teary eyes occurring seasonally or year round	Pollens (tree, grass, and weed), molds, house dust mites, pets, cockroaches, rodents	Environmental control measures; allergen avoidance; antihistamines, decongestants, or both; immunotherapy (desensitization)
Asthma	Impaired breathing, bronchoconstriction, wheezing, shortness of breath, coughing, abnormal breathing sounds, chest tightness	Dust mites, pet dander, pollen, molds, etc.	Antiinflammatory agents, bronchodilators
Food allergies	Tingling sensation in the mouth, swelling of the tongue and throat, difficulty breathing, hives, vomiting, abdominal cramps, diarrhea, drop in blood pressure, loss of consciousness and death	Products in food, food additives, and/or preservatives	Avoidance of the allergy-causing food, treatment of symptoms; no medications are currently available to cure food allergies
Drug allergies	Hives, skin rash, itching of skin or eyes, wheezing, swelling of the lips, tongue, or face; anaphylaxis	A side effect to chemotherapy; antibiotics (most often penicillin)	Avoidance of offending medication; treatment of symptoms, desensitization
Anaphylactic reactions	Dizziness, nausea, difficulty breathing, profound fall in blood pressure, unconsciousness, and sometimes death. Response usually after first exposure	Insect bites, certain foods, medications	Adrenalin, antihistamine, corticosteroids, oxygen when needed. Usual treatment for shock
Type II Hypersensitivity Reactions: Antibody Dependent or Cytotoxic			
Hemolytic disease of the newborn	Jaundice, pallor, enlarged liver and/or spleen, generalized swelling, respiratory distress, death	Sensitized mother against fetal blood (see earlier in this chapter)	*Before birth:* intrauterine transfusion or early induction of labor; plasma exchange in the mother. *After birth:* transfusion with compatible packed red blood; exchange transfusion with a compatible blood type; sodium bicarbonate for correction of acidosis, assisted ventilation
Goodpasture's syndrome	*Lung disease:* dry cough, minor breathlessness, symptoms may last for many years before severe symptoms such as impairment of oxygenation and coughing up blood develop. *Kidney disease:* affects the glomeruli causing a form of nephritis; acute renal failure can occur. Lung and kidney disease may occur alone or together depending on the patient	Unknown	Corticosteroids, immunosuppressant; antibiotic treatment of lung infection

Examples of Hypersensitivity Reactions—cont'd

Allergy	Symptoms	Cause	Treatment
Autoimmune hemolytic anemia (Coombs test positive)	Early destruction of red blood cells; abnormally pale skin, jaundice, dark-colored urine, dizziness, weakness, enlarged spleen and liver, fever, heart murmur, increased heart rate; may be fatal	Chemical agents; drugs (e.g., ibuprofen); infections; spider bites (rare); autoimmune disorders	Intubation, assisted ventilation, and hemodialysis in the acute phase followed by high-dose corticosteroids, immunosuppression with cyclophosphamide; aggressive wound care in case of spider bite
Immune-mediated neutropenia	Fever, rash, lymphadenopathy, hepatitis, nephritis, aplastic anemia	Drugs that act as haptens to stimulate antibody formation (e.g., penicillin)	Offending drugs should be stopped; treatment of symptoms
Type III Hypersensitivity Reactions: Immune Complex			
Serum sickness	Rashes, joint pain, fever, lymph node swelling, shock, decreased blood pressure	Exposure to antibodies derived from animals; some drugs	Symptoms generally disappear on their own; antihistamines and corticosteroids may be prescribed
Rheumatoid arthritis	Fatigue, morning stiffness for more than 1 h, muscle aches, loss of appetite, weakness, eventually joint pain, swollen joints, limited range of motion, deformation of hands and feet, skin redness or inflammation, swollen glands, numbness or tingling	Considered to be an autoimmune disease of unknown origin*	Lifelong treatment, including medications, physical therapy, exercise, surgery if required
Type IV Hypersensitivity Reactions: Cell Mediated or Delayed			
Contact dermatitis	Skin rashes; dry, itchy, scaly skin	Poison ivy, poison oak, poison sumac; exposure to dyes and rubbers, soaps, preservatives, creams, or lotions and other substances at the workplace or home	Topical corticosteroid, oral antihistamines. In severe cases oral or injectable corticosteroids, antibiotics, and other antiinflammatory medications may be necessary
Temporal arteritis	Fever, headache, tenderness and sensitivity on the scalp, blurred vision, sudden blindness	Unknown	Corticosteroids, sometimes aspirin and immunosuppressive medications

*Also see the section Autoimmune Diseases in this chapter.

soluble antigens that combine with an antibody to produce free-floating complexes. These complexes can be deposited in the basement membranes of epithelial tissue or other tissues, causing an immune complex reaction. An example of an immune complex disease is serum sickness, in which a systemic reaction occurs after receiving animal serum or hormones. This condition can cause enlarged lymph nodes, fever, rashes, joint pain, and renal dysfunction. Because of the reduced use of animal serum for immunization, serum sickness is now less common. Type III reactions involve IgG or IgM antibodies, complement proteins, and neutrophils.

Delayed Hypersensitivity (Type IV)

Delayed hypersensitivity (type IV) usually takes more than 24 hours and the reaction occurs when an antigen interacts with antigen-specific lymphocytes that release inflammatory substances. These are cell-mediated immune reactions and therefore part of cell-mediated immunity. The response is caused by T lymphocytes sensitized to an antigen, resulting in the release of lymphokines or other chemical mediators that initiate inflammation followed by destruction of the antigen. An example of this type of allergic reaction is contact dermatitis and the epidermal response often caused by haptens.

TABLE 20.5 Common Autoimmune Diseases

Disease	System	Symptoms	Tests
Myasthenia gravis	Skeletal muscles	Progressive muscle weakness, paralysis, death	Autoantibodies against acetylcholine receptors
Multiple sclerosis	Central nervous system	Problems with coordination and balance, difficulty in speaking and walking; paralysis, tremors, numbness and tingling sensation in extremities	Neurological examinations, MRI, MRS, testing of the cerebrospinal fluid
Graves' disease	Thyroid gland	Insomnia, irritability, weight loss, sweating, muscle weakness, bulging eyes, shaky hands	Blood test for TSH
Hashimoto's thyroiditis	Thyroid gland	Tiredness, depression, cold sensitivity, weight gain, dry hair, muscle weakness, constipation; sometimes asymptomatic	Blood test for TSH
Systemic lupus erythematosus	Affects many organ systems	Swelling and damage to joints, skin, kidneys, heart, lungs, blood vessels, and brain; rash across nose and cheeks ("butterfly rash")	Blood and urine tests
Rheumatoid arthritis	Systemic, mostly affecting joints, but also the nervous system, lungs, and skin	Inflammation of joints, muscle pain, weakness, fatigue, loss of appetite, weight loss	Blood tests

MRI, Magnetic resonance imaging; *MRS*, magnetic resonance spectroscopy; *TSH*, thyroid-stimulating hormone.

Autoimmune Diseases

Autoimmunity occurs when the immune system is unable to distinguish between **self-antigens** and **nonself-antigens** and attacks cells, tissues, or organs of the body. Autoimmune diseases can be subdivided into organ-specific diseases, such as Graves' disease, and nonorgan-specific diseases, such as myasthenia gravis. Autoimmune diseases often occur after an individual has experienced an infection or traumatic injury that activates cytotoxic T cells and antibody production against the body's own cells and/or organs. Exact causes of autoimmune diseases are still unknown, but susceptibility based on genetics and gender is a possibility. This chapter addresses a few of the most common autoimmune diseases (Table 20.5).

Myasthenia Gravis

The autoimmune disease myasthenia gravis is characterized by the presence of autoantibodies against acetylcholine receptors at the neuromuscular junctions. Under normal physiological conditions acetylcholine is released from the presynaptic terminal in response to nerve impulses. Acetylcholine then binds to its receptors on the postsynaptic membrane, resulting in muscle contraction. The binding of autoantibodies with the acetylcholine receptors at the neuromuscular junction interferes with the contraction of the muscle fibers involved. Individuals affected by the disease experience progressive muscle weakness and all other functions involving skeletal muscles become increasingly weak and difficult. Although the disease affects all skeletal muscles, weakness of the muscles of the eyes (high nerve-to-muscle innervation ratio) and throat often rep-

resent the first signs of the disease. As the disease progresses a complete loss of muscle function occurs, eventually leading to paralysis and death.

Multiple Sclerosis

Multiple sclerosis (MS) is a chronic paralyzing autoimmune disease of the central nervous system in which demyelination of axons in both the brain and the spinal cord occurs. Because of the lesions in the myelin sheets caused by T cells and autoantibodies, the capacity of neurons to send impulses is severely compromised. MS can affect any area of the central nervous system (both motor and sensory pathways), resulting in diffuse and varied symptoms. Motor symptoms include but are not limited to muscle weakness, tremors, difficulty walking, lack of coordination, impaired speech, constipation, and problems with control of urination. Sensory symptoms include numbness, itching, tingling, burning sensations, pain, and visual problems. General fatigue is common, combined with depression, mood swings, and sometimes cognitive impairment. Symptoms may last from days to months, and remissions of the symptoms in the early stages of the disease occur in many patients. The cause of MS is still unknown but it has been suggested that the trigger of the disease might be a viral infection, environmental factors, genetic predisposition, or a combination thereof.

Graves' Hyperthyroidism (Graves' Disease)

Graves' disease is caused by autoantibodies that bind to the receptors of thyroid follicle cells. This antigen–antibody reaction stimulates the activity of thyroid cells (thyroxin secreting) in the same manner as thyroid-stimulating hormone, which is produced and released by the anterior pituitary. This abnormal continuous activity of the follicle cells causes an enlargement of the thyroid gland, called a *goiter.*

Systemic Lupus Erythematosus

Systemic lupus erythematosus (SLE) is a chronic, systemic, autoimmune, inflammatory disease that affects many body systems. Organs and structures most often affected by the disease are the kidneys, skin, bone marrow, nervous system, joints, muscles, heart, and gastrointestinal tract. The cause of this disease is not known but it is believed to include genetic predisposition and environmental factors. Females are more likely to develop SLE than males. Signs and symptoms include, but are not limited to, a characteristic rash across the cheeks and nose ("butterfly rash"), slight fever, fatigue, joint pain, oral ulcers, weight loss, enlarged lymph nodes, and spleen. Kidney failure, inflammation of the lungs, and myocarditis can also occur.

Rheumatoid Arthritis

Rheumatoid arthritis is a systemic autoimmune disease that causes progressive, debilitating damage to the joints. On occasion, organs such as the nervous system, lungs, and skin may be involved as well. Autoantibodies form immune complexes that bind to the synovial membrane of the joints, resulting in the activation of phagocytes that stimulate cytokine release. Chronic inflammation due to cytokine release results in the formation of scar tissue and finally joint destruction. Relief from symptoms is usually achieved by antiinflammatory agents or immunosuppressive drugs.

Immune Deficiency Diseases

An immune deficiency disease arises when a specific cell or cells within the immune system do not function properly or if part or all of the system is absent. Primary immune deficiency occurs when the abnormalities of the immune system develop because of an inborn abnormality (genetic defect) of the immune system. Secondary immune deficiencies arise when damage is caused by an environmental factor such as infections, radiation, chemotherapy, or burns.

Primary Immune Deficiencies

More than 70 different types of primary immune deficiencies have been reported. Each type of deficiency results in somewhat different symptoms depending on the part of the immune system affected. Although all immune deficiencies result in high susceptibility to infections, some conditions can be mild whereas others might be lethal. These diseases are complex but can now be traced to the failure of one or more parts of the immune system. They can accordingly be classified as:

- B-cell (antibody) deficiencies
- Combined T-cell and B-cell (antibody) deficiencies
- T-cell deficiencies
- Defective phagocytes
- Complement deficiencies
- Deficiencies of unknown cause

Some cases of primary immune deficiency can be combined deficiencies and nearly any infection is a threat to life.

Severe Combined Immunodeficiency (SCID) Severe combined immunodeficiency (SCID) is a rare disorder in which B cells and T cells are inactive or missing; therefore the body is without an immune response. T-cell deficiencies in infants are usually recognized within days of birth and a variety of infections such as sepsis, pneumonia, and systemic viral infections can occur. Probably the most publicized case of SCID involved a child from Texas who spent his life in an isolation chamber for protection from microbes and was often referred to as "the boy in the bubble."

There are several major causes of SCID, each caused by a different genetic defect. The most common type is caused by a defect in an X-linked gene, resulting in the inability of T and B cells to evoke an immune response. Other types are adenosine deaminase (ADA) deficiencies and purine nucleoside phosphorylase deficiencies, both resulting from lack of an enzyme that helps immune cells remove toxic substances (by-products of cellular metabolism) from their cytoplasm.

Secondary Immune Deficiencies

Acquired immunodeficiency syndrome (AIDS) is a secondary immune deficiency disease caused by human immunodeficiency viruses (HIVs). HIV infection occurs when helper T cells (CD4$^+$), monocytes, and macrophages are infected with the virus. Tests for HIV only disclose antibodies the immune system produces and therefore a negative test for the antibody does not necessarily mean that the virus is not present in the system. The eventual decline in the immune response is believed to be due to the depletion of the helper T cells, which play a major role in the activation of B cells. Once AIDS develops the symptoms vary because the infections that result are caused by different opportunistic organisms such as viruses, fungi, protozoans, and bacteria. Drug "cocktails" are the treatment of choice to inhibit the replication of HIV.

Aging and the Immune System

During the aging process humans become more susceptible to disease, including microbial infections. This is sometimes called *immune senescence,* a description of the progressive decline in immune function with age. The decrease in the functioning of the immune system appears to be a combination of the normal decrease in the metabolic rates of cells combined with stress factors associated with aging.

The decline of immune function during aging may be related to the decline in the production of lymphocytes. In addition, the production of thymosins starts to decline around age 20 years. The thymus gland (responsible for T-cell maturation) atrophies with age and basically is nonfunctional in many people after the age of 60 years. Older adults produce fewer helper T cells, but most of the memory T cells are still present to assist in the immune response.

Summary

- Immunology is the study of the events in the immune system, whereas immunity describes the immune response to invading microorganisms.
- The circulatory system (lymphatic and cardiovascular) helps to facilitate the immune response, by distributing immune system cells and antibodies throughout the body. Antigens and antibodies interact to form antigen–antibody complexes during an immune reaction.
- Tissues and organs of the immune system include the lymphatic vessels, lymphoid tissue, lymphatic nodules, tonsils, adenoids, lymph nodes, spleen, thymus, and red bone marrow. The cells of the immune system are leukocytes, including basophils, eosinophils, neutrophils, monocytes, macrophages, lymphocytes (B and T cells), and dendritic cells. Each of these components fulfills a particular function in the immune response.
- Antigens stimulate phagocytosis, provided by a variety of phagocytes, and the production of antibodies by B cells. The immune response can be nonspecific (innate) and/or specific (adaptive).
- The first line of defense is a nonspecific defense mechanism and consists of physical and chemical barriers. Physical barriers include the skin, mucous membranes, sweat, tears, and urine flow. Chemical barriers include the pH of the skin, fatty acids and lactic acids from sebum, mucus containing lysozymes, and the pH of the stomach.
- The second line of defense is also part of the innate immune system, involving phagocytes (phagocytosis), inflammation, fever, interferons, cytokines, and the complement system.
- The third line of defense is composed of acquired/adaptive defense mechanisms, consisting of cell-mediated (T and B cells) and humoral (antibody-mediated) immune responses.
- Active and passive immunity require the presence of antibodies. In active immunity, B cells produce antibodies, whereas in passive immunity the body receives antibody from an external source. Both active and passive immunity can be naturally or artificially acquired.
- An overactive immune system can cause autoimmune diseases and hypersensitivity reactions. Autoimmune diseases occur when the immune system is unable to distinguish between self and nonself. They are classified as organ specific and nonorgan specific.
- Hypersensitivity reactions are classified as types I, II, III, and IV.
- During the aging process, people become more susceptible to microbial infections and autoimmune diseases because of deficiencies in their lymphatic and immune systems.

Review Questions

1. The antibody found in body secretions is:
   a. IgA
   b. IgD
   c. IgE
   d. IgG

2. An antibody is a:
   a. Substance initiating an allergic response
   b. Marker on the cell surface of macrophages
   c. Protein produced by plasma cells
   d. Marker on the cell surface of mast cells

3. Which of the following cell types secretes antibodies?
   a. Macrophages
   b. T cells
   c. Plasma cells
   d. Monocytes

4. Which of the following provide defense against viral infections?
   a. Histamines
   b. Antibiotics
   c. Prostaglandins
   d. Interferons

5. Which of the following cells is a granulocyte?
   a. Basophil
   b. Monocyte
   c. Lymphocyte
   d. Macrophage

6. Immunity that is a result of an actual infection is called:
   a. Artificially acquired passive immunity
   b. Artificially acquired active immunity
   c. Naturally acquired passive immunity
   d. Naturally acquired active immunity

7. A substance capable of raising the body temperature is:
   a. Heparin
   b. Pyrogen
   c. Serum
   d. Prostaglandin

8. When an organ or tissue is transplanted between genetically different individuals from the same species it is called a(n):
   a. Xenograft
   b. Isograft
   c. Autograft
   d. Allograft

9. Which of the following is a systemic autoimmune disease?
   a. Graves' disease
   b. Multiple sclerosis
   c. Myasthenia gravis
   d. Rheumatoid arthritis

10. Which of the following is *not* part of the second line of defense?
    a. pH of the skin
    b. Cytokines
    c. Phagocytosis
    d. Fever

11. Enzymes that attack the peptidoglycan layer of bacteria and are present in perspiration, nasal secretion, saliva, and tears are _____.

12. Delayed hypersensitivity is a result of _____.

13. B cells are responsible for _____-mediated immunity.

14. Substances that stimulate the production of antibodies are called _____.

15. The body's decreased ability to fight infections is called
    _____.

16. Describe and explain the three lines of host immune defense.

17. Name and describe the steps of inflammation.

18. Describe the structure and function of the various antibodies.

19. Discuss type I hypersensitivity reactions.

20. Name and describe two autoimmune diseases.

Bibliography

Benjamini E, Sunshine G, Coico R: *Immunology: A short course*, New York, 2003, John Wiley & Sons Inc.

Damjanov I: *Pathology for the health professions*, ed 3, St. Louis, 2006, Saunders/Elsevier.

Gould BE: *Pathophysiology for the health professions*, St. Louis, 2006, Saunders/Elsevier.

McCance KL, Huether SE: *Pathophysiology: The biologic basis for disease in adults and children*, ed 5, St. Louis, 2005, Mosby/Elsevier.

Masoro EJ, Austad SN: *Handbook of the biology of aging*, Burlington, San Diego, London, 2006, Academic Press/Elsevier.

Mims C, Dockrell HM, Goering RV, et al: *Medical microbiology*, ed 3, St. Louis, 2004, Mosby/Elsevier.

Thibodeau GA, Patton KT: *Anatomy and physiology*, ed 6, St. Louis, 2007, Mosby/Elsevier.

Internet Resources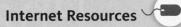

National Institute of Arthritis and Musculoskeletal and Skin Diseases (NIAMS), http://www.niams.nih.gov/hi/index.htm

National Institute of Allergy and Infectious Diseases (NIAID), http://www3.niaid.nih.gov/

Dale and Betty Bumpers Vaccine Research Center (NIH), Vaccine Research Center Journal Publications, http://www.niaid.nih.gov/vrc/publications.htm

National Institutes of Health, Eunice Kennedy Shriver National Institute of Child Health and Human Development, http://www.nichd.nih.gov/

National Cancer Institute, http://www.cancer.gov/

Wikipedia, http://www.wikipedia.org/

healthfinder.gov, http://www.healthfinder.gov/

The Merck Manuals, http://www.merck.com/pubs/

MedlinePlus, http://medlineplus.gov/

MayoClinic.com, http://www.mayoclinic.com/index.cfm

21

Pharmacology

OUTLINE

Introduction
Branches of Pharmacology
Drug Nomenclature
Sources of Drug Information

Principles of Drug Action
Administration
Absorption
Distribution
Biotransformation
Clearance (Elimination)

Responses
Dose Effects
Time Effects
Variability
Toxicity

New Drugs
Development
Public Safety

LEARNING OBJECTIVES

After reading this chapter, the student will be able to:
- Name and explain the various branches of pharmacology
- Discuss drug nomenclature
- Describe administration, absorption, and distribution of drugs in the body
- Explain how biotransformation aids elimination of drugs from the body
- Describe the dose–response curve
- Describe and explain the time–response curve
- Discuss the variability of drug action
- Differentiate between adverse drug response and toxicity
- Describe the steps necessary for the development of new drugs
- Name and describe the schedules used for categorizing drugs

KEY TERMS

analgesics
anesthetic
antidote
bioassays
bioavailability
biotransport
Controlled Substances
    Act
diuretics
dosage
dose
Drug Enforcement
    Administration (DEA)
effective concentration

enteral
first-pass effect
Federal and Drug
    Administration (FDA)
Investigational New
    Drug Application
    (IND)
Kefauver-Harris
    Amendment
latency
New Drug Application
    (NDA)
Orphan Drug Act
orphan drugs

parenteral
peak effect
pharmacodynamics
pharmacokinetics
pharmacotherapeutics
pharmacy
poisons
prodrug
Pure Food and Drug Act
side effects
therapeutic index
toxic effect
toxicology

WHY YOU NEED TO KNOW

HISTORY

"The desire to take medicine is perhaps the greatest feature that distinguishes man from the animals."

Sir William Osler (1849–1919)

Materia medica, in brief terms, is the collected knowledge and use of remedies to treat infection and disease. Most likely it began with the early recorded history of people; attempts to alleviate pain, treat physical maladies, overcome disease, and recover from its effects. Yet, in most cases, causes of the disease were unknown and effective outcome of treatment was uncertain.

Early concepts of disease were markedly influenced by superstitious, primitive, religious fantasies. Some early oral drug candidates persist today from readily available plants— grapes (alcohol) to sedate and poppies (opium) for pain, cinchona bark (quinine) for malaria, saffron (colchicine) for gout, castor beans (castor oil) as a laxative for gastrointestinal tract disturbances, ipecac to treat amoebic dysentery, and willow bark (salicylic acid) as an analgesic for pain remain. Experiences with these remedies formed the folklore basis for the primitive medical practice of witch doctors, and other practitioners. The need of records for medical histories, responses to therapies, preparation procedures, and constituents of medicaments became necessary for continuity, which led to the pharmaceutical and pharmacological sciences.

IMPACT

The history of pharmacology impacts us as an integrated science that continues to evolve with the development of its components:

- *Chemistry:* The chemical composition of a drug
- *Anatomy:* Where in the body the drug acts
- *Physiology:* The body's response to the drug
- *Biochemistry:* A drug's mechanism of action in the body

Pharmacology is further challenged to answer questions concerning what drugs do to the body, what the body does to drugs, and what drugs do to each other. To illustrate the integrated nature of this science, some of the early scientific contributions to the development of pharmacology were made by:

- *Paracelsus* (1493–1541): An alchemist–chemist who introduced chemistry to medicine by proposing that disease results from an imbalance of the body's chemicals that can be treated by chemicals.
- *William Harvey* (1578–1657): An anatomist–physician who demonstrated that blood circulates to reach all cells, which markedly influenced cause-and-effect interpretation and led to the development of the hypodermic needle. This proceeded to the intravenous route of drug administration, which ushered in a new approach to scientific studies of medical sciences in general and drug actions in particular.
- *François Magendie* (1783–1855): A physiologist who used experimental approaches to the study of pharmacological problems to demonstrate that effects of drugs were the result of drug actions within specific body organs.
- *Friedrich W.A. Sertürner* (1783–1841): An apothecary (pharmacist) who was the first to isolate an active constituent—the ammonium salt of morphine—from its botanical source (poppy). This led to the understanding that the therapeutic effects of drugs are due to their active constituents and the value of working with these unadulterated active constituents.
- *Claude Bernard* (1813–1878): A physiologist who demonstrated experimentally in animals specifically how and where drugs act in the body. He interpreted the results of curare's action at the skeletal neuromuscular junction.
- *James Blake* (1815–1893): A physician who proposed that drug effects are determined, after reaching their sites of action, by their chemical structure and time at the site.
- *Paul Ehrlich* (1854–1915): A physician who proposed receptors as the cellular sites for drug action in studies with mercurial compounds to treat syphilis.
- *William Morton* (1819–1868): A dentist who was one of the first to anesthetize a patient with ether for surgical removal of a vascular tumor.

continued.

• *Louis Pasteur* (1822–1895): A microbiologist, who with Koch and others was a major contributor to the germ theory of disease. He demonstrated how to control microbial growth through what is now known as *pasteurization* (see Chapter 1, Scope of Microbiology; and Chapter 19, Physical and Chemical Methods of Control). He also used attenuated toxins to vaccinate.

FUTURE

The goal of medical practice is a rational or reasoned approach to the use of the tools available to the practitioner. Pharmacology is one of these tools. As an integrated science, its future is tied to the development of its parts. It is a dynamic science that continues to evolve at the rate at which scientific disciplines evolve or as new ones are added.

One of the significant challenges for pharmacology is microorganisms that have developed resistance to antimicrobial drugs. In response to this challenge the Food and Drug Administration (FDA), Centers for Disease Control and Prevention (CDC), and U.S. Department of Agriculture (USDA) have developed the National Antimicrobial Resistance Monitoring System (NARMS) to monitor and determine changes in antimicrobial drug resistance. The NARMS identifies antimicrobial drug resistance in humans and animals and provides timely information to physicians and veterinarians about antimicrobial drug resistance patterns. This increased monitoring is essential to keep abreast of changes. There is a need to exercise caution against the inadvertent development of new resistant strains after the introduction of new antibiotics.

Introduction

As already stated, pharmacology (from the Greek *pharmakon* [drug] and *logia* [the study of]) is an integrated medical science. With a few exceptions, such as antibiotics, drugs cannot and do not add any new physiological, biochemical, or other biological functions to living tissues. They alter the rates at which physiological responses can occur, such as adrenaline, which induces an increase in the heart rate.

Branches of Pharmacology

This chapter introduces some fundamentals of "physiological pharmacology" or "pharmacological physiology"—referring to the same anatomy, physiology, and biochemistry discussed in Chapter 2 (Chemistry of Life) and Chapter 3 (Cell Structure and Function). Although all drugs are potential **poisons** (substances that cause severe distress or death), when given in subtoxic doses they are medicinal tools. The goal of rational drug therapy is to aid and maintain the body and its biological systems in healthy working order. In therapy, drugs give living tissues added chemical support to prevent and to meet physical and pathological challenges to which biological systems are exposed. Pharmacology is organized into separate disciplines that describe actions of drugs:

- **Pharmacodynamics** addresses drug-induced responses of the physiological and biochemical systems of the body in health and disease.
- **Pharmacokinetics** addresses drug amounts at various sites in the body after their administration.
- **Pharmacotherapeutics** addresses issues associated with the choice and application of drugs to be used for disease prevention, treatment, or diagnosis.
- **Toxicology** is the study of the body's response to poisons; their harmful effects, mechanisms of action, symptoms, treatment, and identification.

HEALTHCARE APPLICATION

Examples of Drugs Used in the Various Organ Systems

Drug	System/Condition	Effect
Methylphenidate	Central nervous	Stimulant
Digitalis	Cardiovascular	Treats congestive heart failure
Colchicine	Neuromuscular	Analgesic
Quinidine	Cardiovascular	Antiarrhythmic
Procainamide	Cardiovascular	Antiarrhythmic
Phenytoin	Central nervous	Anticonvulsant
Verapamil	Cardiovascular	Antianginal
Nitroglycerin	Cardiovascular	Antianginal
Acetazolamide	Renal	Diuretic
Levothyroxine	Endocrine	Treats hypothyroidism
Barbiturate	Central nervous	Sedative
Benzodiazepine	Central nervous	Antianxiety
Prednisolone	Respiratory	Inhibits inflammatory responses
Sodium bicarbonate	Gastrointestinal	Increases stomach pH
Sildenafil	Reproductive	Treats erectile dysfunction
Sibutramine	Obesity	Inhibits reuptake of serotonin and norepinephrine that regulate food intake
Somatotropin	Endocrine	Antipituitary to block IGF action on liver cells.

IGF, Insulin-like growth factor.

- **Pharmacy,** on the other hand, includes the preparation, compounding, dispensing of, and record keeping about therapeutic drugs, for which drug nomenclature is essential. In addition, pharmacy includes the following:
  - *Pharmacognosy:* The botanical sources of drugs
  - *Pharmaceutical chemistry:* The chemical synthesis and modification of new and existing drugs
  - *Biopharmaceutics:* The effects of formulation of drugs on their pharmacodynamic and pharmacokinetic properties

Drug Nomenclature

Because all drugs are potential poisons, understanding their nomenclature is essential. It is also practical because it specifically identifies the correct drug for the correct use. This starts with their manufacture in the pharmaceutical industry; continues to distribution at pharmacies where drugs are dispensed; and ends with medical personnel who administer them to patients. Moreover, drug nomenclature is needed for a precise chemical description that can help to avoid medical disasters.

In general, therapeutic chemicals are broadly divided into two groups, nonprescription and prescription drugs:

- *Nonprescription:* Over-the-counter (OTC) drugs approved by the Federal Drug Administration (FDA) and herbal supplements, not approved by the FDA
- *Prescription:* Drugs required by law to be prescribed by licensed practitioners (i.e., veterinarians, dentists, and physicians)

Individual drugs have three names: chemical, generic, and proprietary or trade (brand) name (Table 21.1):

- *Chemical:* A single accurate description of the chemical structure, which is often lengthy but is of value to synthetic chemists; for example, 3,5-dihydroxyphenylalanine
- *Generic:* Nonproprietary, a single name, usually indicating the relationship of a drug to a therapeutic class; for example,
  - Antimicrobials (e.g., penicillin)
  - Anticonvulsants (e.g., dilantin)
  - **Analgesics** (e.g., aspirin)
- *Proprietary* or *trade (brand) name:* A legally licensed drug name assigned by manufacturers. If a drug is produced by many manufacturers the list of proprietary names can become lengthy; for example, the local **anesthetic** procaine has at least 24 different names

Sources of Drug Information

Sources for drug information can be people or published information. People who generally have particular drug information include the following:

- Clinicians
- Pharmacists
- Poison control centers
- Pharmaceutical sales representatives

Published information can be found in the following:

- Textbooks
- Newsletters

TABLE 21.1 Examples of Drug Nomenclature

Trade or Brand (Proprietary) Name	Generic (Nonproprietary) Name	Chemical Name	Therapeutic Class
Amoxil, Amoxicot, Trimox, DisperMox ...	Amoxicillin	(2S,5R,6R)-6-[(R)-(–)-2-amino-2-(p-hydroxyphenyl)acetamido]-3,3-dimethyl-7-oxo-4-thia-1-azabicyclo[3.2.0] heptane-2-carboxylic acid trihydrate	Antibiotic
Advil, Motrin, Midol, Nuprin ...	Ibuprofen	(±)-2-(p-Isobutylphenyl) propionic acid	Antiinflammatory
Tylenol, Anacin-3 ...	Acetaminophen	N-Acetyl-p-aminophenol	Analgesic
Dilantin, Dilantin KAPSEALS	Phenytoin	Sodium 5,5-diphenyl-2,4 imidazolidinedione	Anticonvulsants
Allegra	Fexofenadine	(±)-4-[1 hydroxy-4-[4-(hydroxydiphenylmethyl)-1-piperidinyl]-butyl]-α,α-dimethyl benzeneacetic acid hydrochloride	Antihistamines

- Reference books
- Internet

Principles of Drug Action

Drugs alter physiological activity and for them to be effective they must reach their intended target site at the appropriate concentration (Table 21.2). This involves several processes collectively called **pharmacokinetics.** These principles include the following:

- Administration
- Absorption
- Distribution
- Biotransformation
- Clearance (elimination)

MEDICAL HIGHLIGHTS

Physicians' Desk Reference: PDR

The *Physicians' Desk Reference,* or PDR, is a drug reference book that is financed by the pharmaceutical industry and is updated annually. The PDR is the authoritative source of FDA-approved information about prescription drugs. The information about each drug in the book is identical to the information on the package insert. In addition to the text, the PDR provides full-color photos for drug identification.

TABLE 21.2 Drug Losses at Sites of Action Through Administration

Route of Administration	Drug Loss From:
Enteral route only	Degradation in stomach
	First-pass effect
	Small intestine
	Failure to be absorbed
	Binding to food or other contents
	Liver
	Secretion in bile
	Biotransformation
	Tissue binding
Enteral and parenteral routes	
General blood circulation	Biotransformation
	Binding to plasma proteins
Distribution to body tissues	Drug too dispersed, not sufficient at site of action
	Tissue binding
	Biotransformation
	Metabolism
	Excretion

Administration

Drugs are administered **enterally** via the digestive system or **parenterally** via a system other than the digestive system. They are given to affect only the site of administration, or systemically, for distribution to various sites of action via the circulatory system.

For direct local action, drugs may be given (Figure 21.1) in the following ways:

- On the skin
- On mucous membranes (e.g., the nose, mouth, throat, eye, or genitourinary tract)
- Orally (limited to, e.g., osmotic cathartics, osmotic **diuretics,** and antacids for gastrointestinal tract infections)
- By inhalation for some respiratory and lung diseases
- Iontophoretically (in or through the skin via control of ionic [i.e., positive or negative] charges)

For systemic effects, drugs may be given (Figure 21.2) in the following ways:

- Through a *transdermal* therapeutic system (e.g., via a controlled slow-release drug reservoir attached to the skin)
- *Sublingually:* Under the tongue (e.g., nitroglycerine tablets)
- *Orally:* By mouth for absorption via the gastrointestinal tract

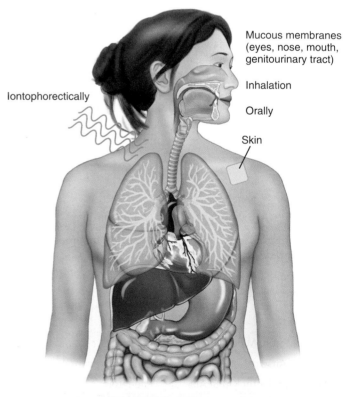

Mucous membranes (eyes, nose, mouth, genitourinary tract)

Iontophorectically

Inhalation

Orally

Skin

FIGURE 21.1 Local drug administration. For direct administration, drugs may be administered to the skin or mucous membranes, orally, by inhalation, or iontophoretically through the skin by electrical charge to the given target.

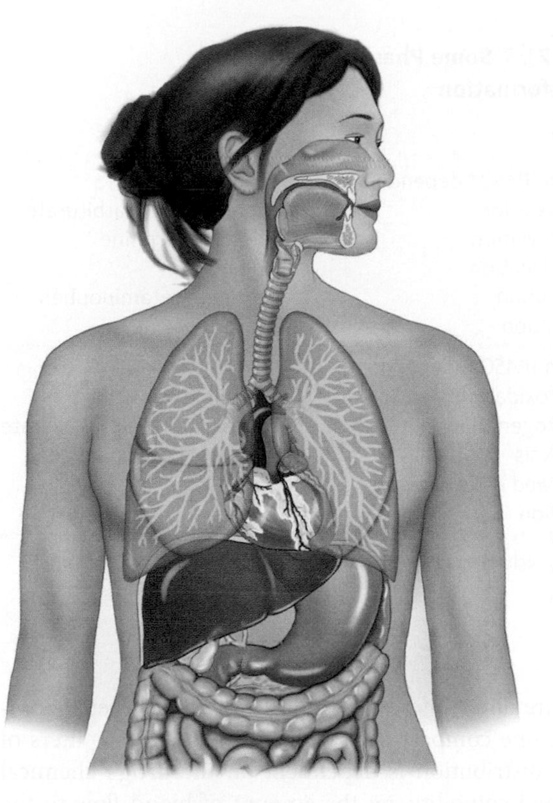

FIGURE 21.2 Systemic drug administration.
Sites through which drugs can be given to achieve
a systemic effect.

- Transdermal therapeutic system
- Sublingually
- Orally
- Rectally
- By inhalation
- Subcutaneously
- Intramuscularly
- Intravenous
- Intrathecally

- *Rectally:* By suppositories in the rectum via the anus into areas of extensive vascularization and rapid blood flow. Useful in infants or in patients with loss of consciousness
- *By inhalation:* Into the lungs; another area of extensive vascularization and rapid blood flow. Good for direct application on huge lung tissue surface (200 m²) vascularly structured to absorb and remove materials. In addition, the lungs receive, in the course of 1 minute, the total amount of blood passing through the rest of the body during the same time interval. In brief, the lungs are the most effective absorptive area of the body
- *Subcutaneously:* Below the cutaneous layer. Good for slow absorption of small amounts of drug
- *Intramuscularly:* Rapid rate of absorption because of extensive vascularization and rapid blood flow, but less than by the intravenous route
- *Intravenously:* Most rapid rate of absorption. Can be modified by a port (cannulation of the great caval veins for repeated drug administrations such as in cancer chemotherapy) or by an intravenous *bolus* (a large volume of fluid given intravenously and rapidly at one time for an immediate effect)
- *Intrathecally:* Administered into the spinal subarachnoid space

Absorption

After administration, drugs must proceed to a site where they can act. *Absorption* describes the rate at which a drug leaves its site of administration and the extent to which it appears at the site of action. Regardless of the route of administration, the drug must be dissolved in body fluids and pass through biologi-

cal barriers before it can arrive at the cellular site of action (Box 21.1). The term used to indicate the extent to which a drug reaches its site of action is **bioavailability.** Drugs are **biotransported** across these biological barriers via mechanisms discussed previously (see Chapter 2 [Chemistry of Life] and Chapter 3 [Cell Structure and Function]). For example, drugs administered orally, dermally, topically, or by inhalation must traverse the epithelium, whereas those given subcutaneously or intramuscularly must traverse the capillary wall. There are three general sites of action:

- *Extracellular:* Such as the decrease in blood clotting by heparin's chemical combination with proteins to remove them from the coagulating mechanism
- *Cellular:* Such as the contraction of skeletal muscle by the action of acetylcholine at the nicotinic, cholinergic skeletal muscle neuromuscular receptor
- *Intracellular:* Such as the inhibition by sulfa drugs of bacterial growth via inhibition of intracellular components needed for bacterial growth

The rate of drug absorption is influenced by the anatomical and physiological properties of the site of administration and the physical and chemical properties of the drug itself. These factors include the following:

- *Surface area:* The larger the surface area is, the faster absorption will occur. For example, the large surface area of the small intestine is conducive to absorption of orally administered drugs.
- *Rate of dissolution:* The rate at which a drug is dissolved will determine the rate of absorption. Drugs with a high

BOX 21.1 Transport of Drugs Through Biological Membranes

Transport of the various forms of drugs can be described by formulas that show:

- The percentage that will be available for successful transport through phospholipid (biological) membranes
- The percentage that will be available for excretion through the kidney
- The amounts of materials that potentially will be available for movement
- Specific information and/or general information about the substances and their mobilities

For example:

- Water-soluble forms of substances:
  - Are ionized (see Chapter 2, Chemistry of Life)
  - Have difficulty passing through biological (phospholipid) membranes such as blood vessels
  - Are readily excreted via an organ system such as the kidney
  - Are transformed in the body from lipid- to water-soluble forms by biotransformation.
- Lipid-soluble forms of substances:
  - Are nonionized
  - Readily pass through biological (phospholipid) membranes such as are found in blood vessels
  - Can be reabsorbed in the kidney, that is, are *not* readily excreted like water-soluble drugs
  - Can be biotransformed to water-soluble (kidney-excretable) forms in the body

The abbreviated relationships that give this information as a percentage are as follows:

$$\frac{I \text{ (ionized percentage) of drug} \times 100}{I \text{ (ionized)} + \text{Nonion (nonionized percentage of drug)}}$$

and

$$\frac{\text{Nonion (percentage)} \times 100}{I \text{ (percentage)} + \text{Nonion (percentage)}} =$$

Percent available for biological transport, respectively

TABLE 21.3 Some Phase I Reactions of Biotransformation

Reaction	Examples of Drugs
Oxidation (P450* dependent)	
Hydroxylation	Amphetamine, barbiturate
N-Dealkylation	Caffeine, morphine
O-Dealkylation	Codeine
N-Oxidation	Nicotine, acetaminophen
S-Oxidation	Chlorpromazine
Oxidation (P450 independent)	
Amine oxidation	Adrenaline
Dehydrogenation	Ethyl alcohol, chloral hydrate
Hydrolysis	Lidocaine, procainamide
Amide and ester oxidation	Aspirin, procaine
Reduction	Chloramphenicol, naloxone

*P450 is a cytochrome capable of catalyzing biotransformation reactions.

Cell Structure and Function). These two compartments combined make one compartment with approximately 40 liters of fluid. Drug distribution is dependent on the drug's chemical properties and solubility, on the amount of blood flow to the target, and on the drug's molecular size and rate of excretion, to name a few. Water-soluble drugs are readily excreted and lost unless bound. Blood flow to the site and molecular size of the drug are additional factors as well. Blood flow to the brain reveals the blood–brain barrier as another obstacle, and blood flow to the fetus must traverse the placental circulation. The placenta presents a pathway for transfer of substances from the mother to the fetus, such as nicotine and marijuana as well as alcohol.

Biotransformation

Biotransformation involves the metabolism of drugs, a mechanism by which the body inactivates drugs and engages phase I and phase II reactions. Phase I reactions convert drugs into more ionized molecules by the introduction of (or by the exposure of) already existing ionized components of the compounds (Table 21.3). Phase II reactions are synthetic reactions in which new compounds are introduced to chemically altered drugs. Some examples include conjugations of moieties with amino (–NH₂), hydroxyl (OH), or sulfhydryl (SH) groups if added to the molecules (Table 21.4).

Although the liver plays the major role in drug metabolism, lungs, kidneys, and adrenal glands contribute as well. The majority of active drugs need high lipid solubility to be transported through bilipid cellular membranes. Drug metabolites also require high water solubility in order to be transported to the kidneys and eliminated in urine formed in nephrons of the kidneys (Figure 21.3). Lipid-soluble drugs can be made more water soluble by metabolic processes such as conjugation, or other metabolic processes that render the metabolite water soluble. Although metabolic processes can inactivate a drug, this is not always the case (see Medical Highlights: Prodrugs).

---

dissolution rate have a faster onset of action than those with a low dissolution rate.

- *Lipid solubility:* Drugs that are highly lipid soluble can more easily cross biological membranes than those with low lipid solubility.
- *Blood flow:* Drug absorption in areas with high blood flow is greater than in areas with decreased blood flow.

Distribution

Distribution is the transfer of drugs across biological membranes into body compartments such as the combined intracellular and extracellular fluid compartments (see Chapter 3,

TABLE 21.4 Some Phase II Reactions of Biotransformation

Reaction	Examples of Drugs
Acetylation	Mescaline, sulfonamide
Conjugation	
Glutathione	Bromobenzene, ethacrynic acid
Glycine	Benzoic acid, salicylic acid
Sulfate	Methyldopa, 3-hydroxycoumarin
Glucuronidation	Digoxin, morphine
Methylation	Dopamine, histamine

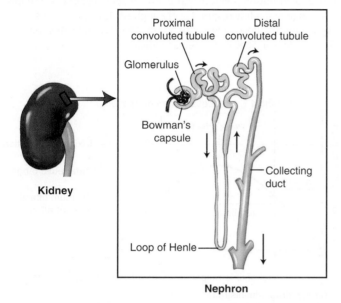

FIGURE 21.3 Nephron. The nephron is the functional unit of the kidney and largely responsible for the elimination of by-products of metabolism and drug metabolites.

MEDICAL HIGHLIGHTS

Prodrugs

A prodrug is a substance administered in an inactive form but that once administered is metabolized into an active metabolite. The quaternary amine dopamine, a drug needed to treat Parkinsonism, cannot enter the brain because of its poor lipid solubility characteristics and the protective membrane property of the blood–brain barrier (BBB) that limits access to lipid-soluble substances. However, L-dopa is a tertiary amine with high lipid solubility that does penetrate the BBB and is a precursor of dopamine. L-Dopa is then metabolized in the brain by dopa decarboxylase to dopamine, the usable therapeutic agent for Parkinson patients. L-Dopa is an example of a **prodrug**—an administered drug that is then activated by endogenous metabolic activity.

Clearance (Elimination)

Drugs are excreted from the body primarily via the kidneys, and this excretion into the urine requires three processes (see Chapter 15, Infections of the Urinary System; and also Figure 21.3):

1. Glomerular filtration
2. Tubular reabsorption
3. Tubular secretion

Some drugs metabolized in the liver are also excreted via bile and the biliary tract as well as via feces. The lungs, in addition to being a route of administration, are also a potential path of elimination for drug metabolites in the expired air. Other paths of clearance include sweat, saliva, tears, and production of breastmilk, which can be a hazard for the newborn if the mother breastfeeds.

Responses

The administration of a drug to the human body evokes a series of responses. These responses are divided into four categories:

1. Dose effects
2. Time effects
3. Variability
4. Toxicity

Dose Effects

Recalling that all drugs are potential poisons depending on the dose given, the effect of a drug depends on the **dose**, and it is essential to determine what a given dose will do to a patient. The dose of a drug is the amount given at a single time. **Dosage** refers to the total amount given over a period of time. For example, say the dose of a drug given to a patient is a 5-mg tablet; if administered for 5 days this equals a dosage of 25 mg. Dose and dosage are not terms to be used interchangeably.

Therapeutic Index

Paul Ehrlich recognized that drugs needed to be judged not only by their useful properties, but also by their toxic effects. The **therapeutic index**, also referred to as the "margin of safety," is the ratio between a drug dose causing undesirable effects and the dose that causes the desired therapeutic response. The therapeutic index is the ratio of a drug's LD_{50} to its ED_{50} and is determined in laboratory animals. The LD_{50} is the lethal dose in 50% of the tested animals and the ED_{50} is the effective dose of the drug in 50% of the treated animals.

$$\text{Therapeutic index (TI)} = \frac{LD_{50}}{ED_{50}}$$

A high therapeutic index indicates that a drug is relatively safe, whereas a low therapeutic index indicates that the drug is relatively unsafe (Figure 21.4). Figure 21.4, *B* shows an overlap

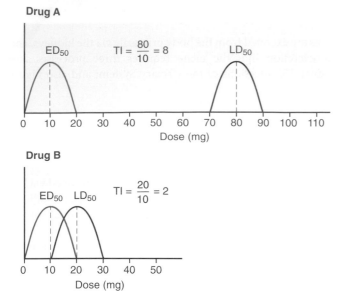

Drug A

$$TI = \frac{80}{10} = 8$$

Drug B

$$TI = \frac{20}{10} = 2$$

FIGURE 21.4 Therapeutic index. A high therapeutic index indicates that a drug is relatively safe, whereas a low therapeutic index indicates that the drug is relatively unsafe. Drug A has a high therapeutic index and is relatively safe. Drug B shows an overlap between the therapeutic effect curve and the lethal effect curve, and therefore this drug is relatively unsafe.

between the curves representing the therapeutic effect and the curve representing the lethal effect. This means that the drug dose needed to produce a therapeutic effect is very high, and may be large enough to cause death in some patients. For a drug to be safe, the highest dose necessary to produce a therapeutic effect must be substantially lower than the lowest dose required to produce death.

Individuals may vary considerably in their responsiveness to a drug. These biological variations among patients lead to pharmacological variations in the dose response of patients. Overcoming pharmacological variation requires quantitation in order to minimize errors of prediction. This begins with sampling of the collected data having a common characteristic such as age, gender, species, strain, weight, and environmental conditions. Because of biological variations patients will not necessarily respond to the same minimal effective dose (ED). However, by use of appropriate statistical methods, generalizations can be drawn with some degree of statistical probability. Normal distribution will predict that a few respond at the low dose range and a few respond at the highest doses, with most responding to a dose range in between (Figure 21.5).

It is essential to know what the response to a given dose of a drug will be. Responses are either:

- *Graded:* For example, the incremental amount of increase or decrease in blood pressure as the dose increases

or

- *Quantal* (all-or-none): The number of patients or animals responding per dose, such as with a drug either inducing sleep or not

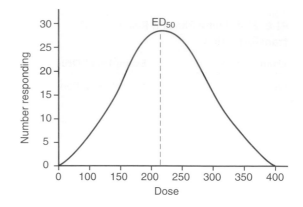

FIGURE 21.5 Biological variations in drug response. This diagram illustrates the biological variations in drug response. Normal distribution predicts that a few persons respond at the low dose range and a few respond at the highest doses, with most responding to a dose range in between. The ED_{50} indicates the effective dose in 50% of the tested individuals.

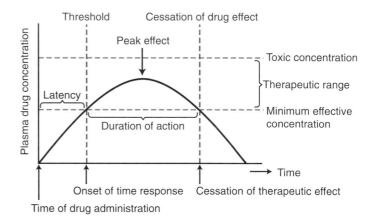

FIGURE 21.6 Time–response curve. The time–response curve indicates the time of drug administration, the onset of time response (the threshold), the peak effect, the duration of action, and the cessation of drug effect. Furthermore, the diagram indicates the toxic concentration of a drug, the therapeutic range, and the minimal effective concentration of that drug.

Time Effects

Dose response includes magnitude of response after a single dose, excluding other factors that affect concentration at the site of action (SOA), such as time. A selected time is chosen and measurements are taken to determine minimal, maximal, or any other chosen level of response for that time (Figure 21.6).

The time response measures the following:

- Time of drug administration
- Onset of time response
- Cessation of drug effect
- Peak effect time
- Duration of action time
- Latency to effect time
- Threshold level

Latency (time 0–1) is regulated primarily by the time a drug takes to get to its SOA (i.e., the rates of absorption, distribution, and focusing after it arrives at the SOA in the target organ). This may also include conversion time from the inactive to active form of the drug.

The **peak effect** occurs when the receptors are maximally activated. This effect is largely determined by the rates of movement of the drug to the SOA and removal of drug from the SOA. It should be noted that with high concentrations of drug the rates of elimination are also high.

The **effective concentration** can be achieved by a single administration or after multiple administrations. The rate of elimination of a drug is a deciding factor in its cessation of action, and biotransformation is a decisive factor within this process. The rate of biotransformation determines the duration of action and effective concentrations are measured by the biological half-life of the drug. The biological half-life is the amount of time needed for the drug concentration in the plasma to be reduced to half the value from the previous measurement.

Antimicrobial drugs (see Chapter 22, Antimicrobial Drugs) are generally given by multiple administrations in order to achieve effective concentrations. Ongoing antimicrobial therapy should be reassessed regularly, and therapy should be appropriately adapted after initial culture results return. Dangerous negative effects can occur after toxic doses of antimicrobial drugs are accumulated or given; therefore, monitoring the patients' vital signs as well as serum levels of drug concentration is essential. Drugs are typically withdrawn after the first sign of toxic or negative effect.

Variability

There are other variables such as age, gender, and species that influence the preparation for excretion or elimination. These include the following:

- *First-pass effect:* The **first-pass effect** is the biotransformation of a drug in the liver or gastrointestinal tract subsequent to oral administration and before entering the general circulation. Actually, the first-pass effect is the combined action of intestinal and hepatic drug-metabolizing enzymes on a drug's bioavailability. **Bioavailability** is the extent to which a drug is absorbed and is available to its site of action.
- *Chemical properties:* Relevant chemical properties of drugs include molecular weight, ionic charge, solubility in water/lipids, and so on.
- *Toxic effects:* Toxic effects typically occur because of depletion of enzymes needed in detoxification reactions subsequent to the administration of a toxic dose of a drug.
- *Liver and kidney diseases:* Liver and kidney diseases result in an inability to metabolize or excrete drugs, respectively.
- *Starvation:* Starvation usually results in a decreased ability to conjugate with glycine because of depletion of that amino acid.
- *Age:* For example, neonates fail to metabolize drugs in the same way as adults or the elderly.

- *Genetics:* For example, some patients are unable to metabolize succinylcholine, resulting in succinylcholine apnea during recovery after surgery.
- *Gender:* For example, young males show increased sensitivity to barbiturates compared to the general population.
- *Species variability:* The responses of experimental animals to drugs are not always the same as those of humans.
- *Circadian rhythm:* The 24-hr cycle in which metabolic cycles repeat themselves. Depending on the time of day administered, a drug can have different effects due to the circadian rhythm.

Toxicity

Toxic, adverse, and/or undesired drug effects are somewhat interchangeable terms. A **toxic effect** is an effect that is harmful to a biological system, whereas an adverse effect may be harmful in some but not all systems. Mild reactions include drowsiness, nausea, itching, and rash, whereas more severe adverse effects include respiratory depression, neutropenia, hepatocellular injury, anaphylaxis, and hemorrhage—all of which may lead to death.

Toxic effects are classified as:

- *Acute:* An effect that occurs within minutes or hours of exposure. An example is carbon monoxide, which, after a single exposure to 1.5% for 5 to 6 minutes, can be lethal
- *Subacute:* An effect that occurs after repeated exposure for days
- *Chronic:* An effect that occurs over months to years, during which time the rate of exposure exceeds the rate of elimination

Toxicology, the study of poisons, includes evaluation of the following characteristics:

- Physiochemical properties
- Routes and rates of administration
- Rates of absorption, biotransformation, and excretion
- Adverse effects of chemicals in air and the environment

Determination of drug safety (drug toxicity) is based on comparisons with other drugs or poisons to measure relative safety levels. For example, penicillin is considered safe compared with the poisonous organophosphate malathion as well as compared with the antimicrobial drug neomycin. Human drug safety evaluated by pharmacological animal testing procedures is shown in Table 21.5.

Nonspecific treatment of suspected poisoning always includes support of respiration and circulation in addition to:

- Removing the patient from exposure to the poison source
- Identifying the poison if possible
- Giving a suitable **antidote**
- Instituting suitable poison elimination procedures
- Instituting supportive measures for the patient

TABLE 21.5 Human Toxicity From Animal LD$_{50}$ Values

Animal LD$_{50}$/kg	Degree of Toxicity	Probable LD$_{50}$/70-kg Human
0.1 mg	Excessive	Simple taste (less than 1mg)
1.0–50 mg	High	1 teaspoon (5.0 ml)
50–500 mg	Average	1.0 fluid ounce
0.5–5.0 g	Slight	1 fluid pint
5.0–15.0 g	Nontoxic	1 quart
15.0 g	Harmless	Greater than 1 quart

LD$_{50}$, Lethal dose in 50% of tested animals.

TABLE 21.6 Specific Treatment for Selected Toxins

Toxic agent	Specific Antidote	Mechanism of Action
Iron (Fe)	Sodium bicarbonate	Forms insoluble ferrous complex
Methanol	Ethanol	No formation of poisonous metabolite
Botulinum toxin	Antitoxin	Complex formed with toxin
Organophosphates	Pralidoxime	Removes poison from cholinesterase
	Atropine	Pharmacological antagonism at site of toxic action
Morphine and other narcotics	Naloxone	Pharmacological antagonism at site of toxic action
Carbon monoxide (CO)	Oxygen (O$_2$)	Pharmacological antagonism at site of toxic action

Specific treatment for poisons (Table 21.6) is as follows:

- In general, increase the rate of elimination of the poison and remove from the SOA via the formation of a water-soluble complex, such as by increasing the rate of bromide removal via NaCl exchange.
- For a specific poison administer the antidote; for example, in the case of cyanide poisoning administer nitrites or thiosulfate.
- For heavy metal poisoning administer a chelator, which will form a complex with the heavy metal that is then excreted; for example, in the case of mercury poisoning, administer dimercaprol (also known as *British anti-Lewisite* [BAL]).
- For lead poisoning administer edetate calcium disodium (CaNa$_2$EDTA), which forms complexes with the lead

Thimerosal: The Heavy Metal Scapegoat

In June of 2007, nearly 5000 families filed a lawsuit against the federal government, claiming that the vaccines being given to children were causing autism. The specific agent being implicated in the vaccines was thimerosal, a mercury-containing compound used as a preservative in the vaccines. Thimerosal has been in use in vaccines since the 1930s and was considered safe until recent claims of a correlation between thimerosal and autism were made by a number of both politically and allegedly science-oriented groups. After extensive reviews of data, both the federal government and science and health agencies have come to the conclusion that there is no solid evidence of any direct connection between thimerosal used in vaccines and the onset of autism. The fervor appears to have been fueled by individuals with political and monetary motivations, and both the Centers for Disease Control and Prevention (CDC) and the American Academy of Pediatrics have generally rejected the studies linking thimerosal to juvenile autism. The agencies concluded that autism should not be included as a risk for those using vaccines with thimerosal (http://www.cdc.gov/vaccinesafety/concerns/thimerosal.htm).

and enhances its excretion 50-fold compared with uncomplexed lead.

New Drugs

Development of new drugs starting at the beginning of the twentieth century did not yield much from natural products. Not until 1928, when Alexander Fleming accidentally discovered the action of the mold penicillin on *Staphylococcus*, was an interest created in antibiotics. In 1952, chemists isolated reserpine as the active constituent of the alkaloid rauwolfia, which had been used in India for centuries as a medication for a number of maladies. The isolation and use of reserpine led to a resurgence of interest in looking to folk remedies as a source for new drugs. However, many plants failed to be of value, such as the periwinkle (*Vinca rosea*), which was originally touted as an effective treatment for diabetes but proved ineffective, yet later was used successfully in some cancers.

Development

Development begins with extraction of the active constituent from the natural product. This active constituent is then tested on a biological system to develop a pharmacological profile. This screening process is time-consuming. For example, even though thousands of soil samples can be screened in the search for therapeutically active antimicrobials, only a few have actually been found. When a pharmacologically active natural compound is found, synthetic chemistry is used to identify a process

New Drug Development: A New Kind of Library

Naturally produced antimicrobial drugs, such as penicillin, continue to be useful as they form the basis of the chemical arsenal in use today against microbial infections. The effectiveness of these compounds and their derivatives makes them important in the treatment of various diseases and infections. However, the production of these natural compounds is generally lengthy and limited in total output. To maximize the effectiveness and increase the availability of these compounds, the pharmaceutical industry has developed various approaches to accomplish these goals. One of the programs developed is the establishment of extensive high-quality natural product libraries. From these libraries samples can be obtained for experimentation and compound development. The types of libraries established include crude extract, semipure mixture, and single purified natural product libraries. Several processes including mass spectrometry and nuclear magnetic resonance are valuable tools in building these libraries and helping in the development of new drugs.

to make it and/or modify the structure to reduce **side effects** that are undesirable or to add structural changes that make the new synthetic compound more therapeutically desirable. Some notable drugs are still feasible to obtain as natural products, such as morphine for pain control or the digitalis glycosides for cardiovascular therapies. Cell cultures from plant sources are also being investigated as potential sources to improve yields from screening procedures.

In addition, these investigations with plants have led to technological advances that:

- Speed the screening of natural products via improvement in separation and identification of active constituents
- Allow chemical manipulation of structures
- Develop new **bioassays** to identify dose–response characteristics
- Allow qualitative pharmacology procedures to identify potential prototypical pharmacological profiles

The development of synthetic chemicals led to the study of structure–activity relationships (SAR) and the evolution of pharmacological prototypes (agents with similar structures that have similar therapeutic properties). With synthetic chemicals and the use of synthetic chemistry, structures of classes of drugs could be manipulated to:

- Improve margins of safety (the range between the effective dose and lethal dose, i.e., LD_{50}/ED_{50})
- Reduce unwanted side effects
- Increase the duration of action
- Improve absorption from the gastrointestinal tract

Many natural products are broken down in the stomach; hence the advent of oral synthetic drugs, such as oral antidiabetics and oral contraceptives, has made a major impact on therapeutic practice. For example, not only have oral contraceptives impacted gynecological medicine but the availability of oral synthetic estrogenic and progestatonal hormones have revolutionized the practice of these medical disciplines as well.

Public Safety

Protection of the public has received the attention of the federal government beginning with federal regulations to guide the manufacture, distribution, and sales of new drugs—and in many instances existing drugs—and through a program of rational tests before permitting use in humans.

The **Pure Food and Drug Act** of 1906 dealt only with drugs already on the market. Basically, it used the Pharmacopeia of the United States and the National Formulary as the official standards of the U.S. government. In addition, the federal government was entrusted with enforcing claims that the purity and strength of drugs were accurate and true.

The **Federal Food, Drug and Cosmetic Act** of 1938 empowered the **Food and Drug Administration (FDA)** to require, for their review and approval, a **New Drug Application (NDA)** that showed the safety of new therapeutic agents. This was prompted by the use of diethylene glycol as a liquid diluent with no toxicity tests. More than 100 fatalities had been reported from severe liver and kidney damage and pulmonary edema linked to diethylene glycol. At present, if the formulation of an existing drug is changed, it becomes a "new drug" for review by the FDA.

The Federal Food, Drug and Cosmetic Act of 1938 was modified by the **Kefauver-Harris Amendment** of 1962 to require proof that a new drug was not only safe but also effective. These substantial requirements to demonstrate evidence of efficacy as well as safety were retroactive to drugs and products marketed between 1938 and 1962. The governmental authority was extended to enforce requirements that preclinical studies be done before clinical testing and distribution of new drugs.

In 1971, the **Controlled Substances Act** became law. This legislation focused on drugs that had the potential for abuse. Those who manufacture, dispense, prescribe, or administer any of these controlled substances must register annually with the Attorney General of the United States. Enforcement is the responsibility of the **Drug Enforcement Administration (DEA)**. The five schedules of controlled substances are as follows:

- *Schedule I:* Drugs and substances with high probability for abuse with no therapeutic use and a lack of safety controls such as opioids, heroin, lysergic acid diethylamide (LSD), marijuana, mescaline, and certain mushroom extracts (peyote).
- *Schedule II:* Drugs and substances with high probability for abuse and are accepted for therapeutic use or accepted for therapy under close restrictions such as raw opium, coca leaves, cocaine, morphine, methadone, amphetamines, and barbiturates.

Drug Development

- Preclinical research and development: 1 to 3 years for synthesis and animal screening. Preclinical testing evaluates new drugs for toxicities, pharmacokinetic properties, and potentially useful biological effects.
- Clinical research and development: 2 to 10 years with phases I to III. In phase I trials drugs are usually tested in normal volunteers, whereas in phases II and III drugs are tested in patients.
- New Drug Application (NDA) review: The time required is 2 months to 7 years, including submission and approval.
- Postmarketing monitoring: This stage is phase IV, in which the new drug is released for general use, permitting observation of its effects in a large population.
  - (+) Accepted for use: Through inspection, reports, surveys
  - (−) Rejected for use: Through sampling and testing

- *Schedule III:* Drugs and substances with less potential for abuse than those of Schedules I and II; therapeutic drugs accepted for treatment in the United States; other agents that may have low potential for physical dependence or high psychological dependence such as nalorphine, combinations of barbiturates, and therapeutic agents with reduced concentrations of morphine, codeine, or opium.
- *Schedule IV:* Drugs in use in the United States with lower potential for abuse than those in Schedule III and may have reduced potential for physical and psychological dependency than those listed in Schedule III such as chloral hydrate, meprobamate, diazepam, and pentazocine.
- *Schedule V:* Drugs in use in the United States with lower potential for abuse (physical or psychological dependency) than those listed in Schedule IV such as codeine dihydro-codeine, opium, or atropinics.

Orphan drugs are those drugs needed to treat diseases affecting fewer than 200,000 U.S. patients, and that fail to receive attention for development primarily because of cost and demand. The Federal Food, Drug and Cosmetic Act of 1938 was amended with the **Orphan Drug Act** of 1983, which gave incentives to develop drugs for rare diseases.

An **Investigational New Drug Application (IND)** is required for approval by the Center for Drug Evaluation and Research of the FDA, and must include specified information required by the Federal Food, Drug and Cosmetic Act. A new drug is:

- Any therapeutic agent to be used in humans to treat a disease

- Any combination of old and new therapeutic agents
- Any use of an approved drug for different therapeutic applications
- Any new dose forms
- Any drugs used as diagnostic agents to evaluate changes in diagnostic procedures or therapeutic treatments for disease in humans

Furthermore, the IND must contain *all* preclinical data (see Life Application: Drug Development).

Summary

- Pharmacology is an integrated medical science of drugs and is organized into several branches: pharmacodynamics, pharmacokinetics, pharmacotherapeutics, toxicology, and pharmacy.
- Because all drugs are poisons the understanding of their nomenclature is essential in order to safely identify the correct drug for the correct use. Therapeutic chemicals are classified into nonprescription and prescription drugs, all of which have chemical, generic, and proprietary (or trade) names.
- Drugs can be administered enterally (via the digestive system) or parenterally (other than via the digestive system).
- After administration it is essential that a drug reach its site of action; therefore the drug must be dissolved in a bodily fluid and pass through biological barriers, before it can get to the cellular site of action. This involves absorption and drug distribution by the body.
- The metabolism of drugs by the body is referred to as biotransformation, which is divided into phase I and phase II reactions. The liver plays the major role in drug metabolism, but the lungs, kidneys, and adrenal glands are also involved.
- Drug clearance follows biotransformation and drugs are excreted primarily by the kidneys through urine formation via glomerular filtration, reabsorption, and tubular secretion.
- Drug administration evokes a series of responses by the human body. The factors affecting these responses include dose, time, variability, biotransformation, and toxicity.
- Dose and time response are determined by the amount of drug given, the time since administration, and the frequency of drug administration. These responses vary with age, gender, and species.
- Toxic or adverse/undesired drug effects are classified as acute, subacute, or chronic, depending on the reaction to the drug.
- Development of new drugs is an extensive process involving research and development, review of new drug application, and postmarketing monitoring, which results in the acceptance or denial of the drug by the FDA.

Review Questions

1. The branch of pharmacology that addresses drug amounts at various sites in the body after drug administration is called:
   a. Pharmacodynamics
   b. Pharmacokinetics
   c. Pharmacotherapeutics
   d. Pharmacy

2. The generic name of a drug refers to its _____ name.
   a. Trade
   b. Proprietary
   c. Chemical
   d. Nonproprietary

3. For a drug to have an almost immediate systemic effect it is usually applied:
   a. On the skin
   b. By inhalation
   c. Rectally
   d. Iontophoretically

4. The decrease in blood clotting by heparin occurs at which general site of action?
   a. Cellular
   b. Extracellular
   c. Neuromuscular
   d. Intracellular

5. Which of the following is a phase I reaction in biotransformation?
   a. Oxidation
   b. Conjugation
   c. Acetylation
   d. Glucuronidation

6. All of the following are ways the kidney can use to achieve urine formation and drug clearance *except*:
   a. Glomerular filtration
   b. Tubular secretion
   c. Tubular filtration
   d. Tubular reabsorption

7. Which of the following is used in the determination of a drug dose response?
   a. Time of administration
   b. Onset of drug effect
   c. Normal frequency distribution
   d. Peak effect time

8. When the drug receptors are maximally activated, this is referred to as the
   a. Threshold level
   b. Peak effect
   c. Cessation effect
   d. Latency time

9. A subacute toxic effect occurs when the adverse drug effect occurs
   a. After 5 minutes of exposure
   b. After 24 hours of exposure
   c. After repeated exposure for days
   d. Over months to years of exposure

10. The specific antidote to botulinum toxin is:
    a. Sodium bicarbonate
    b. Antitoxin
    c. Pralidoxime
    d. Naloxone

11. The body's metabolism of drugs is called _____.

12. The study of the body's response to poisons and their harmful effect is referred to as _____.

13. Drug administration, absorption, distribution, and clearance are collectively called _____.

14. The ED_{50} is a measure of the _____ response.

15. The federal agency that approves the use of a specific drug is the _____.

16. Name and describe five different branches of pharmacology.

17. Compare and contrast dose and time response.

18. Describe five variables that influence drug response.

19. Compare and contrast nonspecific and specific treatments of suspected poisoning.

20. Discuss the public safety measures that need to be taken before a drug is approved.

Bibliography

Clayton BD, Stock YN, Harroun RD: *Basic pharmacology for nurses*, St. Louis, 2007, Mosby/Elsevier.

Hardman JG, Limbird LE, Gilman AG: *Goodman and Gilman's The pharmacological basis of therapeutics*, ed 10, New York, 2001, McGraw-Hill.

Lehne RA: *Pharmacology for nursing care*, St. Louis, 2007, Elsevier/Saunders.

Minneman KP, Wecker L: *Brody's human pharmacology*, St. Louis, 2005, Elsevier/Mosby.

Walsh CT, Schwartz-Bloom RD: *Levine's pharmacology: drug actions and reactions*, ed 7, New York, 2005, Taylor & Francis.

Internet Resources

National Center for Complementary and Alternative Medicine, http://nccam.nih.gov/health/supplement-safety/

MayoClinic.com, Food and Nutrition, Herbal supplements: What to know before you buy, http://www.mayoclinic.com/health/herbal-supplements/SA00044

Coates A, Hu Y, Bax R, et al: *The future challenges facing the development of new antimicrobial drugs*, Nature Reviews Drug Discovery 1:895-910, November 2002 | doi:10.1038/nrd940, http://www.nature.com/nrd/journal/v1/n11/abs/nrd940.html

World Health Organization, Drug Resistance, http://www.who.int/drugresistance/en/

National Institute of Allergy and Infectious Diseases, Antimicrobial (Drug) Resistance, http://www.niaid.nih.gov/factsheets/antimicro.htm

22

Antimicrobial Drugs

[OUTLINE

Mechanisms of Antimicrobial Action
Inhibition of Cell Wall Synthesis
Inhibition of Protein Synthesis
Inhibition of Nucleic Acid Synthesis
Disruption of Plasma Membrane
Inhibition of Metabolic Pathways

Characteristics of Antimicrobial Drugs
Spectrum of Action
Determination of Antibiotic Effectiveness: Efficacy
Side Effects

Resistance to Antimicrobial Drugs
Development/Acquisition of Drug Resistance
Mechanisms of Resistance
Multiple Resistances
Preventing Drug Resistance

Specific Antimicrobial Drugs
Antibacterial Agents
Antiviral Agents
Antifungal Agents
Antiprotozoan Agents
Antihelminthic Agents

[LEARNING OBJECTIVES

- Discuss the general goal of antimicrobial drug actions
- Describe the five basic categories of mechanisms used by antimicrobial drugs
- Explain the various spectra of activity for antimicrobial drugs
- Name and describe factors that need to be considered in selecting an antimicrobial drug
- Explain the therapeutic index and discuss possible side effects associated with antimicrobial therapy
- Discuss the development of drug resistance by microorganisms
- Explain the mechanisms leading to drug resistance, including the development of multiple resistances
- Describe how drug resistance can be controlled
- Name and describe the actions of antibacterial, antiviral, antiprotozoan, and antihelminthic agents

WHY YOU NEED TO KNOW

HISTORY

An antibiotic is a drug, produced by a microorganism, that may be used to inhibit or destroy another microbe when administered at appropriate therapeutic doses that limit harmful effects to the patient. As early as 1877, Louis Pasteur and J.L. Joubert described the competition between microbes and proposed that additional research be undertaken to explore their therapeutic uses.

The term "antibiotic" was coined in 1899 and used to describe this competitive interaction. In 1929, Alexander Fleming (1881–1955) published his findings on the antibacterial properties of *Penicillium notatum*. H.W. Florey and E.B. Chastain, directing a team of investigators at Oxford, began experiments designed to reveal details of the systemic chemical interactions of penicillin. The results of their early work were published in 1940 and this generated interest in the field and promoted work on other antibiotics that might be useful in cases where penicillin was not.

Gerhard Domagk was born in 1895 in Lagow, Brandenburg, which was then part of Germany but now is in Poland. His medical education was interrupted by World War I, but he later completed his studies and the degree was awarded in 1921.

While working on dyes at the I.G. Farbenindustrie he discovered that sulfamidochrysoidine (Prontosil) and Prontosil Red, if injected into mice previously given lethal doses of *Streptococcus* spp., allowed the mice to survive with few or no detrimental side effects. And in 1935, when his daughter became infected with a virulent strain of *Streptococcus*, he gave her Prontosil in doses based on his laboratory results in mice! She recovered and the news triggered a worldwide sensation. In 1939, Domagk was awarded the Nobel Prize in Physiology or Medicine. After initially accepting the award, he was forced to refuse it by the policies of Adolph Hitler. In 1947, after World War II, he accepted the award.

IMPACT

This was the first successful use of a synthetic drug as an antibiotic, originally determined by D. Bovet, in a series of structure–activity relationship (SAR) studies, to be a sulfonamide—a small part of the Prontosil molecule. Bovet's results led to the development of "sulfa" drugs such as sulfanilamide, sulfathiazole, and sulfadiazine as cures for infectious diseases.

However, the success of natural, semisynthetic, and synthetic antibiotics as effective cures has led to their overuse and subsequent emerging problems of drug resistance in humans.

FUTURE

Although overuse of antibiotics by humans has led to our own drug resistance problems, their overuse in agriculture is promoting drug resistance in microbes in that arena as well. Therefore, the need for new antimicrobial drugs is great because of the emergence of multidrug-resistant pathogens, the rapid emergence of new infections, and the potential use of multidrug-resistant microbes as bioweapons. In addition, diagnosis of microbial infections needs to be improved at many levels including new diagnostic tests to facilitate or withdraw antimicrobial therapy immediately after the onset of symptoms.

Mechanisms of Antimicrobial Action

The general goal of any antimicrobial agent is to disrupt the metabolism or structure of an organism to such a point that it can no longer survive or reproduce. The organisms can thus be affected in two different ways: by **microbicidal** action or by **microbiostatic** action. Microbicidal action simply kills the microorganism whereas microbiostatic action reversibly inhibits growth. If the antimicrobial agent is microbiostatic, once it is removed the microorganism will usually recover and grow again normally. Factors that can influence the effectiveness of either type of antimicrobial action include the concentration of the agent as well as the type and nature of the target organisms. An agent that may be microbicidal at a certain concentration may only be microbiostatic at lower levels and one that is lethal to one type of organism may only inhibit another (see Dose Effects in Chapter 21, Pharmacology). The effectiveness of microbiostatic agents may also be dependent on external factors such as the host's own immune system. Because this agent does not directly destroy the target pathogen, the infection must

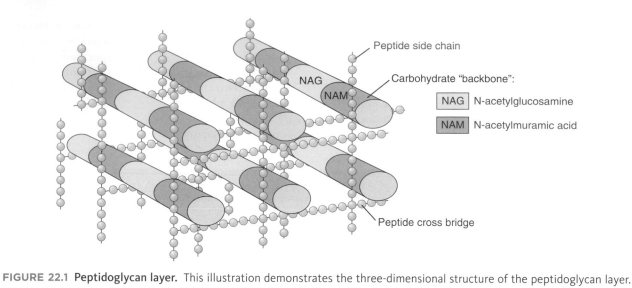

FIGURE 22.1 Peptidoglycan layer. This illustration demonstrates the three-dimensional structure of the peptidoglycan layer.

ultimately be eliminated by the host's own defensive mechanisms.

Regardless of the final result, antimicrobial agents use a number of different mechanisms of action to either kill or inhibit microbial growth. These mechanisms are varied and can target highly specific structures or metabolic functions necessary for the survival of the microorganism. Because of the diversity of microorganisms, which include not only the bacteria but also viruses, fungi, protozoans, and helminths, the variety of agents to control them is equally diverse. Despite the diversity of specific target microorganisms, the general metabolic/structural targets affected are in many cases shared by most antimicrobial agents. Regardless of the target organism, the mechanisms of action can be divided into five basic categories:

1. Cell wall synthesis inhibition
2. Protein synthesis inhibition
3. Nucleic acid synthesis inhibition
4. Cell membrane disruption
5. Metabolic antagonism/disruption

Inhibition of Cell Wall Synthesis

As discussed in Chapter 3 (Cell Structure and Function) and Chapter 6 (Bacteria and Archaea), most bacterial cells contain a rigid cell wall composed of peptidoglycan, which protects the cell from rupturing in hypotonic environments. Young, growing cells must constantly synthesize new peptidoglycan and transport it to the wall (Figure 22.1). Agents such as penicillins and cephalosporins chemically react with the enzymes responsible for completing the peptidoglycan layer, thus preventing the assembly process. This disruption may occur at numerous different sites in the layer and at different points in the process, but in all cases it causes weaknesses at growth points in the layer, which in turn renders the cell vulnerable to lysis. In a hypotonic environment, water then enters the cell and eventually causes it to burst.

Inhibition of Protein Synthesis

Most of the agents that inhibit protein synthesis involve disrupting the process of translation (see Chapter 3, Cell Structure and Function) at the ribosome–mRNA complex (Figure 22.2). The ribosomes of eukaryotic cells are structurally different from those of prokaryotic cells, and because of this human cells are usually not affected by the inhibitory action of these agents because they selectively act against bacteria. The specific chemical reactions that disrupt the translation of the mRNA vary and include the following:

- Prevention of the initiation of synthesis
- Blocking of the formation of peptide bonds between amino acids on the transfer RNAs (tRNAs)
- Prevention of ribosome translocation along the mRNA strand

Whatever the specific point of attack, the result is the same: inhibition of the synthesis of necessary proteins. Antimicrobial agents that affect bacterial protein synthesis include tetracyclines, chloramphenicol, macrolides, and others.

Inhibition of Nucleic Acid Synthesis

The metabolic process involved in the synthesis of DNA and RNA is a long and complex series of enzyme-catalyzed reactions (see Chapter 3, Cell Structure and Function). The complexity of the process lends itself to disruption at many points along the way and inhibition at any point can block subsequent events in the pathway. As with the other mechanisms the specific target within the process is often dependent on the specific antimicrobial agent being used, but the end result is the same no matter where the point of attack is—disruption of the synthesis of nucleic acids. The interference with nucleic acid synthesis by an antimicrobial drug can be due to:

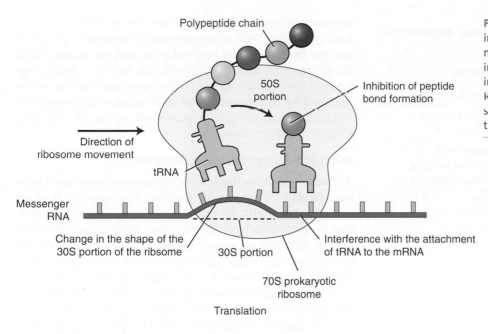

FIGURE 22.2 Inhibition of translation. The inhibition of translation can occur at a number of points, including the following: inhibition of peptide bond formation, interference with the attachment of transfer RNA (tRNA) to mRNA, and changing of the shape of the ribosome, thereby preventing translocation along the mRNA strand.

Labels in figure:
- Polypeptide chain
- 50S portion
- Inhibition of peptide bond formation
- Direction of ribosome movement
- tRNA
- Messenger RNA
- Change in the shape of the 30S portion of the ribsome
- 30S portion
- Interference with the attachment of tRNA to the mRNA
- 70S prokaryotic ribosome
- Translation

- Disruption of synthesis of the nucleotide component
- Inhibition of DNA replication
- Interference with transcription of the RNA

An interesting type of mechanism that is employed by sulfonamides and trimethoprim involves mimicking the normal substrate of an enzyme in a process called **competitive inhibition.** When these agents are supplied to the cell in high concentrations they will substitute for the true substrate of an important enzyme, thus preventing the enzyme from producing a needed product and causing the metabolism of the cell to slow or stop.

Disruption of Plasma Membrane

Damage to the cell membrane is a form of catastrophic damage for any cell. Not only can it affect the transport of substances required for metabolism both in and out of the cell, it is a major factor in the maintenance of the cell's physical integrity. Most membrane–disrupting agents target the different types of lipids in the cell membrane, which lends to their specificity for a particular microbial group. Because all microorganisms (except for viruses) share the same basic plasma membrane structure, these agents are useful against both bacteria and fungi. Unfortunately, they can also be toxic to human cells.

Antibiotics, specifically polypeptides such as polymyxin B, adversely affect the membrane permeability of microbial cells, resulting in a loss of important metabolites. Antifungal drugs that disrupt fungal plasma membranes include nystatin, miconazole, ketoconazole, and amphotericin B.

Inhibition of Metabolic Pathways

Antimicrobial agents not only are able to disrupt the metabolic pathways involved in the synthesis of proteins and nucleic acids, but can affect numerous cellular metabolic processes that can lead to cell death. Disruption of crucial enzyme activity/production as well as blocking the synthesis of other essential metabolic compounds such as NAD or folic acid can be catastrophic to the overall metabolism of any cell, thus allowing use of these agents against a wide variety of microorganisms. The sulfonamides (sulfa drugs) and trimethoprim are broad-spectrum antimicrobial drugs that disrupt the synthesis of tetrahydrofolic acid, a precursor to nucleic acids, necessary for microbial metabolism.

Characteristics of Antimicrobial Agents

Almost all antimicrobial agents share a set of common characteristics that are important to remember when selecting a drug for treatment. These characteristics provide a great deal of information regarding how the agents work, and in some cases why they don't work, in the treatment of an infection. These characteristics of an antimicrobial agent include the following:

- Its selective toxicity
- Whether it is microbicidal rather than microbiostatic
- How readily and easily the agent may be delivered to the site of infection
- Whether it is readily soluble in body fluids and will maintain its potency long enough to be effective
- How long the agent remains active in the body
- The degree of antimicrobial resistance to the agent
- Whether it complements or aids in host body defenses
- Is it nonallergenic?
- Does it have a long shelf life?
- Is it affordable/available to all patients who might need it?

TABLE 22.1 Spectrum of Activity of Some Antimicrobial Drugs

Drug	Activity against:
Penicillin G	Gram-positive bacteria
Streptomycin	Gram-negative bacteria, mycobacteria
Tetracycline	Gram-negative bacteria, gram-positive bacteria, chlamydias, rickettsias
Isoniazid	Mycobacteria
Acyclovir	Viruses
Ketoconazole	Fungi
Mefloquine (malaria)	Protozoans
Niclosamide (tapeworms)	Helminths
Biltricide (flukes)	Helminths

Spectrum of Action

Most antimicrobial drugs do not inhibit the growth of all pathogens. Antimicrobial drugs have a **spectrum of activity,** which is the range of pathogen types against which a given drug is effective (Table 22.1). On the basis of the spectrum of activity, drugs can be classified as antimicrobials with a broad spectrum of activity and those that have a narrow spectrum of activity.

- Drugs with a **broad spectrum** of activity are effective against a large variety of microorganisms. An example would be the sulfonamides, which are effective against both gram-positive and gram-negative bacteria, actinomycetes, chlamydias, and some protozoans. These drugs exert their effects on all cell components of the microbes. An advantage of using broad-spectrum antibiotics is the high possibility of efficacy against an unidentified pathogen. The disadvantage of using such a drug is the likelihood of also destroying the normal flora (see Chapter 9, Infection and Disease). Destruction of the normal flora can lead to disease if one organism of the normal flora is replaced by a pathogen. This then leads to what is referred to as a **superinfection.**
- Drugs with a **narrow spectrum** of activity, such as isoniazid and penicillin G, are effective only against a relatively small number of microbes, and generally avoid destruction of the normal flora. They target a specific component that is present only in certain bacteria.
- Drugs with a **medium spectrum** of activity are effective against some gram-positive and gram-negative bacteria, but not all of them.

Selective Toxicity

An ideal antimicrobial drug will kill harmful microorganisms without significant damage to the host. This principle is referred to as **selective toxicity.** The differences in structure and/or metabolism between the microbe and the host make selective toxicity possible. With greater differences between the pathogen and the host it is easier to develop an effective antimicrobial drug. Regarding toxicity, it is preferable to have a wide range between the toxic dosage level, which can cause damage to the host, and the therapeutic dosage level, which will eliminate the infectious pathogen over a prescribed period of time (see Chapter 21, Pharmacology).

Microbicidal versus Microbiostatic

Antimicrobial drugs that kill microorganisms are referred to as **bactericidal;** if they prevent microbes from growing they are called **bacteriostatic.** Ideally the drug being used would eliminate the pathogens by destroying them. Inhibition of microbial growth does not necessarily eliminate the pathogens already present and may require prolonged use of the drug to ensure that high-enough levels are maintained to keep populations from recovering and increasing. Because of the potential negative effects the drugs may have on the host, the use of a killing agent instead of an inhibitory one is not always a simple decision. Microbicidal agents can also kill natural flora in areas such as the healthy intestine, creating a potential digestion problem because the normal resident flora are vital to proper digestion. The destruction of the normal flora population anywhere in or on the body may also create an advantage for competing pathogens that would normally be kept in check by the resident population (superinfection).

Delivery to the Site of Infection

To be effective, drugs need to be easily and effectively delivered to the site of infection. Therefore, an important criterion for the effectiveness (**efficacy**) of a drug is its ability to cross biological barriers (see Chapter 21, Pharmacology). Potential barriers may be physiological, such as the lining of the body compartments and the blood–brain barrier, or those induced by inflammation and disease. Abscess walls, exudates, and necrotic material are classic examples of host reactions to pathogens and can impede the transport of drugs to the invading microorganisms.

Furthermore, if the antimicrobial drug is not sufficiently soluble or becomes too dilute once in solution, the effectiveness of the drug is greatly diminished. In addition, if the means of delivery and/or transport of the agent does not efficiently and rapidly deliver the antibiotic to the site of infection, the drug will not have the opportunity to fight the pathogen even if it is in solution and in the correct concentration. For example, some agents are effective against a particular infection but are not lipid soluble. Therefore, these compounds are not able to cross the blood–brain barrier, rendering them ineffective against an infection in the central nervous system, such as meningitis. Whereas most antibiotics cannot cross the blood–brain barrier, some third-generation cephalosporins (cefotaxime, ceftizoxime, and ceftriaxone) and metronidazole can.

Time of Activity

It is desirable for an antimicrobial drug to be active over a long period of time for an optimal effect. As covered in Chapter 21 (Pharmacology), the duration of action time is a major consideration when evaluating the overall effect of a drug on an infection/pathogen. If the destruction of a population of pathogens requires a sustained concentration of agent over a specified period of time, any shortening of this time may significantly decrease the effectiveness of the treatment. By subjecting the organisms to the agent for a time that proves to be nonlethal to many of them, the risk of producing a resistant population is increased.

Not Subject to Antimicrobial Resistance

The ideal antimicrobial drug is an agent that is not subject to the development of antimicrobial resistance. If the nature of the agent and its mechanism is such that populations of pathogens are less likely to develop resistance to the agent, its effectiveness and scope of use would be dramatically increased. Because of microbial genetic mutations as well as the acquisition of resistance genes from other cells, viruses, and the environment; it is difficult to develop an antibiotic against which microbes will not eventually develop some resistance (see Resistance to Antimicrobial Drugs).

Complements/Aids in Host's Own Defenses

The natural defenses of a host, including barriers at portals of entry, protective cells and environments within the host, and an acquired immune system (both active and passive), do an excellent job in fighting off infections in the healthy host (see Chapter 20, The Immune System). When these layers of defense are compromised, antimicrobial drugs need to be administered in order to aid the immune system. Any time a foreign substance is introduced into a host there is a risk of upsetting this complex balance of defenses and actually inhibiting the body's natural response to pathogens. For example, if an antibiotic harms an organ or system it may adversely affect the natural defenses of the host, causing such things as excessive damage to the kidneys.

Nonallergenic

Certain antimicrobial agents are capable of inducing a hypersensitivity reaction (Chapter 20, The Immune System) in certain individuals. Patients with allergies to specific agents such as penicillin must be careful to inform medical personnel about their allergy, or the shock that may result from receiving penicillin could be fatal.

Stable with Long Shelf Life

Ideally, an antibiotic should remain chemically stable, thus ensuring the safety and efficacy of the product over a given period of time. The longer the shelf life, the more easily the agent can be stored and made immediately available for use. In addition to the logistical and economic advantages of a long shelf life there may also be a safety consideration: chemical degradation could result in antibiotics with low potency or in chemical products of degradation that may be toxic.

Affordability and Availability

It is obvious that even the most effective agents will not be useful if the product is not widely available to patients in need and, once available, it is also important that the product be affordable.

Determination of Antibiotic Effectiveness: Efficacy

Microorganisms vary dramatically in their susceptibility to different antibiotics. In addition, the susceptibility of a microorganism can change under certain conditions over a period of time. This change can even occur during treatment with a specific drug. Although broad-spectrum antibiotics can be used against a number of different organisms that may be causing an infection, it is more effective to identify the specific pathogen responsible and then to target that organism with a specific antibiotic. There are a number of tests currently in use to determine the most effective antimicrobial against a specific organism, and they include the following:

- The disk diffusion or Kirby-Bauer method
- The dilution or minimal inhibitory concentration (MIC) method
- The serum killing power method

Sometimes two different antibiotics may be given together to achieve a therapeutic effect that is greater than when the drugs are given alone. This phenomenon is referred to as **synergism.** On the other hand, drug combinations may result in **antagonism,** meaning that the drug combination is less effective than when the drugs are administered alone.

Disk Diffusion or Kirby-Bauer Method

In the disk diffusion or Kirby-Bauer method a culture of the pathogen is uniformly spread over the entire surface of an agar plate, using the spread plate method, or in a modified streak pattern, using a sterile swab to literally paint the surface of the plate. Paper filter disks impregnated with specific concentrations of selected antibiotics are then evenly spaced on the agar surface. The inoculated plate with disks is then incubated. As they are incubated the antibiotic in each disk begins to diffuse into the agar. If the antibiotic affects the growth of the organism that has been spread on the surface this will be evident as a clear area of no growth surrounding the disk (Figure 22.3). This area is called a **zone of inhibition** because it delineates the area where the diffused antibiotic inhibited growth of the organism. Because larger molecules diffuse into the agar at a slower rate than smaller molecules, the size of the zone of inhibition is not necessarily a measure of effectiveness. Standard zone diameters have been established for each concentration of antibiotic, as well as approximate number of cells plated on the specific medium being used. The diameter of each individual zone can then be measured and evaluated in order to determine whether the organism is sensitive or resistant to the antibiotic.

Although an effective tool, this method has some shortcomings when being used to find the most effective agent with which to treat an infection. If the organisms causing the infection need to be killed and not just inhibited, this method will not necessarily identify a microbicidal agent. Another potential problem lies in the fact that drugs may act quite differently *in vivo* (in a living organism) than *in vitro* (in a laboratory vessel, such as a Petri plate). Some metabolic processes in the body may inactivate or interfere with the action of the antibiotic and

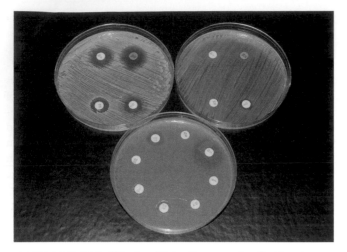

FIGURE 22.3 Disk diffusion (Kirby-Bauer method). The clear areas surrounding the antibiotic disks are called the *zones of inhibition*. The size of these zones can be used to determine the effectiveness of the antibiotic against the selected bacterium.

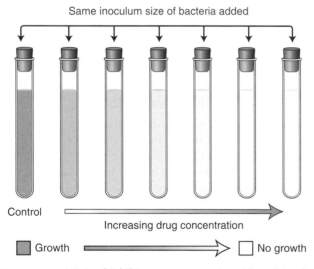

Same inoculum size of bacteria added

Control

Increasing drug concentration

☐ Growth ⟶ ☐ No growth

FIGURE 22.4 Minimal inhibitory concentration. The minimal inhibitory concentration (MIC) for a specific agent is indicated by the absence of growth in the tube containing the lowest drug concentration.

in some cases the antibiotic itself may be harmful to the body systems of the host.

Dilution/Minimal Inhibitory Concentration Method

In the dilution/minimal inhibitory concentration method a given quantity of the pathogen culture is added to a series of tubes containing decreasing concentrations of a specific antibiotic. The tubes are then incubated and examined for growth. Turbidity (cloudiness) indicates bacterial growth; lack of turbidity signifies that bacterial growth is either inhibited or the organisms have been killed by the antimicrobial agent (Figure 22.4). The goal is to identify the tube with the lowest concentration of drug that inhibits visible growth. This concentration is referred to as the **minimal inhibitory concentration** (MIC) for a specific agent acting on a selected microorganism. In the past

this test was performed in individual test tubes. However, kits are now available wherein the test is performed in shallow wells on standard testing plates. This test is widely used in hospitals and clinics today; however, there are also shortcomings with this method. As with the Kirby-Bauer method, the basic test procedure will not indicate whether an antibiotic is microbicidal or microbiostatic. A second test using this method can be added to determine whether the organisms are being inhibited or killed. In this test a sample from the tube with the lowest concentration showing no growth is subcultured in order to see whether there are any organisms still surviving in the tube. This lowest concentration containing no living organisms is called the **minimal bactericidal concentration** (MBC).

Serum Killing Power

In the serum killing power method a sample of a patient's blood is obtained while they are receiving an antibiotic. The blood is then processed to extract the serum, which will contain the drugs that are in the bloodstream. A bacterial suspension is then added to a measured quantity of the patient's serum. If the bacteria grow in the tube of serum this indicates that the antibiotic is ineffective, whereas no growth indicates it is effective. Using serial dilutions, the lowest concentration that still provides effective serum killing power can be easily determined.

Side Effects

All drugs are potential poisons (see Chapter 21, Pharmacology) and the administration of therapeutic drugs can possibly lead to side effects that can be potentially serious. Drugs can adversely affect the liver (hepatotoxic), kidneys (nephrotoxic), gastrointestinal tract, cardiovascular system, red bone marrow (hemotoxic), nervous system (neurotoxic), respiratory system, integument, bones, and teeth. The administration of drugs involves a previous assessment of the risks and benefits. This type of assessment is referred to as the **therapeutic index** (see Chapter 21).

The liver is responsible for the metabolism and detoxification of chemical substances in the blood. Liver damage can occur due to a drug or its metabolic by-products. The kidneys are in charge of the excretion of drugs and drug metabolites. Both drugs and their metabolic by-products have the potential to damage the structures of the nephron and therefore are capable of interfering with the filtration and reabsorption ability of the nephron.

One of the most common side effects to antimicrobial therapy is diarrhea, which may progress to severe intestinal irritation and colitis. Most often these irritations occur because of disruption of the normal intestinal flora. The organisms in the normal flora of the skin, intestine, urogenital tract, and oral cavity are with a few exceptions harmless and also prevent the colonization of potentially harmful organisms. However, with the use of broad-spectrum antibiotics these harmless microbes can be destroyed, allowing resistant organisms to overgrow, resulting in a superinfection.

For example, the use of a broad-spectrum cephalosporin for the treatment of *Escherichia coli*–induced urinary tract infections can also destroy lactobacilli in the vagina. Lactobacilli and *Candida albicans* are both part of the normal vaginal flora. *Lactobacillus* will be killed by the broad-spectrum antibiotic, allowing *Candida albicans* to flourish and cause a yeast infection. Similar superinfections by *Candida* can also occur in the oral cavity (thrush) and the large intestine.

Antibiotic-associated colitis, a serious and potentially fatal condition, can be caused by oral administration of:

- Tetracyclines
- Clindamycin
- Broad-spectrum penicillins
- Cephalosporins

The condition is a result of the overgrowth of *Clostridium difficile,* an antibiotic-resistant and endospore-forming bacterium. The organism invades the intestinal mucosa, where it releases toxins (enterotoxins) that result in diarrhea, fever, and abdominal pain. Other drug-induced side effects may involve the skin, either because of an allergic reaction or by interaction of the drugs with sunlight, causing photodermatitis.

The antibiotic tetracycline is contraindicated in children from birth to 8 years of age, because the drug causes permanent discoloration of tooth enamel in this age group. The drug also should be avoided during pregnancy because of its capacity to cross the placenta, followed by its deposition in the developing fetal bones and teeth.

Certain antiparasitic drugs are potentially toxic to the heart, causing irregular heartbeat and in severe cases even cardiac arrest. Other antimicrobial drugs can directly affect the brain, resulting in seizures. Aminoglycosides and some other antimicrobials can cause nerve damage resulting in dizziness, deafness, and motor and sensory disorders.

When using different drugs at the same time, toxic effects can occur that do not come about when the drugs are given alone. Another possibility is that one drug can potentially neutralize another. For example, it has been reported that certain antibiotics can neutralize the effect of contraceptive pills.

Another example of an unwanted side effect is when an individual develops a hypersensitivity (allergic) reaction. Allergic reactions have been reported for most antimicrobial drugs, with penicillin accounting for the majority of antimicrobial drug–induced allergies, followed by sulfonamides. Individuals allergic to these drugs become sensitized during the first exposure, not showing any symptoms. After sensitizing the immune system, a second exposure will result in hives, respiratory problems, and occasionally anaphylaxis that may become fatal (see Hypersensitivity Reactions in Chapter 20, The Immune System). For pregnant women the U.S. Food and Drug Administration (FDA) has identified and classified antibiotics that present no evidence of risk to the fetus.

Resistance to Antimicrobial Drugs

One of the major challenges in healthcare today is the problem caused by bacteria that are already resistant to antimicrobial drugs as well as those that are acquiring resistance at an alarming rate. The evolution of bacteria toward antibiotic resistance, including multidrug resistance, represents an aspect of the general evolution of bacteria and most likely cannot be stopped. Bacterial drug resistance goes beyond the traditional evolutionary mechanisms, because bacteria can pass on drug resistance without having to inherit it. This process occurs via plasmids, the nonchromosomal DNA of bacteria (see Genetics in Chapter 6, Bacteria and Archaea). Furthermore, these plasmids can also be transferred to different species of microorganisms.

Development/Acquisition of Drug Resistance

Resistance of a microorganism to an antibiotic means that the organism is no longer susceptible to the agent's effects as it had previously been. The development of resistant organisms is a special problem when developing and prescribing microbiostatic agents that are specifically designed not to kill the microbes but just to inhibit their growth.

Microorganisms and specifically bacteria usually acquire their resistance by changes in their genetics, but there are also nongenetic mechanisms that can contribute to resistance. One of these nongenetic means of resistance is a method known as evasion, and is as simple as the pathogens infecting tissue that is out of reach of specific antimicrobial agents (such as the blood–brain barrier). Another method involves alteration of the cell wall into the L-form, (a form of bacterial cell without a developed cell wall), thus modifying the wall enough to prevent antibiotics from attacking the cell wall.

Genetic resistance to antibiotics involves changes in the genes of the microorganisms followed by natural selection favoring these organisms. Those mutations that result in a resistant organism can quickly increase their frequency in a population because many microorganisms have a relatively short generation time and they have a potential survival advantage over organisms that do not have resistance to an antibiotic. The antibiotics themselves do not induce genetic mutations but they instead create a chemical environment that will greatly favor the growth of microbes that have in fact mutated and are resistant.

Any large population of microorganisms, especially bacteria, contains a few cells that are already resistant due to prior transfer of plasmids or by mutation. When the drug is not present in the environment the resistant forms will remain small in numbers, but when the drug is administered, the nonresistant organisms will die and the resistant ones will flourish and multiply (Figure 22.5). This natural selection of drug-resistant forms is common and takes place in a variety of natural habitats, laboratories, and medical environments, as well as in individuals during drug therapy.

In addition to underuse or misuse of antimicrobials, poor patient compliance also adds to the development of resistant strains. The use of antimicrobials for any infection, in any dose, and over any time period, forces microorganisms to adapt or die. This phenomenon is known as **selective pressure** and the organisms that adapt and survive will pass on the resistant gene.

Mechanisms of Resistance

Once a mutation occurs in bacteria that results in a resistance gene or genes, there are a number of natural mechanisms that

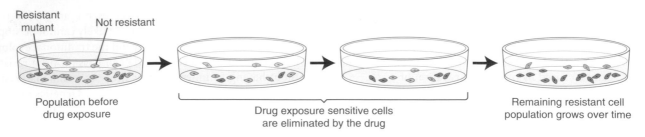

Resistant mutant   Not resistant

Population before drug exposure

Drug exposure sensitive cells are eliminated by the drug

Remaining resistant cell population grows over time

FIGURE 22.5 Acquisition of drug resistance. As drug exposure increases nonresistant cells are eliminated, eventually producing a population consisting only of resistant cells.

can allow the resistance genes to be acquired by nonresistant organisms. The three mechanisms are transduction, transformation, and conjugation (see Chapter 3, Cell Structure and Function). Some cells contain resistance genes on a plasmid called a *resistance* or *R plasmid* and may contain as many as six or seven genes, each of which may confer resistance against a number of different antibiotics. Even plasmids can be transferred from one strain or species to another, widening the distribution of the resistance genes even further. These resistance genes confer a variety of different mechanisms of resistance to the microorganisms that possess them.

Several basic mechanisms have been identified and include the following: change in membrane permeability, increased drug elimination, change in the target of the agent (drug receptors), change in some part of the microbial metabolic pathway, change in a previously inhibited enzyme, and the development of enzymes that can destroy or inactivate antimicrobial agents.

- *Change in membrane permeability:* Changes in the proteins of the plasma membrane interfere with the transport mechanisms and this may prevent some antibiotics from crossing the membrane to enter the cell.
- *Increased drug elimination:* Resistance to tetracycline can arise through plasmid-encoded proteins that pump the drug out of the cell. Aminoglycoside resistance develops through changes in drug permeability caused by point mutation, affecting proteins in the membrane transport system. Many bacteria have multidrug-resistant pumps capable of actively transporting chemicals, including drugs, out of the cell. These protein pumps are encoded in plasmids or chromosomes; they are not selective and are capable of removing a variety of antimicrobial drugs, detergents, and other substances toxic to the microbe.
- *Change in the target (receptor) of the agent:* The majority of antimicrobial drugs act on a specific target (receptor) such as a protein, RNA, DNA, or a structure within the plasma membranes. Microbes can avoid attack by antimicrobials by altering the drug target. In other words a change in the DNA can occur and a protein important to the functioning of the target site is altered and antibiotics can no longer bind to and disrupt this target protein. For example, bacteria can become resistant to aminoglycosides by changing ribosomal binding sites. Alterations of binding sites in the cell wall of a bacterium can result in

resistance to penicillin by *Streptococcus pneumoniae* and methicillin by *Staphylococcus aureus*. Some enterococci have developed resistance to vancomycin by a similar mechanism.

- *Change in a metabolic pathway:* Microbes can develop an alternative metabolic pathway or enzyme that allows the bypassing of a metabolic reaction that could be inhibited by an antibiotic.
- *Change in a previously inhibited enzyme:* Modifying an enzyme that was previously being inhibited may prevent a reaction or series of reactions in a bacterial cell. With modification of the enzyme this inhibition by the antibiotic may be prevented and the reactions may occur unhampered.
- *Development of defensive enzymes:* Bacterial enzymes may be developed that are capable of destroying or inactivating antibiotics before they can act on the bacterial cell. A prominent example of this mechanism is the production of β-lactamase, that is, penicillinase, by some bacteria, which breaks the β-lactam ring in penicillin and destroys its effectiveness. Another β-lactamase, cephaloporinase, disrupts the structure of cephalosporin molecules.

Multiple Resistances

Antimicrobial resistance is a global problem. Historically, antimicrobials were regarded as wonder drugs and have been inappropriately used for infections that did not require the use of antibiotics. Furthermore, antibiotics often were not used for the appropriate length of time to ensure their bactericidal effect. Consequently, antibiotic-resistant bacterial strains emerged. For many years this resistance was overcome by the use of newer, more effective antibiotics. However, the development of new drugs has slowed down and multiple antimicrobial resistant (MAR) strains have emerged. The development of MAR is a serious concern in both human and animal communities as MAR compromises treatment and can potentially lead to increased morbidity and mortality.

The development of multiresistant strains occurs primarily in hospitals, nursing homes, and other healthcare facilities. In these environments the constant use of many different types of antimicrobial agents eliminates sensitive cells while encouraging the development of resistant cells. Multiple drug–resistant strains are often called *"superbugs"* and are usually resistant to three or more antimicrobial agents. At present, multiresistant organisms include strains from *Staphylococcus, Streptococcus, Enterococcus, Pseudomonas, Mycobacterium,* and the malaria-causing protozoan *Plasmodium.* In addition, resistance to only one type of drug unfortunately also may allow resistance to a similar drug by a phenomenon called **cross-resistance.**

Preventing Drug Resistance

Since the discovery of antibiotics and other antimicrobial drugs, they have been widely used for more than 50 years and over time microbes have developed resistance to many of the agents on the market. This resistance has been determined to be one of the world's most pressing public health problems. To prevent the spread of antimicrobial drug-resistant microbes and to minimize the evolution of antimicrobial resistance among pathogens the following guidelines should be considered:

- Healthcare professionals and providers should wash their hands thoroughly between patient visits.
- Physicians should not grant patients' demands for antibiotics when not warranted for the particular infection. Consumers should not demand antibiotics from a physician because the infection may be other than bacterial (e.g., common viral infections).
- Antibiotics when prescribed should target a narrow range of microbes whenever possible.
- Antibiotics may be used in combination in order to kill pathogens that are resistant to one antimicrobial but will be killed by the other (see synergism, discussed previously).
- Hospital and nursing home patients with multidrug-resistant infections should be isolated.

- Physicians should be familiar with local data on antibiotic resistance.
- Patients, when given antibiotics, should take them exactly as prescribed and complete the full course of the treatment to avoid the development of resistant strains.
- Antimicrobials should not be hoarded for later use. Leftover medication should be discarded after completion of the prescribed course of treatment.
- Individuals should not take antimicrobials that have been prescribed to someone else. This may lead to a delay in the correct treatment and also allow bacteria to multiply.
- Antimicrobial soaps and lotions should be used only when protecting a sick individual with a weakened immune system. This will:
  - Prevent disruption of the normal flora
  - Avoid selecting for resistance
  - Prevent the inadvertent selection of naturally resistant bacterial types, which may become emergent pathogens. The human immune system is generally effective at controlling the majority of microbes dominating the environment. The overuse of antimicrobial soaps/lotions may change the composition of microbes in the environment, allowing resistant strains to become dominant.

In 1996 the National Antimicrobial Resistance Monitoring System (NARMS) was implemented to track the emergence of any antimicrobial drug–resistant organisms and strains. Furthermore, the WHO Global Strategy for Containment of Antimicrobial Resistance provides a framework of action for effective containment at various levels.

Specific Antimicrobial Drugs

A great number of antimicrobial drugs are marketed in the United States. Drug companies market the drugs through physicians, and lately also directly to the consumer via television and Internet advertisements. Although a wide variety of commercial names are used, most of them are variants of a small number of drug families. However, different drug companies assign different trade names to the same generic drug (see Chapter 21, Pharmacology). Antimicrobials can be classified as antibacterial, antiviral, antifungal, antiprotozoan, and antihelminthic agents.

Antibacterial Agents

Antibacterial agents can be subdivided into natural antibiotics, semisynthetic drugs, and synthetic drugs.

- A *natural antibiotic* is a chemical substance that is produced by a microorganism and has the capacity to either destroy bacteria or inhibit their growth.
- A *semisynthetic antibiotic* drug is an antibiotic that has been chemically modified for greater efficacy.
- *Synthetic drugs* are agents produced in the laboratory rather than by a microorganism, but can act identically to antibiotics. Sulfonamides, trimethoprim, and quinolones are man-made drugs and therefore are not considered to be antibiotics, but synthetic antibacterial agents.

Synthetic Drugs

Sulfonamides, or sulfa drugs were the first antimicrobial agents that used the metabolic disruption mechanism successfully against bacteria. Since its discovery by Domagk (see "Why You Need to Know") many sulfonamides have been developed including sulfadoxine, sulfadimidine (short acting), sulfamethoxazole (intermediate acting), sulfametopyrazine (long acting), sulfasalazine (poor absorption by the gastrointestinal tract), and sulfamethoxazole in combination with trimethoprim. This group of antibacterial agents is manufactured synthetically The mechanism of action is to compete with a metabolic intermediate in the folic acid synthesis pathway in bacteria. Folic acid is essential to the synthesis of purines and pyrimidines, which are the bases used in the construction of nucleic acids and other cellular components in both bacteria and mammals (see Chapter 2 [Chemistry of Life] and Chapter 3 [Cell Structure and Function]). Sulfonamides are selectively toxic to bacteria, which must synthesize folic acid because they are unable to obtain it from the environment. In contrast, humans acquire folic acid from dietary sources; therefore the disruption of the folic acid synthesis pathway will not affect the host. The effectiveness of sulfonamides has been seeing some decline as more bacteria have been developing resistance. Mild to moderate side effects include nausea, vomiting, headache, and mental depression. Its use is also limited because of some allergenic reactions, which are experienced by about 5% of patients. These side effects may include rashes, fever, or hives.

Trimethoprim was introduced in 1969 as a combination with sulfonamides. The agent synergizes sulfonamide activity and minimizes bacterial resistance. Trimethoprim is chemically related to pyrimethamine, an antimalarial drug. Both agents are folate antagonists. Trimethoprim is given orally and is bacteriostatic against most common bacterial pathogens. Because sulfonamides inhibit the same bacterial metabolic pathway, they can potentiate the action of trimethoprim. Side effects of trimethoprim include nausea, vomiting, blood disorders, and skin rashes. Folate deficiency, a toxic effect of the drug, can be prevented by the administration of folinic acid.

Quinolones, also referred to as *fluoroquinolones,* are broad-spectrum synthetic drugs used to treat a wide variety of bacterial infections. Nalidixic acid was the first quinolone developed but a family of these drugs is being developed, such as ciprofloxacin and doxycycline, which have gained fame as the drugs of choice for treating anthrax. Quinolones are effective against both gram-negative and gram-positive bacteria and are used in treating urinary tract infections, sexually transmitted diseases, gastrointestinal infections, respiratory tract infections, skin infections, and osteomyelitis. The mechanism used by these agents is the disruption of nucleic acid synthesis through binding to the DNA gyrase complex. This enzyme complex is responsible for the unwinding of DNA for replication, repair, transcription, and other DNA cell processes. Quinolones are divided into generations based on their spectrum of activity. In general, the earlier generations have a narrower spectrum of activity than the later generations (Table 22.2). Some side effects may be experienced including gastrointestinal problems and, in some rare cases, seizures or other neural disturbances.

Antibiotic (Nonsynthetic) and Semisynthetic Antibacterials

Antibiotics are chemotherapeutic agents naturally produced by some microorganisms. Semisynthetic agents, on the other hand, are natural products that have been chemically modified in the laboratory to improve the effectiveness (efficacy) of the antibiotic, expand the spectrum of activity, reduce side effects, and decrease the development of drug resistance.

Penicillin, a natural product produced by the fungus *Penicillium chrysogenum,* was the first widely used antibiotic. The discovery of penicillin initiated the development of an extensive family of semisynthetic drugs. Penicillins G and V are the most broadly used natural forms of penicillin. The semisynthetics include drugs such as ampicillin and methicillin. Regardless of the derivative, the functional structure common to almost all is the β-lactam ring, which appears to be crucial to the activity of the molecule. The penicillins are effective against sensitive, gram-positive cocci as well as some gram-negative bacteria. Each member of the penicillin family of drugs each has a specific target, such as penicillin G, which is used against *Streptococcus* and *Staphylococcus,* or ampicillin, which has a broader spectrum of activity against a number of gram-negative bacteria. The mechanism used by the penicillins is the disruption of cell wall synthesis. Although the exact details of the process are

TABLE 22.2 Generations of Quinolones Based on Their Spectrum of Activity

Generation	Generic Name	Trade Name(s)
First generation	Cinoxacin	Cinobac
	Flumequine	Flubactin (veterinary use)
	Nalidixic acid	NegGam, Wintomylon
	Oxolinic acid	Cistopax
	Piromidic acid	Panacid
	Pipemidic acid	Dolcol
Second generation	Ciprofloxacin	Ciprobay, Cipro, Ciproxin
	Enoxacin	Enroxil, Penetrex
	Fleroxacin	Megalone (withdrawn)
	Lomefloxacin	Maxaquin
	Nadifloxacin	
	Norfloxacin	Lexinor, Noroxin, Quinabic, Janacin
	Ofloxacin	Floxin, Oxaldin, Tarivid
	Pefloxacin	
	Rufloxacin	Uroflox
Third generation	Balofloxacin	
	Grepafloxacin	Raxar (withdrawn)
	Levofloxacin	Cravit, Levaquin
	Pazufloxacin mesylate	
	Sparfloxacin	Zagam
	Temafloxacin	Omniflox (withdrawn)
	Tosufloxacin	
Fourth generation	Clinafloxacin	
	Gemifloxacin	Factive
	Moxifloxacin	Avelox
	Gatifloxacin	Tequin (withdrawn), Zymar
	Sitafloxacin	
	Trovafloxacin	Trovan (withdrawn)

TABLE 22.3 Generations of Cephalosporins Based on Their Spectrum of Activity

Generation	Generic Name	Trade Name(s)
First generation	Cephacetrile	Cephacetrile
	Cefadroxil	Cefadroxil; Duricef
	Cephaloglycin	Kafocin
	Cefalonium	Cephalonium
	Cephaloridine	Cephaloradine
	Cephalothin	Cephalothin; Keflin
	Cephapirin	Cephapirin; Cefadyl
	Cefatrizine	Axelorax
	Cefazolin	Cephazolin; Ancef, Kefzol
	Cephradine	Cephradine; Velosef
	Cefroxadine	
	Ceftezole	
Second generation	Cefaclor	Ceclor, Distaclor, Keflor, Raniclor
	Cefonicid	Monocid
	Cefprozil	Cefprozil; Cefzil
	Cefuroxime	Zinnat, Zinacef, Ceftin, Biofuroksym
	Cefmetazole	
	Cefotetan	
	Cefoxitin	
Third generation	Cefcapene	
	Cefdaloxime	
	Cefdinir	Omnicef
	Cefditoren	
	Cefetamet	
	Cefixime	Suprax
	Cefmenoxime	
	Cefodizime	
	Cefoperazone	Cefobid
	Cefotaxime	Claforan
	Cefpimizole	
	Cefpodoxime	Vantin
	Cefteram	
	Ceftibuten	Cedax
	Ceftiofur	
	Ceftiolene	
	Ceftizoxime	Cefizax
	Ceftriaxone	Rocephin
Fourth generation	Cefclidine	
	Cefepime	Maxipime
	Cefluprenam	
	Cefoselis	
	Cefozopran	
	Cefpirome	
	Cefquinome	

not completely understood, the disruption involves blocking the formation of the chemical bonds that cross-link the layers of peptidoglycan in the cell wall. By preventing the complete assembly of the cell wall, the cell becomes vulnerable to osmotic lysis. Unfortunately, an increasing number of bacteria have developed resistance to penicillin drugs. Many of these resistant organisms synthesize an enzyme called *penicillinase*, which hydrolyzes a bond in the β-lactam ring, rendering it ineffective. Penicillins have proven to be a relatively safe family of antibiotics although there is a small percentage of the human population, about 1% to 5%, that is allergic to them.

Cephalosporins are a class of β-lactam antibiotics that are structurally similar to penicillins because of the presence of similar β-lactam rings. They also resemble the penicillins because they also inhibit the successful assembly of peptidoglycan in the cell wall. They tend to be more stable than penicillins and have a broader spectrum of activity. Furthermore, cephalosporins are often given to treat infections in patients with penicillin allergies. Another advantage over penicillin is that they resist hydrolysis by penicillinase, an enzyme secreted by a number of bacteria. Four generations of cephalosporins exist and each generation is more effective against gram-negative bacteria (Table 22.3). In general, each generation has a broader spectrum of activity than the previous one, and typically have improved dosing schedules and fewer side effects.

- First-generation drugs have proven to be more effective against gram-positive than gram-negative bacteria.
- Second-generation drugs are effective against gram-positive as well as many gram-negative organisms.
- The third-generation drugs are particularly effective against gram-negative bacteria and are capable of crossing the blood–brain barrier to treat infections in the central nervous system. Furthermore, this generation shows activity against enteric bacteria that produce β-lactamases.
- Fourth-generation cephalosporins have the widest range of activity, are also effective with both gram-positive and gram-negative bacteria, and are rapidly microbicidal.

Tetracyclines are a family of antibiotics with a common four-ring structure to which a number of different side chains are attached. These are broad-spectrum antibiotics that include both naturally produced and semisynthetic drugs. As broad-spectrum agents, these antibiotics are active against both gram-negative and gram-positive bacteria, chlamydias, rickettsias, and mycoplasmas. The mechanism of action is the inhibition of protein synthesis and is typically bacteriostatic and not bactericidal. The host immune response and resistance to the pathogen is ultimately responsible for eliminating the infection. Possible side effects may include nausea, diarrhea, discoloration of teeth, and damage to the liver and kidneys. The first drug of the tetracycline family was introduced in 1948.

Aminoglycosides antibiotics are naturally produced agents with considerable variation in their structure; however, all contain the common characteristics of amino sugars and a cyclohexane ring. These antibiotics are bactericidal and are primarily active against gram-negative organisms. The mechanism of action is the direct disruption of protein synthesis as well as the misreading of mRNA. Some aminoglycosides such as streptomycin are now less effective because of the development of resistance by some target bacteria. It is still effective against tuberculosis and the plague. The aminoglycosides are rather toxic and side effects may include deafness, kidney damage, loss of balance, nausea, and a variety of allergenic reactions.

Macrolides antibiotics are both naturally produced agents such as erythromycin, as well as semisynthetics such as azithromycin. These drugs are composed of a 12- to 22-carbon ring that is linked to one or more sugars. Macrolides are broad-spectrum, bacteriostatic agents with relatively low toxicity. They are effective against gram-positive bacteria, mycoplasmas, and a few select gram-negative bacteria and are useful when fighting infections in patients who are allergic to penicillins. They are also effective in the treatment of whooping cough, diphtheria, gastroenteritis caused by *Campylobacter,* and pneumonia from *Legionella.* Newly developed macrolides are being used to treat infections caused by *Staphylococcus* and *Bacteroides.* Azithromycin is especially effective against *Chlamydia.* The mechanism of action is the disruption of protein synthesis by preventing peptide chain elongation at the ribosome.

Chloramphenicol is a potent broad-spectrum, bacteriostatic antibiotic. Originally this agent was produced naturally, but is now manufactured through chemical synthesis. Chloramphenicol has a nitrobenzene structure and its mechanism of action is much like that of the macrolide erythromycin in that it disrupts protein synthesis at the ribosome. Because of the toxicity of this antibiotic its uses are restricted. It is used primarily to treat typhoid fever, brain abscesses, and rickettsial and chlamydial infections. The side effects can be severe and may include the following:

- Allergic reactions
- Neurotoxic reactions
- Irreversible bone marrow damage leading to a fatal form of aplastic anemia

***Bacillus* Antibiotics** Bacitracin and the polymyxins are relatively narrow-spectrum peptide antibiotics that are naturally produced by bacteria of the genus *Bacillus.* Both bacitracin and polymyxins are topically applied antibiotics that are effective in combating superficial skin infections by *Staphylococcus* and *Streptococcus.* The mechanism of action for bacitracin is the disruption of cell wall synthesis, and polymyxins disrupt the cell membrane structure, causing leakage of metabolites. These agents are typically used for the treatment of surface infections, but can be administered internally when the patient can be closely monitored, because of the potential for kidney damage or respiratory arrest.

Antiviral Agents

Because viruses depend on host cells for replication, it has been a difficult challenge to develop drugs that will destroy or inhibit a virus without also severely affecting the host cell. However, there has been some promise in the development of antiviral drugs that target specific points in the life cycle of viruses. Although this form of treatment for viral infections has shown some success, the agents developed still are limited in their effectiveness and usefulness. Most of these new compounds have modes of action that involve the following:

- Preventing complete penetration of the virus into the host cell
- Blocking transcription and translation of viral molecules
- Steps to prevent maturation of the virus

Unfortunately, most of these drugs are unable to affect viruses in the extracellular environment or when the virus is in a latent state.

Synthetic Antiviral Agents

The search for antiviral agents has resulted in the discovery and development of a number of drugs, such as acyclovir for the treatment of herpes simplex, and azidothymidine for the treatment of AIDS. Additional molecular targets for chemotherapeutic intervention of viral infections have been identified, and novel classes of synthetic antiviral agents have been and are still being discovered.

Antibacterial Agents

Organism	Infection	Drug of Choice	Commercial (Trade) Name(s)
Escherichia coli	Urinary tract infections	Cefotaxime (cephalosporin)	Claforan
Staphylococcus aureus	Abscess, toxic shock syndrome	Penicillinase-resistant penicillin Vancomycin Cephalosporin	Vancocin, Vancoled, Vancor
Streptococcus pyogenes	Strep throat, rheumatic fever	Penicillin Cephalosporin Erythromycin	Benzamycin, EryDerm, Erycette, Erygel, Erymax, Ilotycin, Robimycin, Sansac, Staticin, Theramycin Z
Streptococcus pneumoniae	Pneumonia	Penicillin Cephalosporin Erythromycin	
Bacillus	Anthrax	Penicillin Doxycycline Ciprofloxacin	Doxycin, Monodox, Apo-Doxy, Vibramycin, Periostat Cipro, Ciloxan
Clostridium	Tetanus, gas gangrene	Penicillin Cephalosporin Clindamycin	Cleocin, Dalacin, Clinda-Derm
Corynebacterium	Diphtheria	Penicillin Erythromycin	
Mycobacterium	Tuberculosis	Isoniazid Rifampin Pyrazinamide Ethambutol Streptomycin	Isotamine, Nydrazid, Rimifon, Laniazid, Stanozide Rifadin, Rifamate, Rifater, Rimactane, Rofact Tebrazid Etibi, Myambutol

Purine and pyrimidine analogs are agents involved in the substitution of normal purines and pyrimidines. The molecular analogs results in erroneous genetic information being incorporated into the nucleic acid being synthesized for viral replication. One of the premier drugs in this group is acyclovir (Zovirax), which is an analog of guanine. The agent is rapidly incorporated into cells that are infected with a virus, and it is less toxic than other analogs. Acyclovir is widely used in the treatment of genital herpes, in which it not only interferes with the replication of the virus but also promotes healing of the lesions produced by herpes and is also effective in reducing pain.

Amantadine, a tricyclic amine, is used to prevent influenza A viruses from penetrating cells. As a drug that blocks penetration and uncoating of the virus, it is usually given prophylactically to prevent disease and has proven to be 50% to 80% effective. Side effects include dizziness, confusion, and insomnia.

Azidothymidine (AZT) is an analog group drug that can be designated in its own group, as it is used primarily in the treatment of AIDS. It is an analog of thymidine that inhibits reverse transcriptase, thus blocking DNA synthesis by the retrovirus HIV. This drug does not cure AIDS and is not able to eliminate the latent HIV DNA that may reside in memory T cells and macrophages. AZT is often used along with other antiviral agents in a "cocktail" that is given in relatively high doses to prevent the development of drug resistance.

Interferons are a group of antiviral drugs consisting of proteins produced by cells that are infected with a virus. These naturally produced chemicals induce neighboring cells to produce antiviral proteins that prevent these cells from becoming infected. Some of them are now being genetically engineered to increase their effectiveness. They have shown some positive results in the control of viral hepatitis, warts, and cancers such as Kaposi's sarcoma and even as a treatment for the "common cold."

Antifungal Agents

Fungal infections are becoming more frequent because of their opportunistic behavior in immunocompromised individuals, such as those with AIDS and those cancer patients receiving chemotherapy. Moreover, the widespread use of broad-spectrum antibiotics causes the elimination or decrease of the normal, nonpathogenic flora that competes with the fungal population.

Because fungi are eukaryotic cells, unlike bacteria, they present a different challenge when combating infections with chemical agents. Antimicrobial agents designed to combat bacteria are usually ineffective against fungi. The similarities between fungal and human cells make it difficult to develop drugs that are toxic to the fungus but not to the human host. The main groups of drugs currently in use against fungal infections include the following:

- Macrolide polyene antibiotics
- Griseofulvin
- Synthetic azoles
- Flucytosine
- Echinocandins

Therapeutic antifungal agents can be broadly classified as naturally occurring antifungal agents and synthetic drugs. Most fungal infections are superficial and therefore many preparations are topical. Antifungal medications are toxic to humans and animals, and therefore when systemic therapy is required these agents are used under strict medical supervision.

Synthetic Azoles

Synthetic azoles are broad spectrum, synthetically produced, and designed primarily for use on superficial fungal infections such as athlete's foot and oral and vaginal candidiasis. The mechanism of action for these agents is the disruption of cell membrane permeability by inhibiting the synthesis of membrane sterols. Some select drugs in this group, such as ketoconazole, can also be administered orally to treat systemic fungal infections. Side effects may include skin irritations when using topical agents, and possible drug interactions with antihistamines and immunosuppressants can occur.

Flucytosine

Flucytosine is a broad-spectrum, synthetic agent that is used to combat systemic fungal infections and some cutaneous mycoses. It can be taken orally and is quickly dissolved in the blood and cerebrospinal fluid. The mechanism of action involves transformation and substitution of flucytosine for uracil in the RNA, thus disrupting RNA function. It is often used in combination with amphotericin B because of the increase in fungi that are resistant to flucytosine. Some side effects may include skin rashes, diarrhea, nausea, aplastic anemia, and liver damage.

Macrolide Polyene Antibiotics

Macrolide polyene antibiotics are naturally produced agents and include amphotericin B and nystatin; the latter are products of the genus *Streptomyces*. Amphotericin B is arguably the most versatile and effective antifungal agent that is commonly used against systemic mycoses. The mechanism of action is the disruption of cell membrane permeability, causing leakage of metabolites by binding to the sterols. This agent is poorly absorbed from the digestive tract and is therefore administered intravenously. Amphotericin is quite toxic and the side effects can be severe. These effects include abnormal skin sensations, fever and chills, nausea and vomiting, headache, depression, kidney damage, anemia, abnormal heart rhythms, and in some cases blindness.

Griseofulvin

Griseofulvin is a naturally produced, relatively narrow-spectrum agent used primarily to combat localized dermatophyte infections such as athlete's foot. It is taken orally; deposits in the hair, nails, and epidermis; and is fungistatic. The agent will accumulate in new replacement cells in the area of infection, thus interfering with any further fungal growth. The mechanism of action involves impairing mitotic cell division by disrupting the mitotic spindle apparatus. The eradication of a fungal infection using griseofulvin usually takes from 4 weeks to sometimes over a year. This agent may damage the kidneys and has additional possible side effects of mild headaches, and some gastrointestinal problems.

Echinocandins

Echinocandins are made of a ring of six amino acids, linked to a lipophilic side chain.

Echinocandins inhibit the synthesis of glucan in the cell wall of fungi; they do not have a target in mammalian cells. Their spectrum of activity is rapidly fungicidal against most species of *Candida,* fungistatic against *Aspergillus* spp., and can be useful as prophylaxis against the cyst form of *Pneumocystis carinii*. Echinocandins are administrated intravenously and do represent a major development in the treatment of systemic fungal infections.

Antiprotozoan Agents

Antiprotozoan agents are used in the treatment of parasitic protozoans, which can infect a number of body systems. Although often effective at controlling or even curing these infections, some of these agents have some dramatic and unpleasant side effects due to the fact that the treatment is against eukaryotes, just like human cells. Another inherent difficulty in treating protozoan infections is that many of the organisms have several stages in their life cycles, which may require treatments involving different agents being administered at different stages of the infection. With the exception of quinine, most antiprotozoan drugs are synthetic.

Chloroquine and Primaquine

Synthetically produced chloroquine and primaquine are derived from quinine, a drug obtained from the bark of the cinchona tree, and are widely used in the treatment of the protozoan parasite *Plasmodium,* which causes malaria. Chloroquine interferes with protein synthesis, particularly in red blood cells, which are the cells infected with the protozoan. The mechanism

Antifungal Drugs

Organism	Infection	Drug of Choice	Commercial (Trade) Name(s)
Aspergillus	Aspergillosis	Amphotericin B	Abelcet, AmBisome, Amphotec, Amphocin, Fungizone
		Azoles	
		Flucytosine	Ancobon, Ancotil
Candida albicans	Thrush, vaginal infections	Amphotericin B	
		Fluconazole	Diflucan
Blastomyces	Blastomycosis	Ketoconazole	Nizoral
		Amphotericin B	
Pneumocystis	Pneumonia	Pentamidine	Nebupent, Pentacarinat, Pentam, Pneumopent
		Sulfamethoxazole-trimethoprim	
Microsporum	Athlete's foot	Griseofulvin	Fulvicin, Grifulvin, Grisactin
Candida spp.	Candidiasis	Echinocandins	Caspofungin
Aspergillus spp.	Invasive aspergillosis	Echinocandins	Micafungin

is not fully understood, but may involve accumulation of the drug in the vacuole of the parasite, which prevents it from metabolizing hemoglobin. A combination of chloroquine and primaquine can be used to protect people who are in regions where malaria occurs by reducing the risk of infection. The regimen involves use of the drugs both before and after entering a malarial zone.

Metronidazole

The synthetic drug metronidazole has been proven to be effective in treating *Trichomonas* vaginal infections as well as gastrointestinal infections caused by amoeba and *Giardia*. Its mechanism of action is to disrupt the helical structure of DNA, subsequently inhibiting transcription and protein synthesis. Although effective, it does exhibit some unwanted side effects such as diarrhea, nausea, and "black hairy tongue." Furthermore, it has been shown to cause some forms of cancer.

Pyrimethamine

Pyrimethamine has been used to both prevent and cure malaria and, when used with sulfanilamide, it can treat other infections such as toxoplasmosis. The mechanism of action involves disruption of the synthesis of folic acid, which is required in the synthesis of DNA and other nucleic acids. Side effects may include nausea, loss of appetite, headaches, dry mouth, and dizziness.

Quinine

Quinine, a nonsynthetic drug, is extracted from the bark of the cinchona tree and has been used for centuries in the treatment of malaria. In the 1940s the widespread use of quinine as a malarial treatment declined because of the development of less toxic agents. It is still in use today in severe cases or when the organism has become resistant to other drugs. The theorized mechanism of action involves the disruption of the parasite's

ability to fully metabolize hemoglobin, which it uses as an energy source. The side effects of quinine may include hearing loss, headaches, nausea, vomiting, diarrhea, confusion, anaphylactic shock, birth defects, and in some cases death due to cardiotoxicity.

Antihelminthic Agents

Numerous helminths can infect humans as pathogenic parasites. The agents used to eliminate these organisms once an infection begins present the same problems faced when using antifungal agents: The agent is aimed at eukaryotic cells, which can have a negative effect on the host body cells. Those agents designed to suppress a metabolic process target those processes that are more important to the helminth than the host. Other agents inhibit the movement of the worm and prevent it from remaining in a specific organ. Some representative agents are presented in the following sections.

Niclosamide

Niclosamide prevents ATP formation and also causes the parasite to release large amounts of lactic acid through interference with carbohydrate metabolism. The lactic acid also appears to inactivate substances made by the worm that resist host proteolytic enzymes.

Mebendazole

Mebendazole blocks the uptake of glucose by the worm. This agent will damage a fetus and is therefore not prescribed for pregnant women.

Piperazine

Piperazine is a strong neurotoxin that paralyzes the body wall muscles of a roundworm, thus paralyzing the worm and allowing it to be expelled in the feces. Typically the drug exerts its

Antiprotozoan Drugs

Organism	Infection	Drug of Choice	Commercial (Trade) Name(s)
Giardia lamblia	Giardiasis	Quinacrine	
		Metronidazole	Flagyl, Helidac, RTU, Metrolotion, Metrogel, Metromidol, Nidagel, Noritate, Protostat, Satric, Trikacide, Novonidazol
Plasmodium	Malaria	Chloroquine	Aralen
		Primaquine	
		Quinine	
Trypanosoma cruzi	Chagas' disease	Nifurtimox	Available only through the CDC
Entamoeba histolytica	Amebiasis	Metronidazole	
		Tetracycline	
		Paromomycin	Humatin
Toxoplasma gondii	Toxoplasmosis	Pyrimethamine	Daraprim, Fansidar
		Sulfadiazine	Lantrisul, Neotrizine, Sulfaloid, Terfonyl, Sulfose
Trypanosoma brucei	Sleeping sickness	Suramin	Available only through the CDC
		Pentamidine	Nebupent, Pentacarinat, Pentam, Pneumopent

CDC, Centers for Disease Control and Prevention.

Antihelminthic Drugs

Organism	Infection	Drug of Choice	Commercial (Trade) Name(s)
Ascaris lumbricoides	Roundworm	Piperazine	Entacyl
Trichuris trichiura	Whipworm	Mebendazole	Vermox
Enterobius vermicularis	Pinworm	Piperazine	Entacyl
Necator americanus	Hookworm	Piperazine Mebendazole	Etacyl Vermox
Strongyloides stercoralis	Threadworm	Thiabendazole	Mintezol
Trichinella spiralis	Trichinosis	Mebendazole	Vermox
Wuchereria bancrofti	Elephantiasis	Diethylcarbamazine	Hetrazan
Schistosoma mansoni	Schistosomiasis	Praziquantel Metrifonate	Biltricide
Taenia	Tapeworm	Niclosamide	Niclocide
Onchocerca volvulus	River blindness	Ivermectin	Mectizan Stromectol

effect in the intestine, but if it is absorbed it can travel into the nervous system. This penetration into the nervous system can cause convulsions, especially in children.

Ivermectin

Ivermectin blocks nerve transmission, thereby paralyzing the worm, and is used to treat heartworm infections in dogs as well as river blindness in humans.

Summary

- The goal of antimicrobial agents is to disrupt the metabolism or structure of a pathogen so that it can no longer survive or reproduce.
- Antimicrobial drugs may inhibit cell wall synthesis, protein synthesis, or nucleic acid synthesis, or disrupt the cell membrane and also the metabolism of the microorganism.

- Antimicrobial drugs have a spectrum of activity indicating the range of pathogens against which a given drug is effective. On the basis of their action, antimicrobials are classified as having a broad, medium, or narrow spectrum of activity.
- Several factors need to be considered before selecting an antimicrobial drug. These include selective toxicity, microbicidal or microbiostatic action, delivery to the site of action, time of activity, antimicrobial resistance, host defense, allergies, shelf life, availability, and affordability.
- A number of tests are currently available to determine the most effective antimicrobial against a specific organism including the Kirby-Bauer method, the minimal inhibitory concentration method, and the serum killing power method.
- The administration of drugs can lead to side effects, and an assessment of risks versus benefits needs to be made.
- A challenge to healthcare is the resistance of microbes to antimicrobial drugs.

- The mechanisms of resistance vary and include change in membrane permeability, increased drug elimination, change in the receptor for the agent, change in the metabolic pathways, change in enzymes, and the development of defensive enzymes.
- Antimicrobial resistance is a global problem, and unfortunately multiresistant strains have developed worldwide. The primary sites for multiresistant strain development seem to be hospitals, nursing homes, and other healthcare facilities.
- The spread and also the prevention of the development of resistant microbial organisms involve the action of physicians as well as individuals treated with antimicrobial drugs.
- Specific antimicrobial drugs are subdivided into antibiotics, semisynthetic drugs, and synthetic drugs. Furthermore, antimicrobials are classified as antibacterial, antiviral, antifungal, antiprotozoan, and antihelminthic agents.

Review Questions

1. All of the following are general metabolic or structural targets for antimicrobial drugs *except*:
   a. Lipid synthesis inhibition
   b. Protein synthesis inhibition
   c. Interference with nucleic acid synthesis
   d. Interference with cell wall synthesis

2. Which of the following is *not* a common characteristic used in the selection of an antimicrobial drug?
   a. Selective toxicity
   b. Ease of delivery to the site of infection
   c. Penetration of the blood–brain barrier
   d. Not causing an allergic reaction

3. The term "bacteriostatic" means that bacteria:
   a. Are killed by the antimicrobial drug
   b. Show continuous growth
   c. No longer can multiply
   d. No longer cause disease

4. When two antibiotics are given together to increase the therapeutic effect the phenomenon is referred to as:
   a. Antagonism   c. Synergism
   b. Mutualism   d. Parasitism

5. All of the following are mechanisms of resistance used by microbes *except*:
   a. Change in ribosome composition
   b. Development of defensive enzymes
   c. Increased drug elimination
   d. Change in membrane permeability

6. Which of the following is a synthetic antimicrobial drug?
   a. Penicillin G   c. Cephalosporin
   b. Penicillin V   d. Quinolone

7. Cephalosporins have _____ generations of developed agents.
   a. 2   c. 4
   b. 3   d. 6

8. Which of the following antimicrobials is effective against mycobacteria?
   a. Penicillin   c. Erythromycin
   b. Rifampin   d. Cephalosporin

9. Which of the following is an antiviral agent?
   a. Amantadine   c. Chloramphenicol
   b. Vancomycin   d. Macrolides

10. Which of the following drugs is effective against *Candida albicans*?
    a. Quinine   c. Piperazine
    b. Echinocandins   d. Vancomycin

11. A drug that kills pathogenic bacteria is referred to as _____.

12. Resistance to only one type of drug may allow resistance to a similar drug. This process is called _____.

13. The range of pathogen type against which a given drug is effective is referred to as the drug's _____.

14. The effectiveness of a drug against a microbe is also referred to as the drug's _____.

15. The zone of inhibition is the result of the _____ method.

16. Describe the five basic mechanisms of action that are targeted by antimicrobial drugs.

17. Name five common characteristics that are considered when selecting an antimicrobial drug.

18. Discuss the three types of activity (spectrum of activity) of antimicrobial drugs.

19. Describe how antibiotic effectiveness (efficacy) can be determined.

20. Discuss the possible side effects that can occur during or after treatment with antimicrobial drugs.

Bibliography

Bauman R: *Microbiology*, ed 2, San Francisco, 2007, Benjamin Cummings/Pearson Education.

Clayton BD, Stock YN, Harroun RD: *Basic pharmacology for nurses*, St. Louis, 2007, Mosby/Elsevier.

Lehne RA: *Pharmacology for nursing care*, ed 6, St. Louis, 2007, Saunders/Elsevier.

Rang HP, Dale MM, Titter JM, et al: *Rang and Dale's pharmacology*, ed 6, New York, 2007, Churchill Livingstone/Elsevier.

Talaro KP: *Foundations in microbiology*, ed 6, New York, 2005, McGraw-Hill.

Totora GJ, Funke BR, Case CL: *Microbiology: an introduction*, ed 9, San Francisco, 2007, Benjamin Cummings/Pearson Education.

Internet Resources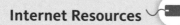

USDA Agricultural Research Service, Bacterial Epidemiology and Antimicrobial Resistance, http://www.ars.usda.gov/research/publications/publications.htm?SEQ_NO_115=135738

Huycke MM, Sahm DF, Gilmore MS: Multiple-drug resistant enterococci: the nature of the problem and an agenda for the future, *Emerging Infectious Diseases* 4(2), April–June, 1998, available at http://www.cdc.gov/NCIDOD/eid/vol4no2/huycke.htm

World Health Organization, Drug Resistance, http://www.who.int/drugresistance/en/

World Health Organization, Regional Office for the Western Pacific, Antimicrobial resistance surveillance, http://www.wpro.who.int/health_topics/antimicrobial_resistance/

World Health Organization, Antimicrobial resistance, http://www.who.int/mediacentre/factsheets/fs194/en/

World Health Organization, Use of antimicrobials outside human medicine and resultant antimicrobial resistance in humans, http://www.who.int/mediacentre/factsheets/fs268/en/

CDC, Antibiotic / Antimicrobial Resistance, http://www.cdc.gov/drugresistance/

CDC, Quinolones and the Clinical Laboratory, http://www.cdc.gov/ncidod/dhqp/ar_lab_quinlolones.html

Contraceptives and Antibiotics, http://www.medicinenet.com/script/main/art.asp?articlekey=7437

Graybill JR: The echinocandins, first novel class of antifungals in two decades: will they live up to their promise? *Int J Clin Pract* 55(9):633–638, Nov 2001, available at http://www.ncbi.nlm.nih.gov/sites/entrez?db=pubmed&uid=11770362&cmd=showdetailview&indexed=google

CDC, Campaign to Prevent Antimicrobial Resistance in Healthcare Settings, http://www.cdc.gov/drugresistance/healthcare/default.htm

U.S. Food and Drug Administration, HHS Response to House Report 106-157- Agriculture, Rural Development, Food and Drug Administration, and Related Agencies, Appropriations Bill, 2000, Human-Use Antibiotics in Livestock Production, http://www.fda.gov/cvm/HRESP106_157.htm

Science Daily: Routine Feeding of Antibiotics to Livestock May Be Contaminating the Environment, *Science Daily* (July 13, 2007), available at http://www.sciencedaily.com/releases/2007/07/070711134530.htm

23

Human Age and Microorganisms

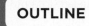

OUTLINE

Perinatal
Introduction
Infections During Pregnancy
Congenital Infections

Infants and Children
Immune System in Infants and Children
Common Microbial Infections in Infants and Children

Young Adults
Immune System in Young Adults
Common Microbial Infections in Young Adults
Environmental Exposures Typical for Young Adults

Older Adults
Immune System in Older Adults
Common Microbial Infections in Older Adults
Factors Influencing Susceptibility to Microbial Disease

LEARNING OBJECTIVES

After reading this chapter, the student will be able to:
- Identify the different effects microorganisms have on the different age groups
- Explain the different immune reactions that occur in the different age groups
- Describe the infections that typically can occur in pregnant women and ultimately can have an effect on fetal development
- Name and describe congenital infections, including causative agent, transmission, symptoms, and treatments
- Discuss the common microbial infections that affect infants and children
- Describe the microbial infections that commonly occur in young adults
- Illustrate the environmental exposures to microbes that are typical for young adults
- Describe the common microbial infections in the elderly and compare these with the other age groups
- Explain the immune system of the elderly and contrast it to the other age groups
- Portray factors that can influence the susceptibility to microbial infections and disease among the elderly

colostrum
congenital disorder
congenital infections
deep folliculitis
embryo
Escherichia coli
fetus
gestation period
group B streptococcal
disease (GBS)

herpes simplex
immune senescence
immune system
immunity
impetigo
perinatal
placenta
pregnancy

sexually transmitted
infections (STIs)
staphylococcal
conjunctivitis
staphylococcal scalded
skin syndrome
toxoplasmosis

WHY YOU NEED TO KNOW

HISTORY

Since ancient times cultures have recognized the problems related to development and aging, including the increased susceptibility to infections and disease, both in the very young and the elderly. From seeking the fountain of youth to cultural banishment of the elderly and sick, civilizations have been attempting to deal with the problems and concerns associated with the human body as it goes through the changes involved in the natural aging process.

IMPACT

Science certainly has progressed and so has the understanding of human aging, and the factors involved in treating diseases and infections during development and aging. Some advances in areas of medical treatments have been presenting new sets of factors in dealing with age-related infection problems. Hormone therapy, particularly in women, is growing in usage to address problems involved in the aging process as it affects the reproductive and related systems. Although this therapy may attenuate the negative effects of changes such as menopause, it also leads to changes of the pH in organs of the reproductive system, which increases susceptibility to both bacterial and fungal infections such as vaginitis. Research has also revealed new disease and infection problems related specifically to youth.

For example, it is now established that there is a direct connection between the consumption of honey and infant botulism. Research has found that an important factor contributing to this problem is the fact that the intestinal tract of infants lacks a normal microflora, which successfully competes against pathogens such as *Clostridium botulinum.* Without such bacterial competition in the digestive system of immature infants, *C. botulinum* is able to thrive in the intestine and produce its lethal toxin. It has now been suggested that infant botulism may be responsible for up to 10% of cases of sudden infant death syndrome (SIDS).

FUTURE

In the last century modern medicine has increased the average human life span from 47 years in 1900 to the present average of 77 years. As the body ages, regardless of the rate of aging, a key factor in fighting disease and infection will be the effectiveness of the **immune system.** Research is underway to bolster the body's immune system to maintain its protective functions longer, and will be the key to maintaining good health in the face of persistent attacks from the microbial world. Research also continues to develop antibiotic therapies that will minimize or eliminate the damage that antibiotics may cause to the organ systems of the very young and the elderly, and in immunocompromised patients.

Perinatal

An infection caused by bacteria or viruses that can be passed from a mother to her baby via the placenta, either during **pregnancy** or delivery, is referred to as a **perinatal** infection. Maternal infections may cause complications at birth, but the mother may or may not experience symptoms of the infection during pregnancy. Many perinatal infections become evident only after birth.

Introduction

The **placenta** is a highly specialized (Figure 23.1) structure that generally is an effective barrier, protecting the fetus from micro-

organisms that may be present in the mother's circulation or in the urogenital tract. Placental tissue normally separates maternal and fetal blood supplies so that no intermixing occurs. Unfortunately, some infectious organisms may penetrate this barrier and injure the developing embryo or fetus.

Infections During Pregnancy

The length of pregnancy in humans is approximately 39 weeks and is called the **gestation period,** divided into three phases referred to as trimesters. The embryonic phase of development extends from fertilization to the end of the eighth week, and the developing individual is referred to as an **embryo.** From the eighth week until birth the developing infant is called a **fetus.** Neither an embryo nor a fetus has a developed immune system

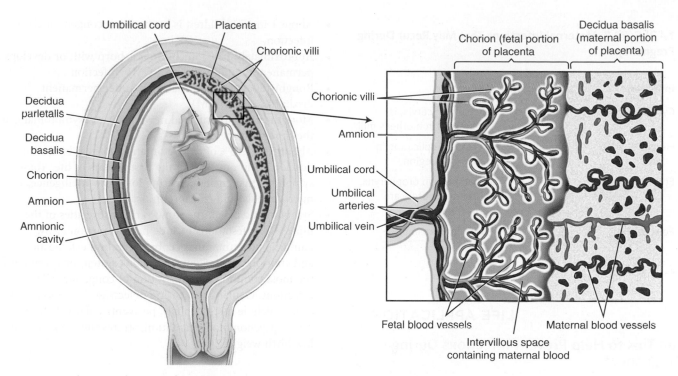

FIGURE 23.1 Schematic drawing of a placenta. The placenta generally is an effective barrier between the maternal and fetal blood supplies, protecting the fetus from most microorganisms that may be present in the mother's bloodstream.

TABLE 23.1 Infections That May Be More Common or Severe During Gestation

Infection	Covered in Chapter(s):	Comments
Urinary tract infections (UTIs)	15	Cystitis; pyelonephritis; atony of the urinary bladder, leading to less effective emptying/flushing
Malaria	14	Probably due to depressed cell-mediated immunity
Viral hepatitis	7 and 12	Probably due to additional stress on metabolic activities
Influenza	11	Higher mortality during pandemics; may be prevented by vaccination
Poliomyelitis	7	Paralysis more common
Coccidioidomycosis	11	Leading cause of maternal mortality in endemic areas in the southwestern United States and Latin America
Candidiasis	10	Vulvovaginitis
Listeriosis	12	Influenza-like disease can cause auto-abortions in pregnant women

(see Chapter 20, The Immune System). IgM and IgA synthesis is limited until the second half of the pregnancy, IgG antibody synthesis is absent, and cell-mediated immune responses are absent or poorly developed. In other words, the embryo/fetus is completely dependent on its mother's immune system. Immunosuppression in the mother will result in a potentially disastrous susceptibility of the unborn to infectious disease. Certain infections can be more common during pregnancy (Table 23.1) and others may recur (Table 23.2), all of which can present a particular risk to the woman and/or her unborn child.

The use of any medication during pregnancy and lactation carries a potential risk for causing birth defects to the developing fetus. For example, the measles-mumps-rubella (MMR) vaccine should not be administered during the first trimester of pregnancy because of an association with fetal defects. Pregnancy and lactation also pose problems in antibiotic treatment, because some of them may cross the placenta. The use of the antibiotic tetracycline by a pregnant woman may cause stained teeth in the child.

Congenital Infections

A **congenital disorder** is any medical condition that is present at birth regardless of its origin and therefore includes a broad category with a variety of conditions. **Congenital infections** are intrauterine infections occurring during pregnancy

TABLE 23.2 Maternal Infections That May Recur During Pregnancy

Infection	Covered in Chapter(s):	Comments
Cytomegalovirus	7	Sheds from cervix, is present in mother's milk
Herpes simplex virus	10 and 12	Increased replication in cervical region
Epstein-Barr virus	14	Virus sheds in oropharynx; antibody titers are increased
Polyomavirus	15	Virus appears in urine

LIFE APPLICATION

Ten Tips to Help Prevent Infections During Pregnancy*

1. Wash your hands often with soap and water.
2. Do not share eating utensils, cups, or food with young children.
3. Cook meat until it is well done.
4. Avoid unpasteurized milk.
5. Do not touch or change cat litter.
6. Avoid wild or pet rodents and their droppings.
7. Get tested for sexually transmitted infections.
8. Check with the physician about vaccinations.
9. Avoid contact with people who have an infection.
10. Ask the physician about group B *Streptococcus*.

*From the Centers for Disease Control and Prevention (CDC) http://www.cdc.gov/Features/Pregnancy/.

when microorganisms enter the blood, subsequently establish an infection of the placenta, and then infect the fetus. These infections may result in the death of the fetus and, if the infection does not result in abortion, it may lead to congenital malformations.

Congenital Cytomegalovirus Infection

Cytomegalovirus (CMV) belongs to the family Herpesviridae and in humans it is commonly referred to as human herpesvirus 5. CMV is a common virus that infects most people at some time during their lives but generally does not cause recognizable illness. According to the Centers for Disease Control and Prevention (CDC, Atlanta, GA), between 50% and 80% of adults in the United States are infected with CMV by age 40 years. Although not highly communicable, it can be spread from person to person through close contact. The virus is present in urine, saliva, semen, and other bodily fluids. Transmission can also occur from an infected mother to her fetus, and CMV is the most common virus transmitted during pregnancy. Reports from the CDC state that:

- About 1 in 150 children is born with a congenital CMV infection
- Approximately 1 in 750 children is born with or develops a permanent disability due to a CMV infection
- Roughly 8000 children each year suffer permanent disabilities due to CMV
- More than 90% of infected newborns are asymptomatic at the time of birth
- About 5% to 15% of asymptomatic babies at birth will develop symptoms within the first 2 years of life. These symptoms may include hearing loss, low intelligence, microcephaly, and chorioretinitis.
- Symptomatic newborns show various severities of the illness. Manifestations include hepatosplenomegaly, jaundice, purpura, microcephaly, cerebral calcifications, and chorioretinitis. Central nervous system involvement is the most common demonstration of congenital CMV infections. Ocular and hearing defects are common, and others include microcephaly, periventricular calcification, severe psychomotor retardation, strabismus, seizures, and low birth weight.

Congenital Rubella

Congenital rubella is caused by the action of the rubella virus when a pregnant woman is infected during the critical time of fetal development, namely during the first trimester of pregnancy. The condition includes a group of birth defects that include but are not limited to:

- Malformations of the heart
- Cloudy corneas and other eye defects
- Deafness
- Developmental setback
- Excessive sleepiness
- Irritability
- Low birth weight
- Mental retardation
- Small head size
- Skin rash at birth: Thrombocytopenic purpura (blueberry muffin rash)
- Hepatomegaly

An infected fetus generally produces its own IgM to the virus, which can be detected in the umbilical cord and in the blood of the infant. Some congenitally infected children will develop insulin-dependent diabetes later in life. The main risk factor for congenital rubella occurs when a pregnant woman who has not been vaccinated comes into contact with a person who has rubella (also called *German measles;* see Chapter 7, Viruses).

Congenital Syphilis

Congenital syphilis is caused by the spirochete *Treponema pallidum* and is passed from an infected mother to the child during fetal development or at birth. Approximately 50% of infected fetuses die shortly before or after birth. Symptoms in infected newborns may include the following:

- Failure to gain weight
- Fever
- Irritability
- No bridge to nose (saddle nose)
- Early rash: Small blisters on palms and soles
- Later rash: Copper-colored, flat or bumpy rash on the face, palms, and soles
- Rash on the mouth, genitalia, and anus
- Severe congenital pneumonia
- Watery discharge from the nose

When a pregnant woman is identified as being infected with syphilis, appropriate treatment regimens, including penicillin, can effectively prevent the development of congenital syphilis in the infant. Patients with penicillin allergies may be desensitized before starting the full treatment. Despite the fact that the disease can be cured with antibiotics if identified early, increasing rates of syphilis among pregnant women in the United States have been reported, resulting in an increased number of infants born with congenital syphilis.

Congenital Toxoplasmosis

Toxoplasmosis is caused by the parasite *Toxoplasma gondii*. The organism can be found in raw meat, and is commonly found in cat litter and contaminated soil. The life cycle of *Toxoplasma gondii* is illustrated in Figure 23.2. Although toxoplasmosis is common in men and women, the infection during pregnancy can lead to congenital toxoplasmosis, which can damage the baby's eyes, nervous system, skin, and ears. Clinical features in the infant include the following:

- Convulsions
- Microcephaly
- Chorioretinitis
- Hepatosplenomegaly
- Jaundice
- Hydrocephaly (later)
- Mental retardation (later)
- Defective vision (later)

Oftentimes there are no detectable abnormalities at birth, but health problems may become apparent in the second or third decade of life. To prevent toxoplasmosis pregnant women should avoid cleaning litter boxes, other areas that have contact with cat litter, and also should cook meat until it is well done. Cross-contamination should be avoided. Treatment is possible for the pregnant mother, usually with spiramycin, and fetal infections diagnosed during pregnancy can be treated with pyrimethamine and sulfadiazine. CDC recommendations to prevent congenital toxoplasmosis are shown in Box 23.1.

Congenital HIV Infection

Clinical symptoms of congenital HIV infections include poor weight gain, susceptibility to sepsis, developmental delays, lymphocytic pneumonitis, oral thrush, enlarged lymph nodes, hepatosplenomegaly, diarrhea, and pneumonia. Some infants develop AIDS by age 1 year. Most infections occur during late

---

BOX 23.1 CDC Recommendations for the Prevention of Congenital Toxoplasmosis

- Cooking meat to safe temperatures—sufficient to kill *Toxoplasma*
- Peeling or washing fruits and vegetables before consumption
- Cleaning cooking surfaces and utensils after they have had contact with raw meat, poultry, seafood or unwashed fruits or vegetables
- Pregnant women should avoid changing cat litter—if no one else is available, gloves need to be used, followed by thorough washing of hands
- Not feeding raw or undercooked meat to cats—keep cats inside to prevent acquisition of *Toxoplasma* by eating infected prey

---

BOX 23.2 Follow-up Care for Babies Born to HIV-positive Mothers

- Routine medical care
- HIV specialty care
- Family planning services
- Mental health services
- Substance abuse treatment
- Case management

---

pregnancy or during delivery; transmission rates can be reduced by lowering the HIV load by using antiretroviral drugs during pregnancy. Elective cesarean section and avoiding breastfeeding may also reduce the risk of infection. The medical and supportive services recommended by the U.S. Department of Health and Human Services after a child is born to an HIV-positive mother are listed in Box 23.2. In developing countries, about a quarter of infants born to HIV-positive mothers are infected.

Vaginal Infections

A common vaginal infection known as bacterial vaginosis (BV) is an imbalance of the normal bacterial flora of the vagina (see Chapter 16, Infections of the Reproductive System). With BV, increased numbers of anaerobic organisms are found, including *Gardnerella vaginalis*, *Mycoplasma hominis*, and *Bacteroides*. Although these organisms are part of the normal vaginal flora, they do cause problems when they outnumber the normal *Lactobacillus* flora. Pregnant women with BV are more likely to give birth to a premature infant with a low birth weight than are women who do not have the vaginal infection.

Vaginal infections caused by the protozoan *Trichomonas vaginalis* also have been associated with preterm labor and preterm birth. The parasite is sexually transmitted and it has been suggested that the infection may spread from the vagina to the uterus. According to the CDC, the prescription drug

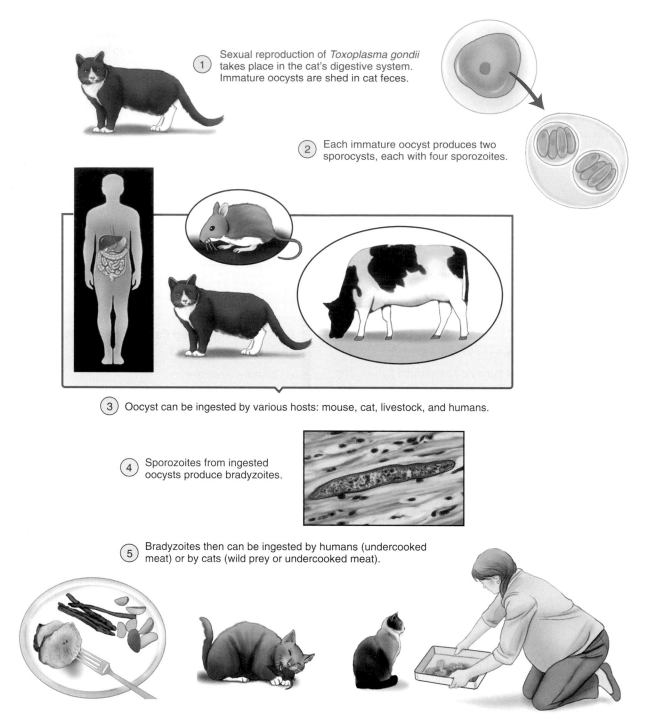

FIGURE 23.2 Life cycle of *Toxoplasma gondii*.

The following labels appear within the figure:

1. Sexual reproduction of *Toxoplasma gondii* takes place in the cat's digestive system. Immature oocysts are shed in cat feces.

2. Each immature oocyst produces two sporocysts, each with four sporozoites.

3. Oocyst can be ingested by various hosts: mouse, cat, livestock, and humans.

4. Sporozoites from ingested oocysts produce bradyzoites.

5. Bradyzoites then can be ingested by humans (undercooked meat) or by cats (wild prey or undercooked meat).

---

metronidazole can be used in the treatment of trichomoniasis in pregnant women; however, some studies indicate an increase in preterm births after treatment. Trichomoniasis also changes the pH balance in the vagina, which then can lead to bacterial vaginosis.

Vaginal yeast infections caused by *Candida albicans* are fairly common during pregnancy, but the infection usually does not travel up to the uterus and therefore does not affect the unborn. Intravaginal treatment is generally preferred over oral treatment with fluconazole, because the orally administered drug will enter the bloodstream. Whereas a single dose of fluconazole does not appear to be a risk to the fetus, high continuous doses may cause birth defects.

Infants and Children

Although many infections and illnesses that occur in infants and young children are due to perinatal infections, others infections may be transmitted to the newborn infant during the first week or two after birth.

Immune System in Infants and Children

The immune system of a newborn is immature and often unable to escalate an effective immune response. At birth and for the next few months the infant is dependent on the passive antibodies received through the placenta before birth, and via **colostrum** and breastmilk after birth. Antibodies that can cross the placenta are IgGs. In addition to IgGs, colostrum and breastmilk also contain IgAs (see Chapter 20, The Immune System) together with a variety of white blood cells. These passive antibodies are the same as the ones circulating in the mother's circulatory system, representing the mother's **immunity** to her environment. Therefore, infants usually have antibodies against microbes in their own home. However, a mother with a compromised or weak immune system will pass fewer antibodies to her child, who will thus have fewer passive antibodies and thus a weaker immune system.

Although there is some protection for an infant in its mother's womb, which contains microbes to which she has developed antibodies, the infant will not be immediately protected against new exposures. The greatest danger of infectious diseases to an infant is caused by microbes against which the mother has no antibodies; she cannot therefore pass on passive immunity to her infant. The hospital environment often contains bacteria that have developed resistance against antibiotics (see Healthcare–associated [Nosocomial] Infections in Chapter 9, Infection and Disease), which can cause a tremendous problem if an infant becomes infected.

The immune system of an infant begins to synthesize IgM antibodies soon after birth in response to the antigenic stimulation of its new environment. About 6 days after birth, the serum concentration of IgM rises sharply and this rise continues until adult levels are reached at about 1 year of age. While maternal passive IgGs will decline during the first 6 months of life, the rate of infant IgG synthesis increases. Furthermore, vaccination is done to stimulate the infant's immune system to certain infectious diseases. Vaccination schedules are available in all doctors' offices. A vaccine can be against a particular microbe, its toxins, or against the symptoms of the disease. Certain vaccinations may be required in order for the child to enter a child care center or, later, school. During childhood children are exposed to a multitude of microorganisms, illnesses, and diseases and therefore actively develop a functioning immune system.

Common Microbial Infections in Infants and Children

Skin Infections

The skin becomes colonized by normal flora during birth. The normal skin flora of an individual is dependent on age. For example, micrococci are more prominent in infants and children than on the adult skin. Skin infections are common during the neonatal period and in preschool age children exposed to contagious organisms. For more details on infections of the skin refer to Chapter 10 (Infections of the Integumentary System, Soft Tissue, and Muscle).

- **Deep folliculitis:** This condition may be extensive, involving a wide area, especially the scalp in infants and young children.
- **Staphylococcal scalded skin syndrome,** caused by group II staphylococci, is more common in infants than in adults.
- **Impetigo:** Three different forms of impetigo are recognized on the basis of clinical, bacteriological, and histological findings. In infants the most common form is impetigo neonatorum, caused by *Staphylococcus aureus*. It is a highly contagious disease and a real problem in nurseries. The illness usually occurs between the fourth and tenth day after birth and if not immediately treated can result in an epidemic in nurseries. Impetigo is also common in older children and usually is not serious; however, if attending a child care center the child may receive antibiotic treatment to be able to return to the center, usually 24 hours after the start of antibiotic therapy.

Other Neonatal Infections

- **Group B streptococcal disease (GBS):** Group B beta-hemolytic streptococci and gram-negative bacilli infection can be acquired by cross-infection in the nursery or transmitted by their mothers during birth. Some of the most common illnesses caused by group B *Streptococcus* are sepsis, pneumonia, and meningitis (also see Chapter 14, Infections of the Circulatory System).
- **Herpes simplex** infections may come from cold sores of attending adults.
- *Escherichia coli* infections are common neonatal infections that can lead to urinary tract infections, sepsis, meningitis, and pneumonia.
- **Staphylococcal conjunctivitis** (sticky eye) can occur through contamination of the infant with staphylococci from the noses and fingers of adult carriers.

Infections in Children

In their first 10 years of life children are constantly exposed to a variety of microbes, especially in day care centers and elementary school. The following is a limited list of common infections in children; a detailed listing and more information can be found on the CDC website: http://www.cdc.gov/ncidod/diseases/children/diseases.htm

- *Sore throat (pharyngitis)* caused by *Streptococcus pyogenes*, which can result in complications (see Streptococcal Infections in Chapter 11, Infections of the Respiratory System).
- *Rheumatic fever* is a childhood disease that does not stand alone. It is always preceded by another streptococcal infection (see Medical Highlights: Complications of Strep Throat [Rheumatic Fever] in Chapter 11).
- *Scarlet fever,* once a serious childhood disease, is now treatable (see Scarlet Fever in Chapter 11).
- *Otitis media:* Ear infections.

- *Chickenpox:* A disease caused by the varicella-zoster virus, causing an itchy skin rash (see Chapter 7, Viruses). Vaccination is available.
- *Rubella:* German measles is a viral respiratory infection and it is recommended by the CDC that children should be vaccinated (see Chapter 7).
- *Common cold:* Caused by human parainfluenza viruses (see Chapter 7).
- *Mumps and measles:* Both are vaccine-preventable diseases (see Chapter 7).

Young Adults

Most infections that occur in young adults can also occur in middle-aged and older adults. The infections listed in the following sections commonly occur during the college years.

Immune System in Young Adults

The immune system of young adults is active and generally has defenses against most childhood diseases, various cold viruses, and other microbes that the individual has been exposed to or has been vaccinated against. The metabolism of young adults is generally high; therefore production of new cells, including those of the immune system, flourishes during young adulthood. However, the immune system still faces major challenges because of the changing environments young adults are experiencing. Also, after puberty the thymus gland, the organ responsible for the maturation of T lymphocytes, starts to show some atrophy (see Chapter 20, The Immune System).

Common Microbial Infections in Young Adults

Infectious Mononucleosis

Infectious mononucleosis is caused by the Epstein-Barr virus and often occurs in young adults, especially during the high school years. It is also called the *"kissing disease"* because it occurs predominantly in high school–aged children. Oftentimes the virus is transmitted by sharing of drinking glasses, bottles, or utensils. For more information refer to Infectious Mononucleosis and Life Application: "Kissing Disease" in Chapter 14, Infections of the Circulatory System.

Sexually Transmitted Infections

Sexually transmitted infections (STIs) are also referred to as sexually transmitted diseases (STDs). There are about 19 million new STIs in the United States each year and almost 50% of these occur among young adults between the ages of 15 and 24 years. Despite awareness efforts, the United States has the highest rates of STIs among developed countries. Common STIs on college campuses are as follows:

- Chlamydia
- Gonorrhea
- Herpes
- Human papillomavirus (HPV)

HIV Infections in Adolescents and Young Adults

The U.S. Department of Health and Human Services expressed rising concern about the occurrence and effects of HIV/AIDS in the United States among adolescents and young adults between the ages of 13 and 24 years. In 2004 the CDC reported 40,049 cumulative cases of AIDS among individuals in this age group. More than 10,000 adolescents and young adults with AIDS have died since the beginning of the epidemic. Because of the average interval between the infection and the development of AIDS, which is 10 years, most adults with AIDS were likely infected as adolescents or young adults. Most of these young HIV-infected individuals are exposed to the virus through sexual intercourse. In addition, there are an increasing number of children who were infected as infants and are now surviving adolescence.

- Syphilis
- Hepatitis B
- Hepatitis C
- HIV

Most college students are or have been sexually active, and many have had multiple partners, increasing the risk for STIs. The rates of chlamydia, gonorrhea, and HPV are highest among female adolescents. For information about specific sexually transmitted infections please refer to Chapter 17, Sexually Transmitted Infections/Diseases.

Influenza

Adolescents and college-age students usually are not considered to be at high risk for serious influenza with resulting mortality. However, because of living in close quarters, they can easily spread the infections. In addition, segments of this population, such as those with asthma, HIV, and those who are pregnant, are at high risk for a serious infection. Influenza vaccination is available on many college campuses not only to high-risk individuals but also to those who want to avoid becoming ill with influenza. Vaccination would greatly reduce the spread of the illness and also lessen the number of days during which students miss classes. For more information about influenza refer to Chapter 11, Infections of the Respiratory System.

Meningococcal Disease

Meningococcal disease may be caused by *Neisseria meningitidis* and can cause both sporadic disease as well as outbreaks. According to the CDC, *N. meningitidis* has become the leading cause of bacterial meningitis in children and young adults in the United States. For more information refer to Meningococcal Meningitis and also to Life Application: Meningitis: The Dorm Disease? in Chapter 13, Infections of the Nervous System and Senses.

Environmental Exposures Typical for Young Adults

During adolescence many individuals become sexually active, exposing themselves to sexually transmitted microorganisms. Many of these microbes will cause infection and show symptoms, and some of them will be asymptomatic (see Chapter 17, Sexually Transmitted Infections/Diseases).

Many young adults also will attend college or join the military, where they usually are in close quarters, which can be breeding grounds for various microorganisms, some of them potentially pathogenic. After finishing college individuals enter the work force, where they are again exposed to new microbes—the immune system being challenged and actively producing antibodies (see Active Immunity [Humoral] in Chapter 20, The Immune System). Another possible exposure to new microbial environments is encountered during the travel many young adults undertake, including international destinations.

Older Adults

The United States population is rapidly aging, leading to the publication of "The State of Aging and Health in America 2007," a report released by the CDC and the Merck Company Foundation in March 2007. According to the report, by 2030 the number of Americans age 65 years and over will be more than 71 million, encompassing about 20% of the U.S. population. This will provide a challenge to the healthcare system to preserve the health of this elderly population. Besides other health challenges for an aging body, it is important to understand that microbes will interact differently in the elderly than in a young adult.

Immune System in Older Adults

Aging brings a decline in immune function, which leads to increased vulnerability to infectious disease as well a delay in recovery after an illness. This progressive dysfunction of the immune system is called **immune senescence.** The changes are generally slight and most people do not notice them. Older people most often notice changes when their immune system is less able to fight infections, when infections linger or become severe. For example, people who were infected with tuberculosis during adolescence or early adulthood may not have symptoms until old age, when the immune system is weakened.

The aging immune system is also often less able to differentiate between the body's own cells and foreign substances, and may start attacking some of the body's own cells. This can result in autoimmune disorders (see Chapter 20, The Immune System), which become more frequent during aging. The immune system is responsible for the destruction of cancer cells, invading microbes, and other foreign substances. The aging immune system is less capable of doing so, which may explain the increased incidence of cancer in the older population. Because of the reduced activity of the immune system, allergic reactions also decline.

Common Microbial Infections in Older Adults

Infectious diseases are a serious concern in the elderly population. It is estimated that infectious diseases are responsible for one third of all deaths in individuals 65 years of age and older. This is in part due to the decline in the immune system response, as well as to the problem of early detection, because the signs and symptoms of an infection are different in the elderly population. Among younger adults the classic indications of infection are fever and leukocytosis, which are present less frequently or not present at all in older infected adults. It has been reported that 60% of older adults with serious infections do develop leukocytosis, but the absence does not necessarily rule out an infection. In addition, frail elderly people generally have a poor temperature body response and elevations in body temperature of only 1.1° C from their normal baseline should be considered a febrile (feverish) response. Therefore, slight increases in body temperature likely indicate a microbial infection, which may even be life-threatening. Some of the most common infections include the following:

- Pneumonia
- Influenza
- Urinary tract infections (UTIs)
- Skin infections

Pneumonia

Although pneumonia (see also Chapter 11, Infections of the Respiratory System) occurs in people of all ages, it occurs more commonly in older people, where it tends to be more serious. Pneumonia is one of the most common and also significant health problems in the elderly, especially those hospitalized or residing in other healthcare facilities. It is often the terminal event after a prolonged serious illness and is the leading infectious cause of death in this age group. The major risk factor for developing pneumonia in this age group is the presence of another serious illness, or it can be a result of a previous illness such as influenza. In 30% to 50% of cases the infectious agent is not identified; the most common identifiable organisms causing the illness are listed as follows:

- *Streptococcus pneumoniae* causes pneumococcal pneumonia and is the most common bacterial cause of community-acquired pneumonia in the elderly. Individuals 65 years of age and older are three to five times more likely to die of this condition than are younger individuals. Drug-resistant strains cause drug-resistant *Streptococcus* pneumonia (DRSP) disease, with the elderly being highly susceptible (see Drug-resistant *Streptococcus pneumoniae* Disease in Chapter 11, Infections of the Respiratory System).
- *Haemophilus influenzae* account for 8% to 20% of pneumonias in the elderly, most frequently in those with chronic bronchitis.
- *Legionella spp.*: The susceptibility to these organisms increases with age.
- *Gram-negative bacilli* are more common in institutional settings and include *Klebsiella, Pseudomonas aeruginosa, Enterobacter* spp., *Proteus* spp., *Escherichia coli,* and others. Gram-negative bacilli often colonize in the pharynx of seriously ill patients and account for approximately 40% to 60% of all culture-diagnosed pneumonias.
- *Anaerobic bacteria* cause 20% of community-acquired infections and 31% of nosocomial cases of pneumonia in the elderly. These microbes usually cause illness among the elderly on aspiration, especially by those with conditions that cause altered consciousness due to medications and medical conditions. The organisms involved may be *Fusobacterium nucleatum,* peptostreptococci, peptococci, and *Bacteroides fragilis.*
- *Viral causes of pneumonia* include influenza and parainfluenza viruses, respiratory syncytial virus, and occasionally adenoviruses.

Influenza

Influenza is caused by one of the influenza viruses and affects the entire body, but its most evident effect is on the airways (see Chapter 11, Infections of the Respiratory System). Influenza affects persons of all ages but is particularly serious in the elderly. In a typical year the illness leads to more than 20,000 deaths, with older people accounting for more than 80% of these. Influenza vaccination is recommended for all older persons. Pneumonia and severe bronchitis commonly accompany influenza in the older population, and the rate of severity increases with age. Pneumonia may be due to primary influenza, other viral infection (e.g., the common cold), or secondary bacterial infection.

Urinary Tract Infections

Urinary tract infections (UTIs) are a common problem in the elderly. Diagnosis, prevention, and treatment can often be a problem because the clinical symptoms may be atypical. Furthermore, the host defenses decrease with age. Common risk factors for urinary tract infections in the elderly are listed in Box 23.3. For more information about urinary tract infections refer to Chapter 15, Infections of the Urinary System.

BOX 23.3 Risk Factors for Urinary Tract Infections in the Elderly

- Atrophic urethritis
- Atrophic vaginitis
- Cancer of the prostate
- Catheter use
- Chronic bacterial prostatitis
- Genitourinary problems
- Perinephric abscess
- Prostatic hyperplasia
- Urinary diversion procedures
- Urethral strictures

HEALTHCARE APPLICATION

Pneumonias in the Elderly*

Organism	Comments	Treatment
Streptococcus pneumoniae	Community-acquired; person-to-person contact or inhalation	Penicillin, first-generation cephalosporin, a macrolide, a fluoroquinolone
Haemophilus influenzae	Mostly in patients with chronic bronchitis; transmitted by aerosol	Cefuroxime, third-generation cephalosporins, trimethoprim-sulfamethoxazole, levofloxacin
Legionella spp.	Susceptibility increases with age; Legionnaire's disease	Erythromycin with or without rifampin, newer macrolide, a fluoroquinolone
Pseudomonas aeruginosa	Institutional setting; colonizes the posterior pharynx of seriously ill patients	Antipseudomonal penicillin or ceftazidime plus an aminoglycoside
Anaerobic bacteria	Community-acquired and nosocomial; usually the result of aspiration	Penicillin or clindamycin
Influenza A virus	Influenza—most important cause of pneumonia in the elderly	Amantadine or rimantadine and an antibiotic

*Also see Healthcare Application: Pneumonias in Chapter 11, Infections of the Respiratory System.

Skin Infections

Aging leads to changes in the skin and its appendages. These changes include dryness, atrophy, and decline in cell replacement, barrier function immunologic responsiveness, thermoregulation, and many more. These changes can cause a variety of skin infections including herpesvirus infections (e.g., varicella-zoster virus and herpes simplex virus [HSV]), cellulitis, erysipelas, necrotizing fasciitis, impetigo, folliculitis, furunculosis, candidiasis, and a variety of rashes. For more detailed information about the various skin infections please refer to Chapter 10, Infections of the Integumentary System, Soft Tissue, and Muscle.

Factors Influencing Susceptibility to Microbial Disease

Biological, cultural, and social factors all influence the susceptibility to infection among the elderly. Biological factors include the decline in defense mechanisms, thinning of the skin, reduced activity of sweat glands, decreased urine flow, and others. All these factors make it easier for microorganism to cause infection and disease. Other factors that increase susceptibility to infections are chronic disease such as heart disease and diabetes.

Elderly individuals in the developed world have more access to good healthcare and therefore are less susceptible to microbial diseases than those in underdeveloped countries. Different lifestyles and behavioral practices also play a major role in the susceptibility of the elderly to infectious diseases. Social factors that play a role in the susceptibility to infectious diseases in the United States include the increasing age of the population, resulting in the increased incidence of some age-related diseases which in turn will increase the susceptibility to infections in this population. Many of the older population spend more time in the hospital/healthcare environment or in nursing homes, thus making them more susceptible to nosocomial infections.

Summary

- Microorganisms affect the various human age groups in different manners because of a variety of factors, one of the most important ones being the functional capacity of the immune system.
- Microbial infections that can be passed on from a mother to a child either during pregnancy or during birth are referred to as perinatal infections. Many of them will become evident after birth.
- A congenital disorder is any medical condition that is present at birth, regardless of the origin. Congenital infections, on the other hand, are intrauterine infections that occur during pregnancy when microorganisms enter the blood, infect the placenta, and ultimately the fetus.
- Many infections and illnesses in infants are due to perinatal infections, but others may be transmitted to the newborn during the first week or two after birth.
- The immune system of the infant is immature and its defense against microorganisms depends on passive antibodies received from the mother during pregnancy and lactation.
- Young children during their day care, preschool, and elementary school years are exposed to a multitude of microbes, infections, and diseases, all of which stimulate the maturation of the immune system. Vaccination also plays an important role in this process.
- Although most infections that occur in young adults can also occur in middle-aged and older adults, certain infections such as mononucleosis and sexually transmitted infections occur more commonly in adolescents and college-aged individuals.
- In general, the immune system of young adults can respond to all the microbes it has previously been exposed to. However, once entering college, the military, or the work environment new microbial environments will challenge the immune systems of young adults to make more antibodies.
- The population aged 65 years and over is constantly increasing in the United States as well as in the rest of the world. Various infectious diseases are of great concern in this population.
- A progressive decline or dysfunction in the aging immune system is referred to as immune senescence, and is responsible for the increased incidence of severe infectious disease in the elderly. The severity of infections often increases with increasing age.

Review Questions

1. The highly specialized structure that protects the fetus from microorganisms is the:
   - a. Uterus
   - b. Placenta
   - c. Vagina
   - d. Mammary gland

2. Congenital CMV infections are caused by:
   - a. Coronavirus
   - b. Herpes simplex virus
   - c. Cytomegalovirus
   - d. Epstein-Barr virus

3. The most common virus transmitted during pregnancy is:
   - a. Cytomegalovirus
   - b. HIV
   - c. Herpes simplex virus
   - d. Epstein-Barr virus

4. A fetus infected with rubella virus produces which of the following antibodies that can then be detected in the umbilical cord?
   - a. IgA
   - b. IgM
   - c. IgG
   - d. IgD

5. The type of antibody that can cross the placenta is:
   a. IgA   c. IgG
   b. IgM   d. IgD

6. Staphylococcal scalded skin syndrome is most common in:
   a. Infants   c. Young adults
   b. Adolescents d. The elderly

7. Infectious mononucleosis most often occurs in:
   a. Infants   c. Young adults
   b. Adolescents d. The elderly

8. Almost half of all the STIs diagnosed in the United States are among:
   a. Infants   c. Young adults
   b. Adolescence d. The elderly

9. Infectious diseases in the adult population are responsible for about one third of all deaths in individuals over the age of:
   a. 50 years   c. 60 years
   b. 55 years   d. 65 years

10. All the following infections may recur during pregnancy *except:*
    a. Epstein-Barr virus infections
    b. Herpes simplex virus infections
    c. Streptococcal infections
    d. Polyomavirus infections

11. A bacterial or viral infection that can be passed from a mother to her child before or during birth is called a(n) _____ infection.

12. Impetigo neonatorum is caused by _____.

13. Infectious mononucleosis is caused by _____.

14. Chlamydia commonly occurring in young adults is a(n) _____ disease.

15. The decline in the functioning of the immune system during aging is referred to as _____.

16. Discuss congenital CMV infections and give three statistics about the infection in the United States.

17. Describe the measures the CDC has recommended to avoid congenital toxoplasmosis.

18. Name the most commonly occurring sexually transmitted infections on U.S. college campuses.

19. Name and discuss the most common microbial infections that occur in the elderly population.

20. Differentiate between the immune systems of the infant, young adult, and older individual.

Bibliography

Beers MH, Berkow R: *The Merck manual of geriatrics,* ed 3, Merck Research Laboratories, 2000–2006, available at http://www.merck.com/mkgr/mmg/home.jsp.

Beers MH, Jones TV: *The Merck manual of health & aging,* Whitehouse Station, NJ, 2004, Merck Research Laboratories.

Masoro EJ, Austad SN: *Handbook of the biology of aging,* ed 6, Burlington, MA, 2006, Academic Press/Elsevier.

Mims C, Dockrell HM, Goering RV, et al: *Medical microbiology,* ed 3, St. Louis, 2004, Mosby/Elsevier.

Murray PR, Rosenthal KS, Pfaller MA: *Medical microbiology,* ed 5, St. Louis, 2005, Mosby/Elsevier.

Internet Resources

CDC Features: *Preventing Infections during Pregnancy,* www.cdc.gov/Features/Pregnancy

CDC, *Sexually Transmitted Diseases, Bacterial Vaginosis - CDC Fact Sheet,* http://www.cdc.gov/std/bv/STDFact-Bacterial-Vaginosis.htm

Medline Plus, Medical Encyclopedia, Congenital Rubella, http://www.nlm.nih.gov/medlineplus/ency/article/001658.htm

CDC, Cytomegalovirus (CMV), http://www.cdc.gov/cmv/facts.htm

National Institute of Allergy and Infectious Diseases, HIV Infection in Adolescents and Young Adults in the U.S., May 2006, http://www.niaid.nih.gov/factsheets/hivadolescent.htm

Jones J, Lopez A, Wilson M: Congenital Toxoplasmosis, *American Family Physician,* May 15, 2003, available at http://www.aafp.org/afp/20030515/2131.html

CDC, Infectious Disease Information: Childhood Diseases, http://www.cdc.gov/ncidod/diseases/children/diseases.htm

CDC, The State of Aging and Health in America 2007 Report, http://www.cdc.gov/aging/saha.htm

24

Microorganisms in the Environment and Environmental Safety

OUTLINE

Normal Environmental Conditions
Microbial Ecology
Biogeochemical Cycles and Microbes
Soil Microbiology
Aquatic Microbiology

Natural Disasters
Floods
Tsunamis
Earthquakes
Hurricanes

Bioterrorism
Category A Agents
Category B Agents
Category C Agents

Role of First Responders in Bioterrorism

LEARNING OBJECTIVES

After reading this chapter, the student will be able to:

- Discuss microbial ecology and describe the levels of microbial relationships within the environment
- Discuss the importance of biogeochemical cycles, including the carbon, nitrogen, sulfur, and phosphorus cycles
- Discuss soil microbiology, with emphasis on the abundance and type of microbes in the soil
- Discuss aquatic microbiology, both freshwater and marine environments, and include the zones observable in these bodies of water
- Describe the characteristics of natural disasters including floods, tsunamis, earthquakes, and hurricanes
- Illustrate the most common infections/diseases associated with natural disasters
- Explain the concepts of biological warfare and bioterrorism
- Describe the initiatives taken to advance national public health capabilities in response to bioterrorism
- Define and describe the three groups of agents that are of concern in bioterrorism
- Discuss the role of first responders in bioterrorism

abiotic
abyssal zone
ammonification
anammox
anthrax
arenaviruses
benthic zone
benthos
biodiversity
biogeochemical cycle
biogeochemistry
biomass
biospheres
bioterrorism
biotic
botulism
Bunyaviridae
carbon cycle
communities
cutaneous anthrax

deamination
denitrification
Division of Bioterrorism
    Preparedness and
    Response
ecosystems
Environmental
    Protection Agency
    (EPA)
eutrophication
Filoviridae
Flaviviridae
free-living
    nitrogen-fixing
guilds
habitats
heterocysts
inhalation anthrax
lichens

limnetic zone
littoral zone
microbial ecology
microhabitats
nitrification
nitrogenase
nitrogen cycle
nitrogen fixation
phosphorus cycle
plague
populations
profundal zone
smallpox
sulfur cycle
symbiotic nitrogen-fixing
tsunami
tularemia
viral hemorrhagic fevers
    (VHFs)

WHY YOU NEED TO KNOW

HISTORY

Floods, tsunamis, earthquakes, hurricanes, fires, and the use of chemical or biological forces are certainly not new to humankind. Some of these can be prevented; others cannot. The biblical story of Noah's ark probably is a description of one major flood in that particular region of the world. Other natural disasters certainly have been described in various ways throughout the history of this planet. In addition to the natural disasters mentioned, humans have also faced attacks by microorganisms, causing major epidemics and pandemics over the centuries.

In the past, humankind has harnessed the destructive power of biology to be used as a weapon in conflict. For example, in ancient times armies would hurl dead or decomposing animals into a city under siege to spread disease. A Tartar attack on a city in 1346 involved catapulting corpses of plague victims into the city, causing the desired epidemic. In more modern times the Japanese army had a specific unit called *Unit 731* during World War II that performed extensive experimentation with biological weapons on prisoners of war. These agents included the causative pathogens of anthrax, botulism, cholera, and the plague, to name but a few. In the most recent past, in October 2001, one month after the 9/11 attack, anthrax spores were sent through the mail, causing 22 infections. Five resulted in death. History is replete with examples of the use of biological agents as weapons, and this tool of warfare will certainly continue to be developed and used in various disputes and conflicts around the world.

IMPACT

Physical science evolved as humans built houses, dams, and other protective structures to help survive natural disasters. At the same time, life science moved forward with the help of philosophers such as Aristoteles (Aristotle), Plato, Socrates, and many others, who studied diverse subjects including biology in order to understand the functioning of the human body and life in general. However, it was not until the merging of physical and life sciences, with the invention of the microscope, that humans could "see" microorganisms and started to understand their power. The physical and biological sciences, combined, have since come a long way to help nations after natural disasters, and to help in the management of epidemics and pandemics.

Since the 9/11 attacks we have also come a long way in our study of potential weapons of terrorism, specifically bioterrorism. Once considered eradicated by the World Health Organization (WHO), the United States is now embarked on a program to produce the smallpox vaccine as it has been identified as a potential bioweapon that could have catastrophic effect if used deliberately against a population. There are numerous groups and agencies recently established or reorganized within the government to deal with a potential bioterrorism threat.

FUTURE

After successfully battling disease-causing microorganisms, new and reemerging ones are challenging today's society. Advances in biotechnology do promise more effective prevention and treatment of infectious diseases. Ongoing climate changes and population movement will also play a role in the occurrence of natural disasters and emerging infectious diseases, respectively.

As new diseases emerge or are added to the list of potential bioweapons, the need for a coordinated and rapidly responding network to deal with the threat is becoming more obvious. The potential for the rapid spread of diseases, the shortage of facilities ready to handle a massive biological crisis, and the psychological impact of mass medical casualties among a civilian population all indicate the need for well-informed and prepared healthcare professionals and "first responders" to help face the increasing bioterrorism threat.

Normal Environmental Conditions

The study of microorganisms in the environment is referred to as *environmental microbiology*. A *habitat* is the physical location where organisms are found. Because of their adaptive capacity to change, microbes can be found in any niches of the environment. The habitats available to microbes include almost every place on earth, including glaciers, Antarctic ice, and hot springs. Depending on their metabolic cycles different microbes will take advantage of different environmental conditions. For example, if a population of aerobic microorganisms in the soil takes up all the oxygen, anaerobic microorganisms will flourish until oxygen is available again and aerobic organisms can emerge.

Microbial Ecology

The study of the interrelationships of microorganisms in their natural environments is referred to as **microbial ecology.** Terms used to describe the levels of microbial relationships in the environment are as follows (Figure 24.1):

- **Populations** are formed by individual organisms through growth and reproduction.
- **Guilds** are populations of microorganisms that perform linked metabolic activities.
- **Communities** are sets of guilds and are characteristically heterogeneous. On occasion, especially in extreme environments, a community can consist of a single population.
- **Microhabitats** are specific small niches in which populations and guilds within a community reside because of optimal conditions for survival.
- **Habitats** are physical locations where organisms are found and they consist of groups of microhabitats. Within habitats the microorganisms interact with larger organisms.
- **Ecosystems** consist of organisms, their abiotic environment, and the relationships between them.
- **Biospheres** are regions of the earth populated by living organisms.

There is no natural habitat on earth that supports higher organisms and not microorganisms, but many microbial

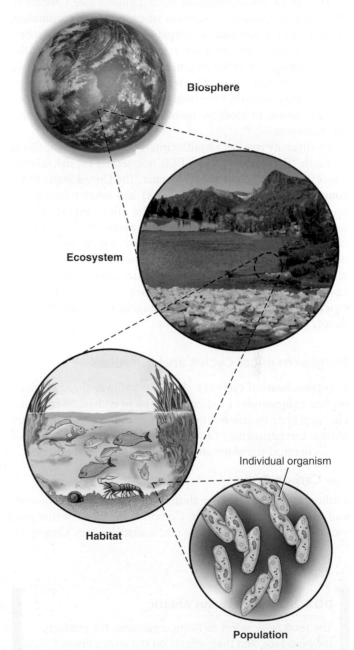

FIGURE 24.1 Example of levels of organization in an ecosystem.

habitats do not support higher organisms. Regardless of their size, microorganisms are responsible for about half of all the biomass on earth. **Biodiversity** refers to the number of species living in a given ecosystem; **biomass** is the quantity of all organisms in an ecosystem. Microorganisms, in their great variety and numbers, represent tremendous metabolic diversity and act as the primary catalyst of many nutrient cycles in nature.

Thriving ecosystems are able to support great biodiversity, but many microbes live in harsh ecosystems where nutrients are limited. Therefore, in order to survive, these microbes must have special adaptation to a given environment. Environments may cycle between excess nutrient availability and depletion. To survive, some microorganisms form biofilms (see Chapter 6, Bacteria and Archaea) on surfaces where nutrients accumulate. Biodiversity is controlled by competition between the microbes, but usually an ecosystem is heterogenic. Microbes often use the waste products of other organisms for their own metabolic activities; in other cases the waste products of one type of microbe may make the environment more favorable for another. The formation of biofilms serves as a good example of this phenomenon.

Biodiversity ensures a healthy interaction between life forms on earth. This complex web of life is essential for the maintenance of sufficient food and freshwater. The United States **Environmental Protection Agency (EPA)** and other national and international organizations recognize the importance of biodiversity for human health and well-being. The EPA in partnership with other organizations implemented the biodiversity-human health project (http://epa.gov/ncer/biodiversity/index.html). One focus of the project is to better understand the relationship of emerging infectious diseases (see Chapter 18, Emerging Infectious Diseases), changing environments, and factors that manipulate biodiversity.

Biogeochemical Cycles and Microbes

A **biogeochemical cycle** is a circuit or pathway through which organic compounds or a chemical element is changed from one chemical state to another by moving through both **biotic** and **abiotic** compartments of an ecosystem (Box 24.1). The study of these chemical transformations is called **biogeochemistry.**

The Carbon Cycle

Carbon is the fourth most abundant element in the universe, and essential to life on earth. Carbon is the element that provides the backbone of all organic molecules (see Chapter 2,

Chemistry of Life). All living organisms from microorganisms, to plants and animals, contain a large number of organic compounds and therefore a large amount of carbon. Thus the **carbon cycle** is considered to be the primary biogeochemical cycle.

For the carbon cycle to start, autotrophic organisms are necessary, either photoautotrophs or chemoautotrophs—organisms that use carbon dioxide as their primary source of carbon. Photoautotrophs are the primary organisms in the carbon cycle and include cyanobacteria, green and purple bacteria (sulfur and nonsulfur), algae, photosynthetic protozoa, and plants. All these organisms convert carbon dioxide (CO_2) to organic molecules via carbon fixation during photosynthesis. Photoautotrophs require sunlight and for that reason are restricted to soil and water surfaces. Chemoautotrophs can also fix carbon dioxide into organic matter, but because they cannot use the energy of the sun, they need to metabolize compounds such as hydrogen sulfide for energy.

The next step in the carbon cycle involves the consumption of autotrophs by chemoheterotrophs such as animals and protozoans, which then catabolize the organic molecules for energy, resulting in the release of CO_2. Some organic molecules produced by the autotrophs may be incorporated into the tissues of heterotrophs, where they remain until that organism dies. Dead organisms are decomposed with the help of microorganisms, metabolizing organic molecules and releasing CO_2 in the process. The release of CO_2 into the atmosphere starts the cycle over again (Figure 24.2).

The Nitrogen Cycle

Nitrogen gas is the most abundant gas in the earth's atmosphere, representing about 79% of all the gases in air. Unfortunately, the nitrogen in the atmosphere is unusable by most organisms. Only about 0.03% of the earth's nitrogen is fixed in the form of nitrates, nitrites, ammonium ion, and organic compounds. Nitrogen is necessary for all living organisms for the synthesis of proteins, nucleic acids, and other nitrogen-containing compounds. The **nitrogen cycle** consists of several steps as illustrated in Figure 24.3.

Nitrogen fixation is a process by which nitrogen gas (N_2) is reduced to ammonia (NH_3), a process catalyzed by the enzyme **nitrogenase.** Only a limited number of prokaryotes are capable of performing this process. Nitrogenase functions only in the complete absence of oxygen, which does not present a problem for anaerobic microbes. Aerobic nitrogen fixers must protect nitrogenase from oxygen, which is done in several ways. Some of these microbes use oxygen at such a high rate that it never enters the cell and therefore does not come in contact with the enzyme. Some cyanobacteria fix nitrogen only at night, when the oxygen-producing cycle of photosynthesis does not occur; other cyanobacteria form nonphotosynthetic cells referred to as **heterocysts** to protect the enzyme from oxygen in the atmosphere as well as from the oxygen produced during photosynthesis. Nitrogen fixers can be free-living or symbiotic.

Free-living, nitrogen-fixing bacteria include aerobic species of *Azotobacter,* aerobic cyanobacteria, and anaerobic species of *Bacillus* and *Clostridium.* They are found in particularly high

---

BOX 24.1 Biotic versus Abiotic

The term *biotic* refers to living organisms, the products they produce, and their effects on the environment. *Abiotic* components are nonliving components in the environment that directly or indirectly affect the environmental conditions, and therefore the biotic components, of the environment.

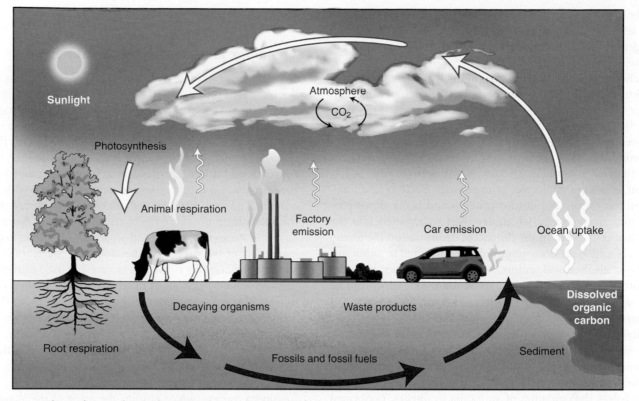

FIGURE 24.2 The carbon cycle. Carbon provides the backbone of all organic molecules necessary for all life forms. This illustration shows the complexity of the recycling/use of carbon from one form to another.

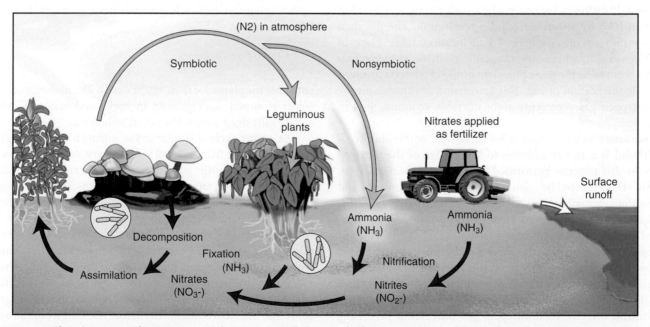

FIGURE 24.3 The nitrogen cycle. Nitrogen is also an essential element for living organisms. Nitrogen from the atmosphere goes through fixation, nitrification, and denitrification and absorption by living organisms. This is then followed by decomposition, ammonification, and then nitrification again.

concentrations in the rhizosphere, a region about 2 mm in diameter around the roots of plants. As these organisms die, they release the fixed nitrogen into the upper layers of the soil, where it then becomes available to plants and to the animals that graze on the plants.

Symbiotic nitrogen-fixing bacteria live in direct symbiosis with plants. The main organism in this category is *Rhizobium,* which is especially adapted to leguminous plant species, on which the organism forms root nodules. Nitrogen is fixed in the nodules, the plant provides an anaerobic environment and nutrients to the bacteria, and the bacteria then provides the plant with usable nitrogen. The nitrogen fixers provide enough nitrogen to the leguminous plants so that the farmer does not have to apply nitrogen fertilizers.

Lichens, which are a symbiotic (mutualistic) combination of a fungus and an algae or cyanobacteria, also play an important role in nitrogen fixation in the forest environment. If the symbiont is a nitrogen-fixing cyanobacterium, the fixed nitrogen will eventually enrich the forest soil.

Ammonification is the process by which amino groups are converted to ammonia. Almost all nitrogen in the soil is present in organic molecules of organisms. Bacteria and fungi decompose wastes and dead organisms and break down proteins into amino acids, which are then transported into the microbial cells. Next, in the process of **deamination** the amino groups of amino acids are removed and converted to ammonia. In dry or alkaline soil ammonia will escape as gas; however, in moist soil it is converted to ammonium ion, which can be absorbed by bacteria and plants and used for amino acid synthesis.

Nitrification involves oxidation of nitrogen in the ammonium ion to produce nitrate (NO_3^-). This is a two-step process involving two genera of autotrophic nitrifying bacteria, which oxidize ammonia or nitrite (NO_2^-) to obtain energy. The first step involves the oxidation of ammonia to nitrites, performed by *Nitrosomonas* spp. Nitrites are toxic to plants, but in the second stage *Nitrobacter* oxidize nitrites into nitrates, which are soluble and can be used by plants.

Denitrification is the process by which nitrate is reduced to nitrogen (N_2) by anaerobic cellular respiration. The gas then escapes into the atmosphere. Denitrification takes place in waterlogged soils where little oxygen is available. *Pseudomonas* species seem to be the most prevalent group of bacteria involved in the denitrification of soil. This conversion of valuable nitrate into nitrogen gas represents a considerable economic loss in agriculture.

Anammox is the acronym for anaerobic ammonium oxidation and is a recent addition to knowledge of the nitrogen cycle. In this process, performed by anammox bacteria (previously thought to be denitrifying bacteria), nitrite and ammonium are directly converted to dinitrogen gas. This process accounts for up to 50% of the dinitrogen gas produced in the oceans. Ammonia is the major source of fixed nitrogen in the oceans and because the anammox bacteria remove ammonia efficiently from those bodies of water, these organisms limit oceanic primary productivity. On the positive side, the ability of anammox bacteria to convert ammonium and nitrite directly to dinitrogen gas provides a promising alternative to current methods of removal of nitrogen from wastewater (see Life Application: Anammox and Wastewater Treatment).

The Sulfur Cycle

Sulfur is the tenth most abundant element in the universe and is present in vitamins, proteins, and hormones. Sulfur is important for the appropriate functioning of proteins and enzymes in plants, as well as in animals that depend on plants for sulfur. Plants absorb sulfur when it is dissolved in water, and animals

Anammox and Wastewater Treatment

The removal of nitrogen is the most complicated factor in the treatment of urban wastewater. Nitrification accounts for more that 50% of the oxygen need and requires long sludge aging. Application of the anammox process is a promising alternative to the current methods used for the removal of nitrogen from wastewaters. Instead of the conventional nitrification–denitrification process, only half the nitrogen needs to be oxidized partly to nitrate with the anammox process. Bacteria that are capable of performing the anammox process are members of the genera *Brocadia, Kuenenia, Anammoxoglobus,* and *Scalindua.* An interesting by-product of this process in the production of hydrazine as an intermediate. This substance is normally used as rocket fuel and is highly poisonous to most living organisms. The running costs of wastewater treatment systems using the anammox process are only about 10% of the cost of the current methods. However, the technique is still young and the first full-scale sludge-water treatment plant using the anammox process was built in Hattingen, Germany, in 2000. The bacteria function in a biofilm system in the treatment process, which ensures the aging of the sludge. As of 2006 there are two full-scale processes in the Netherlands, one municipal treatment plant in Rotterdam and one in an industrial treatment plant. One full-scale plant using this system is a wastewater treatment plant in Strass, Austria.

consume the plants for their sulfur needs. The majority of earth's sulfur is stored underground in rocks and minerals, and as sulfate salts deep within the ocean sediments.

The **sulfur cycle** is similar to the nitrogen cycle, except that sulfur originates from natural sedimentary deposits. The sulfur cycle includes both atmospheric and terrestrial processes (Figure 24.4). The terrestrial process begins with the weathering of rocks, resulting in the release of stored sulfur. Subsequently, the sulfur comes in contact with air and is then converted into sulfate (SO_4). Plants and microorganisms will take up the sulfate and convert it into organic forms. Animals will consume the organic forms via food they consume, thereby moving the sulfur through the food chain. As organisms die, bacteria decompose them, releasing sulfur-containing amino acids into the environment. The sulfur released from the amino acids is converted by microorganisms to its most reduced form, hydrogen sulfide (H_2S). This process is called *sulfur dissimilation.* H_2S is then oxidized to elemental sulfur and then to sulfate by various microorganisms under various conditions. These organisms include nonphotosynthetic autotrophs such as *Thiobacillus* and *Beggiatoa* and photoautotrophic green and purple sulfur bacteria. The cycle starts again with the uptake of sulfate by plants and algae that animals eat. Anaerobic respiration by the bacterium *Desulfovibrio* reduces sulfate back to H_2S.

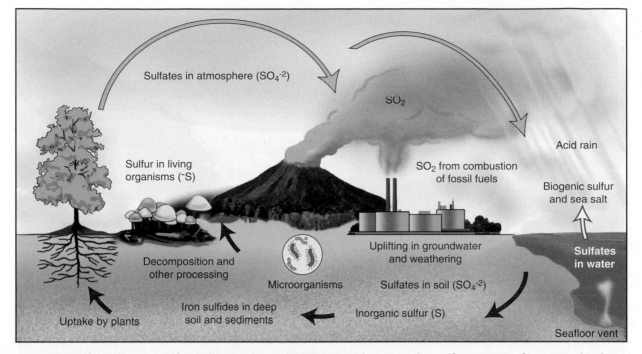

FIGURE 24.4 The sulfur cycle. The sulfur cycle is similar to the nitrogen cycle, except that sulfur originates from natural sedimentary deposits. The sulfur cycle includes both atmospheric and terrestrial processes.

Sulfur can also be found in the atmosphere. A variety of natural sources emit sulfur directly into the atmosphere, including volcanic eruptions, bacterial processes, decaying organisms, and the evaporation of water. When sulfur dioxide enters the atmosphere it will react with oxygen to produce sulfur trioxide gas, or it can react with other chemicals in the atmosphere to produce sulfur salts. Furthermore, sulfur dioxide can react with water to produce sulfuric acid. All these particles will eventually settle back onto the earth, or react with rain and fall back to earth as acid deposition. The particles will then be absorbed by plants, and the sulfur cycle will start over again.

The Phosphorus Cycle

Phosphorus is an essential nutrient for plants, animals, and microorganisms. It is part of nucleic acids (DNA, RNA, ATP, and ADP) and of the plasma membranes (phospholipids). Phosphorus can be found in water, soil, and sediments. Unlike nitrogen and sulfur, phosphorus cannot be found in the atmosphere in the gaseous state. Phosphorus exists in the form of phosphate ion and undergoes little change in its oxidation state. The **phosphorus cycle** (Figure 24.5) involves changes of phosphorus from insoluble to soluble forms that are available for uptake by organisms, and from organic to inorganic forms by pH-dependent processes. Because no gaseous form of phosphorus exists it has the tendency to accumulate in the seas and other bodies of water.

Excess phosphorus can present a problem in a habitat. Agricultural fertilizers rich in phosphate and nitrogen are easily leached from the fields by rain. The resulting runoff into rivers and lakes can cause **eutrophication,** the overgrowth of microorganisms in nutrient-rich waters. The organisms involved include mainly algae and cyanobacteria. Such overgrowth, referred to as a bloom, depletes oxygen from the water, resulting in the death of aerobic organisms such as fish. Anaerobic organisms then take over, leading to increased production of H_2S and resulting in the release of foul odors.

Soil Microbiology

Soil composition such as organic matter, soil structure, nutrient content, nutrient cycling, nutrient availability, and water-holding capacity are influenced by, or dependent on, billions of organisms, microscopic ones as well as fairly large insects and earthworms. All these organisms together form a pulsating, living community in soil. Soil microorganisms can be classified into major groups such as microarthropods, nematodes, protozoa, fungi, algae, and bacteria. The most numerous organisms in the soil are bacteria—each gram of typical soil contains millions of bacteria. The population of bacteria is largest in the top few centimeters of soil and declines rapidly with depth. Organic matter is metabolized by microbes in the soil, and via the biogeochemical cycles, elements are oxidized and reduced (see Chapter 2, Chemistry of Life, for oxidation/reduction reactions) by microorganisms to meet their metabolic needs.

A healthy soil high in humus content provides a rich culture medium for an array for microorganisms. Several environmental factors influence the density and composition of microbes in the soil. These factors include the amount of moisture/water, oxygen content, pH, temperature, and availability of nutrients:

- *Moisture* is essential for the survival of microorganisms. In dry soil microbes will exhibit lower metabolic activity, they

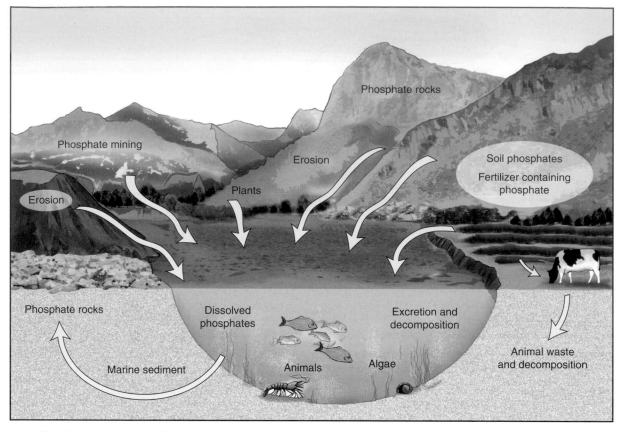

FIGURE 24.5 The phosphorus cycle. The phosphorus cycle involves changes of phosphorus from insoluble to soluble forms that are available for uptake by organisms, and from organic to inorganic forms by pH-dependent processes. Because no gaseous form of phosphorus exists it has the tendency to accumulate in the seas and other bodies of water.

will be less diverse, and lower numbers will be present than in moist soil.

- *Oxygen* dissolves poorly in water; therefore, moist soils are lower in oxygen content than dry soils. Waterlogged soil will result in a decline in microbial diversity and anaerobic organisms will dominate. The presence or absence of rainwater determines moisture, and thus dissolved oxygen.
- The *pH* of soil influences the type of organisms that predominate. It will influence whether the soil is rich in bacteria or rich in fungi. In highly acidic or highly basic soils fungi will predominate, whereas bacteria prefer soil with a pH of about 7.
- The *temperature* of soil determines the types of microbe that can flourish. Most soil organisms are mesophiles and grow well in areas where winters and summers are not too extreme. Psychrophiles grow only in cold environments and cannot survive in areas that experience spring thawing. Thermophiles, on the other hand, grow only in warm environments where winters are not harsh.
- *Nutrient availability* also affects the microbial abundance and diversity of soil. The majority of soil microbes are heterotrophic and utilize the organic matter present in the soil. It is the amount of organic material rather than the kind of organic material that determines the abundance of microorganisms in a microbial community. A continuous influx of organic material (i.e., agricultural land) will

support a wider assortment of microorganisms than soil with low amounts of organic material.

Microbial Populations in Soil

The microbial populations in soil vary depending on the type of soil. Bacteria are the most abundant and diverse soil inhabitants; they are found in all layers and often form biofilms, especially around plant roots. Bacteria are highly adaptable to changing environments, and therefore are plentiful in most soils. Fungi are next in numbers. Both free-living and symbiotic fungi are present only in topsoil, where they can form large mycelia (mats of fibrous hyphae) that potentially cover several acres. Algae and protozoa are also present in soil but in smaller numbers than bacteria and fungi. Soil algae are photoautotrophs and therefore exist on or near the soil surface. Protozoans are mobile and move around the soil feeding on other microbes, especially bacteria. Although viruses are present within microorganisms, they generally are not found free.

Aquatic Microbiology

Water occupies nearly three-fourths of the earth's surface. Aquatic microbiology deals with the study of microorganisms and their activities in freshwater and marine environments, including lakes, ponds, streams, rivers, estuaries, and oceans. Many microorganisms that live in aquatic systems form biofilms attached to surfaces. Biofilms allow these microbes to concentrate enough nutrients to survive and sustain growth. Basically, aquatic habitats are divided into freshwater and marine systems. Natural aquatic systems are affected by the release of domestic water, a result of sewage treatment plants and industrial waste. The amount and quality of domestic water released into the environment greatly affects the chemistry and microbial content of the aquasystem. Large numbers of microorganisms in a body of water indicate a high level of nutrients, often a result of contaminated inflows from sewage systems or from biodegradable industrial organic wastes. Ocean estuaries often have a higher nutrient level than other shoreline waters, and therefore have larger microbial populations.

Freshwater Ecosystems

About 3% of the world's water is freshwater, 99% of which is either frozen in glaciers and pack ice, or is buried in aquifers. The remainder of the freshwater is found in lakes, ponds, rivers, and streams. Microorganisms are dispersed vertically within lake and pond systems, according to the availability of oxygen, light intensity, and temperature. Surface waters are higher in oxygen and light intensity, and warmer than deeper waters. In contrast to stagnant waters where oxygen is readily depleted, in larger lakes the wave action continuously mixes nutrients, oxygen, and organisms, resulting in efficient use of its resources. In stagnant waters, because of the depletion of oxygen, anaerobic organism will dominate and a lesser water quality will be the result. Four distinct vertical zones can be observed in lakes and ponds (Figure 24.6): a littoral zone, a limnetic zone, a profundal zone, and a benthic zone:

- The **littoral zone** (Figure 24.7) is the area along the shoreline with considerable rooted vegetation and good light source. This is the zone where nutrients enter the lake or pond, providing an abundance of food and promoting a high diversity of animals and bacteria in the biotope.

HEALTHCARE APPLICATION

Examples of Soil-borne Diseases

Microorganism	Disease
Bacillus anthracis	Anthrax
Clostridium tetani	Tetanus
Hantavirus	Hantavirus pulmonary syndrome
Histoplasma capsulatum	Histoplasmosis
Blastomyces dermatitidis	Blastomycosis
Sporothrix schenckii	Sporotrichosis

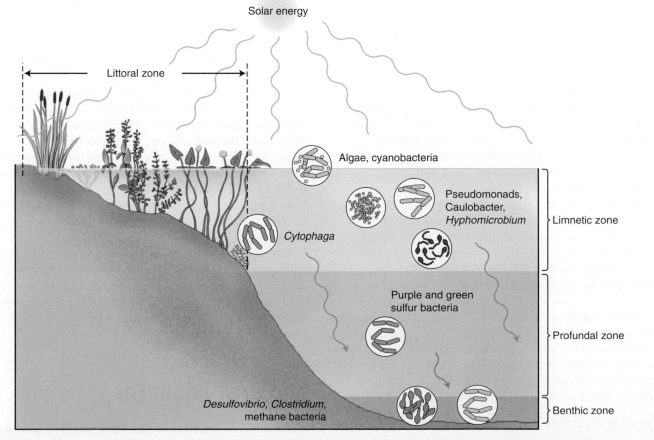

FIGURE 24.6 Zones in a typical lake or pond. Four distinct vertical zones can be observed in lakes and ponds: a littoral zone, a limnetic zone, a profundal zone, and a benthic zone.

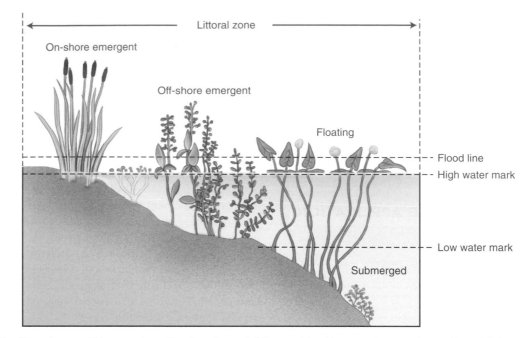

FIGURE 24.7 The littoral zone. This area along the shoreline exhibits considerable rooted vegetation and good light source.

- The **limnetic zone** is the well-lit, upper layer of water away from the shore. This area is occupied by phytoplankton consisting of algae and cyanobacteria, and zooplankton, small crustaceans, and fish. Areas of the limnetic zone with sufficient oxygen supply also contain *Pseudomonas* spp., *Cytophaga, Caulobacter,* and *Hyphomicrobium.*

- The **profundal zone** is the deeper water located below the limnetic zone. It is characterized by limited light penetration (diffuse light), lower oxygen content, and lower temperature. The organisms of this zone depend on import of organic matter drifting down from the littoral and limnetic zones. This zone is inhabited mainly by primary consumers that are either attached to or crawl along the sediments at the bottom of the lake. These bottom-dwelling organisms are referred to as **benthos.** Purple and green sulfur bacteria can also be found in this zone.

- The **benthic zone** consists of the sediments at the bottom of a lake; it includes the sediment surface as well as some subsurface layers. This layer also contains benthos, which generally live in close relationship with the substrate bottom. These life forms can tolerate cool temperatures and low oxygen levels. Bacteria found in this zone include *Desulfovibrio,* methane-producing bacteria, and *Clostridium* species.

Contrary to the vertical stratification of lakes and ponds, rivers and streams lack this stratification because the organisms and nutrients are continuously swept along and mixed. Many organisms live toward the edges, where currents are low and organic material enters the water. Furthermore, biofilms can readily be found on rocks of rivers and streams.

Marine Ecosystems

Marine (saltwater) ecosystems are part of the largest aquatic system on earth, covering more than 70% of the earth's surface. Marine ecosystems host many different species ranging from planktonic organisms that comprise the base of the marine food web, to fish, and large marine mammals. These ecosystems have some unique qualities, specifically the presence of dissolved compounds, particularly salts. As in freshwater systems the oceans can also be divided into layers, but they do have a fifth zone, the **abyssal zone,** which encompasses the deep ocean trenches (Figure 24.8). The majority of marine microorganisms are present in the littoral zone, where light is readily available and nutrient levels are high. The upper 200 m of ocean contains an unseen population of microbes that supports oceanic life. These are photosynthetic organisms called the *marine phytoplankton.* The many kinds of different bacteria among the phytoplankton are a food source for protozoa, which in turn are prey for the multicellular organisms among the zooplankton. The zooplankton is a source of food for the fish. The carbon dioxide and mineral nutrients released as by-products of the metabolic activities of bacteria, protozoa, and zooplankton are recycled into the photosynthetic phytoplankton.

The benthic abyssal zones have sparse nutrients, but they still support microbial growth, especially around hydrothermal vents. These vents release superheated, nutrient-rich water, providing nutrients and energy for thermophilic chemoautotrophic anaerobes. These organisms in turn support a variety of invertebrate and vertebrate animals.

Natural Disasters

Natural disasters are the consequence of natural hazards, including such naturally occurring phenomena as earthquakes, volcanic eruptions, landslides, hurricanes, tsunamis, floods, and

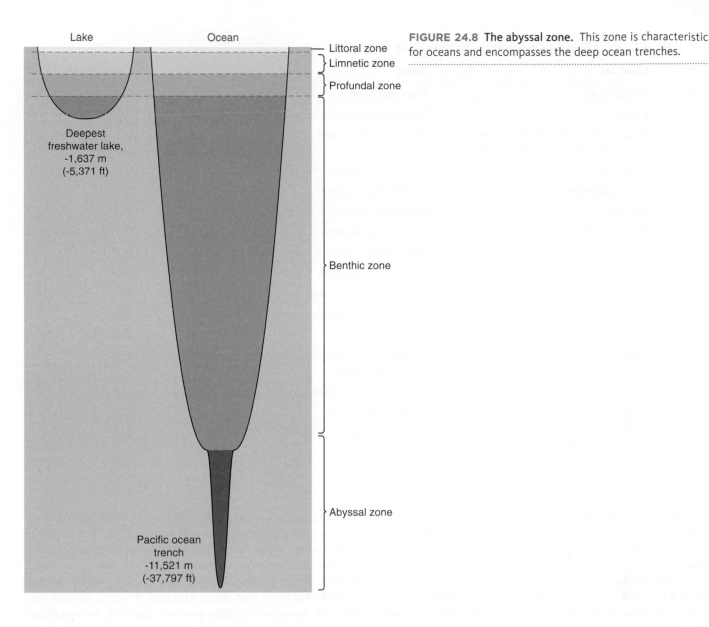

FIGURE 24.8 The abyssal zone. This zone is characteristic for oceans and encompasses the deep ocean trenches.

Lake   Ocean

Littoral zone
Limnetic zone
Profundal zone

Deepest
freshwater lake,
-1,637 m
(-5,371 ft)

Benthic zone

Abyssal zone

Pacific ocean
trench
-11,521 m
(-37,797 ft)

drought. Natural disasters result in a serious breakdown in sustainability of economic and social progress, and also provide a major challenge to public health. The type of medical care required during and after a natural disaster is determined by variables such as the cycle of nature, the type of the disaster, the population, and endemic disease.

During the past two decades, natural disasters have been increasing in frequency, complexity, scope, and destructive capacity. Earthquakes, hurricanes, tornadoes, tsunamis, floods, landslides, volcanic eruptions, and wildfires have killed millions of people, and adversely affected the life of many more due to enormous economic damage. Poor and developing countries show the greatest losses due to the lack of infrastructure, disease prevention, and disaster preparedness and prevention.

Floods

A flood is an overflowing of water onto land that is normally dry. When the volume of water within a body of water, such as a river or lake, surpasses the total capacity of the body, water will flow out of its perimeters, causing a flood. The flood of the Yellow River in 1931 is generally considered to be the deadliest natural disaster ever recorded, certainly in the twentieth century, discounting pandemic diseases such as the influenza pandemic of 1918. The estimated number of people killed in this flood is between 1 and 2 million. Flooding in more recent times is illustrated in Table 24.1.

Worldwide, there is an increased transmission of infectious diseases associated with flooding. The National Center for Medical Intelligence (NCMI, Fort Detrick, MD) is typically interested in the results of flooding, specifically the increased transmission of many infectious diseases, especially in developing countries. Flooding normally does not introduce new diseases to an area but can increase transmission of diseases. Depending on the region of the world affected, this increased transmission may include food-, water-, and vector-borne diseases, respiratory diseases, and water contact diseases. The fecal contamination of drinking water sources, increased direct contact with surface water, and crowding in temporary shelters increase the risk of infectious disease.

TABLE 24.1 Lethal Flooding in the Years 2000 to 2008

Year	Location	Event	Estimated Death Toll
2008	United States	Midwest flooding	17
2007	China	Mountain torrents, mud-rock flows, landslide	1029
2007	Sudan, Nigeria, Burkina Faso, Ghana, Kenya, and other African countries	African Nations Flood	353
2007	Indonesia	Central and East Java torrential monsoon rain, flood	119
2007	United Kingdom	United Kingdom floods	11
2006	Ethiopia	Omo River delta, Dire Dawa, Tena, Gode, flash flood	705
2006	North Korea	North Korea flooding	610
2005	China	Fujian, Anhui, Zhejiang flood	1624
2005	India	Mumbai, Maharashtra, Kamataka, monsoon rain	1503
2005	United States	New Orleans dike failure	70
2004	India, Bangladesh	Eastern India, Bangladesh monsoon rain	3076
2004	Haiti, Dominican Republic	Spring flooding	1605–3363
2003	Indonesia	Sumatra flood, Jambi, Batanghari, Tondano, torrential rain, flash flood	313
2002	Nepal	Nepal flood, Makwanpur, torrential rain	429
2001	Algeria	Algiers, Bab El Oued	827
2000	Mozambique	Mozambique flood	800

Waterborne Diseases

Waterborne diseases that can occur after floods include typhoid fever, cholera, leptospirosis, and hepatitis A (see Chapter 1 [Scope of Microbiology] and Chapter 12 [Infections of the Gastrointestinal System]). Although flooding is associated with an increased risk of infection, the risk is low unless there is a significant population displacement and/or major contamination of the water supply. Therefore a major risk factor for outbreaks associated with floods is the contamination of drinking water facilities. The risk can be minimized once the threat has been recognized and disaster response addresses the provision of safe drinking water as a priority.

Furthermore, an increased risk for waterborne infection and disease exists through direct contact with polluted waters. Such infections include wound infections, dermatitis, conjunctivitis, and ear, nose, and throat infections. However, these conditions generally do not cause epidemics.

A disease that can reach epidemic proportions is leptospirosis, which can be transmitted directly from contaminated water. Transmission occurs by contact of the skin and mucous membranes with water, damp soil or vegetation, or mud contaminated with rodent urine. Flooding facilitates the spread of the organism because of the proliferation of rodents, which shed large amounts of leptospira in their urine.

Vector-borne Diseases

Vector-borne diseases may be indirectly increased after floods because of the increase in the number and range of vector habitats. Standing water caused by overflow of rivers and/or heavy rain are infamous breeding sites for mosquitoes. An increase in the mosquito population enhances the potential for exposure of the disaster-affected population and the emergency personnel. Possible vector-borne infections and disease include dengue, malaria, and West Nile fever. Although flooding initially may flush out mosquito breeding grounds, they will be reestablishing as the floodwaters recede. Malaria epidemics after flooding are a well-known phenomenon in malaria-endemic areas worldwide.

Dead Humans and Animals

Risk posed by corpses exists only for workers who routinely handle corpses. There is no concrete evidence that corpses pose a risk of epidemics after natural disasters. However, workers may have a risk of contracting tuberculosis, blood-borne infections such as hepatitis B/C and HIV, as well as gastrointestinal infections such as rotavirus diarrhea, salmonellosis, *Escherichia coli* infections, typhoid/paratyphoid fevers, hepatitis A, shigellosis, and cholera.

- Tuberculosis can be transmitted if the bacillus is in aerosol form due to residual air in the lungs exhaled, or from fluid from the lungs spurted up through nose and mouth during handling of the corpses.
- Blood-borne viruses can be acquired through direct contact with injured skin, blood, or body fluids, or from exposure to mucous membranes from splashing blood or body fluids.

- Gastrointestinal infections are more common because dead bodies generally leak fecal material. Transmission can occur via the fecal–oral route, by direct contact with the body, soiled clothing, or contaminated equipment. Gastrointestinal infections can also occur if the water supply has been contaminated due to large numbers of corpses.

Other Health Risks

Other health risks associated with flooding include injuries that make people more susceptible to infections. Tetanus boosters may be indicated for people who sustain open wounds. Hypothermia may also be a problem, which increases the risk of respiratory tract infections due to exposure to floodwaters and rain. Furthermore, respiratory diseases are associated with crowded conditions in temporary emergency shelters after flooding.

Tsunamis

When a body of water, such as the ocean, is rapidly displaced, a series of enormous waves are created, called a **tsunami.** Mass movements above or below water such as earthquakes, some volcanic eruptions, underwater explosions, large asteroid impacts, and testing of nuclear weapons at sea, all have the potential to generate a tsunami.

Immediate health concerns after a tsunami include clean drinking water, food, shelter, and medical care for injuries. Floodwaters often contaminate the water and food supplies, generating a high risk for water- and foodborne illnesses. In addition, loss of shelter leaves people in danger of insect exposure, and environmental hazards. The majority of deaths during tsunamis are due to drowning and traumatic injuries.

As with other natural disasters the disaster itself does not necessarily cause an increase in infectious disease outbreak; however, contaminated water and food, and lack of shelter and medical care, generate a secondary effect, worsening illnesses that already exist in the affected region. Whenever water supplies are contaminated and sanitation systems are destroyed, the immediate threat comes from waterborne disease such as shigellosis, typhoid fever, hepatitis A and E, and cholera. Serious outbreaks of diarrheal disease in the aftermath of floods are usual. Crowded settlements of displaced people can bring the risk of outbreaks such as measles, meningitis, and influenza, and increased rates of pneumonia and tuberculosis. Other diseases that can be a potential threat are malaria and dengue fever. Also, trauma wounds can become infected as waves wash tetanus bacteria from the soil. As previously discussed, decaying bodies pose little risk concerning major disease outbreaks, but do present a health risk to those who handle the bodies.

Most of the risks of infectious diseases are similar in river or lake floods and in tsunamis. Some of the more recent tsunamis are listed in Table 24.2.

Earthquakes

An earthquake, the result of a sudden release of the energy in the earth's crust, produces seismic waves that can be measured with a seismometer (seismograph) indicating the strength of the quake. Strong earthquakes can have devastating results. Other

---

TABLE 24.2 Tsunamis in the Twentieth and Twenty-first Centuries

Year	Location	Event (Specific Location)	Estimated Death Toll
2007	Solomon Islands	2007 Solomon Islands earthquake	52
2006	Indonesia	Java earthquake	540
2004	Indian Ocean	Indian Ocean earthquake	>250,000 (sources vary)
1998	Papua New Guinea	1998 Papua New Guinea earthquake (earthquake followed by undersea landslide)	3,000
1993	Japan	Okushiri	202
1983	Japan	Northern Honshu	102
1979	France	Nice	23
1976	The Philippines	Moro Gulf	5,000
1964	United States: Alaska and Hawaii	Good Friday earthquake	131
1960	Chile, United States (Hawaii), the Philippines, and Japan	Great Chilean earthquake	2,000
1952	Russia	Kuril Islands, Kamchatka Peninsula	2,300
1946	United States (Alaska and Hawaii)	Aleutian Island earthquake	173
1944	Japan	Tonankai	1,223
1933	Japan	Sanriku	3,008
1929	Canada (Newfoundland)	1929 Grand Banks earthquake	28
1908	Italy	1908 Messina earthquake	70,000

TABLE 24.3 Earthquakes in the Years 2001 to 2007

Year	Location	Event (Specific Location)	Estimated Death Toll
2007	Indonesia	March 6 earthquake (southern Sumatra)	25
2007	Peru	August 12 earthquake (near central coast)	514
2007	Solomon Islands	April 1 earthquake	52
2007	Indonesia	September 12 earthquake (southern Sumatra)	67
2006	Indonesia	May 2006 Java earthquake	6,234
2005	Pakistan and India	2005 Kashmir earthquake	87,350
2005	Iran	Zarand	564
2004	Indian Ocean	Indian Ocean earthquake	>250,000 (sources vary)
2004	Morocco	Morocco earthquake	571
2003	Iran	Bam earthquake	26,271
2003	Algeria	2003 Boumerdes earthquake	2,266
2001	India	Gujarat earthquake	20,000

than the material losses, the consequences may include a lack of basic necessities, loss of life, and disease. Infectious diseases that may occur after an earthquake include waterborne diseases due to an unsafe water supply, foodborne illnesses due to lack of refrigeration, vector-borne illnesses resulting from standing water, and any disease that might occur because of compromised sanitation and overcrowding of shelters. A listing of some recent earthquakes with lethality is provided in Table 24.3.

Hurricanes

As with other natural disasters, the main threat of infectious disease after a hurricane is based on the associated flooding and includes unsafe drinking water, contaminated food, and crowded shelters. Vector-borne diseases due to standing waters are also a concern. The greatest threat to people in affected areas generally comes from diseases that are endemic to that region.

Bioterrorism

Biological warfare and **bioterrorism** use biological agents to incapacitate or kill civilians or military personnel during a terrorist attack or during war. One of the earliest reported uses of biological weapons goes back to the Assyrians (sixth century

Our First Brush With Bioterrorism

Many Americans are unaware that this country had already experienced a bioterrorist attack 17 years before the anthrax incidents following the 9/11 attacks in 2001. In the small town of The Dalles, Oregon followers of an Indian guru purposely contaminated salad bars at a number of local restaurants with a spray of *Salmonella*. As a result, 752 people were infected, quickly overloading the local hospital and healthcare facilities. The attack was made in an attempt to keep citizens from going to the polls to vote in an election determining whether members of the group could hold positions in the local government thus giving them political leverage. No deaths occurred as a direct result of this attack. The leader of the group was later deported and the group soon thereafter left the area.

BCE), who poisoned enemy wells with rye ergot—a fungal agent that causes convulsions if ingested. Biological warfare is not new and the act of bioterrorism became an issue when terrorists of various kinds decided to kill innocent people to force their political and/or religious points and views.

In 1999, as part of a U.S. Congressional initiative to advance national public health capabilities in response to bioterrorism, the Centers for Disease Control and Prevention (CDC, Atlanta, GA) was designated as the lead agency for overall public health planning. Furthermore, a **Division of Bioterrorism Preparedness and Response** was formed to target several activities including planning, improved surveillance and epidemiologic capabilities, rapid laboratory diagnostics, enhanced communications, and stockpiling of therapeutic agents. In June 1999 national experts met to:

- Review potential general criteria for selecting the biological agents that pose the greatest threats to civilians
- Review lists of previously identified biological threat agents
- Identify those that should be further evaluated and prioritized for public health preparedness efforts

On the basis of the discussions on overall criteria, agents were placed in one of three priority categories for initial public health preparedness efforts: Category A, B, or C.

Category A Agents

Agents in Category A have tremendous potential for an adverse public health impact, including mass casualties. Therefore, these bioterrorism agents are considered high priority in that they pose a risk to national security. Characteristics of these agents are as follows:

- They are easily transmitted from person to person.
- They have a high mortality rate and the potential for a major public health impact.

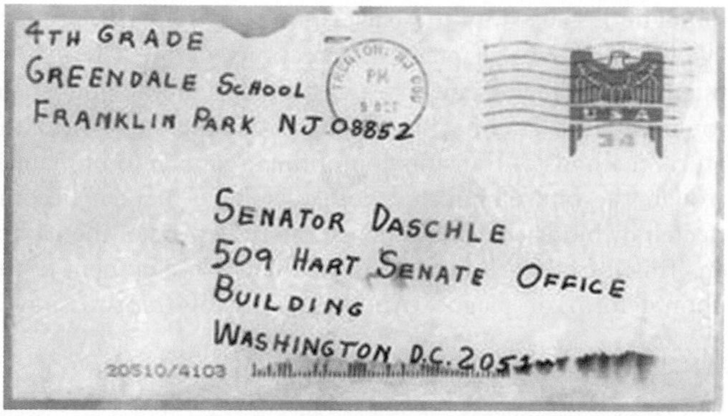

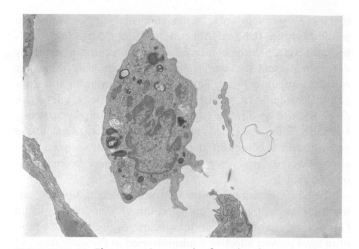

FIGURE 24.9 Letter to U.S. Senator Tom Daschle. This letter contained anthrax spores capable of causing inhalation anthrax.

FIGURE 24.10 Electron micrograph of an alveolar macrophage.

- They have the potential to cause public panic and social disruption.
- They require special action for public health preparedness.

Category A agents are referred to as "the Big Six": smallpox, viral hemorrhagic fevers (VHFs), anthrax, plague, tularemia, and botulism.

Bacterial Agents

Although many microorganisms can serve as biological weapons, most bacteria are easy to grow and therefore are generally most dreaded. These bacterial agents include *Bacillus anthracis, Yersinia pestis, Clostridium botulinum,* and *Francisella tularensis.*

Anthrax is caused by *Bacillus anthracis,* a gram-positive, spore-forming rod. It is a zoonotic disease that can cause three forms of anthrax: cutaneous, gastrointestinal, and respiratory (see section on inhalation anthrax in Chapter 11, Infections of the Respiratory System). Although all forms can lead to dangerous and potentially fatal infections, the forms that best lend themselves to use as bioweapons are the inhalation and cutaneous forms.

Inhalation anthrax is the most lethal form of anthrax. Beginning on September 18, 2001, letters containing anthrax spores were mailed to several news media offices and to two Democratic U.S. Senators (Figure 24.9). In this process, postal workers were also endangered. Among those who developed anthrax during this attack, all who presented the full symptoms of inhalation anthrax before antibiotic therapy was applied, died. The weaponized form of anthrax involved in both inhalation and cutaneous forms of the disease consists of spores that are typically maintained as a powder or are aerosolized. These spores are much more potent than those that occur naturally in the environment. The lethal dose for inhalation anthrax has now been reestimated as several hundred spores instead of earlier estimates of 2500 to 55,000.

The infection process begins when the spores are inhaled into the lungs, where they reach the alveolar spaces. Most are destroyed by alveolar macrophages (Figure 24.10). Surviving spores can move into the lymphatic system and travel to the mediastinal lymph nodes to undergo germination into the veg-

BOX 24.2 Symptoms of Inhalation Anthrax

Early Symptoms
- Fever
- Myalgias
- Nonproductive cough
- Nausea
- Vomiting
- Chest pain
- Chills
- Abdominal pain
- Tachycardia

Symptoms in Late Stages
- Respiratory paralysis
- Acute fever
- Hypotension
- Cyanosis
- Respiratory alkalosis
- Massive lymphadenopathy (swollen lymph nodes)
- Delirium
- Shock
- Hypothermia
- Death (within 24–36 h)

etative bacillus form. Once germination begins toxins are released, causing both local and systemic symptoms. These symptoms include hemorrhagic damage to the lungs and a systemic inflammatory response. The severity of the infection is proportional to the level of toxins in the blood and not the number of bacteria in the blood culture. In other words, a culture negative for the bacterium does not necessarily indicate that the danger of anthrax does not exist. The symptoms of inhalation anthrax change with progression of the disease. Early symptoms and symptoms of late stages (2 to 3 d after the onset of the early stages) of the infection are illustrated in Box 24.2.

Many symptoms of inhalation anthrax are difficult to distinguish from ordinary pneumonias or influenza. Differences that specifically point to anthrax are abnormal lung examination results, dyspnea (labored, difficult breathing), nausea or vomiting, and chest pain or pleurisy. Furthermore, anthrax typically does not present the symptoms of headache, sore throat, or rhinorrhea (runny nose). Because this form of anthrax is difficult to distinguish from other respiratory infections, a definitive diagnosis will require the use of microscopy, sample culturing, and lung radiography. Because early diagnosis is critical for the survival and recovery of the infected patient, anthrax must always be considered when presented with the symptoms previously listed.

The treatment for inhalation anthrax (which is also the treatment for cases of gastrointestinal anthrax) is usually penicillin G procaine, ciprofloxacin or doxycycline, or both. These antibiotics have proven effective if administered in the early stages of the disease. The anthrax vaccination in use in the United States is relatively new and has few clinical data in terms of its effectiveness against inhalation anthrax.

Cutaneous anthrax accounts for 95% of cases of the naturally occurring form of anthrax. Eleven of the 22 cases involved in the anthrax powder attacks after 9/11 were cutaneous forms of the disease. The infection results from spore contact with the skin, particularly in areas where there are abrasions or breaks in the skin. The mechanism of the infection is much the same as for the inhalation form, differing primarily on the tissue being affected. At the infection site, painless, pruritic, papular lesions will form within 1 week of exposure to the spores. Within 2 days fluid vesicles around the papules form, containing numerous bacilli and some white blood cells. These vesicles will enlarge and the site will become edematous (swollen with fluid). Eventually the lesions rupture and become a necrotic ulcer covered by a black eschar (Figure 24.11). Within 2 weeks the eschar will dry up and fall off. On occasion a patient may experience a secondary infection with *Staphylococcus aureus* if the organism is present at the lesion site. In rare cases a systemic infection may occur as a late manifestation of a cutaneous infection. This systemic infection can be manifested as bacteremia, possibly resulting in renal failure, anemia, bleeding, and ecchymoses.

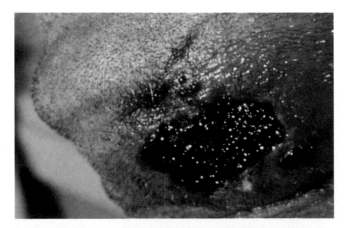

FIGURE 24.11 Typical black eschar, the result of cutaneous anthrax. (From Mims C, Dockrell HM, Goering RV, et al.: *Medical microbiology,* ed 3, St. Louis, 2004, Mosby.)

Plague is caused by the bacterium *Yersinia pestis*, a gram-negative rod (see Chapter 14, Infections of the Circulatory System). The plague can take two forms, bubonic and pneumonic, with the latter having a higher mortality rate. One of the natural methods of transmission of the organism to humans is through the bite of infected fleas that have in turn become infected by biting infected rodents, the reservoirs of the pathogen. This infection route usually results in development of the bubonic form of plague. Another route of transmission is

LIFE APPLICATION

The 2001 Anthrax Attack

The 2001 anthrax episodes focused on inhalation anthrax primarily via spores mailed to Senators Tom Daschle and Patrick Leahy in Washington, DC a week after the 9/11 attack on the World Trade Center in New York, and other mailings to several news agencies made at about the same time. Anthrax, a potentially lethal disease from the germinated spores of *Bacillus anthracis*, appears in three forms: (1) cutaneous, (2) intestinal and (3) inhalation.

- *Cutaneous anthrax* occurs after exposure through cuts or abrasions in the skin. After germination of the spores, it progresses to a characteristic black-centered necrotic ulcer, with about 20% lethality for untreated cases.
- *Intestinal anthrax* occurs after consumption of contaminated meat and then progresses through a series of typical GI tract symptoms that may include vomiting of blood, severe diarrhea, and dehydration. Death occurs in 25% to 60% of cases.
- *Inhalation anthrax* occurs after breathing spores, which germinate in the moist, warm environment of the respiratory tract. Symptoms resemble a common cold, but after several days severe breathing problems develop that progress to shock. It is usually fatal.

Early diagnosis (identification of *B. anthracis* in blood) and treatment with high doses of penicillin, doxycycline, or ciprofloxacin are of value for all but inhalation anthrax. In addition, a vaccine is available that provides protection.

Of the 22 people that developed symptoms, 11 cases were of the deadly inhalation variety, of which five were lethal. An earlier episode with anthrax occurred in 1979 after an accidental release of an airborne cloud of anthrax spores from a military research laboratory in Sverdlovsk in the Soviet Union. There were 79 cases of respiratory infections and 68 reported deaths. In biological warfare, aerosol dispersion of the spores is the desired method of delivery for exposure to the respiratory tract. The size and number of spores determines how deep they go in the respiratory tract and degree of lethality after exposure. To this end, treating bioterrorism-grade samples with a silicone substance prevents an increase in size due to clumping via adhesive van der Waals forces and yields an increase in individual spore numbers or dose.

BOX 24.3 Symptoms of Pneumonic Plague

Symptoms

- Chest pain
- Dyspnea
- Cough
- Bloody sputum
- Nausea
- Vomiting
- Diarrhea

Advanced Symptoms With Sepsis

- Purpura
- Small-vessel necrosis leading to gangrene in the periphery
- Azotemia (presence of increased nitrogenous compounds, usually urea, in the blood)
- Multiorgan failure

BOX 24.4 Clinical Symptoms of Tularemia

Typhoidal

- Fever
- Chills
- Renal failure
- Sepsis
- DIC
- Pneumonia

Pneumonic

- Fever
- Chills
- Renal failure
- Sepsis
- DIC
- Pneumonia
- Inflammation of any part of the respiratory tract

Oropharyngeal

- Exudative pharyngitis
- Swelling of lymph glands in the neck
- Occasional oropharyngeal lesions

DIC, Disseminated intravascular coagulation.

through the inhalation of aerosolized droplets containing the pathogen. In a bioterrorism attack using *Y. pestis,* the most likely means of transmission would be through aerosolization of the pathogen.

Deliberate infection of the natural animal reservoirs in densely populated areas is another possible but rather inefficient means of attempting to spread the plague. The incubation time for the *Y. pestis* organism is between 2 and 7 days. General symptoms for the pneumonic plague and advanced stage symptoms with sepsis are illustrated in Box 24.3.

Diagnosis of plague begins with the confirmation of clinical symptoms, followed by a Gram stain and a Wright, Giemsa, or Wayson stain, which reveals the *Y. pestis* "safety pin" appearance. If plague is suspected at this point, all tests should then be conducted under Biosafety Level (BSL)-2 protocols. Chest x-rays of patients with suspected pneumonic plague will likely show a bilateral pneumonia. A rapid direct fluorescent antibody (DFA) immunoassay is available that can detect *in vivo* antigens associated with the pathogen in a blood sample.

Specific treatment for pneumonic plague varies; however, early antibiotic therapy is necessary in all cases as any delay may increase mortality. The antibiotic of choice is streptomycin or gentamicin. Alternate antibiotics include chloramphenicol, ciprofloxacin, or doxycycline. No vaccine is presently available for the pneumonic form of plague but active research is underway. In cases of pneumonic plague, infection control, particularly in healthcare facilities, is focused primarily on precautions to isolate airborne droplets. Decontamination of surfaces exposed to the pathogen is typically unnecessary because the *Y. pestis* is not a particularly hardy organism and does not survive for long periods of time outside the host.

Tularemia is an infection caused by *Francisella tularensis,* a gram-negative, facultatively anaerobic coccobacillus. It is readily transmitted through direct contact with infected animals, ingestion of contaminated food or water, inhalation of aerosolized bacteria, and through arthropod bites such as those of ticks or mosquitoes. This organism is one of the most communicable bacterial pathogens known. The host reservoirs include rabbits,

rats, and other small mammals. The most commonly occurring cases of tularemia are the result of tick bites. Tularemia is not transmitted by person-to-person contact. For use as a bioweapon the most effective method of transmission would be the use of aerosolized agents. There are six distinct manifestations of tularemia involving different symptoms and organ system targets:

1. Ulceroglandular (80% of cases)
2. Glandular (10% of cases)
3. Typhoidal (10% of cases)
4. Pneumonic (<17% of cases)
5. Oropharyngeal (<5% of cases)
6. Oculoglandular (<1% of cases)

The forms most likely to be encountered in a bioterrorism attack using aerosolized *F. tularensis* would be typhoidal, pneumonic, and oropharyngeal. Of these, the typhoidal form of tularemia would most likely be the dominant form of the disease encountered. Each of these forms has a specific set of clinical symptoms (Box 24.4). Typhoidal and pneumonic forms are the most dangerous, causing the highest mortality rates. These forms of tularemia are especially detrimental in persons with any impaired cellular immunity because this pathogen is an intracellular organism.

Diagnosis of tularemia includes microscopic examination of sputum or blood for the presence of this small coccobacillus. Standard biochemical tests are not always effective because the organism is rather fastidious and slow growing. No readily rapid test for detection is currently available. A more accurate diagnosis will require use of the polymerase chain reaction (PCR), fluorescent antibody testing, enzyme-linked immunosorbent assay (ELISA), and pulsed-field gel electrophoresis (see Chapter 25, Biotechnology) at BSL-2 or BSL-3 laboratories (see Chapter 5, Safety Issues).

The antibiotic of choice for treatment of typhoidal or pneumonic tularemia is streptomycin. Gentamicin is useful in patients with a compromised immune system. Tetracycline and chloramphenicol are alternatives that have proven to be effective. Ciprofloxacin and doxycycline are the preferred antibiotics when treating large-scale outbreaks, with oral administration being the established treatment method.

The U.S. Food and Drug Administration (FDA) is presently assessing the effectiveness of a live attenuated vaccine, but at present vaccination of the general public is not recommended. Strict isolation procedures are not necessary for infection control as tularemia is not transmitted person-to-person. However, the organism is a rather hardy pathogen and areas in contact with infected items should be disinfected. Adequate surface decontamination procedures include washing with 10% chlorine bleach for 10 minutes, followed by washing with a 70% alcohol solution.

Botulism is the result of a potent toxin produced by *Clostridium botulinum,* a gram-positive, spore-forming, anaerobic bacillus (Figure 24.12) (see Chapter 13, Infections of the Nervous System and the Senses). The botulinum toxin is the most potent natural neurotoxin in existence and if dispersed ideally a single gram of this toxin could kill over 1 million people! Botulism is distinct among the Category A agents in that it is the toxin and not the bacterium itself that causes the disease. The means of natural transmission of the organism include consuming contaminated food or to a lesser extent water, and wound-site contact with the organism. The bacterium cannot penetrate through intact skin but can be absorbed through the mucosal linings of the gastrointestinal or respiratory tracts.

In a bioterrorism attack the toxin or organism would most likely be transmitted in an aerosol form, or through contamination of food and water. A number of factors about the toxin limit its effectiveness as a bioweapon. The toxin can be denatured when food is properly cooked. The chlorine levels used in most water treatment plants are also sufficient to denature the toxin, rendering it harmless if used in food or water supplies. Furthermore, the fact that the cells and any aerosolized toxin can be filtered from the air by means of a couple of layers of cloth, and that the toxin itself is denatured by sunlight within 1 to 3 hours of exposure, limits its use in aerosol form. These limitations can be somewhat mitigated by using enormous quantities of the toxin but especially in the case of water supply contamination, the botulinum toxin would be an impractical bioweapon. As previously discussed in Chapter 13 (Infections of the Nervous System and Senses), the botulinum toxin causes a number of symptoms usually associated with the nervous system, with the final stage involving suffocation due to paralysis of the respiratory muscles.

Once symptoms point to botulism, the initial diagnosis involves microscopic examination of serum, stool, gastric juices, and, if possible, vomit and an examination of the patient history and circumstances before the onset of the disease. Because of the quick action of the neurotoxin, it will be impossible to conduct the necessary testing to positively confirm botulism in a laboratory setting. In treating botulism, as soon as the signs and symptoms become convincing, an antitoxin should be administered. The effectiveness of this antitoxin in the case of an aerosol bioterrorism attack is not known because the antitoxin has not yet been tested on inhalation botulism. Even after administration of the antitoxin after the onset of observable symptoms, the patient will still suffer respiratory failure. The antitoxin will prevent only the progression of toxic effects; it will not reverse symptoms that are already present. The antitoxin will be life-saving only if the patient is assisted by mechanical respiration. Improvements in advanced life support and the development of the antitoxin have greatly improved the survival chances of patients with botulism. Long-term problems associated with botulism after recovery are unknown at this time, but survivors often do complain of chronic fatigue and difficult or labored breathing.

Viral Agents

Viruses are true parasites that cannot live on their own; they need a host cell to reproduce and then cause disease (see Chapter 7, Viruses). Although viruses cannot be grown on a plate or in a test tube, their genomes are generally smaller than bacterial genomes, making them easier to manipulate (see Chapter 25, Biotechnology). Because of the available technology, an increasing commercial exploitation of genetic engineering in both agriculture and medicine has occurred. This trend also may have the potential to create viruses and bacteria that are more virulent than nature's worst case. The production of synthetic viruses with the ability to multiply by the millions represents a bioterrorism threat as great as that with natural occurring viruses, or maybe even more.

In 1980 the World Health Organization (WHO, Geneva, Switzerland) declared the **smallpox** virus to be eradicated as a result of a global vaccination program (see Chapter 7, Why You Need to Know and Life Application: Smallpox as Biological

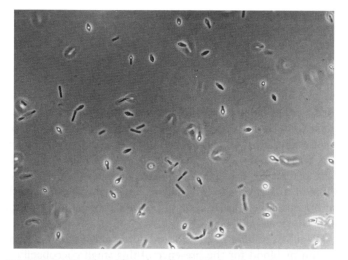

FIGURE 24.12 *Clostridium botulinum. C. botulinum* is a gram-positive, spore-forming, anaerobic bacillus, and the causative agent of botulism. (Courtesy K.M. Marshall, Eric Johnson Lab, University of Wisconsin, Madison.)

Weapon). The smallpox virus is usually inhaled, then taken up by macrophages and transported to lymph nodes where the virus multiplies. This viral increase activates T and B cells and produces a host antibody response (see Chapter 20, The Immune System). Within about 4 days viremia develops and the virus spreads to the spleen, bone marrow, and other lymph nodes. As the infection proceeds the virus infects the dermis and oropharynx, causing the classic skin lesions associated with smallpox. The lesions in the oropharyngeal region form quickly, resulting in the saliva of this region containing large amounts of the virus. Transmission readily occurs through contact with skin lesions before they scab over, or via aerosolized droplets from the oropharynx. Infection can also occur through contact with objects contaminated with the virus including clothes, bedding, and body fluids such as urine, sweat, or sputum.

Symptoms of a smallpox infection include the following:

- Fever
- Malaise
- Headache
- Abdominal pain
- Nausea/vomiting
- Vesicular or pustular poxlike rash: Rash begins at the mouth and face and moves outward to the arms and legs

Diagnosis involves presentation of the symptoms, followed by PCR testing for the definitive diagnosis. Many of the symptoms closely resemble those of chickenpox, produced by the varicella-zoster virus. The main distinguishing features are that the smallpox rash rapidly develops to maturity (1–2 d), whereas the chickenpox rash develops over several days with new lesions appearing as the infection progresses. Furthermore, the lesions of smallpox tend to be deep and concentrated on the face and extremities, whereas chickenpox lesions are superficial and concentrated on the trunk.

At present no chemical agent is approved by the FDA to treat smallpox. Although cidofovir, an antiretroviral agent, has shown some activity against smallpox in the laboratory, including animal studies, there are no human clinical data to support its use in human disease. Prevention through vaccination is still effective and there are ongoing discussions on a potential plan for implementing a large-scale vaccination program. The vaccine is 95% effective and recovery from smallpox confers a lifelong immunity to the disease. Some negative side effects to vaccination include local pain, swelling, and a low-grade fever.

Healthcare workers coming in contact with infected patients should use proper protective equipment such as high-efficiency particulate air (HEPA) filter masks, gowns, gloves, and face shields.

At this time, no naturally occurring smallpox have been reported. There are fears that the virus has been sold on the black market as a result of security problems encountered with the dissolution of the former Soviet Union. Other than laboratory personnel and research scientists, the greatest exposure risk for the general population would be by deliberate release.

Viral hemorrhagic fevers (VHFs) are caused by four families of RNA viruses:

1. *Filoviridae:* Ebola and Marburg viruses
2. *Arenaviridae:* Machupo and Lassa viruses
3. *Bunyaviridae:* Congo-Crimean hemorrhagic fever virus, Rift Valley virus
4. *Flaviviridae:* Dengue fever and yellow fever viruses

With the exception of the filoviruses, all these viruses are zoonotic. The pathogenic mechanism of VHFs is not fully understood; however, all the families display similar symptoms, suggesting similar mechanisms. Several mechanisms including platelet deficiency, direct endothelial and platelet injury, and cytokine dysregulation have been identified and vary somewhat depending on the family. These mechanisms account for the significant bleeding common to all four viral families. Because of the high mortality rate and dangers inherent in working with these viruses, testing for VHFs must be done at a BSL-4 facility (see Chapter 5, Safety Issues).

Filoviridae: Ebola and Marburg viruses can be naturally transmitted in a number of ways including aerosolized animal feces, arthropod bites, contact with contaminated animal carcasses, and person-to-person contact with the skin or oral aerosols of an infected person. As a bioweapon the transmission could be through an aerosol or direct contact with a carrier. Incubation time for Ebola virus is 2 to 21 days, and for Marburg virus it is 2 to 14 days. Both infections include the following symptoms:

- Sudden high fever
- Weakness
- Maculopapular rash
- Hemorrhaging
- Disseminated intravascular coagulation (DIC)

When shock occurs, multiorgan system failure and hemorrhagic complications set in and death follows soon thereafter.

Diagnosis of a specific viral infection is difficult. Healthcare professionals must often rely on patient history and clinical symptoms to determine the possibility of VHF. Nasal, stool, serum, or almost any body fluid of an infected individual will contain the virus and should be sent to a designated BSL-4 facility for definitive diagnosis. These laboratories will then use ELISA, PCR, and viral isolation to confirm a preliminary diagnosis. Through electron microscopy the presence of specific viruses can also be observed. Ebola virus is easily identified by its unique "shepherd's hook" shape (Figure 24.13).

For both Ebola and Marburg viruses no drugs are available for treatment. Supportive management is the only response available, which may include actions such as fluid resuscitation, balancing of electrolytes, dialysis, or mechanical ventilation. Because this type of care will require a patient being placed in a critical care unit, the infection control procedures necessary could lead to significant challenges for the treatment facility regarding transmission management. Because these viruses can be transmitted through aerosols and contact, special precautions such as negative-pressure rooms, strict contact precautions, and patient isolation will be required. At present there are no vaccines for Ebola and Marburg viruses. Mortality rates for filovirus infections are high, ranging from

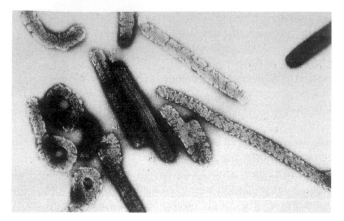

FIGURE 24.13 Electron micrograph of the Ebola virus. (Courtesy Centers for Disease Control and Prevention. In Murray PR, Rosenthal KS, Pfaller MA: *Medical microbiology*, ed 5, St. Louis, 2005, Mosby.)

25% to 70% for the Marburg virus and from 50% to 90% for the Ebola virus.

Arenaviruses: Lassa and Machupo viruses are naturally transmitted through aerosols from infected rodent waste, direct contact via mucous membranes or open skin with the virus, direct person-to-person contact with infected body fluid, and possibly through airborne droplets. As with Ebola and Marburg viruses the most likely method for transmission as a bioweapon would be through person-to-person contact with an infected carrier and possibly through an aerosol. The incubation time for Lassa virus is 5 to 16 days, and for Machupo virus it is 7 to 14 days. Symptoms for these viruses are as follows:

- Gradual onset of fever
- Nausea
- Abdominal pain
- Cough
- Conjunctivitis
- Facial flushing
- Swollen lymph nodes

Specific symptoms for Lassa infections include edema of the head and neck, and pleural and pericardial effusions; specific symptoms for Machupo infections include CNS problems, and local and generalized seizures. Diagnosis of these infections is the same as for all VHFs: initial diagnosis based on history and symptoms and final diagnosis by a designated BSL-4 laboratory through ELISA, PCR, and viral isolation. Lassa virus infection is also distinguished by an elevated white blood cell count.

As with patients infected with Ebola or Marburg virus, the main treatment is supportive care. In the case of an arenavirus infection, if the drug ribavirin is administered just before or just after the infection occurs, the drug appears to be effective by limiting viremia and subsequent liver damage. Mortality rates for arenavirus infections range from 15% to 30%.

Bunyaviridae: Rift Valley and Congo-Crimean fever viruses are transmitted naturally by infected mosquitoes, by inhalation of aerosol from an infected animal, and by direct physical contact with an infected carcass or animal tissue. The potential for infection through the consumption of infected animal milk also exists. At the present time there is no evidence that the viruses can be transmitted by person-to-person contact. As a bioweapon, dissemination would most likely be via an aerosol. The incubation time for these viruses is 2 to 6 days. Symptoms of a Bunyaviridae infection include the following:

- Fever
- Headache
- Retro-orbital pain
- Photophobia
- Jaundice
- Hemorrhaging (rare)
- Retinitis in 10% of cases

Diagnosis for this virus family is the same as for the other VHF families. Treatment involves supportive care and ribavirin, and the mortality rate is low (<1%).

Flaviviridae: Yellow fever and dengue fever viruses are naturally transmitted by mosquito or tick bites. No person-to-person transmission has yet been reported. The incubation time for these viruses ranges from 2 to 9 days. Symptoms of infection include the following:

- Fever
- Facial flushing
- Myalgias
- Conjunctival injection
- Bradycardia
- Jaundice
- Renal failure
- Hemorrhaging

Diagnosis is accomplished by the same methods as for the other VHF families. Treatment for flavivirus infections is strictly supportive and the mortality rate ranges from less than 10% to 20%.

Category B Agents

Category B bioterrorism agents are less virulent than the Category A agents and less likely to be used as bioterrorism weapons of choice. Because of the lesser threat from these organisms/agents they are not as widely studied regarding weapon use, although they all have the potential to be used in a bioterrorism scenario. Moreover, there are indications that some strains of these organisms may have been genetically modified in order to increase their virulence, thus increasing their potential as bioweapons. The list of Category B diseases/agents includes the following:

- Brucellosis (*Brucella* species)
- Epsilon toxin from *Clostridium perfringens*
- *Salmonella* species
- *Escherichia coli* O157:H7
- *Shigella*
- *Staphylococcus* enterotoxin B

Category A Agents/Diseases

Disease	Organism	Transmission (as Bioweapon)	Treatment
Bacterial			
Anthrax	*Bacillus anthracis*	Primarily as aerosol/powder	Ciprofloxacin, doxycycline
Plague	*Yersinia pestis*	Aerosolized droplets	Streptomycin, gentamicin, doxycycline, ciprofloxacin
Tularemia	*Francisella tularensis*	Aerosolized droplets	Streptomycin, gentamicin, doxycycline, ciprofloxacin
Botulism	*Clostridium botulinum*	Toxin dispersed in aerosolized form, also as a food or water contaminant	Botulism antitoxin, supportive measures
Viral			
Smallpox	Variola major virus	Initially dispersed as aerosol, followed by spread through contact	Prevention: Vaccine Treatment: Cidofovir (antiretroviral drug) is being studied
Viral hemorrhagic fevers (VHFs)	*Filoviridae*: Ebola virus and Marburg virus	Aerosol and person-to-person contact	Supportive care
	Arenaviridae: Machupo virus and Lassa virus	Aerosol	Supportive care, ribavirin
	Bunyaviridae: Rift Valley virus and Congo-Crimean fever virus	Aerosol	Supportive care, ribavirin
	Flaviviridae: Dengue fever virus and yellow fever virus	Aerosol	Supportive care

- *Vibrio cholerae*
- Psittacosis (*Chlamydia psittaci*)
- Glanders (*Burkholderia mallei*)
- Melioidosis (*Burkholderia pseudomallei*)
- Q fever (*Coxiella burnetii*)
- Ricin toxin from *Ricinus communis* (castor bean): Sometimes included as a Category A agent
- Typhus fever (*Rickettsia prowazekii*)
- Encephalitis
- Venezuelan, Eastern, and Western equine encephalitis (alphaviruses)
- Cryptosporidiosis (*Cryptosporidium parvum*)

Many of these diseases/agents are discussed in previous chapters. Representative organisms/agents not previously covered in the book are discussed in order to illustrate the diversity of this category and their potential as bioweapons.

***Staphylococcus* enterotoxin B** (SEB) is produced by *Staphylococcus aureus*, a gram-positive coccus. This bacterium is ubiquitous and relatively easy to culture, making it a good candidate for use as an organism for bioterrorism. The toxin is produced in large quantities by the bacterium, is heat stable, and can be denatured only by prolonged boiling. Most of the instances of natural toxin exposure involve the ingestion of food contaminated with the organism or toxin, including meat products, poultry, and baked goods as well as cheese, milk, and egg products. As a bioweapon the toxin would most likely be transmitted as an aerosol, thus entering through the respiratory tract. Contamination of food and water supplies is another possible method of transmission but only on a relatively small scale. Although the same pathogen is involved, the two forms of exposure display somewhat differing symptoms:

- Inhalation (12 h postexposure)
  - Headache
  - High, persistent fever (durations up to 5 d)
  - Chills
  - Myalgia
  - Prostration
  - Shortness of breath
  - Coughing (sometimes productive)
- Ingestion (8 h postexposure)
  - Intense nausea
  - Vomiting
  - Abdominal cramps
  - Diarrhea

Because the illness is caused by a toxin and not by the presence of the organism itself, diagnosis can be difficult. Microscopy alone will not typically reveal the presence of *S. aureus*, and therefore detection of the toxin is accomplished using ELISAs of body fluids or nasal swabs.

Treatment consists of supportive care measures to address the dominant clinical findings in each case. There is no vaccine at the present time for SEB and no antidotes exist for the toxin.

Glanders (*Burkholderia mallei*) is primarily a disease affecting horses, mules, donkeys, and goats. Although humans are not immune to infection with the gram-negative bacillus,

Category B Agents/Diseases

Disease	Organism	Transmission (as Bioweapon)	Treatment
Bacterial			
Brucellosis	*Brucella* species	Aerosol	Doxycycline and rifampin
Gastrointestinal, inhalation, systemic infection	*Clostridium perfringens*	Aerosol, food or water contamination	Supportive care
Salmonellosis	*Salmonella* species	Aerosol, food contamination	Supportive care
Food poisoning/sepsis	*Escherichia coli* O157:H7	Food, water contamination	Supportive care
Shigellosis	*Shigella* species	Food, water contamination	Supportive care
Staphylococcal gastroenteritis	*Staphylococcus aureus*	Aerosol, food contamination	Supportive care
Cholera	*Vibrio cholerae*	Food, water contamination	Doxycycline, trimethoprim-sulfamethoxazole, furazolidone (for pregnant women)
Psittacosis	*Chlamydia psittaci*	Aerosol	Tetracycline, doxycycline
Glanders	*Burkholderia mallei*	Aerosol	Amoxicillin, tetracycline
Melioidosis	*Burkholderia pseudomallei*	Aerosol	Amoxicillin, tetracycline
Q fever	*Coxiella burnetii*	Aerosol	Doxycycline
Plant toxin			
Ricin toxin	Derived from castor bean plant (*Ricinus communis*)	Aerosol, food or water contamination, injection	Supportive care
Viral			
Typhus fever	*Rickettsia prowazekii*	Aerosol	Tetracycline, doxycycline
Alphavirus encephalitides	Alphaviruses	Aerosol	Supportive care
Cryptosporidiosis	*Cryptosporidium parvum*	Food, water contamination	Supportive care

they do not readily acquire the disease. Horses are the primary natural reservoirs of the organism and the common route of transmission is through skin lacerations or breaks in the mucosa of the airways. Although livestock present a viable target for bioterrorism, infection of humans through inhalation of aerosolized organisms is also possible. The resulting symptoms would involve pulmonary problems and generally flulike symptoms. The three acute forms of the disease are as follows:

1. *Focal:* Localized lesions
2. *Pulmonary:* Myalgias, headache, chest pain
3. *Septic:* Sepsis, possible CNS involvement, associated with a high mortality rate

Diagnosis may include microscopic examination of body fluids/lesions to detect the presence of the bacteria; however, the most effective and specific test for the organism is complement fixation. PCR may also be required when attempting to differentiate between glanders, caused by *B. mallei,* and melioidosis, a similar disease caused by *B. pseudomallei.*

Category C Agents

There are a number of agents that could fall into the category C grouping, including newly emerging infectious diseases (see Chapter 18, Emerging Infectious Diseases). Hantavirus and Nipah virus are representatives of the types of agents that may be considered category C agents. Hantavirus is discussed in

Chapter 9 (Infection and Disease) and Chapter 11 (Infections of the Respiratory System) and Nipah virus is briefly covered in Chapter 7 (Viruses). It is anticipated that as bioweapons both of these agents would be transmitted in an aerosolized form. Typically, symptoms for infection by these agents would include the following:

- Hantavirus
  - Initial symptoms
    - Fever
    - Chills
    - Myalgias
    - Malaise
    - Headache
    - Abdominal pain
    - Anorexia
    - Nonproductive cough
  - As it advances
    - Hypotension
    - Tachycardia
    - Bleeding
- Nipah virus
  - Fluctuating body temperature
  - Headache
  - Nausea
  - Vomiting
  - Dizziness
  - Unconsciousness

Category C Agents/Diseases

Disease	Organism	Transmission	Treatment
Hantavirus pulmonary syndrome	Hantavirus (Family Bunyaviridae)	Aerosol	Supportive care
Nipah virus encephalitis	Nipah virus (Family Paramyxoviridae)	Aerosol	Supportive care

- Tachycardia
- Elevated blood pressure
- Occasional neurological symptoms

Diagnosis of these agents is accomplished primarily by PCR coupled with ELISAs to detect the specific antigens. Treatment is primarily supportive; however, the drug ribavirin has shown some promise in reducing the duration and severity of disease. Although research on the drug is continuing, its use has not been approved by the FDA. No vaccines exist for either of these viruses but research is ongoing.

Role of First Responders in Bioterrorism

Hospitals and healthcare facilities will be critical in responding to any bioterrorism event. These facilities will not only be involved in responding to the medical needs of victims but also in the initial identification and isolation of suspected biological agents. This close contact with infected victims and a potentially contaminated environment will invariably place first responders and various healthcare professionals in positions where they may also be affected by the agents. Most facilities and organizations already have procedures and protective measures and equipment in place to handle infectious diseases and hazardous biological agents; however, the rapid response required and proper handling of mass casualties that could spread an infectious agent throughout a facility or population require special awareness and procedures to properly and safely respond to a bioterrorism attack. Healthcare workers must be aware of the emergency response procedures established at an institution, including the following:

- Procedures for handling mail and parcels
- Decontamination
- Chain of command
- Communications protocols within the institution, and with other local/state emergency response agencies
- Communications with and reporting to local/state departments of health and clinical laboratory facilities
- Communications with and reporting to the Federal Bureau of Investigation (FBI), the Department of Homeland Security, and the CDC

Many institutions have an emergency response binder that will provide additional pertinent information, guidance, and established procedures such as those listed previously and others that may be needed in handling a bioterrorism attack. Individual institutions will tailor their procedures to the specific circumstances and roles they would be playing in the response to a bioterrorism attack. Larger institutions and virtually all hospitals, clinics, and laboratories will also have occupational and employee health services. Their staff will play a vital role in planning, preparing, and implementing employee safety programs, which will be important in training and protecting employees who will be handling the victims of bioterrorism.

First responders will also need to be knowledgeable about the requirements for and the proper use and disposal of personal protective equipment that may be needed to respond to a bioweapons attack (see Chapter 5, Safety Issues). Special attention should be given to respiratory and dermal protection as these will be the primary transmission routes for many bioterrorism agents.

If an agency, institution, or laboratory does not have a comprehensive emergency plan or set of emergency procedures, there are a number of publications promulgated by the CDC to provide standards and procedures. These include the following:

- Hazardous Waste Operations and Emergency Response (OSHA 1910.120)
- Hazardous Communication Standard (OSHA 1910.1200)
- Respiratory Protection Standard (OSHA 1910.134)
- Personal Protective Equipment (OSHA 1910.132)
- Maintenance, Safeguards and Operational Features for Exit Routes (OSHA 1910.37)

There are also a number of websites that provide detailed information for emergency planning and procedures:

- www.osha.gov
- www.fema.gov
- www.training.fema.gov
- www.cdc.gov/niosh/topics/emres/responders

In addition to healthcare facilities that will be treating the victims of a bioterrorism, there is also a critical need to quickly identify and evaluate the biological agents used in an attack. Many facilities will not have the equipment, facilities, or expertise to conduct advanced diagnostic testing. In 1999 the federal government created the Laboratory Response Network (LRN) to integrate the efforts of numerous designated clinical laboratories to facilitate the surveillance, detection, identification, and advanced testing of suspected bioterrorism agents. This network is made up of more than 140 government-supported laboratories located in all 50 states as well as in other nations such as Britain, Canada, and Australia. Samples from hospitals and local facilities will be sent to a laboratory in the LRN or evaluated at the facility according to protocols for handling bioterrorism agents as established by the CDC, based on the biosafety level (see Chapter 5, Safety Issues) required to handle the suspected agent.

MEDICAL HIGHLIGHTS

Bioterrorism: Not a Child's Game

By all estimates, the CDC and other agencies studying the aspects of a potential bioterrorism attack warn that a major attack using a biological agent is somewhere in the not too distant future. In addition to the myriad of different problems that will be encountered in dealing with a biological agent attack, the American Academy of Pediatrics has identified children as a particularly vulnerable target group in the case of such a scenario. Because of their metabolism and physiological makeup, children are more likely to be severely affected by a biological agent delivered by aerosol compared with the average adult. A child is shorter and closer to the ground, where heavier aerosols will first begin to accumulate. Children also exchange more cubic feet of air per minute than the average adult, thus potentially taking a greater amount of the agent into their lungs. The outer layer of a child's skin is less keratinized than adult skin and therefore is a less effective physical barrier against droplets of aerosol that may land on the skin. Because children consume, on average, much more liquid than the average adult each day, and because the variety of foods they consume is often greater than that eaten by an adult, they are more vulnerable to agents placed in water or food. Considering physiological factors, behavioral patterns, and even the psychological stability of children, the American Academy of Pediatrics has recommended that all professional healthcare facilities consider these special factors for children when conducting planning and training in preparation for a bioterrorism attack. Recommended actions include specialized training for those working in pediatrics as well as for health professionals in general.

Summary

- The study of the relationships of microorganisms in their natural environments is referred to as microbial ecology. The levels of these relationships are as follows: populations, guilds, communities, microhabitats, habitats, ecosystems, and finally biospheres.
- Biogeochemical cycles are circuits or pathways through which organic compounds or elements are changed from one chemical state to another, by moving through biotic and abiotic compartments of the ecosystem.
- The biogeochemical cycles include the carbon cycle, the nitrogen cycle, the sulfur cycle, and the phosphorus cycle.
- Soil microbiology deals with the microbial abundance and the various microbial populations in the soil. It is dependent on moisture content, oxygen concentration, pH, and temperature of the soil.
- Water occupies nearly three fourths of the earth's surface and aquatic microbiology deals with the study of microorganisms and their activities in freshwater and marine environments.
- Natural disasters such as floods, tsunamis, earthquakes, hurricanes, and others pose a potential threat of infectious diseases due to contaminated water and food. Vector-borne diseases due to natural disasters pose another problem in affected areas.
- The use of biological agents to incapacitate or kill civilians and military personnel is categorized as biological warfare and/or bioterrorism.
- On the basis of potency and various chemical and biological criteria, agents that can be used in biological warfare and/bioterrorism are placed in Category A, B, or C.
- Healthcare facilities are critical in the initial identification and isolation of suspected biological agents.
- The actions of first responders in natural disasters and bioterrorism are regulated and guided by federal, state, and local agencies.

Review Questions

1. A set of guilds is referred to as:
   a. Microhabitat
   b. Biosphere
   c. Community
   d. Population

2. All of the following are free-living, nitrogen-fixing bacteria except:
   a. *Clostridium*
   b. *Bacillus*
   c. *Rhizobium*
   d. *Azotobacter*

3. Which of the following is *not* found in the atmosphere?
   a. Carbon dioxide
   b. Nitrogen
   c. Sulfur
   d. Phosphorus

4. Which of the following zones is present only in oceans?
   a. Abyssal zone
   b. Benthic zone
   c. Littoral zone
   d. Profundal zone

5. Most marine microorganisms are present in the:
   a. Benthic zone
   b. Littoral zone
   c. Profundal zone
   d. Limnetic zone

6. Which of the following is a category A agent?
   a. *Bacillus anthracis*
   b. *Escherichia coli*
   c. *Vibrio cholerae*
   d. *Chlamydia psittaci*

7. Category B agents include:
   a. *Vibrio cholerae*
   b. *Yersinia pestis*
   c. *Francisella tularensis*
   d. *Clostridium botulinum*

8. Which of the following is the fourth most abundant element in the universe?
   a. Nitrogen
   b. Oxygen
   c. Carbon
   d. Hydrogen

9. The process by which nitrate is reduced to nitrogen is called
   a. Nitrification
   b. Denitrification
   c. Anammox
   d. Deamination

10. Eutrophication is a term used in the:
    a. Carbon cycle
    b. Phosphorus cycle
    c. Sulfur cycle
    d. Oxygen cycle

11. A region or regions of the earth populated by living organisms is referred to as _____.

12. The physical location where organisms are found is called a(n) _____.

13. The conversion of CO_2 to organic molecules is called _____.

14. Cholera is considered a Category _____ disease.

15. *Rhizobium* is involved in the _____ cycle.

16. Describe the sulfur cycle.

17. Name the U.S. agency designated as lead agency in overall public health planning in response to bioterrorism and list the activities for which it is responsible.

18. Name and describe the four vertical layers that can be found in lakes.

19. Name and briefly describe the public health concerns regarding disease transmission after a flood.

20. Name and explain the three different categories of agents that could be involved in bioterrorism.

Bibliography

Bauman R: *Microbiology: with diseases by taxonomy*, ed 2, San Francisco, 2007, Pearson/Benjamin Cummings.

Grey MR, Spaeth KR: *The bioterrorism sourcebook*, New York, 2006, McGraw-Hill.

Lindler LE, Lebeda FJ, Korch GW: *Biological weapons defense*, 2005, Humana.

Madigan MT, Martinko JM, Dunlap PV, et al: *Biology of microorganisms*, ed 12, San Francisco, 2009, Pearson, Benjamin Cummings.

Totora GJ, Funke BR, Case CL: *Microbiology: an introduction*, ed 9, San Francisco, 2007, Pearson/Benjamin Cummings.

Internet Resources

History of bioterrorism, http://www.cdc.gov/ncidod/eid/vol8no9/01-0536.htm

Unit 731 http://en.wikipedia.org/wiki/Unit_731

Max-Plank-Institut für Marine Mikrobiologie, Anammox Bacteria Produce Nitrogen Gas in Oceans' Snackbar, 2005, http://www.mpi-bremen.de/en/Anammox_Bacteria_produce_Nitrogen_Gas_in_Oceans_Snackbar.html

Wikipedia, *Anammox*, http://en.wikipedia.org/wiki/Anammox

Environmental Literacy Council, *Sulfur Cycle*, http://www.enviroliteracy.org/article.php/1348.php

UNESCO, Natural Disaster Reduction, http://www.unesco.org/science/disaster/about_disaster.shtml

CDC, Emergency Preparedness and Response: Floods, http://www.bt.cdc.gov/disasters/floods/

Wikipedia, List of Natural Disasters by Death Toll, http://en.wikipedia.org/wiki/List_of_natural_disasters_by_death_toll

CDC, Emergency Preparedness and Response: Immunization Recommendations for Disaster Responders, http://www.bt.cdc.gov/disasters/disease/responderimmun.asp

CDC, http://www.cdc.gov/

Environmental Protection Agency, Biodiversity and Human Health, http://es.epa.gov/ncer/biodiversity/index.html

World Health Organization, Flooding and Communicable Diseases Fact Sheet, http://www.who.int/hac/techguidance/ems/flood_cds/en/

CDC, Emergency Preparedness and Response: Health Effects of Tsunamis, http://www.bt.cdc.gov/disasters/tsunamis/healtheff.asp

MMWR MGuide, Hurricanes, http://www.cdc.gov/mmwr/mguide_nd.html

CDC, Emergency Preparedness and Response: Earthquakes, http://www.bt.cdc.gov/disasters/earthquakes/

U.S. Department of Health and Human Services, Smallpox Vaccine Implementation Plan, http://www.hhs.gov/asl/testify/t030129a.html

CDC Policy on Unused Smallpox Vaccine, October 17, 2005, http://www.bt.cdc.gov/agent/smallpox/vaccination/pdf/storagepolicy.pdf

U.S. Department of Agriculture, Homeland Security, http://www.usda.gov/wps/portal/!ut/p/_s.7_0_A/7_0_CJ?navid=HOMELANDSECU&navtype=CO

Virtual Naval Hospital, http://www.vnh.org

National Institute of Allergy and Infectious Diseases (NIAID), http://www.niaid.nih.gov

World Health Organization, http://www.who.int

25

Biotechnology

OUTLINE

Tools of Genetic Engineering
  Restriction Enzymes
  Gene Libraries
  Plasmids
  Polymerase Chain Reaction

Vectors in Biotechnology
  Plasmid Vectors
  Lambda (λ) Phage Vectors
  Cosmid Vectors

Biotechnology in Human Medicine
  Human Protein Replacements
  Human Disease Therapies
  Vaccines

Biotechnology in Agriculture
  Transgenic Plants
  Transgenic Animals

LEARNING OBJECTIVES

After reading this chapter, the student will be able to:
- Define biotechnology, recombinant DNA technology, and some goals of recombinant technology
- Describe the common steps and tools used in genetic engineering
- Illustrate the structure and function of restriction enzymes, and explain their source and naming; include the description of "blunt" and "sticky" ends, as well as the function of DNA ligase
- Describe gene libraries including the creation and screening of gene libraries, as well as cDNA libraries and synthetic DNA
- Explain the nature of plasmids and their usefulness in recombinant DNA technology
- Discuss the polymerase chain reaction and describe the main three steps of the procedure
- Describe the various types of vectors employed in biotechnology, their usefulness, and the criteria they all have in common
- Discuss human protein replacement, including recombinant insulin, human growth hormone, and factor VIII

- Discuss human disease therapies and vaccine development that have been developed through genetic engineering
- Describe transgenic plants and animals and discuss their usefulness as well as possible problems

KEY TERMS

antisense molecules
bacteriophages
blunt ends
cDNA
clone
conjugation
cosmids
denaturation
DNA ligase
donor
endonuclease
erythropoietin

extension
factor VIII
gene library
genomic library
hemophilia
human growth hormone (HGH)
insulin
interferon
lambda (λ) phage
polymerase chain reaction (PCR)

priming
recombinant DNA
replica plating
restriction enzyme
reverse transcriptase
sticky ends
tissue plasminogen activator (tPA)
transduction
transformation
transgenic
vector

WHY YOU NEED TO KNOW

HISTORY

Traditional biotechnology has been used for thousands of years, most likely from the beginning of civilization. With the domestication of the dog during the Mesolithic Period of the Stone Age, to the time when the first human beings realized that they could breed plants to get their own crops, humans have used biotechnology to survive. The best animals and plants were bred, with each successive generation more likely to carry the traits desired. People discovered that fruit juices could be fermented into wine, milk could be converted into cheese or yogurt, and beer could be made by fermenting malt and hops together. At the end of the nineteenth century microorganisms were discovered, Mendel's work on genetics was accomplished, and institutes for investigating microbial processes were established, including those of Koch and Pasteur.

The term "biotechnology" was created in 1919 by Karl Ereky, a Hungarian engineer. He introduced the term in his book entitled *Biotechnologie der Fleisch-, Fett- und Milcherzeugung im landwirtschaftlichen Grossbetriebe* (Biotechnology of Meat, Fat and Milk Production in an Agricultural Large-Scale Farm). Much later, in 1989, Robert Bud rediscovered this work and acknowledged Ereky as the father of the term biotechnology. During World War I, fermentation processes were developed, and microbes were used to produce chemicals such as acetone, ethanol, and citric acid. Since World War II, microorganisms have been grown on a large scale to produce penicillin.

IMPACT

Modern biotechnology deals more with the treatment of ailments and alteration of organisms to better human life. One of the most important discoveries in biotechnology was the identification and description of DNA structure by Watson and Crick in 1953. In 1973, after the discovery of restriction enzymes and plasmids, Stanley Cohen and Herbert Boyer invented the technique of recombinant DNA, which signaled the beginning of genetic engineering. Today, biotechnology companies are producing recombinant DNA products to be used in human protein replacements, human disease therapies, vaccines, transgenic plants, and transgenic animals.

FUTURE

Recombinant DNA technology will be without question an important science in the twenty-first century. In medicine faster and more efficient diagnosis and treatment will be developed, and in agriculture transgenic plants and animals will be further developed and improved. Promising early results in gene therapy are encouraging scientists to develop methods to successfully alter or remove genes that cause genetic defects. In addition, scientists are investigating the aging process in the hope that recombinant DNA technology may be used to increase the human life span and quality of life. The possible applications for this technology seem endless.

Biotechnology is a subdiscipline of biology that uses microorganisms, cells, or cell components to produce a practical product. Although biotechnology has been a part of human lives for thousands of years to produce products such as bread, cheese, and alcohol, modern biotechnology involves **recombi-** **nant DNA** technology, also referred to as genetic engineering, for industrial, medical, and agricultural purposes.

Humans have used gene manipulations unknowingly for thousands of years by cross-breeding plants as well as animals. For example, a pluot is a cross between a plum and an apricot, and a mule is the result of breeding a female horse to a male donkey. However, genetic engineering should not be confused with this traditional breeding, by which the genes of organisms are manipulated indirectly. The primary goals of recombinant DNA technology include, but are not limited to:

- Removing certain traits in humans, animals, plants, and microorganisms that are undesirable for the specific organism
- Transferring genes from one organism to another in order to improve the quality or survival of the receiving organism
- Creating organisms that are capable of synthesizing products for human use

Tools of Genetic Engineering

Genetic engineering is a sophisticated science performed largely in test tubes. Scientists are now able to take fragments of DNA from different species and splice them together, producing a novel form of DNA that changes the character of the organism. For example, gene-altered, insulin-producing bacteria are no longer identical to their native species, but successfully produce insulin that is harvested for human use.

Although there are several methods/processes to accomplish genetic engineering, all have several steps in common:

- Selection of the organism
- Isolation of the genes of interest
- Insertion of the genes into a vector
- Transformation of cells of the organism to be altered
- Isolation of the genetically modified organism

DNA technology has been made possible by extensive work with viruses, especially bacteriophages, and many bacterial species. The most popular bacterium for use in biotechnology has been *Escherichia coli*, the organism that is considered to be the "workhorse" for experiments in genetic engineering. The bacterial chromosome is ideal for DNA experiments because it consists only of DNA, whereas eukaryotic chromosomes consist of large amounts of proteins, called *histones*, associated with the DNA molecules. Furthermore, eukaryotic DNA exists in pairs and one chromosome can dominate the other, whereas bacterial DNA is a single entity. Also, bacterial DNA floats free in the cytoplasm, whereas eukaryotic DNA is enclosed by the nuclear envelope (membrane).

Because the genetic code is nearly universal, bacteria can express foreign DNA if it is attached to the bacterial DNA. This can be achieved through genetic engineering. Bacteria can also acquire fragments of DNA from the local environment and then express the proteins encoded by the genes in those fragments. This genetic recombination process is called **transformation.** Transformation reportedly takes place in less than 1% of the bacterial population, but it can bring about profound genetic changes. In this process several **donor** bacteria lyse, and their DNA bursts into fragments. If a recipient bacterium is present a segment of double-stranded DNA can pass through the wall and plasma membrane. An enzyme then dissolves one strand of the DNA, and the remaining strand incorporates itself into the recipient's DNA (Figure 25.1). The transformation is complete when the foreign genes are expressed during protein synthesis. This process is one way by which bacteria can obtain drug resistance.

Another process used by bacteria to obtain DNA fragments from other bacteria is **conjugation** (Figure 25.2). This genetic recombination process occurs between two living bacteria: a donor and a recipient. The donor and recipient form a cytoplasmic bridge by which single-stranded DNA of the donor crosses to the recipient. On rare occasions the DNA may be integrated

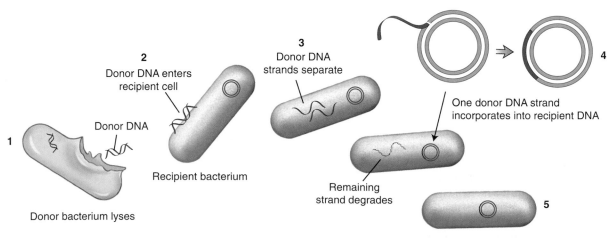

FIGURE 25.1 Transformation in bacteria. *(1)* The donor bacterium lyses and the DNA is released; *(2)* donor DNA enters the recipient bacterium; *(3)* the donor DNA strands separate; *(4)* one donor DNA strand incorporates into the recipient DNA, and the other strand degrades; *(5)* the result is a transformed cell containing recipient DNA and donor DNA.

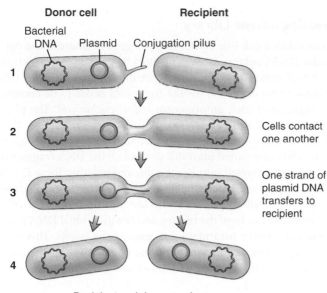

Donor cell   **Recipient**

Bacterial DNA   Plasmid   Conjugation pilus

1

2 — Cells contact one another

3 — One strand of plasmid DNA transfers to recipient

4

Recipient and donor produce
complementary strands to complete plasmid

FIGURE 25.2 Conjugation in bacteria. *(1)* A cytoplasmic bridge forms between the donor cell and the recipient; *(2)* the cells contact each other; *(3)* one strand of donor plasmid DA transfers to the recipient; and *(4)* a strand complementary to the plasmid is formed in both the recipient and donor cells.

TABLE 25.1 Examples of Restriction Enzymes That Produce "blunt" Ends

Enzyme	Source	Recognition Site
*Alu*I	*Arthrobacter luteus*	5′-AG↓CT-3′ 3′-TC↑GA-5′
*Eco*RII	*Escherichia coli* R245	5′-CC↓GG-3′ 3′-GG↑CC-5′
*Hae*III	*Haemophilus aegyptius*	5′-GG↓CC-3′ 3′-CC↑GG-5′
*Hpa*I	*Haemophilus parainfluenzae*	5′-GTT↓AAC-3′ 3′-CAA↑TTG-5′
*Sma*I	*Serratia marcescens*	5′-CCC↓GGG-3′ 3′-GGG↑CCC-5′

into the recipient's chromosome, but most often the DNA remains in the cytoplasm as a free-floating loop, called a *plasmid* (see Chapter 6, Bacteria and Archaea).

A third form of recombination is **transduction,** which involves bacterial viruses called **bacteriophages** (see Chapter 7, Viruses). The virus enters a bacterial cell and integrates its DNA into the bacterial chromosome.

Viruses other than bacteriophages are also useful in genetic engineering experiments. Viruses (see Chapter 7) consist of nucleic acid fragments, either DNA or RNA, surrounded by a protein coat. They can replicate only in living cells, taking over the host cell machinery. Some viruses integrate their own DNA into the host cell's DNA and become part of the cell's genome. An example is herpesvirus, which integrates into a nerve cell genome and remains within that cell for years, causing recurrent herpes infections. DNA technologists realized that this was a way to bring genes into a cell of choice. The tools of genetic engineering include the following:

- Restrictions enzymes
- Gene libraries
- Plasmids
- Complementary DNA (cDNA)
- Polymerase chain reaction

Restriction Enzymes

In the 1950s Salvador Luria and colleagues discovered that *E. coli* could resist destruction by bacteriophages; the organism could "restrict" the replication of the virus. Later, in 1962 Werner Arber and his research group identified the mechanism by which *E. coli* could achieve this restriction. They showed that an enzyme system was able to cleave the phage DNA before it could get to the bacterial cytoplasm. Subsequently they isolated the DNA-cleaving enzyme, which they called **endonuclease,** now known as a **restriction enzyme.** The enzyme is capable of cutting viral DNA but does not cut the host DNA because the organism modifies the bacterial DNA by adding a methyl group to it. Since the work of these two research groups other restriction enzymes have been discovered. More than 800 restriction enzymes have been identified so far, recognizing more than 100 different nucleotide sequences. Restriction enzymes are named after the bacterium from which they have been isolated. The name includes three letters from the bacterium, one from the strain, and roman numerals indicating the order in which enzymes from the same type of bacterium were identified (Box 25.1).

A restriction enzyme scans a DNA molecule, recognizing and cutting DNA only at a particular sequence of nucleotides. Some enzymes cut the DNA straight across both of the strands of the double helix and therefore produce **"blunt" ends** (Table 25.1). On the other hand, many restriction enzymes cut in an offset fashion and the ends of the cut have an overhanging piece of single-stranded DNA. These ends are called **"sticky" ends** (Table 25.2) because they are able to form base pairs with any

DNA molecule that contains the complementary sticky end. Every cleavage performed with the same enzyme will occur at the same restriction site, regardless of the source of the DNA. When such molecules from different DNA sources are mixed together they will join with each other by base pairing between their sticky ends (Figure 25.3, *A*). This combination can be made permanent by **DNA ligase,** an enzyme that forms covalent bonds along the backbone of each strand. The result of this reaction is a molecule of recombinant DNA (rDNA) (Figure 25.3, *B*). The ability to produce rDNA molecules has revolutionized the study of genetics and formed the foundation for the biotechnology industry.

Gene Libraries

A **gene library** is composed of a series of cells or unicellular organisms that are used to store genes that have been obtained from foreign cells. To form a gene library a mass of cells that contain the desired gene must be acquired. The desired gene must then be isolated from the total DNA of the cells. For example, human cells have a total of 100,000 genes and only 1 gene may be the target of interest, such as the gene for insulin (pancreatic cells), or the gene for human growth hormone (anterior pituitary).

TABLE 25.2 Examples of Restriction Enzymes That Produce "Sticky" Ends

Enzyme	Source	Recognition Site
*Bam*HI	*Bacillus amyloliquefaciens* H	5'-G↓GATCC-3' 3'-CCTAG↑G-5'
*Eco*RI	*Escherichia coli* RY13	5'-G↓AATTC-3' 3'-CTTAA↑G-5'
*Hind*III	*Haemophilus influenzae* Rd	5'-A↓AGCTT-3' 3'-TTCGA↑A-5'
*Pst*I	*Providencia stuartii*	5'-CTGCA↓G-3' 3'-G↑ACGTC-5'
*Sal*I	*Streptomyces albus*	5'-G↓TCGAC-3' 3'-CAGCT↑G-5'

Creating a Gene Library

To establish a cell line containing the gene of interest, the particular DNA containing the gene must be isolated. A restriction enzyme is used to cut the cell's DNA into fragments. After this process a host organism for the fragments needs to be chosen. An example of such an organism *is Escherichia coli.* The plasmids of *E. coli* are then isolated and the DNA fragments that were previously obtained are inserted into the plasmids (Figure 25.4). The recombined plasmids contain all the DNA fragments and are then inserted into *E. coli* cells, and together these *E. coli* cells now are a warehouse of all the DNA of the original cell of interest. The cell collection is the library, the individual cells represent the books of the library, and the individual DNA fragments contain the information in each of the books. This type of library is referred to as a **genomic library.** The next step is to find the particular gene of interest and therefore the library must be screened.

Screening the Gene Library

The screening process begins with growing the transformed *E. coli* cells on nutrient agar. Colonies derived from each individual cell will be visible within 24 to 48 hours, and each colony contains cells with the DNA insert. Now each colony needs to be examined for the presence of the insert that contains the gene of interest. To identify the specific colony a copy of the plate must be made for further work. This is done by a process called **replica plating** (Figure 25.5). This technique is performed by pressing a piece of sterile velvet onto the gel containing the colonies, followed by pressing the velvet to a new petri dish of nutrient agar to establish another plate, which then can be used for analysis of the target gene.

The analysis can be done a number of ways, one of which is by using a radioactive mRNA probe to identify the gene of interest. Bacteria from a particular colony are taken; their DNA is fragmented and then separated in a process called *electrophoresis.* The radioactive mRNA probe is then applied to find out whether any of the fragments on the gel contain the DNA (gene) for the complementary mRNA. If no radioactivity occurs, the gene of interest is not present in that particular colony. If radioactivity accumulates at one site, the DNA fragment has been identified and the colony with the DNA of interest has been

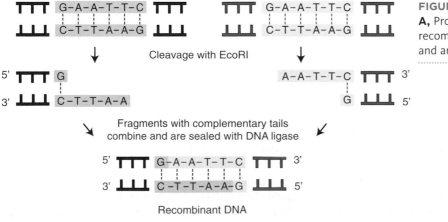

FIGURE 25.3 Action of restriction enzymes. A, Production of "sticky" ends. **B,** Formation of recombinant DNA—the DNA fragments combine and are sealed by DNA ligase.

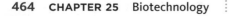

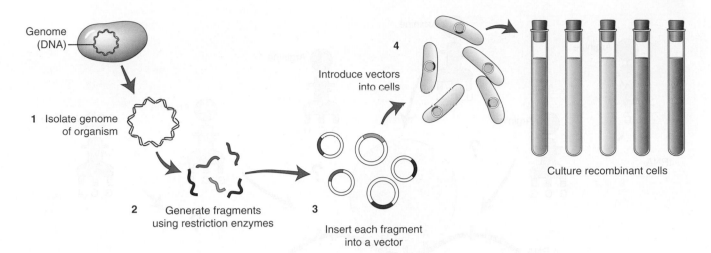

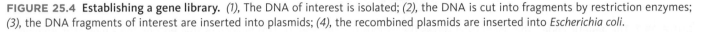

FIGURE 25.4 Establishing a gene library. *(1)*, The DNA of interest is isolated; *(2)*, the DNA is cut into fragments by restriction enzymes; *(3)*, the DNA fragments of interest are inserted into plasmids; *(4)*, the recombined plasmids are inserted into *Escherichia coli*.

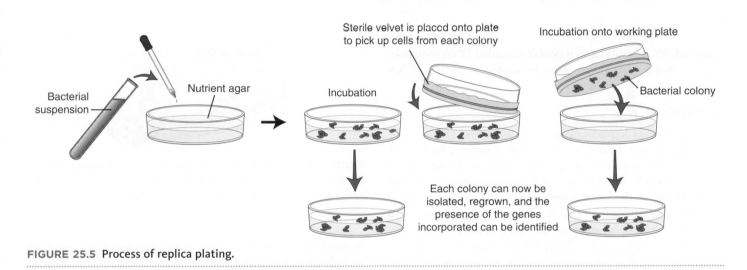

FIGURE 25.5 Process of replica plating.

identified on the working (replica) plate. By working backward the colony in the original plate, the one containing the gene of interest, can be identified and then extracted far more easily than from the original cells (e.g., cells of the pancreas producing the insulin).

cDNA Libraries

Cloning genes from a eukaryotic cell is more problematic than cloning genes from prokaryotes. As described in Chapter 3 (Cell Structure and Function), eukaryotic genes contain exons, the stretches of DNA that encode a protein, and introns, portions of DNA that do not encode a protein and are removed from the mRNA before leaving the nucleus. To clone eukaryotic genes it is best to use a version of the gene that lacks the introns, because once a gene is placed into a bacterial cell, the bacterium will be unable to remove these introns, and therefore will be unable to produce the intended protein. With the advances of genetic engineering it is now possible to create artificial genes that contain only exons. This is achieved with the aid of an enzyme called **reverse transcriptase** to synthesize complementary DNA (cDNA) from an mRNA template (Figure 25.6). This process is

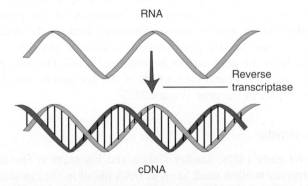

FIGURE 25.6 Complementary DNA. Complementary DNA (cDNA) can be synthesized from an mRNA template with the help of the enzyme reverse transcriptase.

the reverse of the normal interaction between DNA and RNA, in that the isolated mRNA is used to produce a complementary DNA molecule. After the synthesis of the first strand of DNA, the mRNA is digested by reverse transcriptase, and the addition of DNA polymerase will produce the second, complementary

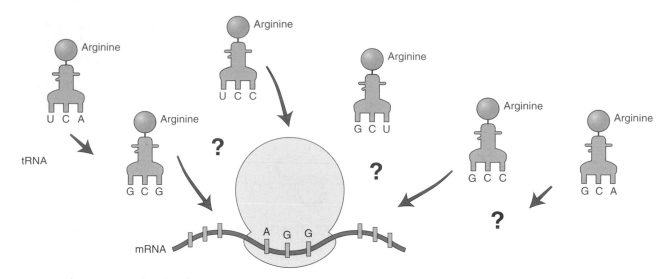

FIGURE 25.7 **The genetic code.** This illustration shows the various transfer RNA (tRNA) molecules that encode the amino acid arginine—only one will base pair with the codon on the complementary mRNA.

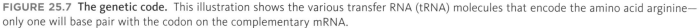

strand of DNA, resulting in a double-stranded DNA molecule. These cDNA molecules can then be cloned to form a cDNA library.

Synthetic DNA

DNA technology has advanced to the point that DNA can be produced in the laboratory with instruments called *DNA synthesis machines*. The nucleotide sequence of the desired DNA is entered via keyboard, and a microprocessor controls the synthesis of the DNA from stored nucleotides and other vital reagents. Because only a relatively small number of nucleotides can be created in this way, several chains may have to be produced and then linked together to form a desired gene. To use this technique the nucleotide sequence of the gene must be known. If the gene has not been isolated previously the technique can still be used by predicting the DNA sequence if the amino acid sequence of the protein product of the gene is known. However, because the degeneracy of the genetic code prevents a definite outcome, the makeup of the gene cannot be 100% predicted. For example, how can it be determined which of the six codons for arginine is part of the gene (Figure 25.7)?

Plasmids

In the early 1970s, Stanley Cohen and his team at Stanford University studied small loops of DNA found in the cytoplasm of bacteria, which are now know as plasmids (Figure 25.8) (see Chapter 6, Bacteria and Archaea). At about the same time Herbert Boyer at the University of California San Francisco studied restriction enzymes found in *E. coli*. In 1973, Herbert Boyer and Stanley Cohen teamed up to produce the world's first recombinant DNA organism, using gene splicing. They removed plasmids from *E. coli* and, using restriction enzymes, they cut the plasmid at precise positions. The segments could then be inserted into a different spliced plasmid and recombined using DNA ligase. The altered DNA (recombinant) could then be

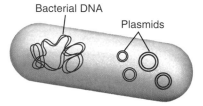

FIGURE 25.8 **Plasmids.** Plasmids are circular nonchromosomal DNA molecules. They can be of different size, and vary in number. Plasmids replicate independently from cell division.

inserted into *E. coli*. With their studies with restriction enzymes and plasmids Boyer and Stanley set the foundation of modern biotechnology/genetic engineering (see Why You Need to Know at the beginning of this chapter).

Once a recombinant plasmid is in the bacterial cell, the single plasmid multiplies itself, independent from the chromosomal DNA, forming dozens of replicas among the normal plasmids. At the time of cell division, the plasmid with the foreign DNA is also copied. In certain bacteria cell division occurs as often as every 20 minutes, and each new bacterium will contain several new plasmids. A single bacterium can breed millions of others—this population is referred to as a **clone.** Because all cells of a clone have the identical plasmids, millions of copies of the foreign gene have been generated. The gene has been cloned.

Polymerase Chain Reaction

The **polymerase chain reaction (PCR)** is a technique, developed in 1986, that can produce DNA copies without a host cell. It is a technique by which small DNA fragments can quickly be amplified to quantities large enough to allow analysis. PCR is used for many applications such as in molecular biology, human genetics, evolution, development, conservation, and forensics. Before starting the PCR process with just one piece of DNA, generally the size of a gene, information concerning the nucleotide sequence of the target DNA is required. This information is necessary to be able to produce two nucleotide primers: one complementary to the 5′ end and one complementary to the 3′ end. PCR can be used to make billions of DNA copies in only a few hours and the amount of amplified DNA produced is limited only to the number of times the steps in the PCR process are repeated. These steps are as follows (Figure 25.9):

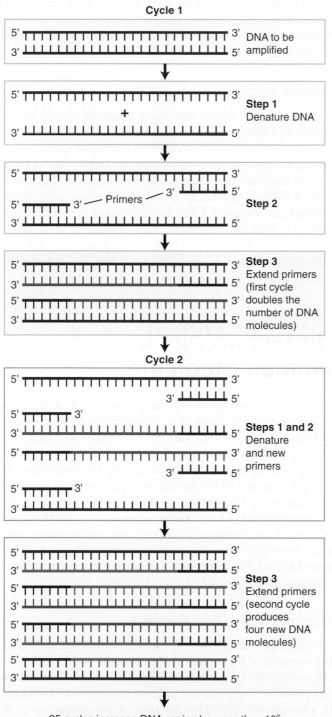

FIGURE 25.9 Polymerase chain reaction (PCR).

25 cycles increase DNA copies by more than 10^6

- **Denaturation:** The double-stranded target DNA to be cloned is denatured into two single strands. This process takes place when heating the double-stranded DNA from 90° C to 95° C for about 1 minute.
- **Priming:** Subsequently the temperature of the reactions is lowered to about 50° C to 70° C, which causes the primers to bind to the single-stranded DNA molecules. These primers, synthetic oligonucleotides, are complementary to the sequences flanking the DNA. They serve as the starting points for the synthesis of new DNA strands, complementary to the original strands.
- **Extension:** A heat-stable DNA polymerase is added and DNA synthesis takes place at temperatures between 70° C and 75° C.

After each cycle the DNA is heated up again to denature all newly formed DNA into single strands and the multiplication can continue. Thirty cycles can be completed in just a few hours and will increase the amount of the original DNA by more than 1 billion times. PCR is applied in many situations, including the identification of infectious agents that would otherwise stay undetected because of low numbers in a sample.

Vectors in Biotechnology

One of the goals of biotechnology is to insert foreign or modified genes into a cell to produce a new phenotype. Various types of DNA molecules can serve as vectors, which are carriers intended to deliver the newly inserted gene into a given cell. All vectors have certain criteria in common:

- Vectors need to be small so that they can be manipulated in the laboratory. A large DNA molecule, such as an entire chromosome, is usually too frail to serve as a vector.
- Vectors need to survive in the target cell.
- Vectors need to contain a recognizable genetic marker so that the biotechnologist can identify the cells that have received the vector and the associated gene of interest.
- Vectors need to provide the required promoters to ensure genetic expression of the target gene in the cell.

Plasmid Vectors

The first vectors developed and still being used were genetically modified plasmids, derived from naturally occurring plasmids. Many plasmids have been genetically modified to serve as vectors and are now commercially available. As previously stated, once a plasmid enters a bacterial cell it will multiply and therefore enhance the number of DNA clones within that cell. In addition, these vectors have been genetically engineered and contain a number of different restriction enzyme recognition sequences, as well as marker genes that can express their presence in the host cell. In general, plasmids that are used in DNA technology should be as small as possible because they are less easily damaged than large plasmids. Furthermore, small plasmids are more easily taken up by the host cell. The ease of

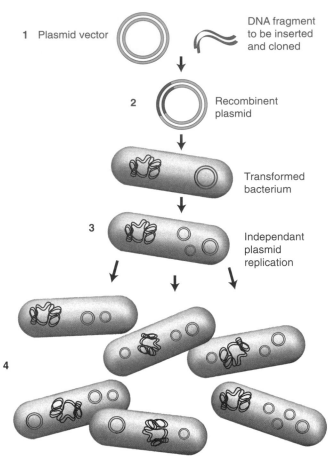

1 Plasmid vector

DNA fragment to be inserted and cloned

2 Recombinent plasmid

Transformed bacterium

3 Independant plasmid replication

4

Cell multiplication

FIGURE 25.10 **Plasmid vector.** *(1)* A plasmid vector is cut by a specific restriction enzyme and the DNA fragment of interest is inserted to form a recombinant plasmid; *(2)* the recombinant plasmid is inserted into a bacterial cell (e.g., *E. coli*) and the bacterium is transformed; *(3)* within the bacteria the recombinant plasmids multiply independent of cell division; and *(4)* as the bacterial cells divide the plasmids continue to multiply and produce the desired gene product.

uptake of a plasmid into the host cell also requires that the inserted cDNA cannot be unreasonably large. A simplified version of the insertion of DNA into a plasmid and subsequent cloning is illustrated in Figure 25.10.

Lambda (λ) Phage Vectors

Plasmid vectors are generally used for cloning small DNA segments consisting of up to about 25 kilobases (kb) of inserted DNA. To prepare a genomic library for a eukaryote, the clone fragments need to be large enough to contain a whole gene. The requirements to clone larger segments of DNA can be fulfilled by both the **lambda (λ) phage** and cosmid vectors; the former allows cloning of segments up to 25 kb and the latter can accommodate segments up to 45 kb.

The lambda phage is a bacteriophage (see Chapter 7, Viruses) that infects *E. coli*. The genome of the phage has been completely mapped and sequenced, and experiments with this

phage have shown that the central part of its chromosome can be replaced with foreign DNA without affecting the phage and its ability to infect *E. coli*. This makes this phage an ideal vector for larger DNA segments. To clone the phage and use it as a vector, the phage DNA needs to be isolated and cut with a restriction enzyme, to produce three chromosomal fragments, with the middle one being replaced by the DNA of another source. Once the foreign DNA has been inserted, DNA ligase is used to produce the recombinant λ vector that is then enclosed into the phage protein head (Figure 25.11). The recombinant phage will then be introduced to a culture of *E. coli*, and once in the bacteria the vectors replicate, forming many phages with the inserted DNA. As the phages reproduce, they lyse their bacterial host cells, and the cloned DNA can be recovered in multiple copies.

Cosmid Vectors

Another class of useful vectors is **cosmids**, hybrid vectors created by combining a fragment of DNA (cDNA) from a virus, usually a bacteriophage, with parts of a plasmid. Cosmids have sequences allowing them to pack phage DNA into the phage protein coat, and the plasmid sequence necessary for replication. A marker, such as an antibiotic resistance gene, is also inserted into the cosmid for identification of the host cell. The cosmid is then packed into the protein head of the bacteriophage and is ready to infect a bacterial cell. Once in the bacterial host cell the linear DNA becomes a plasmid-like loop and replicates as a plasmid.

Biotechnology in Human Medicine

Today's biotechnology allows the production of a variety of pharmaceutical and therapeutic substances to assist in a variety of medical tasks. These include protein replacement such as for insulin, aiding in therapy such as with interferons, vaccines such as the hepatitis B vaccine, screening for genetic diseases, and gene therapy, which for the most part is still in the developmental stage. Traditional biotechnology is now supplemented by recombinant DNA technology to produce a variety of pharmaceutical and therapeutic products, performing many medically important tasks. A summary of products produced by recombinant DNA technology and used in human medicine is shown in Table 25.3.

Human Protein Replacements

Although the Human Genome Project was finished in 2003 and the sequence of the human chromosome is essentially known, the exact number of genes within the genome is still not known. In contrast to the previously believed number of 100,000 genes in a human cell, in 2003 at the time of the completion of the project this number was reduced to 35,000 protein-coding genes. Then, in a National Institutes of Health (NIH) news

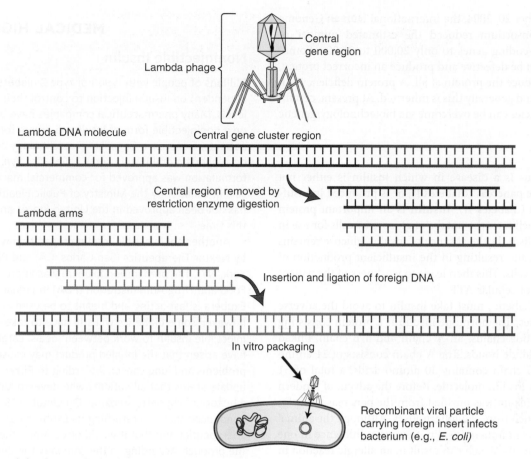

FIGURE 25.11 Lambda phage. The lambda phage can act as a vector once a desired gene has been inserted into its DNA. The recombinant phage will then infect *E. coli* and the bacterium will produce the desired gene product.

TABLE 25.3 Products From Recombinant DNA Technology Used in Human Medicine

Product	Use
Insulin	Treatment for some type 1 and type 2 diabetes mellitus
Human growth hormone (hGH)	Dwarfism, growth hormone deficiency, adult growth hormone deficiency
Factor VIII	Replacement for blood-clotting factor in type A hemophilia
Tissue plasminogen activator (tPA)	Can dissolve blood clots in heart attack and stroke
Interferon	Treatment of viral infections such as hepatitis C and genital warts, some types of cancer, and multiple sclerosis
Interleukins	Cancer treatment
Orthoclone	Immune suppressant in transplant patients
Macrophage colony-stimulating factor	Stimulation of red bone marrow activity after bone marrow grafting
Tumor necrosis factor (TNF)	Treatment of cancer
Granulocyte colony-stimulating factor	Treatment of cancer patients experiencing low neutrophil counts
Antisense molecules	Possible way to treat genetic disorders
Erythropoietin	Treatment of anemia; hormone stimulates red blood cell production
rhDNase	Treatment that can break down thick lung secretions in cystic fibrosis
Antitrypsin	Replacement therapy to benefit emphysema patients
Vaccines	Hepatitis B, *Haemophilus influenzae* type b meningitis, experimental HPV and AIDS vaccine

release on October 20, 2004, the International Human Genome Sequencing Consortium reduced the estimated number of human protein-coding genes to only 20,000 to 25,000. Sometimes a gene can be defective and produce an incorrect protein, or does not produce the protein at all. A protein deficiency can lead to disease and generally this is inherited. At present, certain protein deficiencies can be overcome via biotechnology/genetic engineering.

Insulin

Diabetes mellitus is a disease in which insulin is either not produced by the pancreas (diabetes I), or is produced in insufficient amounts (diabetes II). **Insulin** is an important protein hormone that facilitates the uptake of glucose by cells for use in cellular metabolism. In the absence of insulin, glucose remains in the bloodstream, resulting in the insufficient production of ATP within the cells. This then leads to weakness of the patient due to the lack of cellular ATP.

Millions of diabetics must take insulin to avoid the adverse affects of diabetes. The hormone insulin is a protein consisting of two polypeptide chains, an A chain and a B chain, linked together by disulfide bonds. The A chain consists of 21 amino acids and the B chain contains 30 amino acids, a total of 51 amino acids per insulin molecule. Before the advent of modern biotechnology insulin was purified from the pancreases of pigs and cows, obtained from slaughterhouses. Although the animal insulin is similar to human insulin, there is a difference in one or three amino acids, which can result in an allergic reaction in human patients. With current methods human insulin can now be mass-produced by the application of recombinant DNA technology and with the help of a plasmid from *E. coli*. The steps of insulin production involve the tools of genetic engineering previously discussed:

- Isolation of the human insulin gene
- Preparation of the target DNA, the plasmid
- Insertion of the human gene into the plasmid
- Incorporation of the recombinant plasmid back into the bacteria
- Multiplication of the plasmid
- Target cell reproduction, and production of human insulin
- Harvesting of human insulin

Millions of diabetics now use the human insulin produced by bacteria.

Human Growth Hormone

Human growth hormone (HGH) is a protein hormone of about 190 amino acids, synthesized and secreted by somatotroph cells of the anterior pituitary. The hormone plays a major role in several metabolic processes, including growth and metabolism. It stimulates overall body growth by increasing cellular uptake of amino acids and encouraging protein synthesis.

Dwarfism, a metabolic disorder, occurs when the anterior pituitary fails to secrete sufficient amounts of HGH. Growth hormone deficiency (GHD) in children is also a condition that occurs when not enough HGH is produced and released. Chil-

dren with GHD may grow less than 2 in. per year. Once an adult reaches full height, growth hormone helps to maintain the proper amounts of fat, muscle, and bone. If an adult does not produce enough growth hormone, the individual may have a condition called *adult growth hormone deficiency,* or aGHD.

In the past, generally only dwarfism was treated with growth hormone, which had to be obtained from cadavers. Approximately 80 cadavers had to be used to obtain enough HGH for a year's therapy. This method of treatment unfortunately also brought the risk of the development of Creutzfeldt-Jakob syndrome, a central nervous system disease caused by a prion (see Chapter 7, Viruses). Because of the possibility of transmission of this disease, the use of cadaver tissue in the United States and Britain was restricted in 1985. HGH can now be produced by genetic engineering, using cDNA encoding growth hormone. The cDNA is then expressed in a bacterial expression vector. A problem with producing a short polypeptide hormone such as HGH is its susceptibility to protease digestion. This problem is being resolved by using bacterial host strains that lack several proteases.

Factor VIII

Hemophilia A is the most common inherited blood-clotting disorder in the United States. The defective gene is located on the X chromosome; therefore the disorder occurs primarily in males. This is because females carry two X chromosomes, and if one of them carries the defective gene the other chromosome can pick up the duty to produce **factor VIII** (FVIII). Males carry only one X chromosome and if the gene for factor VIII is defective, the individual will have hemophilia A. One in 5000 males in the United States has hemophilia and all races are affected equally. To restore homeostasis hemophiliacs can receive FVIII concentrated from donated blood plasma or from recombinant sources.

To yield enough clotting factor for a single patient for 1 year, approximately 8000 pints of blood are needed. Any transfer of a blood plasma by-product into a recipient with hemophilia can lead to the transmission of blood-borne infections such as HIV and hepatitis B and C. During the early 1980s, before purification methods were improved and DNA technologists worked to produce synthetic factor VIII, thousands of hemophiliacs became infected with these viruses. In the early 1990s, pharmaceutical companies began to produce recombinant factors and two versions of FVIII were approved by the U.S. Food and Drug Administration (FDA). The recombinant factor now can prevent disease transmission during replacement therapy.

Human Disease Therapies

Biotechnology has also entered into the territory of disease therapy, and biotechnology companies are now able to produce new drugs by recombinant DNA technology.

Tissue Plasminogen Activator

Tissue plasminogen activator (tPA) is a serine protease (enzyme) that is made by endothelial cells to help dissolve blood clots. For many years, coronary thrombosis has been treated with streptokinase, a naturally occurring bacterial enzyme; now, however, recombinant tPA can be used in diseases that feature blood clots, such as heart attack and stroke. To be effective, tPA needs to be administered intravenously within the first 3 hours of the event. After this period of time, but within 6 hours, tPA can still be administered through an arterial catheter, directly to the site of occlusion, and be effective.

Interferon

Interferon is a small protein produced naturally by certain white blood cells and by cells that have been infected with a virus (see Chapter 20, The Immune System). Originally, the interferon system was believed to be a defense system against viruses only, but it is now known to be involved in the defense against other microbes and also in immune regulation. The interferon system consists of three main groups: interferon-α, interferon-β, and interferon-γ. Interferon-α is primarily a product of lymphocytes and macrophages, interferon-β is produced by fibroblasts and epithelial cells, and interferon-γ is produced by T cells, B-cells, and NK cells. Interferon was not readily available until 1980, when the interferon gene was inserted into bacteria by recombinant DNA technology; this allowed mass cultivation and purification from bacterial cultures or from yeast. Synthetic interferons are now used in the treatment of viral infections, multiple sclerosis, and cancer (see Health Care Application: Examples of Interferon Therapy in Humans).

Antisense Molecules

A sense strand is a 5'-to-3' mRNA or DNA molecule. The complementary strand to the sense strand is called **antisense**. Antisense technology uses antisense strands to bind with the sense

Examples of Interferon Therapy in Humans

Generic Interferon	Trade Name	Source	Used in Treatment of:
Interferon alfa-n3	Alferon N	Human leukocytes	Genital warts
Interferon alfa-2b	Intron A	Recombinant (*E. coli*)	Chronic hepatitis C Hairy cell leukemia Malignant melanoma Follicular lymphoma Condylomata acuminatum AIDS-related Kaposi's sarcoma
Interferon alfa-2a	Roferon A (discontinued for the U.S. market in 2008)	Recombinant	Chronic hepatitis C Hairy cell leukemia AIDS-related Kaposi's sarcoma
Interferon beta-1a	Avonex Rebif CinnoVex	Recombinant (*E. coli*)	Multiple sclerosis
Interferon beta-1b	Betaseron	Recombinant (*E. coli*)	Relapsing forms of multiple sclerosis
Interferon Alfacon-1	Infergen	Recombinant (*E. coli*)	Chronic hepatitis C
Interferon gamma-1b	Actimmune	Recombinant (*E. coli*)	Chronic granulomatous disease

strand. When an antisense strand binds to an mRNA sense strand, the cell will identify the now double-stranded RNA as foreign to the cell and degrade the defective mRNA molecule, and therefore prevent the production of the undesired protein.

Antisense therapy is a possible way to treat genetic disorders or infections. If the genetic sequence of a gene is known to be the cause of a particular disease, and antisense molecules can be produced and inactivate the functioning of that gene—the gene is turned "off." Antisense drugs are being investigated to treat cancer, diabetes, amyotrophic lateral sclerosis (ALS), and diseases with an inflammatory component, such as asthma and arthritis. Although many potential therapies are under investigation, most of them have not yet produced significant clinical results. At present, one antisense drug, fomivirsen (Vitravene) has been approved by the FDA as a treatment for cytomegalovirus retinitis in patients with AIDS. This approval is an important step in demonstrating that antisense drugs can be effective in the treatment of specific diseases.

Erythropoietin

Erythropoietin is a hormone produced by the kidneys to stimulate bone marrow stem cells to mature into red blood cells. If erythropoietin levels are low, anemia (low erythrocyte count) will occur. This is especially a problem in patients with kidney failure, in cancer patients undergoing chemotherapy, and in patients who use drugs for the treatment of AIDS.

In 1989 the FDA approved the genetically engineered version of the hormone Epogen produced by Amgen (Thousand Oaks, CA). Another genetically engineered version of erythropoietin, epoetin alfa, received FDA approval in 1997. The drug is marketed as Procrit by Ortho Biotech (Raritan, NJ) and is designed to be an alternative to blood transfusions in anemic patients who undergo noncardiovascular surgery. Because the drug stimulates the production of erythrocytes, the drug is administered before surgery to counteract the effects of blood loss, and therefore limiting the need for preoperative blood transfusions.

Vaccines

Vaccines are preparations that provide/improve immunity against certain infectious diseases (see Chapter 20, The Immune System). Before the development of genetically engineered vaccines, vaccines included attenuated microbes, killed or fragmented microbes, and toxoids. In addition to genetically engineered vaccines, traditional vaccines are still available and in use to this date.

Subunit Vaccines

Subunit vaccines are defined as those containing only a molecule or fragment of a pathogen, but still can stimulate the immune system. Because of the developments in biotechnology these types of vaccines can now be made by genetically modified yeasts.

An advantage of a subunit vaccine is that there is no chance of becoming infected from the vaccine. Subunit vaccines have been developed for a number of infectious diseases, including the hepatitis B vaccine.

Blood Doping

Blood doping is the practice of illegally boosting the number of erythrocytes (red blood cells [RBCs]) in the circulation in order to enhance athletic performance. Because the main function of RBCs is to carry oxygen from the lungs to the muscles, a higher RBC count dramatically improves an athlete's performance by increasing their aerobic capacity and stamina. Blood doping was traditionally done by harvesting red blood cells from the athlete or a compatible donor, freezing and saving the cells until needed, and then transfusing the cells back into the body.

Genetically engineered erythropoietin (EPO) has changed this practice. There now is no need for transfusions, just an EPO shot. For many years accurate testing was not possible because the synthetic EPO is practically identical to the naturally occurring form. However, the testing technology now is improved with an accurate urine test that can detect the differences between normal and synthetic EPO. Blood doping has been especially problematic in professional cycling (for more reading see http://www.rice.edu/~jenky/sports/epo.html).

DNA Vaccines

DNA vaccines consist of genetically modified plasmids injected into humans or animals. The cells receiving the plasmid will then synthesize polypeptides that are characteristic of the pathogen. These polypeptides will stimulate immunologic memory, which is then ready for an intense immune response as a result of invasion by the real pathogen. In contrast to conventional vaccines, DNA vaccines stimulate cell-mediated as well as antibody-mediated immunity. At present, most of the work on DNA vaccines has been done on mice, which have shown protection against tuberculosis, severe acute respiratory syndrome (SARS), smallpox, and other intracellular pathogens. In addition, many other trial DNA vaccines are currently being tested.

Biotechnology in Agriculture

Genetic engineering can be used to modify the genomes of microorganisms, plants, and animals. All genetically engineered products, just like other products, must undergo extensive research and development before they are ready for commercial release. DNA technology has been successfully applied in agriculture to produce recombinant plants and animals. The genes of both plants and animals have been altered for specific purposes by adding genes from other organisms. Through its Biotechnology Regulatory Services program, the U.S. Department of Agriculture (USDA) is responsible for regulating and supporting the safe use of genetically engineered organisms. Within the USDA there are several agencies to investigate new agricultural biotechnology products and make sure that these products are safe. Once approved the USDA supports bringing these U.S. products to the world market.

Transgenic Plants

At present, the most widespread application of genetic engineering in agriculture consists of genetically modified crops. **Transgenic** plants have been enhanced for herbicide resistance, tolerance to salty soils, resistance to freezing and pests, and have improved nutritional value and yield. Furthermore, transgenic plants also can be used to produce medical or industrial products including human or veterinary drugs, industrial or research chemicals, and enzymes. Examples of genetically modified plants that have been used for this purpose include rice, corn, barley, tobacco, and safflower.

Herbicide Tolerance/Resistance

Herbicide tolerance permits plants, specifically crops, to withstand otherwise lethal doses of herbicides. The herbicide glyphosate (Roundup), widely used in gardens to kill weeds, kills all plants, including crops, by blocking a key plant enzyme that is essential for the production of several amino acids. Some bacteria that initially were killed by glyphosate (e.g., *Agrobacterium*) became resistant to the herbicide. The resistant gene was isolated, cloned, modified for expression in plants, and transferred into crop plants. As a result of these transgenic crops, farmers can apply glyphosate to crop fields in order to kill weeds, without damaging the crop. These crops are often referred to as "Roundup Ready."

Insect Tolerance/Resistance

Commercially available insect-tolerant plants contain a protein produced by *Bacillus thuringiensis* (Bt), an organism commonly found in the bacterial flora of soil. When this protein is consumed by insects it is modified by enzymes in the insect's intestinal tract and forms Bt-toxin, causing the tissue to dissolve. Bt-toxin is naturally occurring and harms only insects. Farmers have used this toxin for more than 30 years to reduce insect damage to their crops. The gene for Bt-toxin is now inserted into a variety of crop plants, which then produce the toxin themselves and insects feeding on the plants are killed without harming humans and most animals. The major concern among farmers is that wide use of Bt crops might lead to the development of resistance to the toxin.

Virus Tolerance/Resistance

Viruses also may cause economically important plant diseases, reducing the yield of certain crops up to 50%. Unfortunately, the spread of most plant viruses is difficult to control, and once infection sets in, chemical treatment methods do not exist. Viruses are often transmitted from plant to plant by insects. Biotechnology can be used to produce virus-resistant crops. This generally involves inserting a gene that encodes a viral coat protein. The mechanism of developing resistance to a viral infection by expressing only a single viral protein is called *pathogen-derived resistance*. The plant is then capable of producing this viral protein before the virus attacks and once the virus arrives, it is unable to reproduce, because the production of its essential coat protein is already blocked.

Fungus Tolerance/Resistance

Fungi are the largest group of plant pathogens and are responsible for a variety of plant diseases that kill all kinds of crops, often resulting in heavy losses. In general, these diseases are managed by the application of chemical fungicides or heavy metals. In addition to yield losses, some pathogenic fungi produce mycotoxins that are carcinogenic. Genetic engineering also provides ways of managing fungal infections, using several approaches. These include the following:

- Introducing genes from other plants or bacteria that encode enzymes that break down essential components of fungal cell walls
- Introducing plant genes that enhance innate plant defense mechanisms
- Invoking a plant hypersensitivity reaction, resulting in the death of the infected cell, and thus stopping the fungal infection from spreading to other cells

Transgenic Animals

With the dramatic increase in the world's population from 1.6 billion in 1900, to 6 billion at present, to an estimated 10 billion by 2030, the demand for agricultural animals will also increase. The use of genetic engineering has already impacted domesticated livestock and companion animals. More recently, steps have been taken to create transgenic animals. These animals received genes from other organisms to provide solutions for disease treatment, organ transplant shortage, and food production. Some mammals have been modified to produce therapeutic proteins in their milk for human use. These include agents for the treatment of cancer, heart attacks, hemophilia, rheuma-

LIFE APPLICATION

"Superweeds"?

Genetically modified "Roundup Ready" crops include a variety of crops, some of which are still under development. These modified crops greatly improve the conventional farmer's capacity to control weeds, because glyphosate can be sprayed on the fields without hurting the crop. Critics to the "Roundup Ready System" state that the system relies on herbicide control and that tilling is no longer used to control the growth of weeds. Within the last few years, several reports have identified the emergence of resistant weeds that require much higher doses of glyphosate than the original weeds. This phenomenon is more pronounced in areas where the farmers plant the same genetically engineered crop every year.

toid arthritis, and many other diseases/conditions. Scientists are also attempting to create transgenic pigs for the purpose of transplanting their organs into humans (xenotransplants) (see Chapter 20, The Immune System).

Summary

- Modern biotechnology, a subdiscipline of biology, involves recombinant DNA technology, also referred to as genetic engineering, for industrial, medical, and agricultural purposes.
- The tools of genetic engineering include the use of restriction enzymes, plasmids, the polymerase chain reaction (PCR), and the creation of gene libraries.
- Restriction enzymes are molecular scissors, capable of cutting DNA at specific sites. Plasmids are capable of inserting these pieces of foreign DNA into their own, and PCR can produce multiple copies of DNA without a host cell.
- There are two different types of gene library: cDNA libraries and synthetic DNA. Both of these libraries must be created and then screened before they are usable in the laboratory.
- Vectors in biotechnology serve to insert foreign genes into a host cell to produce a new phenotype. Such vectors include plasmid vectors, lambda phage vectors, and cosmid vectors.
- With the help of recombinant DNA technology, human protein deficits such as insulin deficiency in diabetes mellitus, growth hormone deficiencies, and factor VIII disorder, can be treated.
- The use of recombinant DNA technology has allowed biotechnology companies to produce new drugs for human disease therapies. These include tissue plasminogen activator (tPA), various interferons, antisense molecules, and erythropoietin.
- Vaccines produced by traditional methods can now also be produced by recombinant DNA technology, typically genetically modified subunit vaccines and DNA vaccines consisting of genetically modified plasmids.
- Genetic engineering also has had a great impact in agriculture in the production of genetically modified plants and animals.
- The most widespread application of biotechnology in agriculture involves crops genetically modified to make them tolerant or resistant to herbicides, insects, viruses, and fungi. Moreover, certain mammals have been genetically modified to produce therapeutic proteins in their milk.

Review Questions

1. Which of the following is a true statement about recombinant DNA technology?
   a. It is a single technique for genetic manipulation.
   b. It involves the modification of an organism's genome.
   c. It will replace biotechnology in the future.
   d. It manipulates only the genotype.

2. The genetic recombination process that occurs when bacteria acquire fragments of DNA from the local environment and then express the encoded proteins is called:
   a. Transcription
   b. Transformation
   c. Transduction
   d. Ligation

3. The term *endonuclease* refers to:
   a. Gene libraries
   b. Restriction enzymes
   c. Plasmids
   d. cDNA

4. Small loops of DNA found in the cytoplasm of bacteria are:
   a. cDNA
   b. mRNA
   c. Plasmids
   d. Clones

5. All of the following are steps in the polymerase chain reaction *except*:
   a. Extension
   b. Translation
   c. Priming
   d. Denaturation

6. Which of the following is a vector created by the combination viral DNA fragments and fragments from a plasmid?
   a. Cosmid vector
   b. Plasmid vector
   c. Combined vector
   d. Lambda phage vector

7. A portion of DNA, such as a gene, that is synthesized from an RNA template is:
   a. Recombinant DNA
   b. Probe DNA
   c. Complementary DNA
   d. Reverse transcriptase

8. Which of the following tools of genetic engineering is used to make multiple copies of DNA?
   a. PCR
   b. Gel electrophoresis
   c. Reverse transcription
   d. Recombinant DNA

9. The recombinant protein that is used to help dissolve blood clots such as occur in heart attacks and stroke is
   a. Interferon
   b. Factor VIII
   c. Antisense molecule
   d. Tissue plasminogen activator

10. The synthetic interferon that is used in the treatment of multiple sclerosis is:
    a. Interferon alfa-2b
    b. Interferon beta-1a
    c. Interferon alfa-2a
    d. Interferon gamma-1b

11. Recombinant DNA technology is also referred to as _____.

12. Enzymes that can cleave DNA at a particular site are _____.

13. Enzymes that cut DNA straight across both of the double helix strands produce _____ ends.

14. When a single bacterium can produce millions of identical cells, the population is called a(n) _____.

15. Synthetic proteins that can be used in the treatment of hepatitis C are _____.

16. Describe the steps and tools used in genetic engineering.

17. Describe a gene library and its usefulness.

18. In correct sequence, name and describe the steps used in PCR.

19. Name and describe the various vectors used in biotechnology.

20. Discuss transgenic plants used in the agricultural environment.

Bibliography

Alcamo IE: *DNA technology, the awesome skill*, ed 2, San Diego, 2001, Academic Press.

Bauman R: *Microbiology: with diseases by taxonomy*, ed 2, San Francisco, 2007, Benjamin Cummings/Pearson Education.

Klug WS, Cummings MR, Spencer CA, et al: *Concepts of genetics*, ed 9, San Francisco, 2008, Benjamin Cummings/Pearson Education.

Madigan MT, Martinko JM, Dunlap PV, et al: *Biology of microorganisms*, ed 12, San Francisco, 2009, Benjamin Cummings/Pearson Education.

Totora GJ, Funke BR, Case CL: *Microbiology: an introduction*, ed 9, San Francisco, 2007, Benjamin Cummings/Pearson Education.

Internet Resources

cnet News, "Researchers in Maryland unleash synthetic DNA," by Mark Rutherford, January 27, 2008, available at http://www.cnet.com/8301-13639_1-9859042-42.html

The Washington Post, "Synthetic DNA on the Brink of Yielding New Life Forms," by Rick Weiss, December 17, 2007; A01, available at http://www.washingtonpost.com/wp-dyn/content/article/2007/12/16/AR2007121601900_pf.html

Herbert W. Boyer Biography, http://www.bookrags.com/biography/herbert-w-boyer-woc/

Human Genome Project Information, How Many Genes Are in the Human Genome? http://www.ornl.gov/sci/techresources/Human_Genome/faq/genenumber.shtml

International Human Genome Sequencing Consortium: Finishing the euchromatic sequence of the human genome, *Nature* 431:931-945, October 21, 2004, available at http://www.nature.com/nature/journal/v431/n7011/full/nature03001.html

National Human Genome Research Institute, 2004 Release: IHGSC Describes Finished Human Sequence (NIH News Release), http://www.genome.gov/12513430

FDA News, FDA Approves First Ever Inhaled Insulin Combination Product for Treatment of Diabetes, January 27, 2006, http://www.fda.gov/bbs/topics/news/2006/new01304.html

Diabetes In Control.com, Oral-lyn Insulin: First Non-Injectable Insulin Gets Released this Month, http://www.diabetesincontrol.com/modules.php?name=News&file=article&sid=3276

Massachusetts General Hospital, "Advances in Recombinant Human Growth Hormone Replacement Therapy in Adults," by Steven Grinspoon, M.D., available at http://pituitary.mgh.harvard.edu/e-f-944.htm

Medline Plus, Hemophilia A, http://www.nlm.nih.gov/medlineplus/ency/article/000538.htm

Hemispherx Biopharma Inc., About ALFERON N Injection®, http://www.hemispherx.net/content/products/

RxList, Roferon-A, http://www.rxlist.com/cgi/generic/roferon_ids.htm

Medline Plus, Drugs, Supplements, and Herbal Information, http://www.nlm.nih.gov/medlineplus/druginfo/medmaster/a693040.html

RxList, Vitravene, http://www.rxlist.com/cgi/generic/fomivirsen_ids.htm

"Erythropoietin," COPYRIGHT©2005 Mark Jenkins, http://www.rice.edu/~jenky/sports/epo.html

Finding of No Significant Impact, Animal and Plant Health Inspection Service, Petition for Non-regulated Status for Soybean Line MON 89788 (APHIS 06-178—01p), http://www.aphis.usda.gov/brs/aphisdocs/06_17801p_ea.pdf

California Department of Pesticide Regulation, California Product/Label Database Queries & Lists, http://www.cdpr.ca.gov/docs/label/labelque.htm#regprods

Randerson J: Genetically-modified superweeds "not uncommon," *NewScientist* 15:34 05 February 2002, available at http://www.newscientist.com/article.ns?id=dn1882

SourceWatch (Center for Media and Democracy, Monsanto and the Roundup Ready Controversy, http://www.sourcewatch.org/index.php?title=Monsanto_and_the_Roundup_Ready_Controversy

Biotech Chronicles, http://www.accessexcellence.org/RC/AB/BC/

Bergey's Manual of Systematic Bacteriology

Bergey's Manual (first edition) consists of four volumes. In the following table the volumes are broken down to show the general content of each volume. The second edition of the *Manual,* which at the present time is being completed, will be organized much differently because the most recent classifications are based on nucleotide sequencing of ribosomal RNA.

Volume	General Content	Volume	General Content
1	Spirochetes Aerobic/microaerophilic, motile, helical/vibrioid gram negatives Nonmotile, gram-negative curved rods Gram-negative aerobic rods and cocci Facultatively anaerobic gram-negative rods Anaerobic gram-negative straight/curved/helical rods Dissimilatory sulfate or sulfate-reducing bacteria Anaerobic gram-negative cocci Rickettsias and chlamydias Mycoplasmas Endosymbionts	3	Anoxygenic phototrophic bacteria Oxygenic photosynthetic bacteria Aerobic chemolithotrophic bacteria and associated organisms Budding and/or appendaged bacteria Sheathed bacteria Nonphotosynthetic, nonfruiting gliding bacteria Fruiting gliding bacteria (myxobacteria) Archaeobacteria
2	Gram-positive cocci Endospore-forming gram-positive rods and cocci Regular nonsporing gram-positive rods Irregular nonsporing gram-positive rods Mycobacteria Nocardioforms	4	Nocardioform actinomycetes Actinomycetes with multilocular sporangia Actinoplanes Streptomycetes and related genera Maduromycetes Thermomonospora and related genera Thermoactinomycetes Other genera

Glossary

Abiogenesis the development of living organisms from non-living matter.

Abiotic components that are nonliving chemical and physical factors in the environment.

Abortive infection an infection in which some or all viral components are synthesized but no infective virus is produced.

Abscess a localized collection of pus in an area of tissue that is infected.

Abyssal zone this zone is characteristic for oceans and encompasses the deep ocean trenches.

Accessory glands glandular tissue aiding a particular organ system.

Acetylcholine neurotransmitter used by motor neurons at the neuromuscular junction; also a neurotransmitter in the brain and in the autonomic nervous system.

Active site the site on an enzyme to which substrates bind; is specific for each substrate.

Active transport the transport of substances across a plasma membrane; requires cellular energy (see adenosine triphosphate [ATP]). This transport mechanism often occurs against the concentration gradient.

Acute infections infections that appear rapidly, with pronounced (severe) symptoms, but then rapidly vanish.

Adaptive immune response a response that is specific to a specific antigen and is therefore also referred to as specific defense; represents the third line of defense of the immune response.

Adenosine triphosphate (ATP) a chemical compound (nucleotide) that provides energy for the cell.

Adhesion the first and probably most crucial step in infection, involving the physical attachment of an organism to a tissue surface.

Adoption in microbiology, the establishment and further spreading of a pathogen within a new host population.

Adsorption the first step by which a bacteriophage infects a bacterium; involves attachment to the host cell.

Aerobes bacteria that require oxygen to live.

Aerobic cellular respiration catabolic process that requires oxygen and releases energy.

Aerotolerant anaerobes bacteria that do not require oxygen; its presence neither hinders nor helps the growth of the organisms.

Affinity an attraction or force between particles that causes them to combine.

Agar a gelatinous substance obtained from red algae, used as a solidifying agent in culture media.

AIDS (acquired immune deficiency syndrome) caused by the HIV virus. It is regarded as a secondary immune deficiency. AIDS is not a disease but a syndrome; it has complex signs and symptoms, and a variety of diseases are associated with a common cause. AIDS results in many opportunistic infections due to a severely compromised immune system.

Airborne disease refers to the spread of pathogens by droplet nuclei (droplets of mucus), other aerosols, and dust that travel for more than 1 m from the reservoir to the host.

Aldehydes organic compounds with a terminal carbonyl group ($-HC=O$); in microbiology, aldehydes are used in the control of microorganisms.

Algae large and diverse group of simple organisms, ranging from unicellular to multicellular forms, containing chlorophyll that is needed for photosynthesis. Primarily aquatic organisms.

Algicides substances that kill or inhibit the growth of algae.

Allergen a substance that usually is not harmful to the body but causes hypersensitivity reactions.

Allograft a transplant between genetically different individuals of the same species (e.g., humans) but with different genomes (genetic information).

Allosteric site a site that, when activated by a noncompetitive inhibitor, will change the shape of the active site of an enzyme.

Alternative complement pathway an innate component of the immune system's natural defenses against infection. It can operate without antibody participation.

Amebiasis disease caused by amoebas.

Amensalism an interaction between two species in which one organism can hamper or prevent the growth and/or survival of another, without being positively or negatively affected by the other organism.

Ammonification the process by which amino groups are removed from organic compounds and then converted to ammonia.

Amphitrichous describing a microbial cell with a single flagellum at opposite poles.

Anabolism the synthesis of large molecules from smaller ones. This reaction requires energy.

Anaerobes microorganisms that grow best or only in the absence of oxygen.

Anaerobic cellular respiration catabolic process, part of cellular respiration that does not require oxygen.

Analgesic a medication capable of reducing or eliminating pain.

Analytical epidemiology attempts to demonstrate a probable cause-and-effect relationship, using analysis of data collected by descriptive epidemiology.

Anammox the acronym for anaerobic ammonium oxidation; a recent addition to knowledge of the nitrogen cycle.

Anesthetic a substance that produces anesthesia, a state in which the conscious sensation of pain is blocked.

Animalcules microscopic organisms; *"small animals"* so named by van Leeuwenhoek.

Anions negatively charged ions; they move toward the positive pole or anode of an electric field.

Antagonism describing a drug combination that is less effective than when the drugs are administered alone.

Anthrax a zoonotic disease caused by the bacterium *Bacillus anthracis*. Can manifest itself in three forms: cutaneous, respiratory, and gastrointestinal.

Antibiotics chemotherapeutic agents naturally produced by some microorganisms.

Antibody a protein molecule produced in response to an antigen.

Antibody titer the antibody concentration in serum.

Anticodon trinucleotide sequence of transfer RNA (tRNA) that is complementary to the trinucleotide sequence of messenger RNA (mRNA).

Antidote a remedy to counteract the effects of poison.

Antigen any agent that is capable of inducing a specific immune response.

Antigenic drift small changes in the viral coat (surface proteins) that happen over time. Antigenic drift can produce a new influenza viral strain that may not be recognized by the body's immune system.

Antigenic shift a process involving at least two different strains of viruses, or even different viruses, combining to form a new virus that may then infect different species.

Antigen-presenting cells cells that take in antigens, process them, and then present parts of the antigen to B and T cells to activate them.

Antimicrobial agents agents capable of killing microorganisms or suppressing their multiplication or growth.

Antisense molecules in molecular biology, the strand complementary to the mRNA or DNA sense strand.

Antisepsis disinfection of living tissues.

Antiseptic a growth-inhibiting substance used to disinfect skin.

APIC Association of Professionals in Infection Control and Epidemiology.

Apical complex unique organelle, characteristic of the Apicomplexa, a large group of protozoans.

Apoenzyme the protein portion of an enzyme.

Archaea a group of single-celled microorganisms that are similar to bacteria because they are also prokaryotes, but are evolutionarily different.

Arenaviruses double-stranded RNA viruses that cause human disease including Lassa fever.

Ascariasis an infection caused by *Ascaris lumbricoides*, the most common nematode infection of humans worldwide.

Aseptic free of microorganisms; also, using methods to protect against pathogenic microorganisms.

Aseptic technique method used to protect against contamination/infection by microorganisms.

ASM American Society for Microbiology.

Aspergillosis illnesses caused by the genus *Aspergillus*. *Aspergillus* is a fungus found in soil, food, compost, agricultural buildings, and air vents of homes and offices worldwide.

Atom a unit of matter, the smallest unit of an element.

Atomic nucleus the center of the atom; contains protons (positively charged particles) and neutrons (no charge; the exception is hydrogen, which does not contain neutrons).

Atomic number equals the number of protons in an atomic nucleus.

Atomic weight equals the number of protons and neutrons in an atom.

Autograft tissue transplanted from one site in an individual to another site in the same individual.

Autoimmune disease occurs when the immune system is unable to distinguish between self and nonself-antigens and attacks cells, tissues, or organs of the body.

Autoinoculation a secondary infection caused by self-inoculation.

Autotroph microorganisms that can obtain carbon from atmospheric carbon dioxide.

B cells small lymphocytes with antibodies located in the cell membrane.

Bacilli rod-shaped bacteria, some of which are endospore forming.

Bacteremia the presence of bacteria in the blood.

Bacteria a large group of unicellular, prokaryotic organisms.

Bacterial infection a bacterial invasion and colonization of cells or tissues.

Bacterial intoxication occurs when toxins produced by bacteria contaminate food or water and are then introduced into the human body.

Bactericidal the action of substances that kill bacteria.

Bactericide an agent that destroys bacteria.

Bacteriophage a virus that infects bacteria.

Bacteriostatic substances that interfere with or inhibit bacterial cell growth and reproduction.

Bacteriuria the presence of bacteria in the urine.

Balanitis inflammation of the glans penis.

Baltimore classification system a viral classification system devised by David Baltimore. This system places the virus into one of seven groups distinguishing the viruses on the basis of the relationship between the viral genome and the messenger RNA.

Barophiles microorganisms that grow best under high hydrostatic pressures and live only in the deepest parts of oceans.

Barotolerant microorganisms that can survive under conditions of increased hydrostatic pressure.

Base a chemical compound that dissociates in water and releases hydroxyl ions.

Basophils the least common of the five leukocyte types. They have dark, bluish purple granules that contain chemical mediators promoting inflammation.

Benthic zone consists of the sediments at the bottom of a lake; it includes the sediment surface as well as some subsurface layers.

Benthos organisms that live on, in, or near the ocean floor.

Binary fission form of asexual reproduction involving dividing the cell into two equal, duplicate cells. A method by which all bacteria and most protists reproduce.

Binomial consisting of or relating to two names or terms.

Binomial system the system of nomenclature in which organisms are identified by a two-part latinized name. It was devised by Linnaeus and therefore is also referred to as the Linnaean system.

Bioassay an assay determining the biological activity or potency of a substance by testing its effect on a living organism.

Bioavailability the term used to indicate the extent to which a drug reaches its site of action.

Biodiversity the variation of species/life forms living in a given ecosystem.

Biofilm microorganisms organized into complex communities of different organisms, growing on a surface.

Biogeochemical cycle a circuit or pathway through which organic compounds or a chemical element is changed from one chemical state to another by moving through both biotic and abiotic compartments of an ecosystem.

Biogeochemistry the study of chemical transformations in a biogeochemical cycle.

Biomass the quantity of all organisms in an ecosystem.

Bioremediation any process that uses microorganisms or their enzymes to return the environment altered by contaminants to its original condition.

Biosafety safety precautions to be followed when dealing with or handling biological materials.

Biosphere regions of the earth populated by living organisms.

Bioterrorism the use of biological agents to incapacitate or kill civilians or military personnel during a terrorist attack or during war.

Biotic refers to living organisms, the products they produce, and the effects of these on the environment.

Biotransport the transport of drugs across biological membranes.

Blood–brain barrier an anatomical and physiological barrier between the blood and the brain that inhibits various chemical substances and microscopic objects from entering the brain tissue.

Blunt ends in molecular genetics, the ends of a double-stranded DNA molecule in which both strands are of the same length; there is no overhang.

Bodily fluid fluid such as blood, semen, or saliva.

Boil also called a *furuncle;* an infection that starts in a hair follicle, resulting in localized accumulation of pus and dead tissue.

Botulism a rare, serious paralytic illness caused by a neurotoxin produced by the bacterium *Clostridium botulinum.*

Broad-spectrum activity drugs drugs that are effective against a large variety of microorganisms.

Bronchi part of the airways in the respiratory tract that conducts air to the lungs.

Brucellosis an infectious zoonotic disease that occurs worldwide and is caused by various *Brucella* species.

Bunyaviridae a family of single-stranded, negative-sense RNA viruses that can cause human disease; includes hantavirus and hemorrhagic fever virus.

Campylobacteriosis a bacterial infection that affects the intestinal tract and, rarely, the bloodstream. In humans the illness is usually caused by *Campylobacter jejuni, C. fetus,* and *C. coli.*

Candidiasis a fungal infection, commonly called a *yeast infection,* caused by a species of *Candida.*

Capneic describing bacteria (capnophiles) that require more carbon dioxide than is present in the normal atmosphere.

Capsid or viral coat; consists of proteins that are encoded by the viral genome. It protects the viral nucleic acid.

Capsomeres the protein subunits that make up the capsid.

Carbon a naturally abundant chemical element with the symbol C and the atomic number 6. Carbon provides the backbone of all organic molecules.

Carbon cycle a complex biogeochemical cycle through which all the carbon atoms in existence rotate.

Carbuncle a large infected mass resulting from fusion of furuncles, which may drain through several sinuses or develop into an abscess; usually a result of a *Staphylococcus* infection.

Caries bacterial tooth decay causing cavities or holes in the teeth.

CAS Chemical Abstracts Service; chemical registry number; a unique number assigned to each chemical to aid in searching computerized databases.

Catabolism metabolic pathway that breaks down large molecules into smaller units. These reactions release energy.

Cation an ion with a positive charge.

CDC Centers for Disease Control and Prevention; serves as a central source of epidemiological information.

cDNA complementary DNA formed from an mRNA template with the help of reverse transcriptase.

Cell organelle a specialized subunit within a cell, with a specific function and usually membrane bound.

Cellular respiration the process by which the chemical energy of nutrient molecules is released and captured in the form of ATP.

Central dogma the transcription of DNA to RNA to protein.

Central nervous system that part of the nervous system consisting of the brain and spinal cord.

Cerebrospinal fluid a clear, colorless fluid that fills the brain ventricles, the central canal of the spinal cord, and the subarachnoid space.

Chancroid a bacterial sexually transmitted disease, characterized by painful sores and ulcers in the genital areas.

Chemical bond the result of forces of attraction that hold together atoms in an element or compound, due to the interaction of electrons.

Chemical compound a chemical substance that consists of two or more different elements bonded together.

Chemically defined media media with defined, exact chemical composition; also called *synthetic media*.

Chemical formula the shorthand expression for a chemical compound.

Chemoautotroph uses inorganic chemical compounds as the source of energy and carbon dioxide as the carbon source.

Chemoheterotroph uses organic compounds as both the source of energy and as a carbon source.

Chemotaxis the guided movement of a cell or organism as a result of a chemical attraction caused by chemotactic agents.

Chemotroph an organism that uses energy from the breakdown of nutrient molecules.

Chlamydia a common sexually transmitted disease (STD) caused by the bacterium *Chlamydia trachomatis*.

Chloroplasts cell organelles found in algae and plant cells that are capable of converting sun energy into chemical energy through the process of photosynthesis.

Cholesterol a sterol, a combination of a steroid and an alcohol.

Chromoblastomycosis a chronic localized fungal infection of the subcutaneous tissue characterized by verrucoid lesions of the skin, usually in the lower extremities.

Chromosome in eukaryotic cells, a single DNA molecule that includes proteins called *histones*. In prokaryotic cells the DNA is not associated with histones and the chromosome is usually circular.

Chronic infections infections that persist for long periods of time with usually less severe symptoms than occur in acute infections.

Ciliary escalator ciliated epithelial cells in the mucosa of the upper respiratory tract that move trapped particles cranially, away from the lungs.

Classical complement pathway part of the complement system; becomes activated when an antigen–antibody complex binds to the C1 component, a major complement protein.

Classification the assignment of organisms into taxa on the basis of similarities.

Clonal selection after an antigen has been recognized, B cells become activated and start dividing into clones that produce antibody-producing plasma cells and memory cells capable of recognizing the original antigen.

Clone formed when a single bacterium produces a population of genetically identical offspring.

Cocci spherical bacteria; pleural of *coccus*.

Coenocytic fungal hyphae (filaments) that do not contain septa and therefore appear as long, continuous cells with many nuclei.

Coenzymes nonprotein portions of an enzyme, usually a derivative of a water-soluble vitamin, and often necessary for enzyme activation.

Cofactor nonprotein portion of an enzyme, usually a metal ion.

Colonization whenever one or more species populate a new area, an essential step in the development of a microbial infection.

Colony-forming unit (CFU) a measure of viable bacterial or fungal numbers.

Colostrum a thin yellowish fluid secreted by the mammary glands at the time of parturition. It is rich in antibodies and minerals, and precedes the production of true milk; it is also called *foremilk*.

Commensalism a term used to describe a symbiotic relationship in which one of the organisms benefits and the other is neither harmed nor helped.

Communities sets of guilds and characteristically heterogeneous.

Competition carrier-mediated transport can exhibit competition for binding sites on the carrier molecule when two similarly shaped molecules compete for the same binding site.

Competitive inhibition describing a situation in which a substance similar to the substrate is competing for the active site of an enzyme.

Complex media media containing at least one component that cannot be chemically defined and thus the media cannot be represented by exact chemical formula(s); also called *nonsynthetic media*.

Compound molecules molecules that are made from atoms of different elements.

Compound microscope a form of light microscope with ocular and objective lenses.

Congenital disorder any medical condition that is present at birth regardless of its origin.

Congenital infection an intrauterine infection that occurs during pregnancy when microorganisms enter the blood, and subsequently establish an infection of the placenta and then infect the fetus.

Conjugation the transfer of genetic material during cell-to-cell contact.

Conjunctivitis a viral or bacterial infection of the conjunctiva. It is also referred to as pink eye.

Contaminant a substance that is present in an environment where it does not belong or is present at levels that may cause harmful effects to living organisms or the environment.

Contamination refers to the presence of microbes in or on the body, or on objects.

Controlled Substances Act the federal U.S. drug policy under which the manufacture, importation, possession, uses, and distribution of certain substances are regulated.

Cosmids a class of hybrid vectors created by combining a fragment of DNA (cDNA) from a virus (usually a bacteriophage), with parts of a plasmid.

Covalent bond a form of chemical bonding that results from a sharing of electrons between two atoms of the same element or between atoms of different elements.

Cross-resistance the phenomenon in which bacteria that are resistant to a particular drug also become resistant to a similar drug.

Cryophiles bacteria that are cold-loving and can grow at 0° C or lower with optimal growth at about 15° C; also called *psychrophiles.*

Cryptosporidiosis a parasitic diarrheal disease, also known as "crypto," caused by the protozoan *Cryptosporidium* and spread via the fecal–oral route, through contaminated water, and uncooked or cross-contaminated food.

Culture microorganisms that grow and multiply in a container of culture medium.

Culture medium a liquid or gel that supports the growth of microorganisms or cells.

Cutaneous anthrax the skin form of the disease anthrax, characterized by large deep lesions on the skin called *eschars.*

Cyst a dormant stage of protozoans produced when the environment becomes unfavorable for feeding and therefore growth.

Cystitis an infection that occurs in the urinary bladder and is sometimes simply referred to as a bladder infection.

Cytocidal infection an infection that kills the host cell; also referred to as a lytic infection.

Cytokines small proteins considered to be chemical mediators of the immune response and secreted by cells of the immune system.

Cytopathic effects morphological changes in a host cell caused by certain viral infections and that may result in host cell damage or death.

Cytoplasm a dense, gelatinous matrix composed of 70% to 80% water, located within the plasma membrane.

Cytoskeleton the internal framework of a cell composed of microfilaments, intermediate filaments, and microtubules. It provides support and movement in eukaryotic cells.

Cytosol the liquid portion of a cell's cytoplasm.

DEA Drug Enforcement Administration.

Deamination the removal of an amino group from an amino acid to form ammonia.

Death phase the death phase of bacterial growth begins when growth stops and the number of dead cells is larger than the number of viable cells.

Decimal reduction time (DRT) indicates the time in minutes in which 90% of the bacterial population in question will be killed at a given temperature.

Decontamination the reduction or removal of chemical or biological agents.

Definitive host the host in which sexual reproduction of a parasite occurs.

Degermination the mechanical removal of the majority of microbes in a given/limited area.

Dehydration synthesis the formation of a larger compound (polymer) from smaller ones (monomers); also called *condensation.*

Denaturation the process of partial or total alteration of the structure of a macromolecule. This can occur when proteins or nucleic acids are subjected to elevated temperatures or to extremes of pH, a process that is part of the polymerase chain reaction.

Dendritic cells antigen-presenting cells that arise from monocytes and are characterized by long finger-like extensions; they are found in blood, lymph, and almost every tissue.

Denitrification the process by which nitrate is reduced to nitrogen (N_2) by anaerobic cellular respiration.

Dental plaque a microbial biofilm that attaches to the enamel of teeth.

Deoxyribonucleic acid (DNA) contains the genetic information of a cell; it is a nucleic acid with a double helix structure containing the sugar deoxyribose and 10 bases per turn.

Dermatophytes fungi that cause diseases of the skin, hair, and nails.

Dermis the layer of the skin below the epidermis (outer skin layer).

Descriptive epidemiology the collecting and tabulating of data concerning disease.

Desiccation the removal of water; drying.

Differential media can grow several different organisms that show visible differences. These differences can include variations in colony size, color, change in media color, or the formation of gas bubbles and precipitates.

Diffusion the movement of molecules from an area of higher concentration to an area of lower concentration without the expenditure of cellular energy.

Dikaryon a state in some fungi in which each compartment of a hypha contains two nuclei, each nucleus derived from a different parent cell.

Diplococci round bacteria (cocci) that remain paired after cell division.

Direct contact direct contact transmission involves direct physical contact of the infectious agent between hosts without an intermediate object; for example, person-to-person contact.

Disaccharides compounds formed when two monosaccharides combine with the loss of a water molecule.

Disinfectants antimicrobial chemicals specifically designed to be used on nonliving surfaces.

Disinfection the destruction of vegetative microorganisms via chemical or physical methods.

Disk-diffusion method an agar diffusion method to determine the susceptibility of microbes to a particular chemical agent.

Dissection microscope a low-power microscope designed for observing larger objects such as insects, worms, plants, or any objects that may have to be dissected for further observation.

Diuretic a substance that promotes the excretion of urine.

Division of Bioterrorism Preparedness and Response Office a program administered by the Centers for Disease Control and Prevention (CDC) to assist organizations/governmental organizations in addressing the challenges of bioterrorism.

DNA ligase an enzyme that forms covalent bonds between a carbon atom of one nucleotide with the phosphate of another along the backbone of each DNA strand.

Domain the highest taxonomic rank of an organism.

Donor donor bacteria are bacteria that lyse; their DNA bursts into fragments and can be picked up by other living bacteria (recipients).

Donovanosis a sexually transmitted disease caused by *Klebsiella.*

Dosage the total amount of a drug given over a period of time.

Dose the amount of a drug given at a single time.

DOT U.S. Department of Transportation.

Droplet transmission occurs when infectious agents are transmitted through respiratory droplets that travel a distance of less than 1 m.

Eclipse period in this phase of the lytic life cycle of bacteriophages, no infectious phage particles can be found in the host cell.

Ecosystem consists of the organisms, their abiotic environment, and the relationships between them.

Effective concentration drug effectiveness that can be achieved by a single administration or after multiple administrations.

Efficacy the effectiveness of a drug.

Ehrlichiosis caused by several species of the genus *Ehrlichia,* a gram-negative, obligatory intracellular bacterium. Early signs of the condition are nonspecific and may resemble the symptoms of various other diseases.

Electrolyte a substance that dissociates into free ions when dissolved in a solvent such as water.

Electron negatively charged particle orbiting in the shells of atoms.

Electron microscope uses a beam of electrons rather than light as the source of energy to visualize specimens.

Electron transport chain the last step in aerobic cellular respiration, which takes place in the cristae of the inner mitochondrial membrane and produces most of the energy in aerobic respiration.

Element a type of atom that can be distinguished by its atomic number.

Embryo among animals, an organism in its early stages of development from the zygote until differentiation into a fetus.

Emerging infectious diseases diseases that are newly identified in the population, or have existed but have changed.

Encapsidation the process by which the viral capsid is produced first and serves as an empty shell for the nucleic acid.

Encephalitis inflammation of the brain.

Endemic a disease that is repeatedly present in a given population or geographical area.

Endergonic a chemical reaction that requires energy.

Endocarditis an inflammation of the endocardium.

Endocardium inner lining of the heart.

Endocytosis a transport mechanism used by cells to bring substances into the cell.

Endoenzyme an enzyme that functions within biological membranes.

Endogenous infections infections caused by microbes in the normal flora of a patient, which become pathogenic because of a variety of factors, often associated with the healthcare setting.

Endometritis infection that affects the uterus and can be caused by a number of different organisms.

Endonuclease a DNA-cleaving enzyme; also called a *restriction enzyme.*

Endospore a dormant, tough, nonreproductive structure that some bacteria can produce in response to unfavorable environmental conditions.

Enriched media contain complex organic substances such as blood, serum, hemoglobin, or growth factors for the growth needs of specific species.

Enteral used to describe drugs administered via the digestive system.

Enzyme a biological catalyst that speeds up chemical reactions by lowering the activation energy of a reaction.

Enzyme-linked immunosorbent assay (ELISA) a biochemical technique to detect the presence of a specific antibody or antigen in a sample.

Eosinophils phagocytic white blood cells distinguished by their large reddish-staining granules.

EPA Environmental Protection Agency.

Epidemic a disease that occurs with greater frequency than usual in a population of a given area.

Epidemiology the study of the distribution and causes of diseases in a population; it is the foundation for necessary interventions in the interest of public health.

Epidermis outermost protective layer of the skin.

Epididymitis represents a complication of urethritis or prostatitis; often a complication of a sexually transmitted infection.

Episome a unit of genetic material composed of a series of genes, such as a plasmid; it is capable of integrating itself into the chromosomal DNA of the organism and can be duplicated with every cell division.

Epitope the smallest part of an antigen molecule that can bind with an antibody; also called an *antigenic determinant.*

Erythropoiesis the formation of erythrocytes (red blood cells) stimulated by the hormone erythropoietin, which is produced in the kidneys.

Erythropoietin a glycoprotein hormone produced by the kidneys that promotes the formation of erythrocytes in the red bone marrow.

Etiology the study of the cause of disease.

Eukaryote an organism whose cells contain a DNA-containing nucleus and membrane-bound cell organelles.

Eutrophication the overgrowth of microorganisms in nutrient-rich waters, due to runoff into rivers and lakes.

Evasion of host defenses the ability of a microbe to avoid the host response; can be due to the presence of a capsule, the production of proteins that bind to the host cell antibodies, or mutation of the organism to alter its antigenicity.

Exchange reaction reactions that transfer the same molecules but in a different combination, and therefore the components of the reaction remain the same but their combination results in a different product.

Exergonic describes chemical reactions that give off energy.

Exocytosis a process by which large molecules, such as polypeptides, proteins, and others, may be excreted from the cell.

Exoenzymes secreted by cells into their extracellular environment, where they act to break down large molecules into smaller ones so that they can be taken up into the cells.

Exogenous describing infections that are caused by pathogens in the healthcare environment, generally shed from sick people.

Experimental epidemiology a branch of epidemiology in which a hypothesis about a particular disease is generated, followed by the design of experiments and studies to test the hypothesis.

Exponential growth phase the second phase of bacterial growth, during which the maximal growth rate of a culture occurs.

Extension in molecular genetics, the final step in the polymerase chain reaction (PCR) process, whereby a heat-stable DNA polymerase is added and DNA synthesis takes place at temperatures between 70° C and 75° C.

Factor VIII essential blood-clotting factor.

Facultative anaerobes bacteria that can grow either in the absence or presence of oxygen.

Facultative halophiles salt-tolerating microbes and can live in NaCl concentrations up to 10%.

Fallopian tubes also known as oviducts or uterine tubes; they are structures leading from the ovaries to the uterus.

FDA U.S. Food and Drug Administration.

Fermentation a process of energy production for cells under anaerobic conditions.

Fetus a developing mammal after the first weeks of embryonic development until birth.

FFDCA (Federal Food, Drug, and Cosmetic Act) set of laws that give the FDA the authority to oversee the safety of food, drugs, and cosmetics.

Filamentous describing a chainlike series of cells.

Filoviridae family of single-stranded, negative-sense RNA viruses that cause human disease. Family includes Ebola and Marburg viruses.

Fimbriae hairlike bacterial surface projections that are more rigid than flagella.

First law of thermodynamics states that energy cannot be created or destroyed but only transferred from one form to another.

Flagella hairlike projections that extend from some unicellular organisms.

Flatworm invertebrate organism of the phylum Platyhelminthes.

Flaviviridae family of single-stranded, positive-sense RNA viruses that cause human disease, including dengue and yellow fever.

Fluid compartments the compartmentalization of the body's water into divisions, mainly the intracellular fluid (ICF) and extracellular fluid (ECF) compartments.

Fluid-mosaic the plasma membrane is not solid; its components are freely movable, presenting a constantly changing membrane structure referred to as fluid-mosaic structure/interphase.

Focal infection occurs when a pathogen spreads from a local infection to other tissues.

Folliculitis inflammation of one or more hair follicles.

Fomite an inanimate object or substance that is capable of transmitting infectious organisms.

Foodborne foodborne transmission generally involves pathogens in or on foods that are incompletely cooked, poorly processed under unsanitary conditions, not refrigerated, or poorly refrigerated.

Frameshift mutations genetic mutations that involve the deletion or insertion of one or more nitrogen bases.

Free-living nitrogen-fixing bacteria nitrogen-fixing bacteria that live in the soil independently of other organisms.

Fungi heterotrophic single-celled, multinucleated, or multicellular organisms, including yeasts, molds, and mushrooms.

Fungicides chemical or biological compounds that kill fungi and their spores.

Furuncle skin abscesses caused by staphylococcal infections, involving hair follicles and surrounding tissue.

Fusiform spindle-like shape.

G1 phase the first step in the interphase of the cell cycle. Cells carry out the metabolic activities characteristic of the tissue to which they belong.

G2 phase the third step in the interphase of the cell cycle. The cell continues to grow and its metabolic activities prepare for mitosis.

Gametocyte a cell that develops into gametes by meiotic cell division.

Gangrene a complication of necrosis; the decay and death of tissue, often related to wounds.

Gastroenteritis inflammation of the stomach and intestine that can be caused by microorganisms or ingestion of chemical toxins.

Gastrointestinal (GI) tract represents a system of organs with the purpose of ingestion, digestion, absorption, and defecation. It is a common and easily accessible portal of entry for microbes or their toxins.

Gene a unit, located on a DNA molecule, that encodes particular information.

Gene library composed of a series of cells or unicellular organisms that are used to store genes that have been obtained from foreign cells.

Genomic library a collection of clones made from a set of randomly generated overlapping DNA fragments that correspond to the entire genome of an organism.

Genotype the exact genetic makeup of an organism.

Genus a group of species closely related in structure and evolutionary origin; the level of grouping falls between *family* and *species*. The genus name forms part of the name of an organism according to the Linnaean system (*see* binomial system).

Germicide an agent that kills "germ", especially pathogenic microorganisms.

Gestation period the length of pregnancy, which in humans is approximately 39 weeks and is divided into three phases referred to as trimesters.

Giardiasis a common waterborne gastrointestinal disease. The causative agent is *Giardia lamblia,* which can be present in both drinking and recreational water.

Gingivitis an inflammation of the gums usually caused by bacterial biofilms.

Glomerulonephritis also referred to as Bright's disease; involves inflammation and damage to the glomeruli of the kidneys.

Glycocalyx an extracellular polymeric matrix surrounding the plasma membrane.

Glycolysis also known as the *Embden-Meyerhof pathway,* glycolysis is the two-stage process involving the breakdown of glucose to pyruvate.

Group B streptococcal disease (GBS) a group of neonatal illnesses caused by cross-infection on group B, beta hemolytic streptococci, and gram-negative bacilli. Includes illnesses such as sepsis, pneumonia, and meningitis.

Growth factors compounds that cannot be synthesized by a microorganism but are essential for growth. They are typically essential cell components or precursors of these components.

Guild populations of microorganisms that perform linked metabolic activities.

Habitat the physical location where organisms are found.

Halophiles organisms that are "salt loving" and thrive in environments with a high salt content.

Haptens small molecules that cannot elicit an immune response themselves, but that do so when combined with a carrier protein.

Harmful algal bloom (HAB) algal blooms that occur in both marine and freshwater environments when a particular algal species succeeds in competing with other species and undergoes rapid reproduction, producing toxins harmful to other life forms.

Harmful Algal Bloom–related Illness Surveillance System (HABISS) supports public health decision-making in cases of algal blooms in particular areas in the United States.

Helical virus virus with a protein capsid that appears in a coiled pattern.

Helicase enzymes that use the energy of nucleotide hydrolysis to unwind nucleic acid duplexes.

Hematuria the presence of blood in the urine.

Hemocytoblast pluripotent stem cell in the red bone marrow, capable of giving rise to all other blood cells.

Hemolysins enzymes that lyse erythrocytes.

Hemophilia a common inherited blood-clotting disorder with the defective gene located on the X chromosome; therefore the disorder occurs primarily in males.

Hemopoiesis the process of blood cell formation.

Hepatitis an infection of the liver, capable of causing significant destruction of liver cells.

Herpes simplex a type of virus having two strains, HSV1 and HSV2; HSV1 usually causes infections on the lips and in the mouth, HSV2 is primarily responsible for genital herpes.

Heterocysts specialized nitrogen-fixing cells formed by some cyanobacteria.

Heterotroph a heterotroph uses organic compounds as its source of carbon.

HHS U.S. Department of Health and Human Services.

HICPAC Healthcare Infection Control Practices Advisory Committee.

Holoenzymes enzyme that is combined with one or more cofactors or coenzymes.

Homeostasis the maintenance of a relatively stable internal environment of the body, regardless of environmental changes.

Host range the specificity of viruses to certain hosts.

Human growth hormone (HGH) a protein hormone synthesized and secreted by the anterior pituitary. The hormone plays a major role in growth and metabolism.

Human immunodeficiency virus (HIV) the causative agent of acquired immune deficiency syndrome (AIDS), a secondary immune deficiency.

Hydrogen bond a weak chemical bond between molecules that always involves a hydrogen atom with a slight positive charge and an oxygen or nitrogen atom with a slightly negative charge.

Hydrolases enzymes that catalyze hydrolysis reactions.

Hydrolysis or decomposition; the breaking down of large molecules (polymers) into unit molecules (monomers) in the presence of water.

Hydrophilic "water-loving"/water-soluble compounds.

Hydrophobic molecules held together by nonpolar covalent bonds; they are water repellent and insoluble in water.

Hypertonic a solution that has a higher concentration of solutes than solvent.

Hyphae filamentous, multinucleated fungal structures that form threadlike filaments, many of which collectively form the mycelium and fruiting bodies of a fungus.

Hypodermis also referred to as the subcutaneous layer; it is the deepest layer of the skin, located immediately below the dermis.

Hypotonic a solution that has a lower concentration of solutes than solvent.

Iatrogenic infections caused by the introduction of microorganisms through a medical procedure.

Icosahedrons Viral capsids that are 3-dimensional, geometric figures with 12 corners, 20 triangular faces, and 30 edges.

ICTV International Committee on Taxonomy of Viruses.

Identification in taxonomy, the process of specifying, identifying, and recording the traits of organisms.

IDSA Infectious Disease Society of America.

IEIP International Emerging Infections Program.

IHR International Health Regulations.

Immune senescence a decline in immune function during aging, which leads to increased vulnerability to infectious diseases.

Immune system the major system responsible for a body's immunity, composed of special cells, tissues, and organs as well as a special system of proteins.

Immunity the body's ability to respond to the presence of any foreign substance.

Immunocompetent when the immune system of a person functions properly.

Immunogen a substance that stimulates the production of specific antibodies by the immune system.

Immunoglobulin (Ig) globular protein with known antibody activity.

Immunology the study of the genetic, biological, chemical, and physical characteristics of the immune system.

Immunosuppressed when part or all of the immune system cannot respond appropriately to a challenge by antigens.

Impetigo a superficial bacterial skin infection caused primarily by *Streptococcus pyogenes*.

Inclusion various nonliving structures within the cytoplasm of a cell.

Incubation in microbiology, the placement of inoculated media in a proper environment to facilitate the growth process.

IND Investigational New Drug Application.

Index case the primary case in the population sample of an epidemiological investigation.

Indirect contact a type of transmission that occurs when the pathogen is transmitted from the reservoir to the susceptible host by a fomite—a nonliving object.

Infection the colonization and growth of microorganisms in the body.

Inflammation a response of a tissue to injury, characterized by redness, heat, pain, and swelling.

Inflammatory reflex a response between the nervous system and the immune system via the vagus cranial nerve to create a "neuroimmune axis."

Influenza also referred to as the flu; it is a contagious infection of the respiratory tract, caused by RNA viruses of the Orthomyxoviridae family.

Inhalation anthrax also referred to as respiratory anthrax, this form of anthrax causes lesions and tissue damage to the lungs. Unless treated early, this form of the disease is almost always fatal.

Innate existing naturally rather than acquired.

Inoculation the process of an inoculum being introduced to a culture medium.

Inoculum a small sample of a microorganism.

Insulin an important protein hormone that facilitates the uptake of glucose by cells for use in cellular metabolism.

Integral proteins plasma membrane proteins that extend from one side through to the other side of the membrane.

Interferon a small protein produced naturally by certain white blood cells and by cells that have been infected by a virus.

Intermediate host an organism that hosts a parasite in the nonmature, nonsexual phase.

Intracellular accumulation phase in this phase of the lytic life cycle of bacteriophages, the nucleic acids and structural proteins are assembled into complete infectious phages that accumulate in the host cell.

Invasins proteins produced by pathogens to promote penetration.

Invasion in microbiology, the penetration into a cell or structure by bacteria.

Inversion in genetics, a macrolesion of the DNA in which the order of bases is switched or inverted.

Ion an atom or molecule that has lost or gained one or more electrons, resulting in a positive or negative electrical charge.

Ionic bond formed when one or more electrons from one atom are transferred to another.

Ionizing radiation high-energy radiation capable of ionizing substances through which the radiation passes.

Irreversible inhibition condition in which substances compete with the substrate for the active site of an enzyme, thus inhibiting enzyme action.

Ischemia an insufficient supply of blood to a tissue or organ.

Isograft a tissue or organ transplanted between genetically identical entities, such as identical twins.

Isolation in microbiology, the process of separating a specific colony/organism for further investigation.

Isomerases enzymes that rearrange atoms within molecules, changing the configuration of the atoms.

Isotonic solutions with the same amount of solute and solvent.

Isotope form of an atom of an element with the same number of protons but with a different number of neutrons.

Kefauver-Harris Amendment an amendment to the FFDCA that places controls on human experimentation and the processes used in the approval and regulation of new drugs.

Kidneys the major organs of excretion.

Koch's postulates criteria to establish the causative agent of a specific disease.

Krebs cycle also called the *citric acid cycle* or *tricarboxylic acid cycle* (TCA); it is a series of enzyme-catalyzed chemical reactions in aerobic cellular respiration.

Laboratory safety equipment an integral component of all laboratories and regulated by federal, state, and local laws. The amount of regulation depends on the levels of sophistication and needs of the individual laboratories.

Lag phase that phase of bacterial growth during which the bacteria adapt to a medium before cell division starts.

Lambda (λ) phage a temperate bacteriophage that infects *Escherichia coli*.

Langerhans cells dendritic cells in the epidermis, playing a role in defense against invading microbes.

Larynx air passageway between the lower pharynx and the trachea, containing the vocal cords.

Latency the period of time between the time something has been initiated, and the time when the effect becomes detectable.

LBNL Lawrence Berkeley National Laboratory.

Lectin pathway one of the biochemical pathways that activates the complement system.

Leptospirosis caused by the spirochete *Leptospira interrogans*, a zoonotic organism that can kidney infection and other, nonspecific illnesses.

Leukopoiesis the formation of leukocytes (white blood cells) from hematopoietic stem cells of the red bone marrow.

Lichen an organism consisting of fungus combined with algae or cyanobacteria, living in a symbiotic relationship.

Ligases enzymes that form bonds between individual monomers to form polymers.

Light-dependent reaction the first stage of photosynthesis; it requires solar energy, which is converted to chemical energy.

Light-independent reactions the second stage of photosynthesis, called the *dark reactions;* they take place in the stroma of chloroplasts.

Light microscope microscope that uses the visible light spectrum to visualize a specimen.

Limnetic zone the well-lit, upper layer of water away from the shore.

Liquid media water-based solutions that do not solidify at temperatures above freezing and flow freely in containers when tilted.

Listeriosis an infection caused by ingestion of food contaminated by *Listeria monocytogenes.*

Littoral zone the area along the shoreline with considerable rooted vegetation and a good light source.

Local infection occurs when a microbe enters the body and remains confined to a specific tissue.

Logarithmic growth phase that phase of bacterial growth during which bacterial numbers increase logarithmically; also known as the exponential growth phase.

Lophotrichous describing a bacterial cell with flagella present in tufts at one or both ends of the organism.

Lyases enzymes that remove functional groups from a substrate without adding water, or that add functional groups to a double bond.

Lyme disease a tick-borne illness caused by *Borrelia burgdorferi,* a gram-negative, motile spirochete.

Lymphocytes white blood cells essential in the specific immune response.

Lymphogranuloma venereum (LGV) a sexually transmitted infection involving the lymph glands in the genital area, caused by *Chlamydia trachomatis.*

Lymphopoiesis production of lymphocytes.

Lyophilization a technique that combines freezing and subsequent drying to preserve microbes, other cells, and materials for many years.

Lysis cell "bursting" due to destruction of the plasma membrane.

Lysis and release phase in this phase of the lytic life cycle of bacteriophages, virus-infected bacteria begin to lyse because of the accumulation of phage lysis proteins.

Lysogenic process by which bacteriophages incorporate genes into the bacterial host genome and do not necessarily immediately lyse the cell.

Lysogeny a less deadly form of parasitism, in which the host bacterium carries a prophage without being adversely affected.

Lysozymes enzymes that attack the peptidoglycan layer of the bacterial cell wall.

Lytic infection a type of infection that produces lysis and kills the host.

Macrolesion an injury to the DNA that involves more than one base pair, or several genes.

Macronucleus the larger form of a nucleus found in ciliates.

Macrophages phagocytotic, antigen-presenting cells of the immune system.

Major histocompatibility complex (MHC) membrane protein that can display both self-antigens and nonself-antigens to cells of the immune system.

Mastitis inflammation of the mammary glands.

Matter anything with volume and mass, and that takes up space.

Medium-spectrum activity drugs drugs that are effective against some, but not all, gram-positive and gram-negative bacteria.

Meiosis also called *reduction division,* a special type of cell division in eukaryotic cells. This type of cell division occurs only in the formation of gametes.

Meninges the membranes surrounding the brain and spinal cord.

Meningitis inflammation of the meninges.

Meningoencephalitis inflammation of the brain and its meninges.

Merozoite a daughter cell of a protozoan parasite.

Mesophiles microorganisms that undergo optimal growth in moderate temperature, generally between 25°C and 40°C.

Microaerophiles organisms that require a low concentration of oxygen, about 2% to 10%, which is a much lower concentration than is present in the atmosphere.

Microbemia a term used to describe infections caused by microorganisms that enter the circulatory system through the lymphatic drainage.

Microbial ecology study of the interrelationships of microorganisms in their natural environments.

Microbicidal agents agents that kill all microbes.

Microbiostatic agents agents that prevent or inhibit the growth of microbes.

Microbiota normal flora.

Microhabitat a specific small niche in which populations and guilds within a community reside due to optimal conditions for survival.

Microlesion an injury to the DNA that involves only one base pair.

Micronucleus the smaller of two nuclei in ciliates.

Minerals in biology, inorganic chemical elements required by living organisms.

Minimal bactericidal concentration (MBC) the lowest concentration of an agent that kills all living organisms in a test tube.

Minimal inhibitory concentration (MIC) the lowest concentration of an agent that prevents the growth of a selected microorganism.

Mitosis the usual process of cell division in eukaryotes, with the replicated (daughter) cells containing the same genetic material as the mother cell.

Mitosome an organelle found in some unicellular eukaryotic organisms; mitosomes appear similar to mitochondria but have almost no energy-producing capacity.

Mixed infection occurs when several infectious agents concurrently establish themselves at the same site.

Molecule two or more atoms linked together by chemical bonds.

Monocytes agranular leukocytes that can differentiate into macrophages or dendritic cells.

Monosaccharides simple sugars that contain three to seven carbon atoms and an aldehyde sugar or a ketone sugar (depending on the position of the carbonyl group).

Monotrichous describing a bacterial cell with a flagellum at one end.

Motility the ability of an organism to move by itself.

Motor neuron a nerve cell with a motor function.

MSDS Manufacturer's Material Safety Data Sheet.

Mucosa mucous membranes that line some organs and body cavities.

Mutation changes to the base pair sequence of DNA or RNA, passed on by cell division.

Mutualism a symbiotic relationship in which both organisms benefit.

Mycelium a collective mass of the threadlike hyphae of fungi.

Mycetoma a chronic, granulomatous disease of the skin and subcutaneous tissue, which sometimes involves muscle, bones, and neighboring organs.

Mycology the study of fungi.

Mycoplasma a gram-negative, pleomorphic, faculty anaerobic bacterium that is responsible for causing some infections in the urinary tract and in reproductive organs; usually sexually transmitted and can cause PID in women and urethritis in men.

Mycorrhizae fungi that help the roots of plants to absorb minerals and water from the soil.

Mycoses fungal infections.

Myelopoiesis generally refers to the production of monocytes and granulocytes.

Myocarditis inflammation of the myocardium.

Myocardium the middle layer of the heart, composed of cardiac muscle.

Narrow-spectrum activity drugs drugs that are effective only against a relatively small number of microbes, but that generally avoid destruction of the normal flora.

NCEH National Center for Environmental Health.

NCPDCID National Center for Preparedness, Detection, and Control of Infectious Diseases.

NDA New Drug Application.

Necatoriasis infection caused by hookworm.

Necrotizing infection infection that causes irreversible damage/destruction of tissue.

Necrotizing ulcerative gingivitis a painful infection of the gums, with acute pain, bleeding, and a foul breath.

Nephron the functional unit of the kidney.

Nephrostomy a surgical procedure by which a tube, stent, or catheter is inserted through the skin and into the kidney.

Neuromuscular junction the junction of the axon terminal of a motor neuron and a muscle fiber.

Neurotoxin a substance that damages nervous tissue and interferes with the proper functioning of the nervous system.

Neurotransmitter a chemical substance that transmits impulses across a synapse.

Neutron particle in the atomic nucleus that is without electrical charge.

Neutrophils or polymorphonuclear leukocytes; the most abundant of actively motile phagocytes.

NIAID National Institute of Allergy and Infectious Diseases.

NIH National Institutes of Health.

NIOSH National Institute for Occupational Safety and Health.

Nitrification the oxidation of ammonium to produce nitrate.

Nitrogen an essential element of all life forms, its atomic number is 7.

Nitrogenase the enzyme necessary for nitrogen fixation.

Nitrogen cycle the biogeochemical cycle that involves the transformations of nitrogen-containing compounds in nature.

Nitrogen fixation a process by which nitrogen gas (N_2) is reduced to ammonia (NH_3).

Nomenclature deals with the rules for naming organisms.

Noncompetitive inhibition occurs when a substance binds to the allosteric site of an enzyme, which results in a change of the active site, inhibiting enzyme action.

Nongonococcal urethritis (NGU) an infection of the urethra caused by some agent other than that causing gonorrhea *(Neisseria gonorrhoeae)*.

Nonionizing radiation a type of electromagnetic radiation that does not have enough energy to remove an electron from an atom. It includes sound; ultraviolet, visible, and infrared light; microwaves; and radiowaves.

Nonpermissive cell a cell that does not support the replication of a virus.

Nonpolar without electrical charge.

Nonself antigen an antigen or substance that is foreign to a person's immune system.

Nonsynthetic medium contains at least one component that cannot be chemically defined and thus the medium cannot be represented by an exact chemical formula.

Normal flora microorganisms that are usually found at given anatomical sites in a healthy human body without causing infection or disease.

Nuclear envelope also called the *nuclear membrane,* it is a phospholipid bilayer that surrounds the cell nucleus.

Nucleocapsid represents the viral genome together with the protein coat.

Nucleoid area the area in the cytoplasm of bacteria and archaea where the chromosomal DNA is located.

Obligate aerobes organisms that grow only in the presence of oxygen.

Obligate anaerobes organisms that grow only in the absence of oxygen and are often inhibited or killed by the presence of oxygen.

Obligate halophiles organisms that show optimal growth in salty environments.

Occupational hazard a hazard associated with a specific activity or type of work.

Oncogenic the tendency to give rise to tumors.

Opportunistic pathogens organisms that do not cause disease when the immune system is properly functioning but that may flourish if the immune system or normal flora is out of balance.

Orphan Drug Amendment The amendment to the Federal Food, Drug, and Cosmetic Act of 1938 giving incentives to develop drugs for rare diseases.

Orphan drugs those drugs needed to treat diseases affecting fewer than 200,000 U.S. patients, and that fail to receive attention for development primarily because of cost and perceived lack of need.

OSHA Occupational Safety and Health Administration.

Osmophiles organisms that require a high solute concentration in the environment for optimal growth.

Osmosis the diffusion of water through a selectively permeable membrane, from an area of higher concentration to an area of lower concentration.

Otitis media inflammation of the middle ear.

Ovaries paired female reproductive organ that produces ova, estrogen, and progesterone.

Oxidation occurs when an atom or molecule loses one or more electrons.

Oxidoreductases enzymes that catalyze the transfer of electrons in oxidation–reduction reactions.

Pandemic a worldwide epidemic.

Parasitism a symbiotic relationship wherein one organism benefits and the other is harmed.

Parenteral describing the introduction of a substance into the body by means other than gastrointestinally or via the lungs.

Passive transport the transport of molecules across plasma membranes without using cellular energy.

Pasteurization the process of heating foods at a temperature and time combination intended to destroy harmful bacteria without changing the composition, flavor, or nutrient value of the food.

Pathogen an infectious agent, capable of causing disease.

Pathogenic the ability to cause disease.

Pathogenicity the ability of a pathogen to produce infectious disease in another organism.

Peak effect in pharmacology, occurs when receptors are maximally activated by a drug.

Pellicle a microbial growth pattern in a test tube, characterized by a thick mat of growth at the top of the tube.

Pelvic inflammatory disease (PID) an infection and inflammation of the female reproductive organs.

Peptic ulcers mucosal erosions in the lining of the stomach or duodenum.

Peptidoglycan a large polymer that is a major component of the bacterial cell wall; also known as murein.

Peptone a partially digested protein used in some culture media.

Pericarditis inflammation of the pericardium.

Pericardium the double-walled sac filled with serous fluid that encloses the heart and the roots of the great vessels of the heart.

Perinatal period of time around childbirth.

Periodontitis inflammation of the gums, involving the supporting structures of the teeth.

Peripheral nervous system part of the nervous system that consists of cranial nerves, spinal nerves, ganglia, and sensory receptors located outside of the central nervous system.

Peripheral proteins proteins that are partially embedded on one side of the plasma membrane.

Peritrichous describing a microbial cell with flagella distributed over the general cell surface.

Permissive cells in virology, cells that provide the biosynthetic machinery to support the complete replication cycle of a virus.

Persistent infection infections that do not cause cell death.

Pertussis also known as whooping cough; a highly contagious disease caused by *Bordetella pertussis*.

Phagocytosis ingestion of solids by eukaryotic cells through the process of engulfment.

Phagosome a membrane-bound vesicle in a phagocyte, containing phagocytosed material.

Pharmacodynamics addresses drug-induced responses of the physiological and biochemical systems of the body.

Pharmacokinetics addresses drug amounts at various sites in the body after their administration.

Pharmacotherapeutics addresses issues associated with the choice and application of drugs to be used for disease prevention, treatment, or diagnosis.

Pharmacy the preparation, compounding, dispensing of, and record keeping about therapeutic drugs.

Pharyngitis also referred to as strep throat; an inflammation of the throat or pharynx caused by Group A streptococcal bacteria.

Pharynx a muscular passageway shared by the digestive and respiratory systems, generally referred to as the throat.

Phenotype the observable characteristics or traits of an organism.

Phosphogluconate pathway also called the *pentose phosphate pathway*; it is an alternate catabolic pathway followed by some bacteria.

Phospholipids polar lipids and the main component of plasma membranes.

Phosphorus cycle a biogeochemical cycle that involves changes of phosphorus from insoluble to soluble forms that are available for uptake by organisms, and from organic to inorganic forms by pH-dependent processes.

Photoautotrophs organisms that use sunlight as an energy source and atmospheric carbon dioxide as their carbon source.

Photoheterotrophs organisms that use sunlight for energy and organic compounds as their source for carbon.

Photosynthesis fundamental biochemical process that converts light energy into chemical energy.

Phototrophs organisms that use sunlight for photosynthesis and release energy during the process.

pH scale scale based on the hydrogen ion concentration of a solution and is used to measure the acidity or alkalinity of a solution.

Phylogeny deals with the evolutionary relationship between organisms.

Phylum the taxonomic rank below Kingdom and above Class.

Pili also called *fimbriae*; bacterial surface projections that are more rigid than flagella.

Pinocytosis a form of endocytosis by which small particles or liquid are transported into a cell.

Placenta a vascular organ that develops during pregnancy, lining the uterine wall and joining mother and fetus.

Plague a life-threatening disease caused by *Yersinia pestis*.

Plants a major division of living organisms generally composed of eukaryotic cells capable of photosynthesis.

Plasma membrane a phospholipid bilayer surrounding living cells.

Plasmid a circular nonchromosomal DNA molecule in bacteria.

Plasmodium a protozoan parasite.

Pleomorphic describing organisms that exhibit variations in size and shape.

Pneumonia an inflammation of the lungs, usually caused by an infection.

Point mutation a mutation in which a single nucleotide base is altered.

Poison any substance that is harmful to the body.

Polymerase chain reaction (PCR) a technique that can produce DNA copies without a host cell and by which small DNA fragments can quickly be amplified to quantities large enough to allow analysis.

Polysaccharides complex carbohydrates such as starch, glycogen, and cellulose.

Population in ecology, a collection of interbreeding organisms of a particular species.

Pour plate a culture technique whereby bacteria are inoculated into a tube of cooled but still melted agar, and then mixed and poured into a sterile Petri plate.

Pregnancy the period from conception to birth.

Primary infection an initial infection that may be followed by complications caused by another microbe.

Primary response the response of the immune system when exposed to a specific antigen for the first time.

Primer RNA a short strand of RNA initiating DNA synthesis.

Priming in molecular genetics, a step in PCR during which the temperature of the reaction is lowered so that the primers can bind to the single-stranded DNA molecules.

Prions infectious proteinaceous particles that are neither cellular organisms nor viruses.

Prodrug a substance administered in an inactive form but that once administered is metabolized into an active form.

Profundal zone deeper water located below the limnetic zone, characterized by limited light penetration (diffuse light), lower oxygen content, and lower temperature.

Prokaryote an organism, typically unicellular, that does not have a nucleus or membrane-bound organelles. Bacteria and archaea are prokaryotic.

Promoter a unidirectional sequence on one strand of DNA that tells the RNA polymerase where to start transcription and in which direction to continue synthesis.

Prophage a latent form of a bacteriophage with the viral genes incorporated into the bacterial chromosome without disruption of the bacterial cell.

Prostaglandins hormone-like substances derived from arachidonic acid. They participate in a wide range of body functions including contraction and relaxation of smooth muscle, dilation and constriction of blood vessels, and modulation of inflammation.

Prostate gland an accessory organ of the male reproductive system producing a milky-colored fluid that is part of the semen.

Prostatitis a painful infection and inflammation of the prostate gland.

Protective gear gloves, respiratory protection, eye protection, protective clothing, and any other protective gear as needed in a given laboratory environment.

Protomeres individual subunits of a viral capsid.

Proton positively charged particles in the atomic nucleus.

Prototype in microbiology, the originally described bacterium of a species.

Protozoans unicellular, eukaryotic, usually chemoheterotrophic organisms that live in environments with an ample water supply.

Provirus a viral genome that has integrated itself into the host cell DNA.

Psychrophiles cold-loving organisms that can grow at 0° C or lower, with optimal growth at about 15° C.

Psychrotrophs organisms that grow very slowly at 0° C but have an optimal growth range of 25° C to 30° C.

Pure Food and Drug Act enacted in 1906, entrusting the federal government with testing drugs on the market for accuracy regarding claims of purity and strength.

Pyelonephritis an infection of the kidney and ureters.

Pyogenic exudates drainage of a lesion; also called *pus*.

Pyrexia fever; a systemic response to extensive inflammation or microbial invasion.

Pyrogens fever-producing substances released from white blood cells in response to microbial invasion.

Radioactivity the spontaneous emission of energy and/or particles from an unstable atom.

Receptor-mediated endocytosis a transport process in which a substance binds to a receptor on the plasma membrane, which invaginates, surrounding the substance and pinching off inside the cell.

Recombinant DNA DNA consisting of DNA from two or more sources.

Redox a reduction–oxidation reaction.

Reduction the gaining of an electron(s) by an atom or molecule.

Reemerging infectious diseases older diseases thought to be under control but that are reemerging.

Replica plating a plating method by which the patterns of colonies are precisely duplicated on another plate.

Resident flora populations of microorganisms that are always present on or in an organism.

Restriction enzymes enzymes that cleave specific DNA sequences.

Reverse transcriptase an enzyme that transcribes RNA into DNA.

Reversion a change in a point mutation that restores the original phenotype.

Rheumatic fever a complication/disorder that can follow an infection by *Streptococcus pyogenes* and affects numerous body systems.

Ribonucleic acid (RNA) nucleic acid that is transcribed from DNA and directs/participates in protein synthesis.

Rocky Mountain spotted fever disease caused by the bacterium *Rickettsia rickettsii*, transmitted by ticks.

Roundworm also called a *nematode*, a cylindrical worm with an unsegmented body. Some are human parasites (e.g., pinworms).

RTECS Registry of Toxic Effects of Chemical Substances.

Salmonellosis a disease affecting primarily the gastrointestinal tract; caused by species of the genus *Salmonella*.

Sanitization removal of debris, organic material, microorganisms, and toxins.

Saprobes free-living microorganisms that feed primarily on organic material from dead organisms.

Sarcina a bacterial arrangement in which cocci are grouped in a 3-dimensional cube of 8, 16, or more cells.

Satellites viruses and bacteria that rely on the presence of unrelated organisms to help them grow.

Saturated fat triglycerides containing only saturated fatty acids. Saturated fatty acids do not have double bonds between the carbon atoms in the carbon backbone chain.

Scarlet fever serious infection caused by Group A *Streptococcus*, characterized by redness, shedding of the skin, and high fever.

Schizogony fission process in which first the nucleus divides multiple times, and then the cytoplasm is divided for each new nucleus.

Scolex anterior end of a tapeworm, equipped with hooks/suckers for attachment to the host.

Secondary immune response occurs when the body is exposed to the same immunogen weeks, months, or years later.

Secondary infection when a primary infection is complicated by another infection by a different microorganism.

Sediment solid particulate matter that eventually settles out of a solution, in bodies of water; the materials that form at the bottom.

Selective media media designed to favor the growth of a specific microorganism and inhibit the growth of others.

Selective pressure process by which organisms are forced to adapt or die when exposed to antimicrobial agents.

Selective toxicity in which an agent is toxic to the target microorganism but far less toxic to cells of the host.

Self-antigens specific molecules on a cell surface that allows the body's immune system to recognize it as a "normal" host component.

Semisolid media media that have the physical properties of a loose gel.

Sepsis the growth of microorganisms in blood and other tissues.

Septate hyphae fungal hyphae divided into segments by cross-walls.

Septic condition involving the growth of unwanted microorganisms.

Septic shock shock and dangerously low blood pressure cause by bacterial endotoxins.

Septicemia a systemic infection in which microorganisms multiply in the bloodstream.

Severe acute respiratory syndrome (SARS) an emerging respiratory disease caused by viruses of the genus *Coronavirus*.

Sexually transmitted disease (STD) a disease transmitted by sexual activities. Symptoms and damaging effects are observable.

Sexually transmitted infection (STI) an infection transmitted by sexual activities. Refers to the presence of pathogens, although symptoms/effects may be absent.

SHEA Society for Healthcare Epidemiology of America.

Shell in atoms, the discrete energy regions occupied by the electrons orbiting around the nucleus.

Shigellosis a gastrointestinal disease caused by strains of the genus *Shigella*.

Side effect unintended, usually negative effect resulting from the pharmacological treatment of disease.

Smallpox a highly contagious, often fatal disease caused by a poxvirus.

Solid media media in a solid physical state. Agar is a type of solid medium.

Solute dissolved particles in a solution.

Solution a homogeneous mixture of solvent and solutes that will not separate out on standing.

Solvent a liquid capable of dissolving a substance.

Species a biological taxonomic grouping below genus in which all organisms bear a close resemblance to each other in essential features and sexually can produce fertile progeny.

Specific carrier in carrier-mediated transport, these are protein molecules with binding sites for a particular molecule that will be transported across the plasma membrane.

Spectrum of activity the range of microorganisms against which an agent is effective.

S phase phase of the cell cycle during which DNA is replicated in preparation for cell division.

Spikes in virology, glycoprotein projections on a viral capsid or envelope. Used for attachment or fusion to the host cell.

Spirals occur as vibrios, spirilla, or spirochetes.

Spirilla bacteria with a coiled, "snakelike" shape. Flagella often provide the mechanism for motility.

Spirochetes bacteria with a coiled, helical, "snakelike" shape. An axial filament provides a mechanism for motility, allowing the bacteria to move by flexing or bending.

Sporadic occurring randomly or infrequently.

Sporangia a fungal structure in which asexual spores are formed.

Sporozoite a malarial trophozoite in the salivary glands of infected mosquitoes.

Spread plate an agar plate onto which a small amount of liquid inoculum had been plated and spread out evenly over the whole surface.

Spreading infection Concerning bacterial infections of the skin, soft tissue, and muscle, spreading infections are those limited to the epidermis (e.g., impetigo) or that involve the subcutaneous fat (e.g., cellulitis).

Staphylococcal conjunctivitis a neonatal staph infection that can occur through contamination of the infant with staphylococci from the noses and fingers of adult carriers. Also known as "*sticky eye*".

Staphylococcal scalded skin syndrome infection caused by group II staphylococci; more common in infants than adults. Infected skin looks scalded and will die and slough off, leaning skin open to secondary infections.

Staphylococci cocci arranged in irregular clumps or grapelike clusters.

Stationary phase the third phase of bacterial growth, in which the production of new cells equals the rate of cell death.

Stereomicroscopes low-power microscopes designed for observing larger objects such as insects, worms, plants, or any objects that may need to be dissected for further observation.

Sterile in which no living organisms are present on or in a material.

Sterilization the destruction/removal of all microorganisms and their spores.

Steroid a lipid with a four-ring structure.

Sticky ends in molecular genetics, the ends of a double-stranded DNA molecule in which one end is longer than the other, creating an overhang; the staggered ends are the result of restriction enzyme action; they are called "*sticky*" because these ends can form complementary bonds with another strand of DNA with sticky ends.

Strain in taxonomy, a subgroup of a species with characteristics that distinguish it from other subgroups of that species.

Streak plate a plating method used primarily to produce isolated colonies.

Streptococci cocci arranged in a string or chain.

Stroma the matrix of a chloroplast. The site of the dark reactions of photosynthesis.

Stromatolites masses of cells or microbial mats made up of fossilized photosynthetic prokaryotes.

Subclinical infection an infection that does not produce symptoms.

Subcutaneous layer layer beneath the skin.

Sulfur an essential life element with the atomic number 16.

Sulfur cycle the biogeochemical cycle that involves the transformations of sulfur-containing compounds in nature.

Superinfection a secondary infection that occurs when normal microflora are removed, thus allowing pathogens to colonize.

Symbiosis describing two different kinds of organisms living together.

Symbiotic nitrogen-fixing bacteria nitrogen-fixing bacteria that live in a symbiotic association with plants or other organisms.

Synergism the effect produced in a relationship in which two chemicals or organisms work together to produce an effect greater than could have been achieved individually.

Synthesis chemical reaction in which reactants bond together to form a new molecule.

Synthetic media media prepared from materials of precise or well-defined composition.

Syphilis a sexually transmitted disease caused by *Treponema pallidum*.

Taeniasis infection by a tapeworm of the genus *Taenia*, usually *T. saginata* or *solium*.

Tapeworm large flat parasitic worm belonging to the class Cestoida and found in the intestinal tract.

Taxon a group of related organisms; pleural, *taxa*.

Taxis an innate behavioral response to a directional stimulus.

Taxonomy the practice and science of classification of living things.

T cells a class of lymphocytes involved in a variety of cell-mediated immune responses.

Temperate phage a bacteriophage existing in a bacterial cell but seldom causing immediate lysis.

Terminator sequence a nucleotide sequence that marks the end of a gene to stop transcription.

Testes two egg-shaped male reproductive organs, located in the scrotum, and responsible for sperm and hormone production.

Tetanus disease caused by *Clostridium tetani,* in which the skeletal muscles are in a constant state of contraction. Also called "*lock jaw.*"

Tetrads in microbiology, a bacterial arrangement in which the cells are grouped in squares of four.

Thallus undifferentiated structure of many fungi that does not possess distinct parts such as leaves, stems, or roots.

The five "I's" Inoculation, Incubation, Isolation, Inspection (observation), Identification: the five basic procedures for examining and characterizing microbes.

Therapeutic index ratio comparing the drug dose that produces an undesired toxic effect with the dose that produces a desired positive (therapeutic) effect.

Thermal death point (TDP) the lowest temperature required to kill a population of microorganisms in liquid suspension in 10 minutes.

Thermal death time (TDT) the shortest time required to kill a population of microorganisms at a specific temperature.

Thermophiles microorganisms whose optimal growth temperature is relatively high, usually between 45° C and 80° C.

Thylakoid membrane membrane covering of the thylakoid, where the light reactions of photosynthesis take place.

Tineas superficial fungal infections of skin, nails, and hairs.

Tissue plasminogen activator (tPA) a protein that activates plasmin, a proteolytic enzyme that dissolves blood clots.

Titer the reciprocal of the highest dilution of antiserum and that produces a positive test reaction.

Toxemia the presence of toxins in the blood.

Toxic effect physiological or physical effect that is caused by a substance.

Toxicology study of the body's response to poisons, their harmful effects, mechanisms of action, symptoms, treatment, and identification.

Toxic shock syndrome (TSS) a relatively rare but life-threatening illness usually caused by *Staphylococcus aureus*.

Toxin a poisonous substance produced by living organisms.

Toxoplasmosis disease caused by protozoan parasite *Toxoplasma gondii.* Common in men and women; infection during pregnancy can lead to serious damage to the baby's eyes, nervous system, skin, and ears. Parasite can be found in raw meat and is commonly found in cat litter and contaminated soil.

Transduction in virology, a method of gene transfer in which genes are transported into a bacterial cell by a bacteriophage.

Transferase an enzyme that catalyzes the transfer of a functional group from one molecule to another.

Transformation a method of gene transfer in which a piece of free DNA is taken into a bacterial cell and integrated into its genome.

Transgenic describing an organism that has acquired new genes by the insertion of foreign DNA.

Transient flora microorganisms that are present on/in the host for a short period without becoming permanently established.

Transposons sequences of DNA that can move around to different positions in the genome.

Trichomoniasis a urogenital disease caused by *Trichomonas vaginalis;* primarily sexually transmitted.

Triglycerides lipids composed of fatty acids and glycerol; they are neutral fats.

Trophozoite vegetative form of a protozoan.

Tsunami wave that is created when a large amount of water is rapidly displaced; sometimes referred to as a "tidal wave."

Tuberculosis (TB) a serious disease of the respiratory system caused by bacteria, with members of the genus *Mycobacterium,* particularly *M. tuberculosis,* causing the vast majority of cases.

Tularemia a zoonotic disease of mammals cased by *Francisella tularensis;* most often associated with rabbits.

Turbidity in microbiology, cloudiness in liquid due to microbial growth.

Typhoid fever a highly contagious, enteric infection caused by *Salmonella typhi.*

Uncoating in virology, removal of the viral coat by proteolytic enzymes in the host cell.

United Nations an international organization that aims to facilitate cooperation between countries regarding international law and other topics to achieve world peace.

Urbanization a process by which large numbers of people become concentrated in smaller areas, forming cities.

Ureters tubes that carry urine from the kidneys to the urinary bladder.

Urethra channel from the urinary bladder to the outside of the body for elimination of urine; in males the urethra also acts as a genital duct carrying sperm.

Urethritis infection of the urethra.

Urinary bladder muscular sac that stores urine before urination.

Urinary system the body system that regulates the volume and composition of body fluids and secretes the waste products of metabolism from the body.

Use-dilution test method of evaluating the effectiveness of antimicrobial agents, using standard cultures of test bacteria.

Uterus pear-shaped female reproductive organ where the embryo implants and further develops into a fetus.

Vaccine a preparation of either killed or weakened microorganisms, or of inactivated bacterial toxins, that when administered will cause an immune response and protect the individual from future attacks by the pathogen or toxin.

Vagina female genital canal, from the cervix to the outside of the body.

Vaginitis infection of the vagina.

Valence electrons the electrons in the outermost shell of an atom that can be gained or lost in a chemical reaction.

Van der Waals forces weak attractions between molecules that have a small degree of polarity.

Vector in microbiology, an organism that transmits pathogenic organisms from host to host; in molecular genetics, an agent, often a virus or plasmid, that transfers genetic material from one organism to another.

Vibrios simple curved, rod-shaped bacteria.

Viral envelope the flexible outer covering of some viruses that begins as some membrane taken from the host cell but is modified significantly by the virus.

Viral hemorrhagic fevers a group of febrile illnesses that range in severity from relatively mild to life-threatening, and can result in severe multisystem problems.

Viremia an infection in which a virus is present in the blood but does not replicate there.

Virion a complete virus, including the envelope (if it has one).

Viroid a single-stranded RNA molecule, lacking a capsid, that is an infectious agent in plants.

Virucide an agent that inactivates viruses.

Virulence the capacity of a pathogen to infect and harm host cells.

Virulence factor a microbial product or characteristic that aids a pathogen in infecting or harming the host.

Virulent the ability to invade host tissue and cause disease.

Virusoids circular, single-stranded RNA similar to viroids but require that the host cells is infected with a specific helper virus. Also referred to as "satellites."

Waterborne disease spread or sustained by water.

Western blot an immunologic technique involving electrophoresis of a protein followed by transfer to nitrocellulose where they are treated with enzyme tagged antibodies, allowing visualization of the protein bands.

WHO World Health Organization.

Xenograft a tissue graft between animals of different species.

Zone of inhibition area of no bacterial growth surrounding an antibiotic disk on a Kirby-Bauer plate.

Zoonosis any disease and/or infection that can be transmitted from vertebrate animals to humans.

Index

A

abiogenesis, 7
abiotic components of ecosystems, 438, 438b
ABO blood typing, 366, 366t
abortions, 282–283, 425t
abortive infections, 149
ABPA (allergic bronchopulmonary aspergillosis), 232–233
Academy of Dentistry, 243b
acetylcholine, 406
acidity, 28, 28f, 123, 358. *See also* alkalinity; pH environment/values
acids, 27, 27b, 38
ACIP (Advisory Committee on Immunization Practices), 229–230
acne (*Propionibacterium acnes*), 206, 206f, 207t
actin filaments, 51
active site (enzyme binding), 61
active transport mechanisms. *See under* transport mechanisms
acute necrotizing fasciitis (flesh eating bacteria), 203, 205, 205b, 207t
acute respiratory distress syndrome (ARDS), 230
adaptive immune system, 375–376
adenosine monophosphate (AMP), 38
adenosine triphosphate (ATP), 38, 38f
    cellular respiration, 64
    description, 38
    formation of, 48, 54, 64–65, 67f, 69, 69f, 75–78
adenoviruses, 150, 150t, 250, 303–304
adhesion, 186–188, 187t, 377–378
adipose (fat) tissue, 58, 202
adolescents/young adults, 430. *See also* infants and children
    acne, 206
    environment of, 431, 433
    HIV, 430b

adolescents/young adults (*Continued*)
    immune system of, 430
    infectious mononucleosis, 430
    influenza, 430
    meningococcal diseases, 262b, 430
    puberty, 371–372, 430
    sexually transmitted infections (STIs), 321, 429–430
    warts, 207–208
Advisory Committee on Immunization Practices (ACIP), 229–230
Advisory Committee on Variola Virus Research (WHO), 210
aerobic bacteria. *See under* bacteria
aerobic cellular respiration, 67t
African trypanosomiasis (sleeping sickness), 271
agar cultures
    blood agar plates (BAPs), 91–92, 299, 299f
    chocolate agar (CHOC), 91–92
    colony morphology on, 92f
    composition of, 84
    disk diffusion test (Kirby-Bauer method), 354f
    hemolysins, 91–92
    Kligler's iron agar, 93
    Koser's citrate medium, 93
    MacConkey agar (MAC), 91–92
    mannitol salt agar (MSA), 91–92
    Mueller Hinton agar, 354f
    nutrient agar, 91–92
    phenylethyl alcohol agar (PEA), 91–92
    plates, 86–87
    Sabouraud dextrose agar, 328
    Simmons citrate agar, 93
    slants, 92
    sulfur reduction, indole, production, and motility (SIM), 93
    Thayer-Martin agar (TM), 91–92

agar cultures (*Continued*)
    tryptic (Trypticase) soy agar, 91–92
    types, 91
    xylose lysine deoxycholate (XLD) agar, 91–92
agar slants, 92
aging process/human life stages
    adolescents (*See* adolescents/young adults)
    body water content, 58
    children (*See* infants and children)
    effect on drug absorption of, 399
    future concerns, 461b
    immune system throughout, 387–388, 424b, 433
    infants (*See* infants and children)
    older adults (*See* older adults/elderly)
    respiratory tract infections, 233 (*See also* respiratory tract)
    "The State of Aging and Health in America 2007", 431
    tuberculosis and, 223
    water distribution in the body, 58f
agranulocytes, 374–375, 374f
agriculture, 15, 334. *See also* environment(s); plant entries; plants; soil entries; U.S. Department of Agriculture (USDA); water entries
    agricultural inoculants, 128b
    biotechnology in, 472–474
    denitrification, 440
    emerging/reemerging diseases related to, 334
    microbes in, 15
    nitrification, 440
    rhizobia, 128b
    runoff water, 166, 441
    transgenic plants, 473

---

f, Figures; t, tables; b, boxes.

AIDS, 186t, 318b, 324–326, 387. *See also* HIV
  antiviral agents for, 416
  Health and Human Services (HHS) concerns, 430b
  in health care settings, 111t
  in HIV-infected infants, 427
  molluscum contagiosum, 209
  opportunistic infections related to, 325b
  skin infections, 202
  stages of infection, 326t
  surface antigens in blood cells, 375
  tuberculosis and, 223
airborne diseases, 14, 14t, 195–196, 222–223
alcoholic beverage production, 14–15, 15b
aldehydes, 356–357
algae, 11, 166–169, 440
  blooms, 441
  brown, 167–169
  cell wall structure, 46
  characteristics of, 167
  classification of, 167–169
  green (chlorophyta), 167–169
  growing cultures, 91
  harmful algal blooms (HABs), 167b
  life cycle of, 167
  medical concerns about, 166
  red (rhodophyta), 167–169
  reproduction methods, 167–169, 168f
  in soil, 441–442
  Spirogyra, 169f
  summary of, 168t
  taxonomy, 167
  toxin-producing, 159b–160b, 166
algicides, 353, 356
alkalinity, 28, 28f, 93, 123. *See also* acidity; pH environment/values
alkaliphiles, 123
alkylating agents, 355t
allergens, 364–365, 383, 383t. *See also* immune response
allergic bronchopulmonary aspergillosis (ABPA), 232–233
allergy/hypersensitivity reactions, 383–385, 388. *See also* antigen-antibody response; immune system response
  to antimicrobial agents, 409
  cytotoxic hypersensitivity (type II), 383
  delayed hypersensitivity (type IV), 385
  immediate hypersensitivity (type I), 383
  immune complex hypersensitivity (type III), 383–385
  to molds, 165b
  National Institute of Allergy and Infectious Diseases (NIAID), 103, 337
  prostaglandin actions in, 36b
  responses/symptoms/causative allergens, 383t
  skin manifestations, 384t–385t
  symptoms/treatment of, 383
allografts, 365
allosteric site of an enzyme, 63–64
alphavirus encephalitides, 456t

alternative complement pathway, 380
Altman, Richard, 43t
alveolar macrophages, 374, 449f
amantadine, 417
amensalism, 182, 182t
American Academy of Pediatrics, 458b
American Academy of Periodontology, 241
American College Health Association (ACHA), 262b
American National Standards Institute (ANSI), 107
American Society of Microbiology (ASM), 103
American trypanosomiasis (Chagas' disease), 272, 290t, 292
amino acids, 33f, 38, 71t, 75–78, 440
  base triplets, mRNA codons, and their, 71t
  cysteine, 93
  description, 32
  encoding of, 71, 71t
  multiple mRNA codons, 71t
  naturally occurring, 32t
  phenylalanine, 93
  structure of, 32f
  for synthesis of polypeptide chains, 70–71
aminoglycosides, 416
ammonia, 27b, 440
ammonification/deamination
  ammonification process, 440
amoebae/amoebic infections, 159b–160b, 172, 173f, 174, 252
amoebozoa, 172
AMP (adenosine monophosphate), 38
anabolic steroids, 35–36
anabolism/anabolic reactions, 25, 25f, 38, 61
anaerobic ammonium oxidation (anammox), 440
anaerobic cellular respiration, 64, 67, 70–71
anaerobic microorganisms, 281, 444
  aerotolerant, 123, 123t
  bacteria, 123t, 127–129, 128f, 128t, 265b, 432, 432t
  facultative, 123
  obligate, 123, 123t
  water-related, 441
anaerobic wounds, 264
analytical epidemiology, 191–192
anaphylactic reactions, 383t–385t
anatomy. *See specific body area or system*
anemia, 253–254
animalcules, 3, 7, 41b–42b, 115b, 181b
animal health, 282b
animal populations, 334
animal reservoirs, 192, 194t, 252, 284
animals. *See also* transmissible spongiform encephalopathies/prion diseases (TSEs); vectors; vector-transmitted infections/diseases; zoonoses
  antibiotic use in livestock, 413b
  bites of, 154
  diseases of, 166
  rat-bite fever, 282t
  transgenic, 473–474
animal vectors, 210–211, 283–284, 287t, 290t, 291–292, 446

animal viruses
  Eastern/Western equine encephalitis (EEE), 270
  enveloped viruses, 137, 141–142, 142f, 144t, 148f
  glanders, 455–456
  multiplication of, 148f
    adsorption, 147
    assembly, 149
    host cell machinery/metabolism, 145
    penetration, 147
    release, 149
    replication, 148–149
    uncoating, 147
  naked viruses, 142f, 148f
  structure of, 141f
anions, 22, 23t, 28, 29t
ANSI (American National Standards Institute), 107
antagonism (drug interactions/combinations), 409
anthrax
  as biological weapon, 8–9, 81b, 95b, 226, 436b–437b, 449, 449f, 455t
  cutaneous, 450, 450f
  inhalation, 449, 449b
antibacterials, 414–416
  overuse of, 413
  semisynthetic, 414–416
    aminoglycosides, 416
    cephalosporins, 415–416, 415t
    chloramphenicol, 416
    macrolides, 416
    tetracyclines, 416
antibiogram pattern method, 126
antibiosis, 15
antibiotic-producing microorganisms, 15
antibiotic-resistant bacterial infections, 147b. *See also* drug resistance
antibiotics, 414–416
  in aquatic microbiology, 413b
  Bacillus antibiotics, 416
  care in prescribing, 413
  cell defenses against, 45–46
  drugs of choice, 417t
  effectiveness of, 19b–20b
  first use of term, 81b, 405b
  macrolide polyene, 418
  natural, 414
  nonsynthetic and semisynthetic, 414–416
    aminoglycosides, 416
    cephalosporins, 415–416, 415t
    chloramphenicol, 416
    macrolides, 416
    penicillins, 414–415
    tetracyclines, 416
  overuse of, 413b (*See also* drug resistance)
  pathogenic spirochetes, 127t
  patient noncompliance with treatment, 223
  penicillins, 46b
  resistance to, 413b
  for sexually transmitted infections, 329
  streptomycete sources, 132t
  subdivisions of, 414
  success of early, 332b
  synthetic

antibiotics (*Continued*)
  quinolones (fluoroquinolones), 414, 415t
  sulfa drugs (sulfonamides), 414
  trimethoprim, 414
  for urinary tract infections (UTIs), 301
  use in livestock, 413b
antibodies/immunoglobulins (Igs/gammagobulins), 50b, 364, 366–368, 367f, 383, 388. *See also* allergy/hypersensitivity reactions
  basic structure, 367f
  classification of, 367–368
  IgE and IgG production, 383 (*See also* allergy/hypersensitivity reactions)
  IgG/IgA/IgM/IgD/IgE, 367–368
  lack of, 297b
  passive, 429
  summary of classes of, 367t
  titering, 94–95
antibody-antigen complexes, 299
antibody dependent hypersensitivity reactions, 384t–385t
antibody titer, 381–382
anticodons, 38, 72
antidotes, 399, 400t
antifungals, 418. *See also under* fungal infections/diseases
  drugs of choice, 417t
  echinocandins, 418
  ergosterol inhibitor compounds, 36b
  flucytosine, 418
  griseofulvin, 418
  groups of, 418
  intravenous (IV), 233
  macrolide polyene antibiotics, 418
  oral, 328
  plasma membrane disrupters, 407
  for sexually transmitted infections, 328
  synthetic azoles, 418
  topical, 328
antigen-antibody response, 94–95, 363–364
antigenic determinants, 364f
antigenic shift/drift, 335b
antigenic stimulation, 429
antigen-presenting cells, 374, 380, 380f
antigens, 45–46, 50b, 364–366, 388. *See also* allergy/hypersensitivity reactions
  autoantigens, 364–365
  binding actions, 381f
  blood groups/types, 366
  classification of, 364
  D antigen (Rh factor), 366, 366b
  definition, 364
  H antigen, 47–48
  immune system reactions, 45–48, 50b, 364–366
  immunogenic, 47–48, 364–365
  self-antigens, 363–365
  self-/non-self antigens, 386
  surface, 375
  tumor, 364–365
antihelminthics, 419–420
  drugs of choice, 420t
  ivermectin, 420
  mebendazole, 419
  niclosamide, 419
  piperazine, 419–420
antiinflammatory drug actions, 36b

antimicrobial agents
  broad-spectrum, 408–411
antimicrobials (in general)
  administration of, 399
  alcohols, 356
  alkylating agents, 356–357
  allergy/hypersensitivity reactions to, 409
  for assisting host defense mechanisms, 409
  bacterial ribosomes and, 56b
  biofilms and, 50b
  broad-spectrum, 408–411
  as cause of infection, 196
  characteristics of, 407–411
  chemical, 354–357
  classification of, 420–421
  for control measures, 347
  cross-resistance, 412–413
  denaturing of proteins, 33
  dilution/minimal inhibitory concentration method, 410, 410f
  disk diffusion (Kirby-Bauer method), 410f
  drugs of choice, 417t
  efficacy, 353, 359, 409–410
  ergosterol inhibitors, 36b
  goal of, 420–421
  halogens, 355–356
  heavy metal compounds, 356
  iodine, 356
  mechanisms of action
    disruption of plasma membrane, 407
    inhibition of cell wall synthesis, 406
    inhibition of metabolic pathways, 407
    inhibition of nucleic acid synthesis, 406–407
    inhibition of protein synthesis, 406
    inhibition of translation, 407f
    microbicidal or microbiostatic, 406
  medium spectrum, 408
  microbicidal/microbiostatic actions of, 405–406
  phenols/phenolics, 354–355
  quaternary compounds, 356
  resistance to (*See* drug resistance)
  risk factors of, 420–421
  selection of, 420–421
  serum killing power, 410
  serum killing power method, 410
  side effects, 410–411, 420–421
  spectrum of activity, 408–409, 408t, 415t
    affordability/availability, 409
    complements/aids in host's defenses, 409
    delivery to site of infection, 408
    microbicidal versus microbiostatic, 408
    nonallergenic, 409
    not subject to antimicrobial resistance, 409
    selective toxicity, 408
    stability/shelf life, 409
    time of activity, 408–409
  sulfa drugs (sulfonamides), 63b
  surfactants, 356
  synthetic drugs
    quinolones (fluoroquinolones), 414, 415t

antimicrobials (in general) (*Continued*)
    sulfa drugs (sulfonamides), 414
    trimethoprim, 414
  vulnerability of microbes to, 346b
antimicrobial soaps/lotions, 201b, 413
antiprostaglandins, 36b
antiprotozoals, 170t, 418–419
  chloroquine and primaquine, 418–419
  drugs of choice, 420t
  metronidazole, 419
  pyrimethamine, 419
  quinine, 419
antisepsis/antiseptics, 83, 346t, 353
antitoxins, 452
antivirals
  for herpes simplex virus (HSV), 327
  for HIV, 326
  modes of action of, 416
  for smallpox, 453
  synthetic, 416–417
  virucides, 353, 356, 473
apical complex, 172–173
Apicomplexa, 172–173, 173f
apoenzymes, 63
applied microbiology, 14–16
aquatic microbiology, 458. *See also* algae; water entries
  agricultural runoff, 166
  benthos/benthic zone, 443–444, 443f, 445f
  contamination of, 442–443, 445, 447, 455
  description, 29–30
  freshwater environments/ecosystems, 442–444, 443f
    lakes/ponds, 443–444, 443f
    ponds/lakes, 443–444, 443f
    profundal zone, 443–444, 443f
    properties of, 30b
    remediation of, 50
    sanitation of, 252
    states of, 29
  marine (saltwater) environments/ecosystems, 441–444, 447
    abyssal zone, 444, 445f
    Dead Sea, 133
    Great Salt Lake, 133
    hydration spheres, 31f
    hydrogen concentration of, 27
    hydrolysis, 25f
    limnetic zone, 443–444, 443f
    littoral zone, 443–444, 443f–444f
    plankton, 167–169
    red tides, 166
Arber, Werner, 463
arborescent growth, 92
arboviruses, 269–270, 270f
archaea, 10–11, 10f, 46
  cell lines, 9, 10f
  classification of, 10–11, 125–133 (*See also* Bergey's *Manual of Systematic Bacteriology*)
  description, 125
  halophiles, 133
  methanogenic, 9b, 125, 132
  pH environment for, 123
archaezoa, 171–172
ARDS (acute respiratory distress syndrome), 230

arenaviruses, 453–454, 455t
Aristotle, 41b–42b, 436b–437b
arrangements/shapes. *See* morphology/
    morphological identification
arthropod vectors, 195b, 269–270, 288–289
arthrospores, 164–165
Ascaris lumbricoides (roundworms/
    ascarids), 177–178, 177b, 253, 253f
ascomycota, 165–166
asepsis, 346t. *See also* control methods;
    laboratory aseptic techniques
asexual reproduction (microbes). *See under*
    reproduction methods (microbes)
Asian (Russian) flu, 153t, 229b
ASM (American Society of Microbiology),
    103
Aspergillus, 232–233, 233f, 251, 325b
aspirin, 383
astroviruses, 250
asymptomatic carriers. *See* carriers of
    disease
athlete's foot, 211t, 212, 212b, 212f
atmosphere (planetary), 9b, 441
atmospheric conditions. *See under*
    microbial growth
atomic nucleus, 20
atomic numbers, 20–22
atomic structures, 20–22, 21f
atoms, 20–22
    definition, 20, 38
    electric state of, 25–26
    microscopes for observing, 91b
    motion of, 58
    nuclei of, 20–21
    reaction with each other of, 21
ATP. *See* adenosine triphosphate (ATP)
autism, 400b
autoclaves, 83, 83f, 107, 109f, 348t, 350, 350f
autografts, 365–366
autoimmune diseases, 364–365, 386–388.
    See also main entries for specific diseases
    Graves' disease, 386–387, 386t
    Hashimoto's thyroiditis, 386t
    hemolytic anemia, 384t–385t
    immune complex diseases, 383–385
    multiple sclerosis, 386, 386t
    myasthenia gravis, 386, 386t
    rheumatoid arthritis (RA), 384t–386t, 387
    systemic lupus erythematosus (SLE),
      386t, 387
autoinoculation (self-inoculation), 194–195
autopsies, 8, 201b, 272
autotrophs, 121–122, 438, 440
avian influenza (influenza A/H5N1), 145b,
    229b, 337b, 341t
axon terminals, 260f
azidothymidine (AZT), 417
azoles, synthetic, 418
AZT (azidothymidine), 417

B
babesiosis, 287t, 290t, 291–292
bacilli (rods). *See under* bacteria (in general)
Bacillus infections, 118t, 119f, 416
    antibiotics for, 416
    B. anthracis, 226f
    B. cereus, 131f, 248–249
    dysentery, 13t
    intoxication, 248–249

back mutation (reversions), 125
bacteremia, 190, 221, 280
bacteria (in general), 10–11, 10f, 116–118.
    *See also Bergey's Manual of Systematic
    Bacteriology*; taxonomy
    adhesion to host receptors, 187t
    aerobic, 64, 66–67, 67f, 123, 123t,
      126–127, 127f, 127t, 438–439, 441
    anaerobic, 123t, 127–129, 128f, 128t,
      265b, 432, 432t
    arrangements, 117–118
    bacilli (rods), 116–117, 131, 131t
      aerobic, 126–127, 127f, 127t
      anaerobic, 123t, 127–129, 128f, 128t
      cell division, 117–118
      irregular nonsporulating, 131, 132t
      regular nonsporulating, 131
    bioterror agents (*See* bioterrorism/
      bioweapons)
    blooms, 441
    capneic, 123
    categorization of, 133
    cell lines of, 9, 10f
    cell walls, 46f
    characteristics of, 124–125 (*See also*
      genetics)
    classification of, 125–126, 133
    cocci (spherical), 116–118, 119f, 131,
      131t (*See also* staphylococcal
      infections/agents; streptococcal
      infections/agents)
    coliform, 129b
    conjugation in, 463f
    description, 133
    diplobacilli, 117–118
    donor, 462
    evolutionary branches of, 10
    factors influencing, 121–123
    first descriptions of, 41b–42b
    gram-negative (*See* gram-negative
      bacteria)
    gram-positive (*See* gram-positive
      bacteria)
    measurement of, 121, 121f, 126
    origin of word, 115b
    pathogenic agents, 10, 44, 84b
    placenta-crossing, 186t
    pleomorphic, 118t
    population in soil, 441
    probiotics, 184b
    in soil, 442
    uses of, 115b
    viral attacks on, 136b
bacterial infections/diseases, 56b. *See also*
    antibiotics; main entries *for specific
    infections or agents*
    circulatory system, 280–287
    description, 243–244
    disease-causing organisms (summary),
      237t–239t
    drugs of choice for, 417t
    emerging/reemerging, 115b, 338t
    endocarditis, 278, 293
    food intoxications (*See under* foodborne
      diseases/infections)
    food-related (*See food entries*)
    gastrointestinal (GI) tract, 244–247
    global spread of, 334b
    nervous system, 272–273

bacterial infections/diseases (*Continued*)
    opportunistic infections related to AIDS,
      325b
    reproductive tract, 312t, 313–314, 315t
    respiratory tract, 219–226, 219t
    sexually transmitted, 319–324, 324t
    skin, 203–207, 203t, 207t, 213–214
    tonsillitis, 369t
    zoonotic, 194t
bacterial invasins, 188t
bacterial ribosomes, 56b
bacterial toxins, 188
bactericidal substances, 83, 353, 356
bacteriocidal/bacteriostatic antimicrobial
    agents, 408
bacteriophages (phages), 137, 143, 463
    groups of, 144t
    lambda, 468
    multiplication of, 137, 145–147, 146f
    phage typing, 126
    structure of, 143f
    therapeutic, 147b
    unassigned, 138b
    virulent (lytic), 146–147
bacteriostatic substances, 83
bacteriuria, 299
Baker, Josephine, 100b
Balamuthia, 172
balanitis, 314, 315t, 328
Balantidium coli, 172, 252
Baltimore classification system, 137, 138b.
    *See also Bergey's Manual of Systematic
    Bacteriology*; kingdoms of life
barotolerant/barophilic microorganisms,
    123
bases, 27, 27b, 38
base sequences, 125
base triplets. *See* codons
basidiomycota, 165–166
basophils, 373–374, 383
Benda, Carl, 43t
Bergey's Manual of Systematic Bacteriology,
    11, 91, 125–133. *See also* Baltimore
    classification system; taxonomy
    aerobic/microaerophilic helical vibroid
      gram-negative bacteria, 126, 127t
    anaerobic gram-negative rods, 129
    chlamydias, 129
    cocci, 129–131, 130t
    extreme halophiles, 133
    extreme thermophiles, 122t, 132–133
    facultatively anaerobic gram-negative
      rods, 123t, 127–129, 128t
    irregular nonsporulating gram-positive
      rods, 131
    methanogens, 132
    mycobacteria, 131–132
    mycoplasms and ureaplasmas, 130
    nocardioforms, 132
    regular nonsporulating gram-positive
      rods, 131
    rhizobia, 128b
    rickettsias, 129, 129f, 129t
    rods and cocci, 126–127, 127t, 131
    spirilla, 117f, 118t
    spirochetes, 117f, 118t, 126
    streptomycetes, 132, 132t
    vibrios, 117f, 118t
Bernard, Claude, 41b–42b, 391b–392b

beverage production, 15, 15b
β-lactams, 46b, 412, 415–416
binary fission, 42, 54, 73, 74f, 120, 120f, 133
binding actions
    active site (enzyme binding), 61
    antigen, 381f
    enzyme inhibition, 64f
    of enzymes, 62f
    sites of, 58
binomial system of nomenclature, 11, 133
bioassays, 401
bioavailability, 399
biochemical characteristics of microorganisms, 93–94
biochemical conversion processes, 68–69, 75–78
biochemical pathways, 379–380
biochemistry, 391b–392b
bioconversion, 16
biodiversity, 437–438
biofilms, 50b, 75–78
    aquatic, 442–444
    catheter-related, 299–300
    damage caused by, 50
    definition, 12
    formation of, 49–50, 50f
    growth of, 49
    infectious diseases and, 50b
    locations of, 49
    oral/dental bacteria, 119b
    positive uses of, 50
    recruitment, 49
    replication methods, 49
    in wastewater treatment, 440b
biogeochemical cycles
    carbon cycle, 438, 439f
    definition, 458
    nitrogen cycle, 438–440, 439f
    phosphorus cycle, 441, 442f
    sulfur cycle, 440–441, 441f
biogeochemistry, 438
biohazard symbol, 102f
biological agents, guidelines for working with, 100
biological vectors, 195, 195b
biomass, 16, 437–438
biopharmaceutics, 393. See also pharmacology
bioremediation, 15
biosafety levels (BSLs) and guidelines, 101–102, 101b. See also safety issues
    BSL-1, 101–102, 102b
    BSL-2, 101b, 102
    BSL-3, 102–103, 102b
    BSL-4, 103, 103b, 104t
    prion foods and drugs, 272
    risk group levels, 101t
    for specific organisms, 101b
    testing for plague, 451
    training program, 100–101
biosphere, 437, 437f
biotechnology. See also technology/industry
    in agriculture (See agriculture)
    genetic engineering, 462–467
    goals of, 467
    history of, 461b
    in human medicine, 468–472
    transgenic animals, 473–474

biotechnology (Continued)
    vaccines (See vaccine-related entries)
    vectors in, 467–468
Biotechnology Regulatory Services (USDA), 472–473
bioterrorism/bioweapons
    anthrax, 8–9, 81b, 95b, 226, 449, 449t, 455t
    Bioterrorism Preparedness Response, 448
    botulism, 452, 455t
    brucellosis, 456t
    Category A agents, 448–454, 455t
        bacterial, 449–452
        viral, 452–454
    Category B agents, 454–456, 456t
    Category C agents, 456–457, 457t
    cholera, 456t
    definition, 458
    earliest use of, 436b–437b, 448
    first attacks in United States, 448b
    first responder roles, 457–458, 458b
    hantavirus, 230
    microorganisms of concern, 16, 236b
    neurotoxins, 257b
    9/11 attacks, 436b–437b
    plague, 450–451, 455t
    potential for, 458b
    Salmonella, 448b
    smallpox, 152b, 210, 452–453, 455t
    stockpiling of therapeutic agents, 448
    treating victims of, 457–458
    tularemia, 283, 451, 455t
    viral, 455t–456t
    zoonoses, 454–455
biotic components of ecosystems, 438, 438b
biotyping, 126
birth defects, 426–427. See also congenital infections/disorders
BK polyomavirus, 303
bladder infections. See urinary tract infections (UTIs)
Blake, James, 391b–392b
Blastomyces dermatidis, 203t, 232, 232f
blastospores, 164–165
bleach, 26b
blindness. See eyes/eye infections
blood
    clots, 190b, 470–471
    hemocytoblasts, 372
    role of, 276b
    transfusions, 292
    typing/blood groups, 366, 366t
bloodborne pathogens/infections. See also HIV
    Bloodborne Pathogens Standard, 110
    bloodborne training program, 100–101
    in health care settings, 111t
    hepatitis, 326–327
    HIV, 325
    infectious diseases, 280
    nosocomial, 196
    toxic shock syndrome (TSS), 309
    viruses, 111t, 446–447
blood-brain barrier, 272–273, 368, 406, 408
blood cells, 41b–42b, 366, 372, 373f
    red blood cells
        blood doping, 472b
        blood groups, 366
        discovery of, 276b
        formation of, 297

blood cells (Continued)
    surface antigens with AIDS, 375
    white blood cells (WBCs), 49, 372, 471
blood donations, 366
blood doping, 472b
blood infections/disorders. See under circulatory system infections
bloodletting, 276b
blood pressure, 59
bloodstream. See circulatory system
bloodsucking bugs, 195b
body chemistry, 19b–20b, 58f
body fluids, 195, 269, 283, 287–288, 288b, 288t. See also blood; water (human body)
body humors, 276b
bonds, molecular. See molecular bonds
Bordatella pertussis (whooping cough), 222f
botanical sources of drugs, 391b–392b
Botox, 266b
botulism, 247, 265–266, 272–273, 424b
    as biological weapon, 257b, 452, 455t
    cosmetic use of (Botox), 266b
    inhalation, 247
    types of, 265
Bovet, D., 405b
bovine spongiform encephalopathy (BSE), 11b, 358
Boyer, Herbert, 461b, 466
brain, 258–259, 258f–259f, 272–273, 368, 406, 408
breastfeeding, 282, 325, 382
breast infections, 307b, 310, 312t
Bright's disease (glomerulonephritis), 299
bronchial tree, 217
broth. See culture media under laboratory testing/techniques
Brownian movement, 58
brucellosis (undulant fever), 282–283, 282t, 454–455, 456t
BSE (bovine spongiform encephalopathy), 11b, 272, 358
BSLs. See biosafety levels (BSLs) and guidelines
buboes, 283–284. See also plague (Yersinia pestis)
Buchan, William, 217b
Bud, Robert, 461b
buffers, 27b, 28, 38
building blocks of cells, 118–120
Bunyaviridae, 152, 153t, 453–454, 455t

C

caliciviruses, 250
Calvin-Benson cycle, 70, 70f
Calvin cycle, 69–70
Cambridge Instrument Company, 43t
campylobacteriosis, 246
cancer
    breast, 307b
    cervical, 307b, 327
    Kaposi's sarcoma, 324
    leukemia, 372t
    non-Hodgkin's/Hodgkin's lymphomas, 370t
    use of radioisotopes in treating, 22b
    viruses that cause, 151t

Candida albicans (candidiasis), 211t, 212–213, 250–251, 251f, 298, 311, 312t, 314–315, 325b, 328, 425t
capillary action, 29b, 378
capnophiles, 123t
capsids, 133, 137, 143
capsomeres, 137
capsule staining, 89
carbohydrates (sugars), 31–32, 31t, 32f, 38, 44f. *See also* glucose
   description, 31–32
   disaccharides/polysaccharides, 32f
carbolic acid, 201b
carbon, 30–31, 38, 133, 438
carbon atoms, 21f, 23, 32f, 121–122
carbon cycle, 438, 439f
carbon dioxide (CO_2), 27, 438
carbonic acid (H_2CO_3), 28
carbon monoxide (CO), 27
carbuncles, 203–204, 207t
cardiovascular system, 368. *See also* circulatory system
   blood pressure, 59
   carditis, 220b, 281
   congestive heart failure, 220b
   endocarditis, 277–278, 282–283, 293
   heart anatomy, 277, 279f
   myocarditis, 277–278, 293
   myocardium, 277
   oral cavity infections and, 276b
   overview of, 277f–278f
   parasitic myocarditis, 293
   relationship to lymphatic system, 279f
cardiovascular system infections/diseases, pericarditis, 277, 280
caries, dental, 240. *See also* oral cavity
carrier-mediated transport mechanism, 60f
carriers of disease
   asymptomatic, 192–194, 244, 245b
     infectious mononucleosis, 287
     Streptococcus agalactiae, 310b
     toxoplasmosis, 292
     trichomoniasis (infected males), 315t
   definition, 192–194
   human, 192–194
CAS (Chemical Abstracts Service), registry numbers, 103–105
catabolism/catabolic reactions, 25–26, 25f, 61
catalysis/catalysts, 62, 75–78
catheter-related infections, 12t, 298–301, 304
cations, 22, 23t, 28, 29t
cat scratch disease, 282t, 283
causative agents/organisms. *See also specific infection or disease*
   allergens, 383t
   etiology of infectious diseases, 189–191, 197–198
   Koch's postulates, 190–191
   malaria, 174f, 290f
   meningitis, 405–406
   nosocomial infections, 196
   pneumonias, 217b, 432
   poliomyclitis, 268f
   reservoirs of, 192–194
   urinary tract infections (UTIs), 297–299
CDC. *See* Centers for Disease Control (CDC)

CD system, 375
cell absorption, 47
cell biology, 43t
cell counts, 121
cell cycles, 74–75, 74f
cell doctrine of life, 41b–42b, 42, 81b
cell mass, 121
cell membrane damage, 407
cell morphology. *See* morphology/morphological identification
cell replication methods. *See also* reproduction methods (microbes)
   binary fission, 42, 54, 73, 74f, 120, 120f, 133
   cell division, 42, 75–78
     appearance during, 91
     bacilli, 117–118
     of biofilms, 49
     cell cycles and mitosis, 74–75
     fungal mycelia, 165
     meiosis, 75
     processes for, 75–78
   chromosomes/chromatids, 75f
   DNA synthesis, 71f, 74f, 75–78
   meiosis, 77f
   mitochondrial, 54
   mitosis, 75f–76f
   self-, 54
   viruses (*See* viral multiplication)
cells (in general), 75–78
   attachment of, 47
   B cells, 324, 380–381, 381f, 388
   categories of, 75–78
   cell-surface markers, 363–364
   cellular respiration, 62, 64–70
   comparative sizes, 5t
   dry weight measures, 121
   environment for survival of, 57
   evolutionary lines, 9
   first description of, 41b–42b
   function of, 41b–42b, 70–71
   Hooke's discovery of, 42
   membrane damage, 407
   metabolic pathways, 64
   metabolism of, 61–72, 75–78
     cofactors/coenzymes, 63
     enzymes, 61–64
     enzyme specificity, 62
     exoenzymes/endoenzymes, 62
   nucleus of, 52, 52f
   organelles, 50–57
   prokaryotic and eukaryotic, 42–57
   replication of, 74f
   response to pathogens, 377
   rupture of, 59
   sensory capacity, 47–48
   sugars in, 31
   surface appendages, 47–49
   types of, 42
   walls, 42–43, 45–46, 46f, 75–78, 161–162, 406
cellular respiration, 64
cellulitis, 204, 204f, 207t
Centers for Disease Control (CDC), 14, 99b, 391b–392b
   Advisory Committee on Immunization Practices (ACIP), 229–230
   bioterrorism issues, 152b, 458b
   bloodborne pathogens, 280

Centers for Disease Control (CDC) (*Continued*)
   congenital toxoplasmosis, 427b
   drug-resistant *Streptococcus pneumoniae* (DRSP) statistics, 221b
   emergency response standards/procedures, 457
   emerging/reemerging infectious diseases, 337
   epidemiology information, 192
   eradication of smallpox, 210
   guidelines for protection/prevention, 101b, 111b, 197, 340
   incidence of sexually transmitted infections, 319b
   level 4 biosafety laboratories in U.S., 104t
   malaria risk map, 291b
   meningitis vaccinations, 262b
   mold-related health problems, 165b
   mosquito bite prevention, 337b
   overuse of antibacterial products, 413, 413b
   responsibilities of, 337, 339
   rodent control guidelines, 230
   salmonellosis incidence, 244
   Special Pathogens Branch (SPB), 287–288
   stages of HIV infection, 324
   statistics on cryptosporidiosis, 252
   symptoms of toxic shock syndrome, 323b
   "The State of Aging and Health in America 2007", 431
   transmission of infections to fetuses, 426
   trichomoniasis treatment in pregnant women, 427–428
   use of antibiotics for strep throat, 220
   vaccination issues, 400b
central nervous system (CNS), 272–273, 368, 386. *See also* nervous system
   anatomy, 258–259, 258f
   brucellosis, 282–283
   congenital diseases of, 426
   listeriosis, 247
   multiple sclerosis, 386
   pharmacology for, 392t
   protozoan parasites, 170t
centrioles, 51–52
centrosomes, 51–52
cephalosporins, 415–416, 415t
cerate (cold cream), 19b–20b
cerebrospinal fluid (CSF), 258–259, 259t
cestodes (tapeworms), 176, 177f
CFUs (colony-forming units), 302
Chagas' disease (American trypanosomiasis), 272, 290t, 292
Chamberland, Charles, 136b
chancroid, 323, 323f, 324t
Chastain, E. B., 405b
cheese production, 15b
Chemical Abstracts Service (CAS) registry numbers, 103–105
chemical bleaches, 26b
chemical bonds, 21, 23–27
   breaking, 26
   covalent, 23–24, 23f
     carbon formation of, 30–31
     coordinate, 23–24
     definition, 23

chemical bonds (*Continued*)
    nonpolar, 23, 23f
    polar, 23–24, 23f
    and forces, 23–25
    formation and classification of, 23–25
    hydrogen, 24–25
    ionic, 24, 24f
    octet principle, 23
    types of, 23
    van der Waals forces, 23, 25
chemical compounds, 20, 27
chemical drugs, 393
chemical equations, 27b
chemical formulas, 20
chemical imbalance, 19b–20b
chemical mediators of inflammation, 373–374
chemical molecular structure (CMS), 19b–20b
chemical notations, 26–27, 27b, 61
chemical reactions, 38
    of atoms, 21
    cellular metabolism, 75–78
    contribution of water in, 29
    energy level for, 62f
    pathways of, 25
    responses to pathogens, 377
    types of, 25–26
chemicals
    information for registered, 103–105
    safe handling guidelines, 103–105, 112
    toxic/adverse affects, 399–400
chemistry, 391b–392b
chemoautotrophs, 121–122, 133, 438, 444
chemoheterotrophs, 121–122, 133, 169, 438
chemotaxis, 48, 377–378
chemotherapy, 202
chemotrophs, 38, 61, 121
chickenpox (*Varicella zoster*), 151, 207, 208t, 209, 429–430
childbed fever (puerperal sepsis), 100b, 201b
children. *See* infants and children
chitin synthesis, 161–162
Chlamydia, 324t, 430
    C. trachomatis, 321
    diagnosis of, 322b
    pneumonia, 219t, 222
    in pregnancy, 322
    sexually transmitted, 129, 129t, 321–322, 322b
    spread of, 318b
chlamydospores, 164–165
chloramphenicol, 416
chlorine, 355t, 356
chlorophyll, 68–70, 69f, 356
chlorophyta, 167–169
chloroplasts, 54–55, 55f, 68–69
chloroquine, 418–419
cholera, 2b–3b, 13–14, 13t, 115b, 236b, 249, 249b, 454–455, 456t
cholesterol, 36, 36b, 38, 43, 44f
chromatin, 52
chromoblastomycoses, 211t, 213
chromosomes, 37–38, 75, 75f, 120, 124
chronic infections, 190
chronic wasting disease, 272
chrysophyta, 167–169, 169f

cilia, 47, 47t, 49
ciliary escalators, 217–219, 376, 377f
Ciliophora (ciliates), 171–172
circulatory system infections
    bacterial, 280–287, 280t
    bacterial proliferation in bloodstream, 407
    bloodborne infectious diseases, 280
    blood infections/disorders
        hemoflagellates, 172
        hemolytic diseases, 366, 366b, 384t–385t
        hemophilia, 470–471
        hemorrhagic fevers (*See under* viral infections/diseases)
    cardiovascular system (*See* cardiovascular system)
    discovery of circulation, 41b–42b
    drugs used for, 392t
    fungal, 289, 289t
    immune response and, 388
    lymphatic system (*See* lymphatic system)
    microbemia, 280
    protozoan, 170t, 289–293, 290t
    responsibilities of, 276b
    role of blood, 276b
    Trypanosoma, 172f
    vector-transmitted, 283–287
    viral, 287–289, 288t
    zoonotic, 282–283, 282t
circumcision, 301b, 307b
cisternae, 52
citrate use test, 93
citric acid cycle (Krebs cycle), 26, 64, 66, 66f, 70
CJD (Creutzfeldt-Jakob diseases), 272
class (life hierarchy), 10f
classical complement pathway, 380
classification systems. *See* taxonomy
clearance (excretion, elimination) of drugs, 394, 399, 402, 412
climate change, 335
clonal selection, 380–381
clones/cloning, 465–468, 473
Clostridium, 281
    C. sporogenes, 348t
    C. tetani, 264, 264f
clot-dissolving enzymes, 190b
clothing, protective, 110
CMS (chemical molecular structure), 19b–20b
CMV. *See* cytomegalovirus (CMV)
CNS. *See* central nervous system (CNS)
cocci. *See under* bacteria (in general)
Coccidioides immitis, 232f
coccidioidomycosis, 231–232, 325b, 425t
coccobacilli, 117f, 118t
codons, 32–33, 37–38, 71t. *See also DNA and RNA entries;* genetics-related entries
    amino acid, 71
    mRNA, 71t
    silent mutations, 124–125
    stop, 73f
    translation of, 72, 73f
    tRNA, 72f
coenocytic hyphae, 163, 164f
coenzymes, 63

cofactors, 63
Cohen, Stanley, 461b, 466
cohesion-tension theory, 29, 29b
Cohn, Ferdinand, 8
colds. *See* common cold
cold sores, 208t, 209f
Coliform Index (EPA), 129b
colitis, 252, 411
colonization, 187
colony characteristics, 91–92
colony-forming units (CFUs), 302
colony isolation, 86–87, 91
color (inflammation), 378b
colostrum, 382, 429
commensalism, 12, 182, 182t
commercial sterilization, 346
common cold, 14t, 154, 217b, 226–228, 228t, 233, 429–430
community-acquired infections, 221, 224, 413b, 432t
competition, microbial, 58, 182–185
competitive enzyme inhibition, 63, 407
complement proteins, 379–380
complement system, 379–380
complex viruses, 137, 142–143, 143f
compounds
    chemical, 20, 27
    for control of microbes, 355t
    definition, 23
    dissociation of chemical, 27
    ergosterol inhibitor, 36b
    hazardous, 15
    heavy metal, 356
    inorganic, 27–30, 38
    nitrogen, 27b
    organic, 122
    quaternary, 356
    toxic, 83, 103–105, 399–400
compromised immune system. *See under* immune system response
congenital infections/disorders, 425–426, 433
    of central nervous system (CNS), 426
    cytomegalovirus (CMV), 426
    dwarfism, 470
    ears/eyes, 426
    HIV, 427
    perinatal, 426–427
    during pregnancy, 424–425
    rubella, 426
    syphilis, 320, 426–427
    toxoplasmosis, 427, 427b
    vaginal infections, 427–428
conidia, 164–165
conjugated proteins, 33
conjugation of genetic material, 125, 133, 170f, 462, 463f
conservation medicine, 282b
contaminants/contamination
    of culture media, 82, 87
    definition, 185, 197–198
    detection of food/water through DNA technology, 95b
    of food products, 236b
    organic, 354–355
    soil, 247–249, 251, 253, 427
contraceptive use, 299–300, 318b
controlled substances, 401–402
Controlled Substances Act, 401–402

control methods, 348t. *See also*
    antimicrobials; bioterrorism/
    bioweapons; laboratory aseptic
    techniques; natural disasters
  breakdown of, 335
  chemical control, 352–357, 355t
  choosing a method, 345, 347
  containment, 413, 413b
  death curves, 347f
  decontamination, 345, 452
  degermination, 83, 346, 346t
  detection of food/water contaminants,
    95b
  disinfection procedures (*See*
    disinfection/disinfectants)
  efficacy of, 345, 347, 353–354
  emerging/reemerging diseases/
    infections, 339
  for emerging/reemerging diseases/
    infections, 339
  food irradiation, 243b (*See also* food
    preservation)
  in healthcare settings, 197
  history of, 344b
  infectious disease control, 335, 453–454
  laboratory (*See* laboratory aseptic
    techniques)
  microbial death, 347
  microbicidal/microbiostatic agents, 347
  Nationally Notifiable Diseases, 337
  pasteurization, 8, 8b, 346, 357–358, 358b
  pharmacology-related, 401–402
  physical control, 347–352
    boiling water, 351
    desiccation and lyophilization, 351
    dry heat, 349–350
    filtration, 352, 352f
    membrane filters, 353t
    moist heat, 350–351
    osmotic pressure, 351
    radiation, 351–352
    refrigeration and freezing, 351
    steam sterilization, 350–351
    summary of, 348t
    temperature, 348–351
  refrigeration, 348, 348t, 351
  resistance of microbes, 345
  sanitization, 83, 95, 346
  sterile environment, 12 (*See also*
    sterilization methods)
  surveillance, 337–340
  terminology for, 346–347, 346t
  vector control, 339
coronaviruses, 152–153
corpses, health risks of, 446–447
cosmid vectors, 468
covalent bonds. *See under* chemical bonds
cowpox, 9, 152b
Coynebacterium diphtheriae, 225f
Cramer, Carl, 43t
crateriform appearance, 92
Creutzfeldt-Jakob diseases (CJD), 272
Crick, Francis, 71, 461b
cross-resistance (antimicrobial agents),
    412–413
cross-species infections, 229. *See also*
    zoonoses
cryophiles (psychrophiles), 122
cryptococcosis, 271

Cryptococcus neoformans, 203t
cryptosporidiosis, 144t
Cryptosporidium/cryptosporidiosis, 144t,
    252f, 454–455, 456t
culture media. *See under* laboratory
    testing/techniques
cutaneous candidiasis, 211t, 212–213
cyanobacteria, 440–441
cyclic photophosphorylation, 69f
cystitis, 298, 302t
cysts
  amoebic, 172
  Giardia lamblia, 171–172
  hydatid, 237t–239t
  protozoal, 169, 178, 251
  Toxoplasma gondii, 271, 428f
  Trypanosoma cruzi, 271
cytochemistry, 41b–42b
cytocidal (lytic) infections, 149
cytogenetics, 41b–42b
cytokines/cytokinesis, 74–75, 379, 379t,
    382
cytology, 41b–42b
cytomegalovirus (CMV), 143, 151,
    287–288, 288t, 303, 325b, 426t
  congenital, 426
  excretion of, 143, 151, 426t
cytopathic effects (CPEs), 149, 150t
cytoplasm, 56–57, 75–78. *See also*
    plasmids
cytoplasmic streaming, 174
cytoskeleton, 50–57, 51f
cytosol, 50–51
cytotoxic hypersensitivity, 383, 384t–385t

D

deamination, 93
dairy products
  bacteria in, 15b
  brucellosis in, 282
  mastitis in cows, 310b
  milk production, 474
  nonpathogenic microorganisms used in,
    14–15
  pasteurization, 8, 8b, 346, 357–358, 358b
  probiotics in, 184b
  unpasteurized, 128b
dark (light-independent) reactions, 70
Daschle, Tom, 449f
daughter cells, 73, 74f, 77f, 120, 170f
DCs (dendritic cells), 374, 375f
DDT (dichlorodiphenyltrichloroethane),
    159b–160b, 291b. *See also* safety issues
DEA (Drug Enforcement Agency),
    401–402
dead organisms, 201b, 347, 347f, 351–352,
    438, 440–441, 446–447
deamination ammonification process, 440
deaths. *See* mortality rates
decay/decomposition, 7, 12, 25, 165–166,
    201b, 438
decimal reduction time (DRT), 349
decontamination, 345, 346t
dccp folliculitis, 429
deep mycoses, 231
defense mechanisms. *See* host defense
    mechanisms
defensive enzymes, 412
degermination, 83, 346, 346t, 356

dehydration, 22b, 25, 25f, 154
delayed hypersensitivity (type IV), 385
demographics, 333–334, 333t. *See also*
    population (human); public health
denaturation, 33, 348t, 358b, 452, 467
dendritic cells (DCs), 374, 375f
dengue fever, 453
denitrification, 27b, 440
deoxyribonucleic acid. *See* DNA
    (deoxyribonucleic acid); DNA viruses
Department of Transportation (DOT),
    103–105
dermatitis, 384t–385t
dermatomes, 209, 209f
dermatophytes, 210
dermis, 202
descriptive epidemiology, 191–192
desiccation, 348t, 351
detection of emerging/reemerging
    infectious diseases, 339
Deuteromycota, 165–166
diabetes, 299–301, 474
  insulin production, 470–471, 474
  noninjectable insulin, 470b
  skin infections, 202
diagnosis of infections/diseases. *See specific
    infection or disease*
diarrhea. *See under* gastrointestinal (GI)
    tract
diatoms, 167–169, 169f
dichlorodiphenyltrichloroethane (DDT),
    159b–160b, 291b. *See also* safety issues
diffusion, 58–59, 59f
digestion process, 377–378. *See also*
    gastrointestinal (GI) tract
dikaryons, 165
dimorphism, 161
dioecious worms, 175
diphtheria, 219t, 224–225
diploid offspring, 75
direct contact transmission, 195
disaccharides, 31, 32f
disasters. *See* natural disasters
discovery of circulation, 41b–42b
diseases (in general). *See also specific
    infection or disease*
  causes of specific, 8–9, 118t, 237t–239t
  classification of, 192
  detection/surveillance for, 337, 339
  early concepts of, 391b–392b
  eradication of, 99b, 152
  incidence of, 197–198
    determining, 192
    morbidity rates, 192
    recurring urinary tract infections
      (UTIs), 304
  reemerging bacterial, 115b
  virulence/pathogenicity (*See* virulence
    and pathogenicity)
disease therapies, 471–472
disinfection/disinfectants, 83, 346t, 353
  evaluation of, 354, 354f, 359, 409–410,
    410f
  future concerns, 344b
  in laboratory settings, 83
  microbial control using, 346, 354
  microbial resistance to, 353
  procedures for, 82–83, 95, 346
  toxic compounds as, 83

disk diffusion test (Kirby-Bauer method), 354, 354f, 359, 409–410, 410f
dissolution rate of drugs, 395–396
dissolved (dissociated) solutes, 30f
distilled beverages, 15b
diuretics, 394
DNA (deoxyribonucleic acid), 32–33, 38, 42, 75–78, 467. *See also genetics-related entries*
  bacterial mutations, 73
  blunt end strands, 463–464, 463t
  central dogma of, 71, 71f
  chromatins, 52
  chromosomal, 133
  complementary (cDNA), 465f
  description, 37
  gene libraries, 474
  genetic code, 36–37, 466f
  inheritance testing, 54b
  mitochondrial DNA (mtDNA), 54, 54b
  mRNA made from, 32–33
  nuclear, 54b
  organism classification by, 95
  radiation damage to, 351–352
  recombinant, 15, 170f, 461–462, 461b, 466, 469t, 471, 474
  replication, 74f, 120
  ribosomal (rDNA), 95
  single-stranded (ssDNA), 137–140
  sticky end strands, 463–464, 464t
  structural characteristics/arrangements, 37f
  synthesis of, 72–73, 466–467
  transcription of, 71f
  transduction of, 125, 133
  transformation of, 125, 133, 462, 462f
  translation of, 71f, 72
  vaccine development, 472, 474
  vector molecules, 467
DNA ligase, 463–464
DNA probes, 95
DNA tests, 328–329
DNA vector molecules, 467
DNA viruses, 143, 150–152
  adenoviruses, 150, 250
  classification of, 138b
  hepadnaviruses, 150–151
  herpesviruses, 151
  medically important, 139t–140t
  papillomaviruses and polyomaviruses, 151
  parvoviruses, 151
  placenta-crossing, 186t
  poxviruses, 151–152
Domagk, Gerhard, 405b
domains (life hierarchy), 9, 10f
donor bacteria, 462
donor cells, 125
donovanosis (granuloma inguinale), 323–328, 324t
DOT (Department of Transportation), 103–105
droplet transmission, 195
DRT (decimal reduction time), 349
drug absorption, 394–396
  absorption time (latency), 399
  blood flow and, 395–396
  cellular, 47
  cellular/extracellular, 395

drug absorption (*Continued*)
  effective concentration, 399
  effect of circadian rhythm on, 399
drug abuse, 333
drug actions
  adverse effects/drug interactions, 393b, 409
  biotransformation, 394, 396, 402
  clearance (excretion, elimination), 394, 399
  distribution, 396
  time of, 408–409
drug administration methods, 394–395, 394t
  dosage, 19b–20b, 397
  dose effects, 397–398
  drug losses at sites of, 394t
  enteral route, 394, 394t
  local routes, 394f
  oral route, 394–395
  parenteral route, 394, 394t
  risk assessment for, 420–421
  on the skin, 394
  systemic, 394–395, 395f
  time-response curve, 398f
drug categories/nomenclature, 393, 393t
  chemical, 393
  generic, 393
  nonprescription/prescription categories, 393
  proprietary (trade, brand) name, 393
  therapeutic class, 393
drug development, 362b–363b, 400–402, 401b
  antimicrobials, 420–421
  information required for approval of, 400–401
  monitoring, 402b
  public safety issues, 401–402
drug efficacy
  antimicrobial agents, 408–410, 420–421
  dilution/minimal inhibitory concentration method, 410, 410f
  disk diffusion test (Kirby-Bauer method), 409–410
  formal testing of, 359
  response categories (*See* drug response categories)
  serum killing power, 410
  tests to determine, 409
Drug Enforcement Agency (DEA), 401–402
drug-receptor interactions, 25
drug resistance, 197, 262, 264, 332b, 335, 411–413, 412f, 413b, 420–421. *See also* microbial resistance
  biofilms and, 50b
  cause of, 405b, 413b
  development/acquisition of, 411
  drug-resistant *Streptococcus pneumoniae* (DRSP), 219t, 221b, 222
  in healthcare settings, 197
  mechanisms of, 411–412
  microorganisms not subject to, 409
  MRSA (methicillin-resistant *Staphylococcus aureus*) infections, 111b, 413b
  multidrug-resistant pathogens, 224b, 405b, 411–413

drug resistance (*Continued*)
  multiple antimicrobial resistance (MAR), 412–413
  National Antimicrobial Resistance Monitoring System (NARMS), 391b–392b
  overuse of antibiotics, 413b
  prevention guidelines, 301, 413
  Salmonella strains, 244
  sexually transmitted infections, 318b
  use of antimicrobial soaps/lotions, 201b
drug response categories, 397–400, 402
  biological variations in, 398f
  dose effects, 397–398
  therapeutic index, 397–398
  time effects, 398–399
  toxicity, 399–400
  variability, 399
drugs. *See also* pharmaceutical agents; pharmacology
  antimicrobial (*See* antimicrobials)
  biotransformation of, 394, 396, 396t–397t, 402
  biotransport of, 395
  cellular absorption of, 395
  chemical, 393
  chemical names of, 393t
  chemical properties of, 399
  distribution of (systemic), 396
  information required for approval of, 400–401
  lipid solubility of, 395–396
  PDR (*Physician's Desk Reference*), 394b
  postmarketing monitoring, 402b
  public safety issues, 401–402
  side effects, 400–401, 410–411, 416, 420–421
  site of action (SOA) of, 398
drugs of choice
  for gastrointestinal (GI) tract infections, 392t
  for organ systems, 392t
  prostatitis, 313
  protozoal infections, 170t
drug toxicity, 399–400, 402
  classification of, 399
  human toxicity from animal values, 400t
  selective, 408
  therapeutic index (drug safety), 397f
  treatment for, 400t
dyes, composition of, 28
dysentery, 13t, 245

E

E. coli. See Escherichia coli
ears/ear infections
  congenital disorders, 426
  ear anatomy, 263f
  meningitis-related loss of hearing, 262
  otitis media, 262, 429–430
earthquakes, 447–448, 448t
Ebola virus, 334, 453, 454f
EBV (Epstein-Barr virus), 151, 287–288, 288b, 371t, 426t, 430
ECF (extracellular fluid), 42, 57–58, 58f, 75–78
echinocandins, 418
echinulate growth, 92

ecological changes, 334. *See also* microbial ecology
ecosystems, 437–438, 437f
efficacy
  of control methods (*See under* control methods)
  of drugs (*See* drug efficacy)
effuse growth, 92
egg fertilization, 75
EHEC (enterohemorrhagic *E. coli*), 128b
Ehrlich, Paul, 391b–392b
ehrlichiosis, 284t, 286, 287t
elderly. *See* older adults/elderly
electric fields, 22
electricity, 16, 28
electrolytes, 22, 22b, 28, 35–36, 57–58
electron (orbital) clouds, 20
electron micrographs, 7
electrons, 20–21, 21f, 23f, 24–26
electron transfer reactions, 26f, 69–70
electron transport chain, 26, 64, 66–68, 67f
electrostatic forces, 62
elements, 19b–20b, 20, 20t
elimination/excretion of drugs, 394, 399, 402, 412
ELISA test, 325–326, 453–454, 457
embryos/fetuses. *See* pregnancy
emergencies/emergency response systems, 111. *See also* bioterrorism/ bioweapons; control methods
  for bioterror agents, 457
  CDC, 457
  first responder roles, 457–458
  laboratory safety issues, 111
  Material Safety Data Sheet (MSDS), 106f
  microbial control methods (*See* control methods)
  newly emerging known diseases, 336
  OSHA, 111, 457
  procedures for, 112
  severe malaria, 291
  smallpox outbreaks, 210
  Web sites, 457
emerging/reemerging diseases/infections
  antigenic drift, 335b
  avian influenza, 337b
  bacterial, 115b, 338t
  CDC guidelines for protection/ prevention, 340
  detection of, 339
  factors of, 340–341
    bioterrorism/biowarfare, 335
    breakdown of public health measures, 335
    climate/weather/natural disasters, 335
    ecological changes/agricultural development, 334
    human demographics and behavior, 333–334, 333t
    human susceptibility to infection, 335
    international travel/commerce, 334
    introduction of pathogens (adoption), 333
    microbial adaptation/change, 335
    poverty, 335
    urban/rural populations, 333f
    war/famine, 335

emerging/reemerging diseases/infections (*Continued*)
  fungal, 339t
  global concerns, 339–340
    ease of transport, 334b
    geographic distribution of malaria, 336f
    global surveillance, 340
    prevention/protection, 340
    spread of HIV, 336f
    U.S. global public health, 340
  groups of, 340–341
  history of, 332b
  introduction of known agents to new areas, 336
  mosquito bites and, 337b
  Nationally Notifiable Diseases, 337
  newly emerging known diseases, 336
  old diseases, 336
  overview/definitions, 332
  pathogen groups, 337
  prevention/response to, 337–341
  protozoan, 339t
  reemerging old diseases, 336
  steps involved in, 340–341
  study of, 289b
  surveillance for, 339
  swine flu, 337b
  tuberculosis, 223
  types of, 336–337
  viral, 337b, 338t
emulsifying agents, 35b
encephalitis, 272–273
  arboviral, 269–271
  description, 406
  Eastern/Western equine encephalitis (EEE), 270
  West Nile virus, 270
endemic infections, 159b–160b, 192, 229b, 233
endergonic/exergonic reactions, 25
endocarditis, 277–278, 282–283, 293
endocardium, 277
endocrine system, 392t. *See also* hormones
endocytosis, 60, 61f, 147
endoenzymes, 62
endogenous infections, 196, 308
endometritis, 310, 312t
endonuclease, 463
endoplasmic reticulum (ER), 52, 53f, 55–57
endospores, 8–9, 356
endotoxins, 43, 188–189, 189f, 190t
endotoxin shock, 44b
end-product inhibition, 63–64
energy, 16, 35, 61, 68–69, 118–120
energy transfers, 38
Entamoeba histolytica (amebiasis), 172, 252
enteral administration of drugs, 394
enteric fever, 203t, 245
Enterobacteriaceae (enteric) bacteria, 93, 127
Enterobius vermicularis (pinworms/ seatworms), 176, 253, 253f
enteroviruses, 154
environmental health issues, 99b. *See also* public health; safety issues
environmental microbiology. *See* microbial ecology

Environmental Protection Agency (EPA), 129b, 354, 359, 438
environment(s). *See also* temperature (of environment)
  acidic, 358
  aquatic, 442–443
  differences in conditions in, 437
  effects on antimicrobial effectiveness of, 353
  exposures in, 431
  for fungi, 161
  individual responses to, 19b–20b
  of infants/children, 433
  laboratory, 82
  microbes in, 12
  new teachers effect, 430b
  normal conditions of, 437
  normal microorganisms in, 345
  pH changes in, 28
  for protozoa, 171
  relationship between genotypes, phenotypes and, 124
  separation of cells from external, 57
  soil, 441–442
  solute concentrations in, 30
  temperature of, 348
  uses for biofilms, 50
  for yeast infections, 311b
  of young adults, 431
enzyme-linked immunosorbent assay (ELISA) test, 325–326, 453–454, 457
enzymes, 61–64, 75–78. *See also metabolism* entries
  allosteric site of, 63–64
  bacterial production of, 122
  clot dissolving actions of, 190b
  cofactors/coenzymes, 63
  concentration of, 63
  defensive, 412
  DNA ligase, 463–464
  hemolysins, 91–92
  holoenzymes, 63f
  inhibition, 64f, 412
  mechanism for chemical reaction, 62f
  oxidative, 54
  regulation of, 63–64
  restriction, 95, 463b, 463t–464t, 464f
  RNA polymerase, 71
  structure and, 62f
  temperature and, 63
enzyme specificity, 62
eosinophils, 373
epidemics/pandemics, 192. *See also* outbreaks
  after floods, 445
  alerts/responses to, 341t
  antibiotic resistance and, 147b
  avian influenza, 229b, 337b
  cholera, 13–14, 236b, 249b
  detection of, 339
  global concerns, 334b
  HIV, 324
  H1N1 influenza, 337b
  influenza, 2b–3b, 153, 153t, 159b–160b
  leptospirosis, 446
  plague, 332b
  polio, 257b
  potential, 145b

epidemics/pandemics (*Continued*)
   respiratory tract infections, 233
   typhus, 286
epidemiology, 191–195, 249b. *See also*
      global concerns; public health
   adenoviruses, 250
   definition, 191–192, 197–198
   diseases in populations, 192
   modes of transmission, 194–195
   nosocomial infections, 196–197
   reservoirs, 192–194
epidermis, 183f, 185, 202, 375f
epididymitis, 313–314, 315t
episomes, 124
epithelial cells, 49
epitopes, 364, 364f
Epstein-Barr virus (EBV), 151, 287–288,
      288b, 371t, 426t, 430
equine encephalitises, 454–455
equipment safety, 105–108, 112
ER (endoplasmic reticulum), 52, 53f, 55–57
eradication of diseases, 99b, 152, 159b–
      160b, 181b, 206b
Ereky, Karl, 461b
ergosterol, 36b, 161–162
ergosterol inhibitors, 36b
ergotism, 251, 257b
erysipelas, 204–205, 205f, 207t
erythroblastosis fetalis (hemolytic disease),
      366, 366b
erythropoiesis, 372, 472b
erythropoietin (EPO), 472
Escherichia coli (*E. coli*), 13t, 116f, 246, 298,
      301b, 348t, 429, 454–455, 463
   enterohemorrhagic *E. coli* (EHEC), 128b
   gastrointestinal (GI) tract, 246
   lambda phage vectors and, 468
   prevention, 247b
   statistics on infections from, 247b
ethanol production, 16
ethylene oxide (ETO), 356–357
etiology of infectious diseases, 189–191,
      197–198. *See also* causative agents/
      organisms
Euglenozoa, 172
eukaryotes, 9–11, 10f, 42, 57, 75–78
   algae (*See* algae)
   cell cycle phases, 74–75
   chromosomes in, 37–38, 75
   cytoskeleton of, 51, 51f
   division process of, 73
   endomembrane system, 52
   flagella, 49f
   fungi (*See* fungi)
   metabolism of, 64
   Penicillium, 166f
   photosynthesis in, 68f
   phylogenetic tree, 161f
   plasma membranes, 44f
   prokaryotes compared to, 10, 43t, 52
   protozoa (*See* protozoa)
   ribosomes in, 55–56
   slime molds (*See* molds)
   structure of, 42–57
   surface appendages, 47t
   toxicity of, 289
   toxin-producing bacteria that damage,
      57t
   vacuoles, 56–57

eutrophication, 441
evaporation, 29b
evolution, 9, 75, 161f, 332b, 335
exchange reactions, 26
excretion of drugs, 394
exocytosis, 60–61, 61f
exoenzymes, 62
exogenous infections, 196
exotoxins, 188, 189f, 189t–190t, 264
experimental epidemiology, 191–192
extermophiles, 84b
extracellular fluid (ECF), 42, 57–58, 58f,
      75–78
extreme thermophiles, 132–133
eyes/eye infections
   anatomy, 267f
   causes of blindness, 267
   congenital disorders, 426
   conjunctivitis (pink eye), 183–185, 267,
      429
   normal flora of, 184t
   protection of, 107, 108f, 110, 110f
   rabies infection with corneal transplants,
      269
   silver nitrate treatment of newborns,
      356

F

facilitated diffusion, 58
factor VIII (FVIII), 470–471
facultative halophiles, 122
family. *See under* kingdoms of life
fatal familial insomnia, 272
fats, 34–35, 34f
fat (adipose) tissue, 58, 202
fatty acids, 34, 376. *See also* fats; lipids
FDA. *See* Food and Drug Administration
      (FDA)
fecal bacteria, 128b–129b, 446
fecal-oral route of transmission, 176, 177b,
      249–252, 268
Federal Food, Drug and Cosmetic Act, 401
FEMA (Federal Emergency Management
      Agency), 457
females. *See also* pregnancy; reproductive
      tract infections (RTIs); sexually
      transmitted infections (STIs); urinary
      tract infections (UTIs)
   anatomy, 300f, 309f, 314–315
   hormonal changes, 311b
   mastitis, 307b, 310, 312t
   trichomoniasis treatment in pregnant
      women, 427–428
fermentation, 7, 14–15, 64, 75–78
   discovery of, 461b
   end products, 68
   enzyme action in, 190b
   ethanol production during, 16
   hydrogen production, 16
   process of, 67–68
   yeast, 15
fertilization of eggs, 75
fetuses. *See* pregnancy
fever (pyrexia), 379, 379b, 431
fibronectin, 382
filiform growth, 92
Filoviridae, 453, 455t
filtration (biological), 59, 297, 371. *See also*
      lymphatic entries

filtration (mechanical), 136b, 352, 352f,
      353t
fimbriae (pili), 47–48, 47t, 49f, 75–78
first-pass effect, 399
fission. *See* binary fission
flagella, 47t, 75–78
   amphitrichous, 47–48, 48f
   bacterial, 47–48, 48f
   eukaryote, 49f
   of gram-negative bacteria, 47f
   hemoflagellates, 172
   lophotrichous/monotrichous, 48f
   parts of, 47
   peritrichous, 48f
   of prokaryotic cells, 48
   protozoal, 172
   types of, 47–48
flagellar staining, 89
flaviviruses, 155, 453–454, 455t
Fleming, Alexander, 15, 332b, 400, 405b
flesh eating bacteria, 203, 205, 205b, 207t
floods, 13–14, 165b, 445–447, 446t. *See also*
      natural disasters
flora. *See* normal flora
Florey, H. W., 405b
flu, stomach. *See* gastrointestinal (GI) tract
      infections; influenza
flucytosine, 418
fluid compartments, 42, 57–61
fluid-mosaic membrane structure, 42–43
flukes (trematodes), 176, 176f, 253f
fluoroquinolones (quinolones), 414, 415t
focal infections, 190
folate synthesis, 63b
folic acid, 63b
folliculitis, 203–204, 207t
fomite transmission, 82, 195–196, 207, 210,
      212
food allergies, 383, 383t
Food and Drug Administration (FDA),
      334, 382b, 391b–392b, 401. *See also*
      U.S. Department of Agriculture
      (USDA)
   Botox, 266b
   disinfectant efficacy, 354
   drug efficacy testing, 359
   genetically engineered drugs, 472
   listeriosis testing, 247
   use of antibiotics with livestock, 413b
   vaccine for tularemia, 452
foodborne diseases/infections. *See also*
      gastrointestinal (GI) tract; main
      entries for specific infections
   after natural disasters, 447–448
   animal-related, 335
   aspergillosis, 251
   bacterial food intoxications, 247–249,
      254
      Bacillus, 248–249
      botulism, 247
      cholera, 249
      food poisoning, 357, 456t
      imported foods/vector hitchhikers,
         334
      shellfish poisoning, 166
      staphylococcal intoxication, 248
   cholera, 249
   cryptosporidiosis, 252
   description, 12–13

foodborne diseases/infections (*Continued*)
  gastroenteritis, 243
  listeriosis, 247, 262–264
  organisms responsible for, 248t
  prevention of, 12–13
  psittacosis, 225–226
  raw milk products, 358b
  salmonellosis, 244
  shigellosis, 245–246
  staphylococcal, 248, 248f, 455
  symptoms of infections, 13t
  toxoplasmosis, 292, 427
  tracing outbreaks, 16, 357t
  transmissible spongiform
      encephalopathies/prion diseases
      (TSEs), 257b
  transmission of, 195, 253
  from unpasteurized dairy products, 128b
  yersiniosis, 246
food preservation, 357–359
  first understanding of spoilage, 344b
  irradiation, 243b, 358
  pasteurization, 8, 8b, 346, 357–358, 358b
  storage methods, 191, 358–359
food products/production. *See also*
      fermentation
  additives, 36b
  alcoholic beverages, 14–15, 15b
  bread molds, 165–166
  commercial sterilization, 346
  contamination of, 236b, 455
  irradiation of, 236b, 243b
  Pure Food and Drug Act, 401
  spoilage, 165–166
  use of microorganisms in, 14–15, 14b
forensics, 16, 54b
fossilized microbes, 9
four humors, 19b–20b
free-living nitrogen fixing bacteria,
      438–439
freezing for microbial control, 351
freshwater environments. *See under* aquatic
      microbiology
fuel sources, 16
fume hoods, 106–107
functional groups, 23, 23t
fungal infections/diseases, 231–233. *See
      also* antifungals; main entries for
      specific infections
  circulatory system, 289
  disease-causing organisms (summary),
      237t–239t
  emerging/reemerging, 339t
  fungal endocarditis, 278, 293
  gastrointestinal (GI) tract, 250–251
  meningitis, 165–166
  mycoses (fungal skin infections), 164,
      213–214, 254
    chromoblastomycoses, 213
    cutaneous candidiasis, 212–213
    deep, 231
    description, 210
    manifestations of, 203t
    mycetomas, 213
    sporotrichosis, 213
    subcutaneous, 213–214
    superficial/deep, 163b
    systemic, 289, 289t
    Tinea species, 210–212, 211t

fungal infections/diseases (*Continued*)
  nervous system, 271–273
  nosocomial, 304
  opportunistic, 162t, 271, 311b, 325b
  pulmonary aspergillosis, 232–233
  reproductive tract, 311, 312t, 314–315,
      315t
  respiratory tract, 231–233, 231t
  sexually transmitted, 328
  skin, 210–213
  transmission of, 162t, 339t
  urinary tract infections (UTIs), 304
  vaginal, 428
  yeast, 312t
    Candida albicans (candidiasis), 163b,
        212–213, 250–251, 251f, 298,
        311, 312t, 314–315, 325b, 425t
      environment(s) for, 311b
      in males, 314, 315t
  zoonotic, 194t
fungal spores, 356
fungi, 11, 160–166
  beneficial actions of, 190b
  cell walls, 46, 161–162
  characteristics of, 161–164, 163f
  classification of, 164–166
  dimorphic, 163–164
  disease-causing, 163b
  existence types, 163f
  habitats, 210
  hyphae, 161
  life cycle of, 164–165
  molds/slime molds (*See* molds)
  morphologic groups, 161
  mycorrhizae, 160–161
  portals of entry for, 293
  reproduction, 165–166
  reproduction methods, 164–165, 164f
  resistance to osmotic pressure, 161
  in soil, 441
  symbiotic relationships of, 440
  yeasts, 14, 161–165
    characteristics of, 162–163
    fermentation, 15
    in humans, 165–166
    opportunistic, 314
    reproduction methods, 163f
    START, 74–75
fungicides, 353, 356, 473
fungus balls (aspergilloma), 232–233
furuncles (boils), 203–204, 207t
future concerns
  aging process, 461b
  bacterial infectious diseases, 115b
  bioterrorism, 436b–437b
  bloodborne diseases, 276b
  climate change/natural disaster
      management, 436b–437b
  disinfection techniques, 344b
  embryonic stem cells, 41b–42b
  emerging/reemerging infectious diseases,
      332b
  endemic diseases, 159b–160b
  gastrointestinal (GI) tract infections,
      236b
  laboratory techniques, 81b
  pharmacology, 391b–392b
  prion-related diseases, 257b
  progenitor pluripotent cells, 41b–42b

future concerns (*Continued*)
  reproductive tract infections, 307b
  safety issues, 99b
  Semmelweiss reflex, 201b
  spread of disease, 181b
  technology and chemistry, 19b–20b
  urinary tract infections (UTIs), 297b
  uses/prevention of viruses, 136b
  vaccines/immune system, 362b–363b
  viral respiratory infections, 217b

G
Galen, 19b–20b
galenicals, 19b–20b
GALT (gut-associated lymphoid tissue),
      368
gametes, 75
gametocytes, 290–291
gangrene, 205b, 280t, 281, 281f, 293
gastrointestinal (GI) tract, 237–243. *See
      also* foodborne diseases/infections;
      waterborne diseases/infections
  components of, 240b
  enteral administration of drugs, 394
  intestines, 240, 240b
    absorption of materials from, 49f
    large, 240
    lymphoid (lymphatic) tissue, 369f
    normal flora, 93
    parasites, 171b
    small, 240
  microbial growth in, 237–239
  mucous membrane of, 183f
  normal flora of, 184t
  overview of, 241f
  as portal of entry, 183–185
  stomach, 240
gastrointestinal (GI) tract infections. *See
      also* foodborne diseases/infections;
      gastrointestinal (GI) tract infections;
      main entries for specific infections or
      agents
  bacterial, 244–247
    campylobacteriosis, 246
    Escherichia (E. coli), 128b, 246
    gonorrhea of rectum, 319
    Helicobacter (peptic ulcers), 123b, 240,
        244
    listeriosis, 247
    salmonellosis, 244
    shigellosis, 245–246
    typhoid fever, 244–245
    yersiniosis, 246
  bacterial food intoxications (*See under*
      foodborne diseases/infections)
  from contact with dead humans/
      animals, 446–447
  diarrhea, 410
    Bacillus cereus, 248–249
    campylobacteriosis, 246
    cryptosporidiosis, 252
    giardiasis, 251
    Vibrio cholera, 249
    viral causes, 154
  disease-causing organisms (summary),
      237t–239t
  drugs used for, 392t
  E. coli strains, 246
  enteric fever, 203t, 245

gastrointestinal (GI) tract infections
(*Continued*)
enterobacteriaceae (enteric) bacteria, 93,
127
enteroviruses, 154
fungal infections, 250–251
gastroenteritis, 13t, 242–243, 254
helminths, 252–254
history of diseases of, 236b
oral cavity infections related to, 240–242
parasitic, 171b, 251–254
protozoal, 26, 144t, 170t, 172, 251–252
transmission of, 254
viral infections, 249–250
gated channels, 58
gelatinase, 92
gelatin stabs, 92, 93f
gender, 58, 399. *See also* females; males
gene libraries, 464–466, 465f, 474
generic drugs, 393
generic names of drugs, 393, 393t
genes, 124, 365
genetic analysis, 2b–3b, 37–38, 75, 75f, 95,
120, 124
genetic defects, 387
genetic diversity, 75
genetic drug resistance, 411
genetic engineering, 14, 462–467, 472b, 474
genetic markers, 467–468
genetic material, 125, 133, 137–140, 170f,
462, 463f. *See also* DNA
(deoxyribonucleic acid); RNA
(ribonucleic acid)
genetic predisposition, 241, 383
genetics, 124–125
effects of drug absorption on, 399
genetic transfer in prokaryotes, 125
genotypes/phenotypes, 124
mutations, 124–125
genetic sensors, 95b
gene transfers, 184b
genitals. *See* reproductive tract infections
(RTIs); sexually transmitted infections
(STIs)
genome changes, 148
genomes
bacteriophage, 144t
influenza, 229
mitochondrial, 54
sequencing of, 95
virus, 143–145 (*See also* DNA viruses;
RNA viruses)
genomic libraries, 464
genotoxic effects, 150
genotypes, 95, 124, 126
genus. *See under* kingdoms of life
German measles (rubella), 154, 186t, 207,
426, 429–430
germicidal agents. *See* antimicrobials
germ theory of disease, 2b–3b, 8–9, 81b,
115b, 190–191, 201b, 217b, 249b,
391b–392b
Gerstmann-Sträussler-Scheinker syndrome
(GSSS), 272
gestation. *See* pregnancy
Giardia lamblia/giardiasis, 13t, 171–172,
171b, 171f, 251
gingivitis, 240–241
GI tract. *See* gastrointestinal (GI) tract

glaciers, 9b
glanders, 454–455, 456t
Global Alliance for Vaccines and
Immunization, 250
global concerns for infectious diseases,
339–340. *See also* bioterrorism/
bioweapons; emerging/reemerging
diseases/infections; natural disasters;
public health
antimicrobial drug resistance, 413b,
420–421
bacterial pneumonia, 221
brucellosis, 282
ease of transport, 334b
geographic distribution of malaria, 336f
global surveillance, 340
HIV/AIDS, 318b
immune system response to infections/
diseases, 362b–363b
prevention of reproductive tract
infections, 307b
prevention/protection, 340
reproductive tract infections, 308
severe acute respiratory syndrome
(SARS), 230
sexually transmitted infections, 329
spread of HIV, 336f
tuberculosis, 224b
U.S. global public health, 340
glomerulonephritis (Bright's disease), 299
glucocorticoids, 35–36
glucose, 65f, 67. *See also* carbohydrates
(sugars)
aerobic cellular respiration per, 67t
breakdown of, 67
formation of/conversion to, 70f
glycocalyx, 43–44, 45f
glycolysis, 64–66, 65f, 68f
glycoproteins, 33
Golgi, Camillo, 43t
Golgi apparatus (or complex), 52, 53f, 57,
61f
gonorrhea, 318b–319b, 319–320, 320f,
324t, 356, 430
gram-negative bacteria, 44b, 45–46, 46b,
46f, 129, 432
aerobic/microaerophilic helical vibroid,
126, 127t
aerobic rods and cocci, 126–127, 127f,
127t
anaerobic rods and cocci, 123t, 127–129,
128f, 128t
endospore-forming, 131
flagella of, 47f
gram-positive bacteria, 45, 130t
cocci (sphere-shaped), 130–131,
130t–131t
endospore-forming, 131, 131t
irregular nonsporulating rods, 131
regular nonsporulating rods, 131
Gram stain technique, 45, 75–78, 88–89,
89b, 89f, 451
granulocytes (neutrophils), 372–374, 374f
granuloma inguinale (donovanosis),
323–328, 324t
Graves' disease (Graves' hyperthyroidism),
386–387, 386t
greenhouse gases, 9b
griseofulvin, 418

growth conditions (microbial). *See*
microbial growth
guilds, 437
gut-associated lymphoid tissue (GALT),
368

H

habitats, 210, 437–438, 437f, 441
Haemophilus influenzae. See under
influenza
Haemophilus pneumoniae. See under
pneumonias
HAGs (harmful algal blooms), 167b
HAIs. *See* nosocomial/iatrogenic infections
halogens, 355t
halophiles, 122, 125, 133
hand-borne diseases, 35b, 100b, 201b
hand washing, 332b
first practice of, 8, 100b
guidelines for, 101b
nosocomial infections and, 197
soap, 35b
Hansen's disease. *See* leprosy
hantavirus pulmonary syndrome (HPS),
230, 339, 456–457, 457t
haploid cells, 165
haploid gametes, 75
haptens, 364–365, 365f
harmful algal blooms (HAGs), 167b
Harvey, William, 276b, 391b–392b
Hashimoto's thyroiditis, 386t
hay fever (allergic rhinitis), 383t
Hazard Analysis and Critical Control
Points program, 243b
hazardous materials/compounds, 15, 108,
109f, 355
Health and Human Services (HHS), 99b,
427, 430b
health care facilities. *See also* nosocomial/
iatrogenic infections
bloodborne pathogens in, 111t
emergency response procedures, 457
hospitals, 110
nursing homes/personal care facilities,
110–111
physician's offices/clinics, 110
safety issues, 110–111, 111b, 111t
types of, 110
hearing. *See* ears/ear infections
heart/heart diseases. *See* cardiovascular
system; circulatory system
heat-resistant bacterial endospores, 8
heat stability, 188–189
heat sterilization. *See under* sterilization
methods
heavy metals, 355t, 400b
helical viruses, 137–140
helicase enzyme, 72–73
Helicobacter (peptic ulcers), 123b, 240,
242f, 244
helium, 21
helminths/helminthic infections, 174–178,
252–254. *See also* antihelminthics;
main entries for specific helminths or
infections
cestodes (tapeworms), 176, 177f
characteristics of, 175
classification of, 176–178
cystitis, 298

helminths/helminthic infections
    (*Continued*)
    description, 252, 254
    dioecious worms, 175
    disease-causing organisms (summary),
        237t–239t
    hermaphroditic (monoecious) worms,
        176
    life cycle of, 175–176
    necators (hookworms), 176, 177f,
        253–254
    nematodes (roundworms), 177–178,
        253–254, 441
    nervous system, 272–273
    platyhelminths, 176
    portals of entry for, 185
    taeniasis, 253
    trematodes (flukes), 176, 176f, 253f
    zoonotic, 194t
helper T cells, 324, 380
hematuria, 304
hemocytoblasts, 372
hemoflagellates, 172
hemolytic diseases, 128b, 247b, 366, 366b,
    384t–385t
hemophilia, 470–471
hemopoiesis processes, 372
hemorrhagic cystitis, 303–304
hemorrhagic fevers. *See* viral hemorrhagic
    fevers (VHFs) *under* viral infections/
    diseases
hepadnaviruses, 150–151
hepatitis infections, 13t, 111t, 149, 153t,
    155, 250, 325b, 326–327, 425t, 430
hepatocytes, 379–380
herbicide tolerance/resistance, 473
hermaphroditic (monoecious) worms, 176
herpes viruses, 151, 209, 287, 325b
    antiviral agents for, 327
    herpes simplex virus (HSV), 150t, 151,
        208–209, 209f, 327, 426t, 429–430
    neonatal infections, 327
    varicella-zoster virus (VZV)
        chickenpox, 151, 207, 208t, 209,
            429–430
        shingles, 207, 208t, 209, 209f
heterocysts, 438
heterolactic fermentative bacteria, 68f
heterotrophs, 121–122, 161
hexose monophosphate shunt. *See*
    phosphogluconate pathway
HHS. *See* Health and Human Services
    (HHS)
HICPAC (Hospital Infection Control
    Practices Advisory Committee), 100
Hippocrates, 19b–20b, 159b–160b, 217b,
    297b
histamines, 383. *See also* allergy/
    hypersensitivity reactions
Histoplasmosis capsulatum, 231, 231f, 325b
HIV, 150t, 324–326, 387, 430. *See also*
    AIDS
    congenital infections, 427
    global spread of, 336f
    mothers with, 427b
    spread of, 276b
    stages of infection, 326t
    transmission of, 427
    tuberculosis and, 223

hives, 383t
HIV-PCR (HIV polymerase chain
    reaction), 325–326
HIV polymerase chain reaction (HIV-
    PCR), 325–326
H1N1 (swine flu), 337b
Holmes, Oliver Wendell, 8, 100b
holoenzymes, 63, 63f
homeostasis, 57, 297
Hong Kong flu, 153t
Hooke, Robert, 2b–3b, 3, 5t, 41b–42b, 42,
    43t
hookworms (necators), 176, 177f, 253–254
hopanoids, 43
hormones
    denatured, 33
    endocrine system, 392t
    female, 311b
    growth deficiencies, 470
    human growth hormone (HGH), 470
    reproductive system, 307b
    synthesis of steroid, 36
hormone therapy, 424b
hospice care, 111–112
Hospital Infection Control Practices
    Advisory Committee (HICPAC), 100
host cells
    damage to, 149–150
        biochemical effects, 150
        genotoxic effects, 150
        morphological effects, 149–150
        physiological effects, 150
    machinery/metabolism of, 145
    for viruses, 145, 416
host defense mechanisms, 388, 409. *See
    also* immune system response;
    immunity
    antimicrobial agents for assisting, 409
    blood-brain barrier, 272–273, 368, 406,
        408
    complements/aids in, 409
    evasion of, 187
    first line of defense, 376–377
    of gastrointestinal tract, 236b
    host-antibody response, 452–453
    innate defense mechanisms, 375–376
    levels of, 376f
    of reproductive tract, 307–308
    of respiratory tract, 217–219
    second line of defense, 377–380
        complement system, 379–380
        cytokines, 379
        fever, 379
        inflammatory response, 378–379
        interferons, 379
        phagocytosis and phagocytes,
            377–378
    skin/integumentary system, 213–214,
        376
    third line of defense, 380–383
        active immunity (humoral), 381–382
        antibody-mediated immunity,
            380–381
        cell-mediated immunity, 380
        passive immunity, 382–383
    tonsils, 368
host-microbe relationships, 182–185,
    197–198
host range, 147, 147b

host receptors, 187t
hosts
    animal, 292
    dead end, 175f
    definitive, 175
    human, 176, 177b
    intermediate, 175, 289
    parasitic, 175–176
HPS. *See* hantavirus pulmonary syndrome
    (HPS)
HPV. *See* human papillomavirus (HPV)
HSV. *See under* herpes viruses
Human Genome Project, 468–470
human medical technology, 468–472
    disease therapies, 471–472
    factor VIII (FVIII), 470–471
    human growth hormone (HGH), 470
    human protein replacements, 468–471
    insulin, 470
    recombinant DNA products, 469t
    vaccines (*See* vaccine-related entries)
human papillomavirus (HPV), 207, 307b,
    327, 327b, 430
human prion diseases. *See* transmissible
    spongiform encephalopathies/prion
    diseases (TSEs)
human protein replacements, 468–471
humans
    age of (*See* aging process/human life
        stages)
    demographics, 333t (*See also* population
        (human))
    effects of behavior of, 333–334, 333t, 339
    susceptibility to infection, 335
humors, body, 276b
hurricanes, 165b, 448
HUS (hemolytic uremic syndrome), 128b,
    247b
hybrid vectors, 468
hydration spheres, 31f
hydrocarbon backbone, 30–31
hydrogen, 16, 21–22, 22f, 28f
hydrogen atoms, 21f
hydrogen bonds, 23–25, 29
hydrogen peroxide, 26b
hydrogen sulfide production, 93
hydrolases, 62
hydrolysis, 7, 12, 25, 25f, 201b, 438
hydrostatic pressure, 59, 122–123
hydrothermal vents, 444
hypersaline environments, 133
hypersensitivity. *See* allergy/
    hypersensitivity reactions
hypertonic environment, 30, 59
hyphae, 163, 164f, 165–166
hypodermis, 202
hypotonic environment, 30, 31f

I

iatrogenic infections. *See* nosocomial/
    iatrogenic infections
ICF (intracellular fluid), 42, 57–58, 58f,
    75–78
icosahedral viruses, 137, 140–141, 142f
identification. *See* morphology/
    morphological identification;
    taxonomy
identification of cells. *See* morphology/
    morphological identification

identification of microbes. *See* laboratory testing/techniques; morphology/morphological identification

IDLH list of chemical concentrations, 103–105

IEIP (International Emerging Infections Program), 340

IHR (International Health Regulations), 340

immune response, 50b, 94–95, 236b, 280–281. *See also* allergens; allergy/hypersensitivity reactions; vaccinations

immune senescence, 431

immune system response, 383–387. *See also main entries for specific infections/disorders*

  allergies/hypersensitivity (*See* allergy/hypersensitivity reactions)

  antibodies, 50b, 94–95, 366–368, 429

  antigen-antibody response, 94–95

  antigenic shift/drift, 335b

  antigenic stimulation, 429

  autoimmune diseases (*See* autoimmune diseases)

  cells of, 372–375

  compromised/suppressed immune system, 12–13, 271, 304, 364

    cat-scratch fever, 283

    HIV/AIDS patients, 326

    leprosy infections, 206

    opportunistic pathogens and, 183–185

    protozoal infections, 169, 172

    Salmonella in, 245b

    skin infections, 202

    systemic mycoses, 289

    yeast infections in, 314

  embryos/fetuses, 424–425

  fever/febrile response, 431

  first understanding of, 276b

  host defenses (*See* host defense mechanisms)

  immune complex diseases, 299, 383–385

  immune deficiency diseases, 387 (*See also* AIDS; HIV)

  immune-mediated neutropenia, 384t–385t

  infants, 429

  over life span, 387, 424b, 431, 433

  overstimulation of, 184b

  tissue/organs of, 388

    lymphatic nodules, 368

    lymphatic vessels, 368–372

    lymph nodes, 369–370

    lymphoid (lymphatic) tissue, 368

    red bone marrow (myeloid tissue), 372

    spleen, 371

    thymus gland, 371–372

    tonsils, 368–369

immunity, 364

  active (humoral), 381–382, 388

  antibody-mediated, 380–381

  cell-mediated, 380, 380f, 385, 472

  discovery of, 9

  of infants, 382, 429

  passive, 268, 382–383, 388

  recovery from illness as, 284

immunization. *See* vaccinations (immunization)

immunocompetent immune system, 364

immunoglobulins. *See* allergy/hypersensitivity reactions; antibodies/immunoglobulins (Igs/gammagobulins); immune system response

immunological tolerance, 365

immunology, 9, 22b, 94–95, 363–364, 388

impetigo, 205f, 207t, 429

impetigo (pyoderma), 204

IMViC tests, 93

incidence of diseases. *See under* diseases

incinerators/incineration, 348t, 349, 349f

inclusions (inclusion bodies), 50–57

IND (Investigational New Drug Application), 402

index cases, 191–192

indicator bacteria, 15

indirect contact transmission, 195–196

induced mutations, 124

industrial development, 334–335

industrial hygiene, 110

industrial uses of microorganisms, 68

industrial waste, 442–443

inert gases, 21

infants and children. *See also* congenital infections/disorders

  childhood infections, 2b–3b, 429–430

  circumcision, 301b, 307b

  common cold in, 226–228

  erythroblastosis fetalis (hemolytic disease), 366b

  group B streptococcal (GBS) infections, 366

  growth hormone deficiencies, 470

  immune system/response, 429, 433

  infant botulism, 247, 424b

  influenza, 407

  listeriosis in, 264

  molluscum contagiosum in, 328

  neonatal infections, 327, 429

  newborns' first contact with microorganisms, 182–183, 197–198

  passive immunity in, 268, 382

  rheumatic fever/carditis, 281

  roseola infantum, 209

  silver nitrate treatment of newborns, 356

  skin infections, 429–430

  tinea capitis, 210

  urinary tract infections (UTIs) in, 299–301, 301b

  vaccines for, 356b (*See also* vaccinations (immunization))

  varicella-zoster virus (chickenpox), 209

  warts, 207–208

infections/infectious diseases (in general)

  agencies combating, 99b

  bacterial (*See* bacterial infections/diseases)

  biofilms, 50b

  classifications of, 190

  competitive enzyme inhibition, 63

  definition, 12, 189–190

  etiology of, 189–191

  patterns of, 190, 197–198

  portals of entry, 185–186

infections/infectious diseases (in general) (*Continued*)

  slow, 149

  types of, 190

  viral (*See* viral infections/diseases)

  virulence/pathogenicity (*See* virulence and pathogenicity)

  weather effects on, 335

Infectious Disease Society of America, 100

infectious mononucleosis, 287–288, 288b, 288t, 293, 371t, 430

infertility, 322

inflammation/inflammatory response, 257b, 373–374, 378–379

  of brain, 406

  chemical mediators of, 373–374

  signs of, 378b

  steps of, 378, 378f

  systemic, 44b

  to tissue damage, 36b

inflammatory diseases

  amyotrophic lateral sclerosis (ALS), 471–472

  antiinflammatory drug actions, 36b

  endocarditis, 277–278

  myocarditis, 278

  rheumatic fever, 281

  rheumatoid arthritis (RA), 387

influenza, 228–230

  adolescents/young adults, 430

  avian influenza, 145b, 229b, 337b, 341t

  epidemics/pandemics, 2b–3b, 153, 153t, 159b–160b, 337b

  genome, 229

  Haemophilus influenzae, 14t, 142f, 150t, 219t, 224, 225f, 228t, 229f, 261–262, 406–407, 432, 432t

  older adults/elderly, 431–432

  pregnancy, 425t

  risk factors, 430

  serotypes of influenza A virus, 229b

  strains of, 229

  vaccinations for, 86b, 224, 229–230, 230b, 335b, 407, 430

  viral, 228–230

infundibular appearance, 92

ingestion process, 377–378

inhalation administration of drugs, 394–395

inhibition of enzyme actions, 63, 64f, 412

innate defense mechanisms, 375–376

inoculation, 82f, 84, 86–87, 128b, 194–195, 204, 209

inorganic compounds, 27–30, 38

insecticides, 473

insect vectors. *See under* vectors

insertions, 125

inspection (observation) of microbes, 84

insulin, 470–471, 470b, 474. *See also* diabetes

integral proteins, 42–43

integumentary system. *See* skin/integumentary system

intercalating agents, 125

interferons, 379, 417, 471, 474

interferon therapy, 471t

intermediate filaments, 51

intermediate hosts, 175, 289

International Emerging Infections Program (IEIP), 340
International Health Regulations (IHR), 340
interphase (nondividing) stage of cell cycle, 74–75, 74f
interrelationships between microbes and environment, 11
interstitial fluid (ISF), 58f
interventions for emerging/reemerging infectious diseases, 339
intestines. *See under* gastrointestinal (GI) tract
intracellular fluid (ICF), 42, 57–58, 58f, 75–78
intramuscular administration of drugs, 394–395
intrathecal administration of drugs, 394–395
intrauterine devices, 12t
intravenous (IV) administration of drugs, 394–395
introduction of known agents to new areas, 336
introduction (adoption) of pathogens, 333
invasion/invasins, 187, 188t
inversion macrolesions, 125
Investigational New Drug Application (IND), 402
iodine, 355t, 356
ionic bonds, 23–24, 24f
ionic liquids, 28
ionizing radiation, 351, 358
Ion Power Inc., 16
ions, 20–22, 30
    active transport of, 59–60
    bicarbonate, 28
    definition, 22
    hydrogen, 27, 28f
    hydroxyl, 27
    in living organisms, 23t
    polarity of, 30
irradiation of food, 236b, 243b
ischemia, 281
ISF (interstitial fluid), 58f
isografts, 365–366
isolation technique (laboratory), 91
isomerases, 62
isotonic environment, 30, 59
isotopes, 22, 22f
Ivanovski, Dimitri, 136b
ivermectin, 420

J
Janssen, Hans, 3
Janssen, Zaccharias, 3, 5t
JC polyomavirus, 303
Jenner, Edward, 9, 136b, 152b, 332b, 382b
jock itch, 211–212, 211t, 328
Joubert, J. L., 81b, 405b
jumping genes (transposons), 125

K
Kaposi's sarcoma, 324
Katrina, Hurricane, 165b
Kefauver-Harris Amendment, 401
kidneys. *See* renal system; urinary tract entries

kidney stones, 303b
kingdoms of life, 137
    Baltimore classification system, 138b
    family, 10f, 137
        bacteriophages, 144t
        medically important viruses by, 139t–140t
        of viral hemorrhagic fevers, 288
        -*viridae*, 137
        virus groups, 138b
    genus, 10f, 11, 137
        bacteriophages, 144t
        viruses, 138b
        -*virus* suffix, 137
    order, 10f, 137, 138b
    phyla, 10f, 11
    species, 10f, 11, 125–126, 137 (*See also* taxonomy)
    subfamily, 137, 139t–140t, 155t
Kirby-Bauer method (disk diffusion test), 354, 354f, 359, 409–410, 410f
Klebsiella pneumoniae, 219t, 224
Koch, Robert, 5t, 8–9, 43t, 81b, 181b, 190–191, 391b–392b
Koch's postulates, 2b–3b, 5t, 8–9, 9b, 181b, 190–191, 191f, 197–198
KOH (potassium hydroxide), 328
Krebs cycle (citric acid cycle), 26, 64, 66, 66f, 70
Kupffer cells, 374, 375f
kuru, 272

L
laboratory aseptic techniques, 8, 81b, 82–83, 82f, 95–96. *See also* control methods
    autoclaves, 83, 107, 109f
    disinfection, 83
    dry/moist heat sterilization, 83t
    first use of, 344b
    media for raising bacteria, 82f
    sanitization, 83
    sterility, 83
    sterilization, 82–83, 82f–83f, 95
    tunneling microscopes, 91b
    vaccine development, 86b
laboratory identification techniques, 90–95
    cultural characteristics, 91–93
    growth patterns in broth, 93
    manual and automated systems for, 94t
    molecular analysis, 94–95
    morphology, 91
    physiological/biochemical characteristics, 93–94
    rapid identification tests, 93–94
Laboratory Response Network (LRN), 457–458
laboratory safety issues, 100–110
    autoclaves, 107
    biosafety levels (BSLs) and guidelines, 101–103
        BSL-1, 101–102, 102b
        BSL-2, 101b
        BSL-3, 102b
        BSL-4, 103b, 104t
        OSHA's guidelines, 101b
        risk group levels, 101t
        training program, 100–101
    chemical handling, 103–105

laboratory safety issues (*Continued*)
    emergency response procedures, 111, 457
    equipment, 105–108
    eyewashes and safety showers, 107
    fume hoods, 106–107
    hazardous waste disposal, 108
    Material Safety Data Sheet (MSDS), 106f
    protective equipment/gear, 108–110
    refrigerators/freezers, 107–108
    regulations for, 112
laboratory testing/techniques. *See also specific infections or diseases*
    broth cultures, 8f
    contaminants, 82
    culture media, 95, 335b
        agar (*See* agar cultures)
        broth, 8f, 93, 93f, 121
        chemical classification of, 85
        contaminated, 82, 87
        egg cultures, 362b–363b
        functional types of, 85
        gelatin, 93f
        incubation/isolation of, 86–87
        inoculation of, 85–86
        liquid, 84
        litmus milk, 93, 94t
        live, 85–86
        nutritional requirements for microorganisms, 84t
        physical states of, 84
        raising bacteria, 84b
        for raising bacteria, 84b, 86t
        semisolid, 84
        soil, 441–442
        solid, 84
        sterilization of containers, 82f
        sterilizing containers, 82f
        turbidity of, 93, 121
        types of, 84–85, 85f, 87f
    culture plates, 82, 91–92
    culturing techniques, 81b, 82, 84–87
        cell mass, 121
        cell numbers, 121
        disk diffusion test (Kirby-Bauer method), 410f
        incubation/isolation, 86–87
        Kirby-Bauer (disease diffusion) method, 409–410
        pellicle growth (culture tubes), 93
    history of, 81b
    incubation of bacterial cultures, 84, 86, 92
    influenza identification, 229
    pour plate technique, 86–87, 87f
    specimen preparation, 88f
        cryofixation, 90
        for electron microscopy, 90
        fixation and staining methods, 87–90
        freeze-fixing samples, 90
    spread plate technique, 86–87, 87f
    stain techniques, 88f
        acid-fast stain, 88–89, 89f
        differential stains, 88–89
        for electron microscopy, 90
        Giemsa stain, 451
        Gimenez stain, 88f, 129f
        Gram stain, 45, 75–78, 88–89, 89b, 89f, 451

laboratory testing/techniques (*Continued*)
negative stains, 88–90, 88f
simple stain, 88–89, 88f
special staining procedures, 89–90
unstained specimens, 6
Wayson stain, 451
Wright stain, 89, 90f, 451
Ziehl-Neelsen acid-fast staining, 89b
streak plate technique, 86–87, 87f
tissue sample preparation, 89
types of, 84–85, 85f, 87f
vaginal cultures, 328–329
venereal disease tests, 321
lactic acid, 67, 376
lactoferrin, 382
lactose, 31, 93
lakes. *See* aquatic microbiology
lambda phage vectors, 468, 469f
landfills, 16
Langerhans cells, 202, 375f
larynx, 217
Lassa virus, 453–454
latent infections, 149, 208–209
Lawrence Berkeley National Laboratory
(LBNL), 100–101
LBNL (Lawrence Berkeley National
Laboratory), 100–101
lectin pathway, 380
leeching, 276b
Legionella (Legionnaire's disease/
legionellosis), 14t, 219t, 225, 432,
432t
legislation
Controlled Substances Act, 401–402
Federal Food, Drug and Cosmetic Act,
401
Orphan Drug Act, 402
Pure Food and Drug Act, 401
leishmaniasis, 290t, 293
lenses
magnification power of, 4–5
objective, 4–5
ocular, 4–5
refraction, 5
leprosy (Hansen's disease), 85–86, 206–207,
207t, 266–267, 267b, 272–273
classifications of, 206
elimination of, 206b
multibacillary, 206f
leptospira/leptospirosis, 13t, 126f, 127t,
302t, 446
leukemia, 372t
leukocytes. *See* white blood cells (WBCs)
leukopoiesis, 372
LGV (lymphogranuloma venereum), 321,
322b
library of natural products
(pharmaceuticals), 401b
lice, 286–287
lichens, 165–166, 167f, 440
life cycles
algae, 167
Babesia microti, 175f
cellular slime mold, 176f
Cryptosporidium, 252f
fungi, 164–165
helminths, 175–176
malaria parasites, 290–291
phages, 145

life cycles (*Continued*)
Plasmodium species, 159b–160b, 174f,
290f
protozoans, 169–171, 289, 293
Toxoplasma gondii, 425f
life hierarchy. *See* kingdoms of life
life stages. *See* aging process/human life
stages
ligases, 62
light, ultraviolet, 26b
light-dependent/independent reactions,
69–70, 70f
Linnaeus, Carolus, 11, 125–126, 126f,
171
lipids, 31t, 34–36
for energy storage, 35
glycolipids, 43
lipid solubility of drugs, 395–396
phospholipids, 35, 35f, 38, 42–43, 44f
plant lipids (oils), 34–35
prostaglandins, 36, 36b, 38, 378–379,
383
lipopolysaccharide bacterial endotoxins,
43
lipopolysaccharides, 45
lipoproteins, 33
liquefaction configurations, 92
liquid water, 29
Lister, Joseph, 5t, 8, 201b
listeria meningitis, 262–264
listeriosis, 186t, 247, 425t
live cultures, 85–86
liver enzymes tests, 327
liver/liver diseases, 13t, 170t, 250, 287, 292,
326, 396, 399
live viruses, 152
living cells, 26
living systems, 21f
lock and key concept of reactants/
receptors, 25
lockjaw (tetanus), 264–265, 265b, 272–273
LTLT (long temperature, long time), 348t
lungs/lung infections, 217, 233
lyases, 62
Lyme disease, 284t, 285–286, 285f–286f,
287t
lymphatic system. *See also* circulatory
system
lymphatic nodules, 368
lymphatic vessels, 368–372
lymph capillaries, 368, 368f–369f
lymph glands, 287
lymph nodes, 369–370, 370f
microbemia, 280
overview, 363f
poliomyelitis, 268
relationship to cardiovascular system,
279f
treatment of infections of, 293
lymphocytes (mononuclear leukocytes),
374–375
lymphogranuloma venereum (LGV), 321,
322b
lymphoid (lymphatic) tissue, 368, 369f
lymphopoiesis, 372
lyophilization, 348t, 351
lysis, 43, 91–92, 146–147, 147b, 188–189,
189f, 462
lysogenic (temperate) phages, 146–147

lysogeny, 146–147
lysosomes, 52, 54, 54f
lysozymes, 307, 377, 382
lytic (cytocidal) infections, 149
lytic (virulent) phages, 146–147

M

Machupo virus, 453–454
macroconidium, 164–165
macrolide polyene antibiotics, 418
macrolides, 416
macronuclei, 170–171
macrophages, 264, 324, 374. *See also* white
blood cells (WBCs)
mad cow disease. *See* transmissible
spongiform encephalopathies/prion
diseases (TSEs)
Magendie, François, 391b–392b
maggots, 7
major histocompatibility complex (MHC),
365
malaria, 159b–160b, 173, 174f, 289–291,
290f, 290t, 291b, 336f, 425t
males, 297b. *See also* reproductive tract
infections (RTIs); sexually transmitted
infections (STIs); urinary tract
infections (UTIs)
anatomy, 300f, 314–315
bacterial infections, 313–314, 315t
chlamydial infections, 322b
circumcision, 301b, 307b
fungal infections, 314, 315t
gonorrhea, 319b
infections of penis, 314, 328–329
nonsexually transmitted diseases of,
315t
normal flora of, 307
prevention of infections, 301
prostate gland, 313
prostatitis, 313, 315t
protozoan infections, 314, 315t
risk factors, 299–300
urinary tract infections (UTIs), 304
yeast infections, 315t
Mallon, Mary (Typhoid Mary), 236b, 244,
245b
MALT (mucosa-associated lymphoid
tissue), 368
maltose, 31
MAR (multiple antimicrobial resistance),
412
Marburg virus, 334, 453
marine (saltwater) microbiology. *See under*
aquatic microbiology
masks (respiratory protection), 109
mast cells, 383
Mastigophora, 171
mastitis, 307b, 310, 312t
Material Safety Data Sheet (MSDS), 105,
106f
maternal inheritance, 54b. *See also*
pregnancy
matter, definition, 20, 38
MBC (minimal bactericidal concentration),
410
MCV (molluscum contagiosum virus),
208t, 209, 328
measles (*Morbillivirus*), 154, 207, 429–430
mebendazole, 419

mechanical vectors, 195, 195b
medically important microorganisms
  bacteria, 127t–128t
    Bacillus species, 131
    endospore-forming gram-positive
      rods and cocci, 131t
    gram-positive cocci, 130–131, 130t
    growth environments of, 122
    irregular nonsporulating rods, 132t
    mycobacteria, 132t
    mycoplasms, 130t
    rickettsias/chlamydias, 129, 129t
  viruses, 139t–140t
medical negligence, 16
medical practice, 19b–20b
medicaments, 19b–20b
meiosis, 42, 73, 75–78, 77f, 165
melioidosis, 454–455, 456t
membrane-bound compartments, vesicles,
  57
membrane filters, 353t
membrane proteins, 43
membrane transport mechanisms, 57–61
meninges, 258–259, 259f
meningitis, 272–273, 430
  bacterial, 260–264
  causative organisms, 406
  changes in cerebrospinal fluid (CSF) in,
    259t
  on college campuses, 262b
  cryptococcal, 271
  fungal, 165–166
  H. influenzae, 261–262
  listeria, 262–264
  meningococcal, 261
  meningoencephalitis, 406
  outbreaks, 261t
  pneumococcal, 262
  primary amoebic meningoencephalitis,
    172
  septic, 405
  summary of, 263t
  viral (aseptic), 268, 405
menopause, 307b
mercury, 400b
merozoites, 173
mesangial cells, 374
mesophiles, 122, 122t, 133
metabolic disorders, 470
metabolism/metabolic processes
  cellular, 42, 50, 61–72, 75–78
    cofactors/coenzymes, 63
    enzymes, 61–64
    enzyme specificity, 62
    exoenzymes/endoenzymes, 62
  of drugs, 396–397, 399, 402
  fungi, 161–162
  metabolic pathways, 63, 407, 412
  prodrug activation, 397b
  requirements for microbial, 407
  for viral multiplication, 145
  water needed for, 29
metabolites, 54
methane, 16
methane-producing bacteria, 9b
methanogens, 132
methicillin-resistant *Staphylococcus aureus*
  (MRSA), 111b, 413b
metronidazole, 419

MHC (major histocompatibility complex),
  365
MIC (minimal inhibitory concentration),
  410
microaerophiles, 123, 123t
microarthropods, 441
microbe-environment relationship, 11
microbemia, 280
microbial adaptation/change, 335
microbial antagonism, 81b
microbial competition, 182–183
microbial ecology, 11, 437–438
  aquatic microbiology (*See water entries*)
  biogeochemical cycles, 438–441
  bioterrorism (*See* bioterrorism/
    bioweapons)
  definition, 458
  ecological interactions between
    organisms, 11–12
  natural disasters (*See* natural disasters)
  soil (*See soil entries*)
microbial forensics. *See* forensics
microbial growth, 84b, 86t, 92, 118–123,
  133. *See also* reproduction methods
  (microbes)
  bacteria, 86t
  beaded growth, 92
  control of (*See* control methods)
  culturing (*See under* laboratory testing/
    techniques)
  environmental pH, 123, 348t
  experiments proving, 7–8
  in gastrointestinal (GI) tract, 237–239
  growth curves in human populations,
    120–121, 120f
  hydrostatic pressure for, 122–123
  measuring, 121
  of medically important bacteria, 122
  nonpathogenic microorganisms, 123t
  nutritional requirements for, 121–122
  organic compounds, 122
  osmotic pressure for, 122
  overgrowth of, 308
  pathogenic microorganisms, 84b, 123t
  prokaryotic cells, 123
  requirements for, 84t, 118–120
  temperatures for optimal, 122, 122t, 133,
    349f
  water's effect on, 29
microbial resistance, 345. *See also* drug
  resistance
  to antimicrobial agents, 335
  to chemical disinfectants, 353
  cross-resistance, 412–413
  fungal resistance to osmotic pressure,
    161
  Global Strategy for Containment of
    Antimicrobial Resistance (WHO),
    413
  nonresistant microbes, 409
microbicidal agents. *See* antimicrobials
microbiology, 2b–3b, 3–9, 5t, 14–16
microbiota (normal flora). *See* normal flora
microconidium, 164–165
microglial cells, 374
Micrographia (Hooke), 3
micrographs (photomicrographs), 4–5
microhabitats, 437
micronuclei, 170–171

micronutrients (trace elements), 84t
microorganisms (in general), 9
  airborne, 8
  in alcoholic beverage production, 15
  associated with medical devices, 12t
  beneficial, 68
  biochemical characteristics, 93
  bioremediation, 15
  classification/identification of, 95
  classification of, 10–11
  evolution of, 9
  in food production, 14–15
  in health and disease, 11–14
  human use of, 14–16
  identification of, 93–94 (*See also*
    laboratory identification
    techniques)
  nutritional requirements for, 84t
  origin of, 9
  prokaryotes versus eukaryotes, 10
  size comparisons of bacteria/viruses/
    viroids/prions, 141f
  spread of infectious, 334b
  in water supply, 15
microscopes
  bright-field, 3–7, 5f
  confocal, 6–7
  dark-field, 6, 6f
  electron, 7
  first use of, 81b
  fluorescence, 6, 6f
  phase-contrast, 6, 6f
  resolving powers, 41b–42b
  tunneling, 91b
  types of, 2b–3b, 3–7
microscopy, 3
  electron microscopy (EM), 2b–3b, 7, 95,
    136b
  scanning electron microscopy (SEM), 7,
    7f, 90, 91b
  scanning tunneling electron microscopy
    (STEM), 91b
  transmission electron microscopy
    (TEM), 7, 7f, 90, 91b
microspora, 172
microtubules, 51
microvilli, 47, 47t, 49, 49f, 75–78
milk. *See* dairy products
mineralocorticoids, 35–36
minerals, 122
minimal bactericidal concentration (MBC),
  410
minimal inhibitory concentration (MIC),
  410
Minsky, Marvin, 6–7
mitochondria, 54, 55f, 172
mitosis, 42, 73, 75–78, 75f–76f, 151
mitosomes, 171
mobility/motility/locomotion
  amoebas, 172
  bacteria, 48, 48f
  cell, 47–48
  cilia, 49
  cytoplasmic streaming, 174
  Giardia lamblia, 171f
  molecules, 58
  protozoans, 171
modes of transmission. *See* transmission of
  infections

moisture, 441–442
molds, 161, 163
  bread, 165–166
  health problems related to, 165b
  slime molds, 173–174
    cellular, 174, 176f
    plasmodial, 174
molecular analysis, 94–95, 303
molecular bonds, 62
molecular structure, 19b–20b, 29, 36f–37f
molecules (in general), 23–27
  active transport of, 59–60
  antisense, 471–472
  carrier, 67f
  definition, 23
  FAD, 66–67
  formation of, 38
  glucose (See glucose molecules)
  hydrophilic, 30, 42
  hydrophobic, 30
  inorganic, 38
  microscopes for observing, 91b
  movement of, 58
  nicotinamide adenine dinucleotide
      (NAD), 38, 66–68
  nicotinamide adenine dinucleotide
      phosphate (NADP), 69
  number of atoms in, 27b
  organic, 30–38, 31t, 32f, 63
  polar/nonpolar, 42
  protein carrier, 58
  receptor, 19b–20b
  solubility of, 30
  tRNA, 72f
  water soluble/insoluble, 30
molluscum contagiosum virus (MCV),
    208t, 209, 328
monomers, 25, 25f, 31–32, 31t, 38
mononuclear leukocytes (lymphocytes),
    374–375
mononucleosis. See infectious
    mononucleosis
monosaccharides, 31
morbidity. See incidence under diseases
Morbidity and Mortality Weekly Report
    (MMWR), 192
Morbillivirus (measles), 154
morphological effects, 149–150
morphology/morphological identification,
    91. See also laboratory identification
    techniques; taxonomy
  bacteria, 42–57, 90–95, 116–118, 116f,
      118t
  bacteriophages, 144t
  Baltimore classification system, 137
  cestodes, 177f
  cultural characteristics, 91–93
  culture plates, 91–92
  fungi, 161
  growth patterns in broth, 93
  manual and automated systems for, 94t
  methods for, 126
  molecular analysis, 94–95
  physiological/biochemical
      characteristics, 93–94
  viruses (See under viruses)
Morrocci, 130–131
mortality rates, 12–14, 100b, 153t, 192.
    See also specific infection or disease

Morton, William, 391b–392b
motor neurons, 406
MRSA (methicillin-resistant Staphylococcus
    aureus) infections, 111b, 413b
MS (multiple sclerosis), 386
MSDS (Material Safety Data Sheet), 105,
    106f
mucosa, stomach, 240
mucosa-associated lymphoid tissue
    (MALT), 368
mucous membranes, 183f, 185–186
mucus, 190b, 376
multicellular organisms, 75–78
multidrug-resistant pathogens, 224b, 405b,
    411–413
multiple antimicrobial resistance (MAR),
    412
multiple sclerosis (MS), 386, 386t
multiplication, viral. See viral
    multiplication
mumps, 14t, 154, 228t, 429–430
mushrooms, 161, 165–166, 166f
mutagens, 125
mutations
  bacterial DNA, 73
  causes of, 125
  classifications of, 124–125, 133
  drug-resistant organisms due to,
      411–412
  frameshift, 124–125
  genetic, 124–125
  of HIV virus, 318b
  lethal, 125
  point, 124–125
  radiation-related, 351–352
  RNA viruses, 335
  silent, 124–125
  vaccines and, 362b–363b
  viruses of respiratory tract, 233
mutualism, 12, 128b, 167f, 182, 182t
myasthenia gravis, 386, 386t
myceliums, 161
mycetoma, 211t, 213
mycobacteria, 131–132
Mycobacterium
  M. avium, 325b
  M. leprae, 206, 207t, 266f (See also
      leprosy (Hansen's disease))
  M. smegmatis, 223f
mycology, 160. See also fungi
Mycoplasma, 298
  M. pneumoniae, 222f
mycoplasmal and ureaplasmal
      nongonococcal urethritis, 322–323
mycoplasms, 130
mycorrhizae, 160–161
mycoses. See under fungal infections/
    diseases
myelopoiesis, 372
myocardium/myocarditis, 277–278, 293

N

NADH, 66–67
NAD (nicotinamide adenine dinucleotide)
    molecules, 38, 66–68
NADPH, 68f, 70
NADP (nicotinamide adenine dinucleotide
    phosphate) molecules, 69
Naegeli, Carl, 43t

naked viruses, 142f, 148f
naming systems. See nomenclature;
    taxonomy
napiform appearance, 92
NARMS (National Antimicrobial
    Resistance Monitoring System),
    391b–392b, 413
narrow spectrum antimicrobial agents,
    408
National Antimicrobial Resistance
    Monitoring System (NARMS),
    391b–392b, 413
National Center for Environmental Health
    (NECH), 167b
National Center for Infectious Diseases
    (NCID), 339–340
National Center for Medical Intelligence
    (NCMI), 445
National Center for Preparedness,
    Detection, and Control of Infectious
    Diseases (NCPDCID), 339–340
National Institute for Occupational Safety
    and Health (NIOSH), 103–105
National Institute of Allergy and Infectious
    Diseases (NIAID), 103, 223, 337
National Institutes of Health (NIH), 50b,
    101, 382b
Nationally Notifiable Diseases, 192, 193b,
    337
natron, 28
nattokinase, 190b
natural disasters, 335, 444–448
  earthquakes, 447–448, 448t
  emerging/reemerging infectious diseases
      during, 335
  floods, 13–14, 165b, 446–447, 446t
  hurricanes, 165b, 448
  threats from, 458
  tsunamis, 447, 447t
natural selection, 411
NCID (National Center for Infectious
    Diseases), 339–340
NCMI (National Center for Medical
    Intelligence), 445
NCPDCID (National Center for
    Preparedness, Detection, and Control
    of Infectious Diseases), 339–340
NDA (New Drug Application), 401, 402b
necatoriasis (hookworms), 176, 177f,
    253–254
NECH (National Center for Environmental
    Health), 167b
necrosis, 212, 281, 293
necrotizing skin infections, 203, 205, 205b,
    207t
Needham, John, 7–8
negative feedback mechanisms, 63–64, 64f
Neisseria
  N. gonorrhoeae, 356 (See also gonorrhea)
  N. meningitidis, 203t, 406 (See also
      meningitis)
Nelmes, Sarah, 136b
nematodes (roundworms), 177–178,
    253–254, 441
neonatal infections. See infants and
    children
nephrons, 297, 298f, 397f. See also
    urinary-related entries
nephrostomy tubes, 304

nervous system
    anatomy/overview, 258–259, 258f–260f
    bacterial infections, 260–267
    central nervous system (*See* central
        nervous system (CNS))
    cerebrospinal fluid (CSF), 258–259, 259t
    fungal infections, 271
    nerve cells, 51f
    peripheral, 258f
    prion-associated diseases, 272
    protozoal infections, 271–272
    viral infections, 268–271
neuroimmune axis, 257b
neuromuscular system, 260f, 386, 392t,
        406. *See also* nervous system
neurotoxins, 159b–160b, 247, 264–265, 452
neurotransmitters, 406
neutrons, 20
neutrophils (granulocytes), 372–373, 374f
newborns. *See* infants and children
New Drug Application (NDA), 401, 402b
NGU (nongonococcal urethritis), 321–323,
        322b, 324t
niclosamide, 419
NIH (National Institutes of Health), 382b
NIOSH. *See* National Institute for
        Occupational Safety and Health
        (NIOSH)
Nipah virus, 456–457, 457t
nitrates, 27b, 438
nitrification, 440
nitrites, 438
Nitrobacter, 348t
nitrogen (N), 27b, 36–37, 37f, 122,
        438–441, 439f
nitrogenase, 438
nocardioforms, 132
nomenclature, 11
    binomial system of, 11, 125–126, 126f,
        133
    definition, 11
    drug, 393, 393t
    nucleic acids, 36–37
    patterns of infection, 189–190
    surface antigens, 375
noncompetitive inhibition, 63–64
noncyclic photophosphorylation, 69, 69f
nondividing (interphase) stage of cell cycle,
        74–75, 74f
nongonococcal urethritis (NGU), 321–323,
        322b, 324t
nonionizing radiation, 351
nonmicrobial antigenics, 365
nonpermissive cells, 149
nonprescription/prescription drugs, 393
normal flora, 12, 129, 182, 197–198,
        250–251
    antimicrobial effects on, 408, 410–411
    changes in, 196
    fungal, 311b
    gastrointestinal (GI) tract, 93, 237t–239t
    host-microbe relationship, 182–183
    as opportunistic pathogen, 183–185
    in regions of human body, 184t
    reproductive system, 307
    respiratory tract, 217–219, 224, 233
    skin, 429
    of soil, 473
    types of, 182–183

normal flora (*Continued*)
    urinary tract, 299–300
    vaginal, 309
noroviruses, 249–250
nosocomial/iatrogenic infections, 197–198,
        308, 314–315
    control/prevention, 197
    examples of, 197t
    fungal, 304
    transmission of, 196
    types of, 196, 196b
notations. *See* chemical notations
notifiable diseases, 192, 193b
nuclear envelope, 52
nucleic acids, 31t
    adenosine triphosphate (ATP), 38f
    copying of, for phage multiplication, 145
    description, 36–38
    monomers of, 38
    nucleic acid amplification system, 322b
    nucleic acid sequence analysis, 95
    nucleotides, 36–37
    synthesis, 406–407
nucleocapsids, 137
nucleoid area, 124
nucleoproteins, 33
nucleotides, 36–37, 37f
nucleus, cell, 52, 52f, 75–78
nursing homes, 110–111, 111b, 111t
nutrients, 12, 64, 75–78, 161, 165–169, 174,
        441–442
nutritional requirements (microbial), 84,
        84t, 121–122

O

obesity, 58, 392t
objective lenses, 4–5
obligate halophiles, 122
observation (inspection) of microbes, 84
occupational hazards, 100
Occupational Safety and Health
        Administration (OSHA), 99b, 100
    Biosafety Program, 100–101
    Bloodborne Pathogens Standard, 110
    bloodborne training program, 100–101
    emergency response standards/
        procedures, 457
    ergonomic guidelines, 110
    hospital safety, 110
    "On-line" Exposure Control Plan
        development tool, 100–101
    State Plan partners (emergency
        response), 111
oceans. *See* aquatic microbiology
octet principle, 23
oil (sebaceous) glands, 376
oils. *See* fats; lipids
older adults/elderly
    immune system/response, 387, 431, 433
    infections of, 431–433
    influenza, 432
    mental difficulties/dementia and UTIs,
        302–303
    pneumonia, 431–432, 432t
    skin infections, 433
    susceptibility to microbial disease of, 433
    tuberculosis, 223
    urinary tract infections (UTIs), 432,
        432b

oligosaccharides, 382
oncogenic transformation, 149
oncogenic viruses, 151t
"On-line" Exposure Control Plan
        development tool, 100–101
opportunistic infections
    bacterial vaginitis, 308
    description, 183–185
    diphtheria, 224–225
    fungal, 162t, 271, 311b
    HIV/AIDS-related, 271, 325b, 326
    host-microbe relationship, 183–185
    Klebsiella pneumoniae, 224
    normal flora as, 183–185
    respiratory tract, 217–219, 224–226, 233
    sexually transmitted, 318b
    tuberculosis, 223
oral cavity, 240, 240b, 276b
    bacteria of, 119b, 241
    candida infections, 250–251, 251f
    chancres, 323
    dental caries, 240–241
    disease-causing organisms (summary),
        237t–239t
    gingivitis, 240–241
    gonorrhea in, 319
    normal flora of, 184t
    periodontal disease, 241–242
    saliva, 288b
    systemic infections from, 243b
    teeth, 240, 242f–243f
    tongue, 220, 220f
orbital (electron) clouds, 20
organelles, 50–57
organic contaminants, 354–355
organic molecules. *See under* molecules
organ transplants
    classification of, 365
    fungal urinary tract infections (UTIs)
        after, 304
    liver, 327
    rabies transmission through, 269
    rejection of tissues/organs, 365–366
    success of, 365
    toxoplasmosis transmission, 292
    viral urinary tract infections (UTIs)
        after, 303
    xenotransplants, 473–474
Orphan Drug Act, 402
orthomyxoviruses, 153
OSHA. *See* Occupational Safety and Health
        Administration (OSHA)
osmophiles, 122
osmosis, 58–59, 60f
osmotic gradients, 22
osmotic pressure, 58, 122, 161, 347, 348t
otitis media, 262, 429–430
outbreaks. *See also* epidemics/pandemics
    after natural disasters, 447
    Bacillus cereus, 249
    bioterrorism threats, 152b
    botulism, 247
    dysentery, 245–246
    E. coli, 128b
    Ebola virus, 334
    hantavirus, 339
    influenza, 229
    investigation of, 16, 339, 357t
    listeriosis, 247

outbreaks (*Continued*)
 Marburg virus, 334
 meningococcal diseases, 261t, 407, 430
 Outbreak and Response Protocol
  (OPRP) guidelines, 101b
 prevention, 339
 SARS, 217b, 230t
 smallpox, 210
 sporotrichosis, 213
 toxic shock syndrome (TSS), 307b
 viral hemorrhagic fevers (VHFs),
  288–289
 West Nile virus, 339
oxidation, 25–26, 68–70, 355, 440
oxidation-reduction reactions, 26, 26f
oxidative enzymes, 54
oxidoreductases, 62
oxygen, 67, 441–444

P

pain, 19b–20b, 378–379, 378b
pandemics. *See* epidemics/pandemics
papillomaviruses, 151
Pap testing, 327
papules, 328
Paracelsus, Aureolus, 19b–20b, 41b–42b,
 391b–392b
Paramecia, 170f
Paramyxovirus, 154
paramyxoviruses, 154
parasitic hosts, 175–176, 177b
parasitic infections, 452. *See also*
 helminths/helminthic infections;
 protozoan infections
parasitism, 12, 182, 182t
paratyphoid (enteric) fever, 245
parenteral administration of drugs, 394
Paramecium, 172
parvoviruses, 151
PASS (fire extinguisher use guidelines),
 106b
passive transport mechanisms. *See under*
 transport mechanisms
Pasteur, Louis, 2b–3b, 5t, 8–9, 8b, 15, 81b,
 100b, 115b, 154, 181b, 190–191,
 391b–392b, 405b
pasteurization, 8, 8b, 346, 357–358, 358b
paternity testing, 54b
PATH (Program for Appropriate
 Technology in Health), 250
pathogen groups, 101, 337
pathogenicity. *See* virulence and
 pathogenicity
pathogens (in general), 12–14. *See also*
 biosafety levels (BSLs) and guidelines;
 specific pathogen group or
 microorganism
 adoption (introduction) of, 333
 airborne, 14
 definition, 182
 discovery of new, 2b–3b
 growth conditions, 122t–123t
 immune system response to, 362b–363b
  (*See also* immune system response)
 mechanisms of, 236b
 NIH classification of, 101
pathways, biochemical, 380
PCR. *See* polymerase chain reaction (PCR)
 detectors

PDR (*Physician's Desk Reference*), 394b. *See
 also drug entries;* pharmacology
pelvic inflammatory disease (PID), 310,
 312t, 321, 322b
penetration stage of viral multiplication,
 147
penicillins, 405b, 414–415
 discovery/production of, 332b, 400
 periplasmic space, 46b
 production of, 461b
Penicillium, 15, 165–166, 166f
penis, 301b, 307b, 314, 319b, 328–329
Pennsylvania State University, 16
pentose phosphate pathway. *See*
 phosphogluconate pathway
peptic ulcers (*Helicobacter*), 123b, 240,
 242f, 244
peptide bonds, 73f
peptidoglycan, 45, 45f–46f
Peptococcus/Peptostreptococcus, 130–131
peptone, 84
pericarditis, 277, 280
pericardium, 277
periodontal disease, 241–242
peripheral nervous system, 258f. *See also*
 nervous system
peripheral proteins, 42–43
periplasmic space, 45–46, 46b
permissive cells, 149
peroxisomes, 54
persistent infections, 149
personal protective equipment. *See* safety
 issues
perspiration, 376
pertussis (whooping cough), 219t, 222–223
Petri plates, 84, 91–92
Peyer's patches, 368
phages. *See* bacteriophages (phages)
phagocytes/phagocytosis, 50b, 60, 61f, 172,
 187, 377–378, 377f, 388
phagosomes, 377
pharmaceutical agents, 15, 356b, 401b
pharmaceutical chemistry, 393
pharmacodynamics, 392–393
pharmacognosy, 393
pharmacokinetics, 392–394
pharmacology, 392. *See also* antimicrobials;
 drug entries
 adverse effects/drug interactions, 393b
 branches of, 392–393
 brand names of drugs, 393
 description, 392
 history of, 391b–392b
 PDR (*Physician's Desk Reference*), 394b
 prodrugs, 397b
 public health control measures, 401–402
 respiratory infections, 392t
 shelf life of drugs, 409
 sources of drug information, 393–394
 therapeutic index (drug safety), 410
 toxic/adverse effects, 399, 402
 vaccinations, 400b (*See also*
  vaccinations)
pharmacotherapeutics, 392–393
pharmacy, 392–393
pharyngitis, 219–220, 219t, 429–430
pharynx, 217
phases of cell cycles, 74f
phenols/phenolics, 355t

phenotypes, 124, 126
pH environment/values, 27b, 28, 297–298,
 347
 acidity, 28, 28f, 123, 358
 alkalinity, 28, 28f, 93, 123
 archaea, 123
 bacteria growth, 348t
 buffers, 28
 changes in, 28
 enzyme action and, 63
 hydrogen value, 28f
 microbial growth, 123
 skin/integumentary system, 376
 soil, 441–442
 urine, 303b
phenylalanine deamination test, 93
phialospores, 164–165
phosphates, 441
phosphogluconate pathway, 67
phosphogluconate pathways, 68f
phosphoproteins, 33
phosphorus cycle, 441, 442f
photoautotrophs, 121–122, 133, 169, 438
photoheterotrophs, 121–122, 133
photomicrographs (micrographs), 4–5
photophosphorylation, cyclic and
 noncyclic, 69f
photosynthesis, 55f, 68–70, 75–78
 Calvin-Benson cycle, 70f
 categories of processes, 69
 chloroplast function in, 54–55
 in eukaryotic and prokaryotic cells, 68f
 light-dependent reaction of, 69f
 oxygen-generating, 68–69
 stages of, 69–70
photosynthetic organisms, 444
phototaxis, 48
phototrophs, 38, 61, 121
phyla. *See* kingdoms of life
phylogeny, 9, 161f. *See also* evolution
physiological/biochemical characteristics,
 93–94
physiology, 391b–392b
phytoplankton, 167–169, 444
phytosterols, 35–36, 36b
picornaviruses, 154
pigments, 28, 68–69
pili (fimbriae), 47–48, 47t, 49f, 75–78
pink eye (conjunctivitis), 183–185, 267,
 429
pinocytosis, 60, 61f
pinworms/seatworms, 176, 253, 253f
piperazine, 419–420
placenta/placenta-crossing pathogens, 186,
 186t, 264, 327, 424, 425f, 429
plague (*Yersinia pestis*), 283–284, 284t,
 332b
 as biological weapon, 451, 455t
 bubonic, 159b–160b, 284f, 284t, 450–451
 pneumonic, 284t, 450–451, 451b
plankton, 166–169, 444
plant cells, 46, 56–57, 56f
plant microbiology, 15
plants. *See also* agriculture
 cells of, 46, 56–57, 56f
 fungus tolerant/resistant, 473
 genetic engineering of, 472–473
 herbicide tolerance/resistance, 473
 inoculation of roots, 128b

plants (*Continued*)
    insect-tolerant, 473
    macroscopic structures of, 41b–42b
    nitrites/nitrates, 438
    as pharmaceutical sources, 391b–392b, 400
    pharmacological research, 400
    phytosterols, 35–36
    symbiotic nitrogen-fixing bacteria in, 439–440
    uptake of sulfates by, 440
    virus tolerance/resistance, 473
plant toxins, 257b, 456t
plasma membrane, 42–43, 56–57, 75–78
    addition of material to, 60–61
    description, 42–46
    disruption of, 407
    permeability changes, 412
    of prokaryotic and eukaryotic cells, 44f
    transport across, 75–78
plasmids, 37–38, 50, 95, 124, 133, 466–468, 466f, 468f, 474
Plasmodium, 159b–160b
    P. vivax, 174f (*See also* malaria)
platyhelminths, 176
pleomorphic bacteria, 91
pneumococcal meningitis, 262
pneumonias, 221–222, 230
    bacterial, 221
        features/transmission/treatment/
            prevention (summary),
            227t–228t
        mycoplasmal, 219t, 222
        staphylococcal, 224
        streptococcal, 221–222
        Streptococcus pneumoniae, 221, 432, 432t
        summary of, 219t, 227t–228t
    causative organisms, 217b
    chlamydial, 219t, 222
    community-acquired, 221
    drug resistant, 222
    fungal, 232–233
    H. pneumoniae, 224
    Klebsiella pneumoniae, 224
    in older adults/elderly, 217b, 431–432
    risk factors, 221, 431–432
    staphylococcal, 219t
    vaccinations, 222
    viral, 227t–228t, 230, 432
Pneumovirus, 154
PNS (peripheral nervous system). *See*
    nervous system
poisons/poisoning, 19b–20b, 166, 392–393,
    399–400. *See also* foodborne diseases/
    infections; toxins/toxic compounds
poliomyelitis (polio), 150t, 257b, 268–269,
    268f, 272–273, 425t
pollution, 50, 446
polymerase chain reaction (PCR) detectors,
    95b, 325–326, 453, 456–457, 466–467,
    467f
polymerase III, 72–73
polymers, 25, 25f
polyomaviruses, 151, 303, 426t
polypeptides, 33f, 38, 70–72
polyribosomes, 38
polysaccharides, 31–32, 32f
ponds. *See* aquatic microbiology

Pontiac fever, 225
population (human). *See also* global
    concerns; public health
    diseases in, 192
    growth curves (bacterial), 120–121,
        120f
    incidence/prevalence of disease in,
        197–198
    infectious diseases and, 333
    poverty in, 335
    urban/rural, 333f
populations (animal), 334
populations (microbial), 437f
    antimicrobial effectiveness and, 353
    formation of, 437
    overgrowth of bacterial, 308
    soil bacteria, 441–442
porospores, 164–165
portals of entry, 185–186, 185f, 197–198,
    254
    for allergens, 383
    for anthrax, 225–226
    conjunctiva, 183–185
    for fungi, 289, 293
    gastrointestinal (GI) tract as, 183–185
    for helminths, 185
    infections (in general), 185–186, 254
    mouth, 201b
    mucous membranes, 185–186
    for nosocomial infections, 196
    parenteral route as, 186
    placenta, 186
    respiratory tract as, 183–185
    skin, 185–186, 213–214, 264, 272–273,
        283, 328, 378
    urinary/urogenital tract, 183–185
    for viruses, 213–214, 269
portals of exit, 189
postexposure prophylaxis (PEP), 269
poststreptococcal glomerulonephritis
    (PSGN), 220b
postsurgical infections, 8
postulates, 190–191. *See also* Koch's
    postulates
potassium hydroxide (KOH), 328
potential hydrogens. *See* pH environment/
    values
poxviruses, 133, 142–143, 151–152, 209
PPD test (tuberculosis), 223–224
prefixes (chemical notations), 27b
pregnancy. *See also* reproductive tract
    infections (RTIs)
    embryos/fetuses
        embryonic stem cells, 41b–42b
        immune system/responses, 424–425
        infections of, 264
        Rh factor, 366
        sexually transmitted infections of,
            329
    infections during, 424, 426t
        chlamydial, 322
        gonorrhea, 356
        influenza, 425t
        periodontal disease, 241
        polio, 268, 425t
        syphilis in, 321
        toxoplasmosis, 271, 292, 427b
        urinary tract infections (UTIs), 303,
            425t

pregnancy (*Continued*)
        vaginal infections, 427–428
    placenta/placenta-crossing pathogens,
        186, 186t, 264, 327, 424, 425f, 429
    transmission of infections
        in childbirth, 208–209
        HIV, 325
        Streptococcus agalactiae, 310b
    trichomoniasis treatment, 328–329,
        427–428
prescription/nonprescription drugs, 393
prevalence of diseases, 192, 197–198
prevention. *See also* safety issues
    decontamination of surfaces, 452
    drug resistance, 413
    E. coli infection, 128b, 247b
    emerging/reemerging diseases/
        infections, 337–341
    foodborne diseases, 12–13
    fungal infections, 231
    gastrointestinal (GI) tract infections,
        12–13
    hand washing, 35b
    in healthcare settings, 197
    new strategies for biofilm-derived
        diseases, 50b
    postexposure prophylaxis (PEP), 382b
        (*See also* vaccinations
        (immunization))
    reproductive tract infections, 307, 309
    salmonellosis, 244
    tuberculosis, 223
    urinary tract infections (UTIs), 304
    waterborne diseases, 13–14
    zoonotic diseases, 12
primaquine, 418–419
primary fungal pathogens, 162t
primary immune responses, 381
prion diseases. *See* transmissible
    spongiform encephalopathies/prion
    diseases (TSEs)
prions, 11, 155
probiotics, 184b
prodrugs, 397b
product concentration, 63
progenitor pluripotent cells, 41b–42b
Program for Appropriate Technology in
    Health (PATH), 250
prokaryotic cells, 9, 10f, 42, 75–78
    atmospheric requirements for, 123
    classification of bacteria and archaea,
        125–133
    division process of, 73
    environmental requirements for, 121
    eukaryotes versus, 10
    eukaryotic compared to, 43t, 52
    flagella of, 48
    genetic transfer in, 125
    gliding, 48
    inclusions, 57
    metabolism of, 64
    photosynthesis in, 68f
    plasma membranes, 44f
    ribosomes in, 55–56
    structure of, 42–57
    surface appendages, 47f, 47t
prokaryotic transcription, 71–72
promotor sequence, 71
prophages, 146–147

prophylaxis. *See* prevention
Propionibacterium acnes (acne), 206, 207t
proprietary (trade, brand) drugs, 393
prostaglandins, 36, 36b, 38, 378–379, 383
prostate gland, 313
prostatitis, 313, 315t
protective equipment/gear. *See under* safety issues
proteinaceous infectious particles. *See* prions
proteins, 31t, 38, 44f
  amino acids, 32
  for cellular function, 70–71
  complement, 379–380
  composition of, 75–78
  conjugated, 33
  denaturation of, 33
  description, 32–33
  encoding of, 54
  exocytosis, 61f
  functions of, 32–33, 33b
  integral, 42–43
  membrane, 43
  peripheral, 42–43
  production of, by viruses, 155
  structural arrangement of, 33, 33f
protein synthesis, 38, 42, 70–72, 71f, 75–78, 118–120, 406
Proteus mirabilis, 303b
protomeres, 137
protons, 20–21, 21f–22f
prototypes, 125–126
protozoa, 11, 169–173
  Apicomplexa, 173f
  characteristics, 169
  classification of, 171–173
  cyst formation by, 169, 178, 251
  intestinal, 170t
  life cycle of, 169–171
  placenta-crossing, 186t
  in soil, 441
  survival of, 171
protozoal infections, 159b–160b, 169, 170t. *See also* antiprotozoals; main entries for specific infections
  circulatory system, 289–293
  disease-causing organisms (summary), 237t–239t
  emerging/reemerging, 339t
  gastrointestinal (GI) tract, 26, 170t, 251–252
  Giardia lamblia/giardiasis, 13t, 171–172, 171b, 171f, 251
  human, 172–173, 254
  nervous system, 272–273
  reproductive tract, 312t, 314–315, 315t
  sexually transmitted, 171–172, 328–329
  skin, 170t
  transmission of, 170t, 339t
  trichomoniasis, 311, 328–329
  Trypanosoma, 172f, 271–272
  urinary tract, 298
  zoonotic, 194t
proviruses, 154
Prusiner, Stanley, 11b
Pseudomonas, 440
  P. aeruginosa, 203t, 348t, 432t
  P. folliculitis, 203–204, 204f
pseudopods, 172, 173f

PSGN (poststreptococcal glomerulonephritis), 220b
PSI I and II, 69–70
psychotrophs, 122, 122t
psychrophiles (cryophiles), 122
puberty, 371–372, 430
public health. *See also* bioterrorism/ bioweapons; global concerns; natural disasters
  bacterial growth curves, 120–121, 120f
  control (*See* control methods)
  epidemiology (*See* epidemiology)
  infectious diseases and population, 333
  threats, 81b, 152b, 236b, 412–413, 458
  urban/rural populations, 333f
puerperal sepsis (childbed fever), 100b, 201b
pulmonary aspergillosis, 232–233
pump transport, 59–60
puncture wounds, 213, 265b
Pure Food and Drug Act, 401
purine and pyrimidine analogs, 417
purines, 37f
pyclonephritis, 302t
pyogenic exudate (pus), 203–204
pyrexia (fever), 379, 379b, 431
pyrimethamine, 419
pyrimidines, 37f
pyrogens, 44b, 379
pyruvic acid, 67–68

Q

Q fever, 219t, 226, 454–455, 456t
quarantines, 245b
quaternary compounds (quats), 355t, 356
quinine, 419
quinolones (fluoroquinolones), 414, 415t

R

rabbit fever. *See* tularemia (rabbit fever)
rabies, 150t, 154, 269, 269f, 272–273
radiation, 351–352
  food irradiation, 243b, 358
  ionizing, 348t
  mutations due to, 125, 351–352
  nonionizing, 351
radioactive isotopes (radioisotopes), 22b
radioactivity, 22
radioisotopes, 22
raising bacteria. *See* culturing entries under laboratory testing/techniques; laboratory testing/techniques; microbial growth
rashes
  Chagas' disease, 292
  Lyme disease, 285
  measles (*Morbillivirus*), 207
  meningitis, 407
  rat-bite fever, 283
  Rocky Mountain spotted fever, 285, 285f
  roseola infantum, 209
  syphilitic, 320–321, 321f
  typhus, 286
rat-bite fever, 282t, 283
RBCs. *See* red blood cells
receptor-mediated endocytosis, 60, 61f
recipient cells, 125
reclamation procedures, 15
rectal administration of drugs, 394–395

red blood cells, 276b, 297, 366, 472b
red bone marrow (myeloid tissue), 372
Redi, Francesco, 5t, 7
redox (reduction-oxidation), 25–26
red tides, 159b–160b, 166
reduction, 26
reemerging infectious diseases. *See* emerging/reemerging diseases/ infections
Registry of Toxic Effects of Chemical Substances (RTECS), 103–105
rehydration therapy, 22b
relapsing fever, 284t, 287, 287t
renal system. *See also* urinary tract infections (UTIs)
  drug-related kidney diseases, 399
  erythropoietin, 472
  kidney failure, 220b
  kidney filtration function, 59
  nephrons, 397f
  pharmacology, 392t
replica plating, 464, 465f
reportable diseases, 192, 193b
reproduction methods (microbes), 42. *See also* cell replication methods
  algae, 167–169
  asexual, 73, 164–165, 168f, 172, 175f–176f
  Babesia microti, 175f
  cestodes, 177f
  fertilization process for production of offspring, 75
  fungi, 163f–164f, 165–166
  helminths, 175
  hookworms, 177f
  Paramecia, 170f
  Penicillium and *Saccharomyces*, 166f
  sexual, 75, 165, 168f, 172, 175f–176f
  sexual reproduction, 165
  slime molds, 176f
  viruses (*See* virus multiplication)
reproductive tract infections (RTIs), 307b. *See also* females; males; sexually transmitted infections (STIs); urinary/ urogenital tract entries
  categories of, 308
  contraceptive use, 299–300, 318b
  female-specific
    anatomy, 309f, 314–315
    bacterial, 308–310, 312t
    candidiasis, 251f, 328, 371, 428
    chlamydial, 322b
    fungal, 311, 312t, 314–315
    gonorrhea, 319b
    mastitis, 307b, 310, 312t
    nonsexually transmitted (summary), 312t
    normal flora of vagina, 309
    pH of vagina, 307b
    in pregnancy, 427–428
    protozoan, 311, 312t, 314–315
    Streptococcus agalactiae, 310b
    Trichomonas vaginalis, 311f, 328–329
    vaginal infections, 307b, 427–428
    vaginitis, 308–309, 312t
  global burden of, 308
  iatrogenic, 308
  impact of, 308
  male-specific

reproductive tract infections (RTIs)
(*Continued*)
    anatomy, 314–315
    bacterial infections, 313–314
    fungal infections, 314
    infections of penis, 314, 319b,
      328–329
    prostate gland, 313
    prostatitis, 313, 315t
    protozoan infections, 314
    treatment of, 392t
    urinary tract infections (UTIs), 314–315
rER (rough endoplasmic reticulum), 52,
    55–56
reservoirs, 192–194
    animal, 192, 194t, 252, 284
    bacterial, 118t
    fungal pathogens, 162t
    histoplasmosis, 231
    human, 192–194
    nonliving, 194
    tick-borne infections, 287t
    viral hemorrhagic fevers (VHFs), 288
resident flora, 182–183
residual bodies, 54, 54f
resistance, drug. *See* drug resistance
resistance, microbial. *See* microbial
    resistance
resistant microorganisms, 345
respiration, 64–70, 75–78
respiratory tract
    anatomy, 183f, 217, 218f, 233
    asthma, 226–228
    defense mechanisms of, 217–219
    normal flora, 217–219, 224, 233
    as portal of entry, 183–185
respiratory tract infections
    bacterial, 219–226, 429–430, 455
    drugs used for, 392t
    endemic, 233
    first identification of, 217b
    flood/rain-related, 447
    fungal, 231–233, 231t
    global concerns, 230
    lung, 217, 233
    opportunistic, 217–219, 224–226, 233
    rare, 224–226
    transmission of, 220–221, 233
    viral, 154, 217b, 226–230, 407
response systems. *See* bioterrorism/
    bioweapons; Centers for Disease
    Control (CDC); control methods;
    emergencies/emergency response
    systems; public health; World Health
    Organization (WHO)
restriction enzymes, 95, 463–464, 463b,
    463t–464t, 464f, 474
retroviruses, 143, 149, 150t, 154, 155t
reverse-transcribing viruses, 144
reverse transcriptase, 465–466
reversible chemical reactions, 26–28
reversions (back mutation), 125
R group, 32f
rhabdoviruses, 154
rheumatic fever, 220b, 280t, 281, 293,
    429–430
rheumatoid arthritis (RA), 384t–386t, 387
Rh factor (D antigen), 366, 366b
rhinoviruses, 154

rhizobia, 128b
rhizoid growth, 92
rhoptries, 172–173
ribonucleic acid. *See* RNA (ribonucleic
    acid); RNA viruses
ribosomal synthesis, 162
ribosomes, 55–56, 56b, 56f
ribotyping, 95
ricin toxin, 454–455, 456t
Rickettsia, 129, 129f, 129t
    R. prowazeki, 203t
    R. typhi, 203t
ringworm *(Tinea)*, 210–211, 212f
risk factors. *See also* biosafety levels (BSLs)
    and guidelines
    antimicrobial drugs, 420–421
    bacterial pneumonia, 221
    brucellosis infection, 282
    dead humans/animals after natural
      disasters, 446–447
    floods, 445
    of floods, 447
    group B streptococcal infections, 310
    HIV in infants, 427
    influenza, 430
    mastitis, 310
    microbial diseases, 433
    occupational, 100–101
    oral cavity infections/diseases, 241, 243b
    pinworm infestation, 253
    pneumonia, 431–432
    poliomyelitis, 268
    rabies exposure, 154
    skin infections, 202
    tsunamis, 447
    urinary tract infections (UTIs), 299–300,
      301b, 304, 432, 432b
    waterborne diseases, 13–14
risk group levels for biosafety response,
    101t
RNA (ribonucleic acid), 38, 42, 71, 75–78.
    See also genetics-related entries
    description, 38
    messenger RNA (mRNA), 32–33, 38,
      55–56, 71–72, 71t, 72f
    negative/positive sense classification, 144
    organism classification by, 95
    primer RNA, 72–73
    ribosomal RNA (rRNA), 9, 38, 52,
      54–56, 95
    sense strands, 462
    single-stranded (ssRNA), 137–140
    transcription of, 149
    transfer RNA (tRNA), 54–56, 72,
      72f–73f
    translation of viral RNA, 149
    translation/transcription of DNA by, 71f,
      72
RNA polymerase enzyme, 71
RNA viruses, 143–144, 152–155. *See also
    main entries for specific viruses/
    infections*
    astroviruses and caliciviruses, 250
    Bunyaviridae, 152
    classification of, 138b
    coronaviruses, 152–153
    flaviviruses, 155
    hepatitis viruses, 153
    influenza, 228–229

RNA viruses (*Continued*)
    medically important, 139t–140t
    mutations, 335
    noroviruses, 250
    orthomyxoviruses, 153
    paramyxoviruses, 154
    picornaviruses, 154
    placenta-crossing, 186t
    poliovirus, 268, 268f
    rabies, 269f
    retroviruses, 154
    rhabdoviruses, 154
    taxonomy, 138b
    togaviruses, 154
    transcription, 149
    transcription of, 148
    viral hemorrhagic fevers (VHFs), 288,
      453
    virus genome types, 143–144
Rocky Mountain spotted fever, 284–285,
    284t, 285f, 287t
rodents, 283–284, 287t, 291–292, 446
rods (bacilli). *See under* bacteria (in
    general)
roseola infantum, 208t, 209
Roslin Institute, 43t
Ross, Sir Ronald, 159b–160b
Rotary Foundation, 268–269
rotaviruses, 249–250
Rotavirus Vaccine Program (RVP), 250
rough endoplasmic reticulum (rER), 52,
    55–56
Roundup Ready superweeds, 473, 473b
roundworms, 177–178, 253–254, 253f, 441
RTECS (Registry of Toxic Effects of
    Chemical Substances), 103–105
RTIs. *See* reproductive tract infections
    (RTIs)
rubella (German measles), 154, 186t, 207,
    426, 429–430
rubor, 378b
Ruska, Ernst, 43t
Russian (Asiatic) flu, 153t
Russian Vector Institute for Virology, 210
RVP (Rotavirus Vaccine Program), 250

S

Sabin vaccine, 257b, 268–269
saccate appearance, 92
Saccharomyces cerevisiae, 14, 166f
safety issues, 110–111, 111b. *See also*
    Centers for Disease Control (CDC);
    hand washing; Health and Human
    Services (HHS); Occupational Safety
    and Health Administration (OSHA)
    autoclave bags, 109f
    biosafety guidelines, 101b
      level 1 organisms, 102b
      level 2 organisms, 101b
      level 3 organisms, 102b
      level 4 organisms, 103b
    bloodborne pathogens, 111t
    drug administration, 397, 399
    emergency response systems, 111
    eye protection, 110f
    fire extinguishers, 105–106, 106b, 107f
    freezers, 107–108, 108f
    glass containers, 108f
    hand protection, 109

safety issues (*Continued*)
  in health care facilities (*See under* health care facilities)
  home environment, 111–112
  Hospital Infection Control Practices Advisory Committee (HICPAC), 100
  hospitals, 110
  laboratory settings (*See* laboratory safety issues)
  Material Safety Data Sheet (MSDS), 105, 106f
  nursing homes/personal care facilities, 110–111
  physician's offices/clinics, 110
  protective equipment/gear, 108–110, 112, 457
  recommended exposure limits (RELs), 103–105
  refrigerators, 107–108
  respiratory protection, 106–107, 109, 376
  sharps containers, 109f
  showers/eye washes, 108f
  therapeutic index (drug safety), 410
  workplace, 99b
saliva, 269, 283, 287–288, 288b, 288t
Salk vaccine, 257b, 410
Salmonella, 236b, 245b, 448b
  S. typhi, 203t
  salmonellosis, 13t, 244, 325b, 456t
salts, 28, 29t, 38
saltwater (marine) environment/ecosystems. *See under* aquatic microbiology
sanitization, 83, 95, 346, 346t
saprobes, 165–166
saprophytes, 210
sarcinae, 117–118
Sarcodina, 171
SARS (severe acute respiratory syndrome), 217b, 228t, 230
  outbreak of, 230t
SAR (structure-activity relationship) studies, 405b
satellites (virusoids), 155
saxitoxin, 159b–160b
scarlet fever, 203t, 219t, 220, 220f, 429–430
schistosomiasis, 304
schizogony, 169–170
SCID (severe combined immunodeficiency), 387
scientific names, 11
scolex, 176
scrapie, 272
sebaceous (oil) glands, 376
sebum, 376
secondary immune responses, 381
secretory vesicles, 53f, 57
sediment pattern (culture tubes), 93
selective pressure, 411
self-inoculation (autoinoculation), 194–195
semisynthetic agents. *See* antibacterials
Semmelweis, Ignaz, 5t, 8, 35b, 100b, 201b, 332b, 344b
Semmelweis reflex, 201b
sensitivity tests, 299
sensory receptors, 258f

sepsis, 190, 280–281, 283, 451b, 456t
septate hyphae, 163, 164f
septicemia, 190, 196, 203–204, 203t, 280–281, 407
septicemic plague, 284t
sER (smooth endoplasmic reticulum), 52
serologic analysis/diagnosis, 94–95
serotypes/serotyping, 126, 229b, 244–245, 268–269
Sertürner, Friedrich W. A., 391b–392b
serum sickness, 384t–385t
severe acute respiratory syndrome (SARS), 217b, 228t, 230, 230t
severe combined immunodeficiency (SCID), 387
severe malaria, 291
sex pili, 48
sex steroids, 35–36
sexually transmitted infections (STIs). *See also* reproductive tract infections (RTIs)
  bacterial, 319–324
  chancroid, 323
  donovanosis (granuloma inguinale), 324–328
  effects of human behavior on, 333
  females, 329
  fungal, 328
  genital warts, 207
  gonorrhea, 319–320, 320f
  human papillomavirus (HPV), 207, 307b, 327, 327b, 430
  males, 329
  molluscum infections, 209
  mycoplasmal and ureaplasmal nongonococcal urethritis (NGU), 322–323
  overview, 319
  prevalence/incidence of, 319b
  protozoan, 171–172, 328–329
  of reproductive tract, 308
  syphilis, 320–321, 426–427
  testing systems, 322b
  trichomoniasis, 311
  urinary tract infections (UTIs), 301, 314–315
  viral, 324–328
  in young adults, 429–430
sexual reproduction (microbes). *See under* reproduction methods (microbes)
shapes/arrangements. *See* morphology/morphological identification
SHEA (Society for Healthcare Epidemiology of America), 100
shells (energy levels), 20–21, 23
Shigella/shigellosis, 13t, 245–246, 454–455, 456t
shingles (*Varicella zoster*), 207, 208t, 209, 209f
shorthand, chemical. *See* chemical notations
side effects of drugs, 400–401, 410–411, 416, 420–421
SIDS (sudden infant death syndrome), 424b
sister cells, 75f
skin infections/diseases, 433
  abscesses, 203–204
  allergic, 384t–385t

skin infections/diseases (*Continued*)
  bacterial, 203–207, 203t, 207t
    classification of, 203, 213–214
    staphylococcal, 203–204
    streptococcal, 204–205
  bacterial lesions, 293
  burns, 202
  causes of, 202
  contact dermatitis, 201b
  fungal, 164, 203t, 211t, 213–214, 254
    cutaneous/subcutaneous, 212–213
    deep, 231
    description, 210
    manifestations of, 203t
    subcutaneous, 213–214
    superficial/deep, 163b
    systemic, 289, 289t
    Tinea species, 210–212, 211t
  necrotizing, 203, 205, 205b, 207t
  in older adults, 431
  protozoan parasites, 170t
  risk factors for, 202
  viral, 207–210, 208t, 213–214
  wounds
    anaerobic, 264
    puncture, 213, 265b
    treatment of, 344b
    wound botulism, 247
skin/integumentary system
  anatomy, 185, 202, 202f
  as defense mechanism, 213–214, 376
  degermation of, 83
  of infants/children, 429–430, 458b
  normal flora of, 184t
  pH of, 376
  as portal of entry, 185–186, 205b, 213–214, 264, 272–273, 283, 378
SLE (systemic lupus erythematosus), 386t, 387
sleeping sickness (African trypanosomiasis), 271
slime molds. *See* molds
smallpox (variola virus), 150t, 152, 208t, 209–210, 210f
  Beijerinck, Marinus Willem, 136b
  as biological weapon, 152b, 452–453, 455t
  vaccinations for, 332b
smoking/tobacco use, 241
smooth endoplasmic reticulum (sER), 52
Snow, John, 2b–3b, 249b
SOA (site of action) of drugs, 398
Society for Healthcare Epidemiology of America (SHEA), 100
sodium, 28, 29t, 38
sodium hypochlorite (NaOCl), 26b
soft tissue, 267b, 281. *See also skin* entries
soil-borne diseases, 213, 265b, 281, 292, 427, 443t
soil microbiology, 15, 441–442, 458
  agricultural inoculants, 128b
  classification of microorganisms in, 441
  Clostridium spores in, 264
  contaminants, 247–249, 251, 253
  definition, 458
  denitrification of, 440
  microbial populations, 442
  nitrogen in, 440
  remediation of, 50

solid state of water, 29
solubility, 30, 396
solutes, 30, 30f, 60f
solutions, 30, 30f
solvents, 30, 30f
Spallanzani, Lazzaro, 5t, 7–8
Spanish flu, 153t, 229b
Speaker, Andrew, 224b, 245b
species (in general), 10f, 11
  cross-species infections, 229
  definition, 125–126
  grouping, naming, classifying, 11 (*See also* taxonomy)
  medically important viruses by, 139t–140t
  species-specific toxins, 188
  -virus suffix, 137
species variability, 399
specimen preparation. *See under* laboratory testing/techniques
spectrum of activity. *See under* antimicrobials
spikes, 137
spinal cord, 258–259, 258f–260f, 268
spirilla, 117f, 118t
spirochetes, 117f, 118t, 126, 127t, 287, 320
Spirogyra, 169f
spleen, 287, 292, 371, 371f, 371t
spontaneous generation of life, 7–8
spontaneous mutations, 124
sporadic diseases, 192
sporangia, 164–165
spore development, 164–165
spores, fungal, 164f
sporotrichosis, 211t, 213
Sporozoa protozoa, 171
sporozoites, 173, 290–291
spreading skin infections, 203
spread of diseases. *See* transmission of infections
stages of infection. *See under* infections/ infectious diseases (in general)
stain techniques. *See under* laboratory testing/techniques
Stanley, Wendell, 136b
staphylococcal infections/agents (*Staphylococcus*), 130–131, 203–204, 248, 248f. *See also* bacterial infections/ diseases; main entries for specific infections
  cellulitis, 204
  conjunctivitis, 429
  furuncles (boils), 203–204
  impetigo (pyoderma), 204
  nonpathogenic *Staphylococcus*, 118
  pneumonia, 219t, 224
  S. aureus, 116f, 203–204, 203t, 207t, 224f, 248f, 307b, 429
  S. epidermidis, 130f
  skin, 203–204
  staphylococcal scalded skin syndrome, 429
  Staphylococcus enterotoxin B (SEB), 455
  staphylo- prefix, 117–118
starvation, 399
steam (gas state of water), 29
steam state of water, 29
stem cells, 41b–42b, 303–304, 372
sterile environment, 12

sterility, 83
sterilization methods, 82–83, 82f–83f, 95, 346. *See also* control methods; laboratory aseptic techniques
  autoclaves, 350f
  boiling water, 351
  commercial, 346
  culture media containers, 82f
  definition, 82–83, 346t
  dry heat, 83t, 349–350
  flowing steam, 351
  methods for, 125
  moist heat, 83t, 350–351
  steam sterilization, 350–351
  temperatures for, 348t, 349f
steroids, 35, 36f, 38
Stewart, William H., 332b
STIs. *See* sexually transmitted infections (STIs)
stomach, 123b, 240, 240b, 242–243. *See also* gastrointestinal (GI) tract
strains, 125–126, 229, 244, 246, 335b
stratiform appearance, 92
streptococcal infections/agents (*Streptococcus*), 204–205, 219–222. *See also* bacterial infections/diseases; main entries for specific infections
  acne, 206
  acute necrotizing fasciitis (flesh eating bacteria), 203, 205, 205b, 207t
  complications of, 281, 293
  drug-resistant *Streptococcus pneumoniae* (DRSP), 219t, 221b, 222
  erysipelas, 204–205
  group A streptococci (GAS), 204, 205b, 207t, 220
  group B streptococci (GBS), 309–310, 314–315, 366, 429
  leprosy (Hansen's disease), 206–207
  Peptococcus/Peptostreptococcus, 130–131
  poststreptococcal glomerulonephritis (PSGN), 220b
  S. agalactiae, 310b
  S. pneumoniae (pneumonia), 221–222, 221f, 432, 432t
  S. pyogenes, 203t, 207t, 220, 220f
  S. salivarios, 240
  scarlet fever, 220
  skin, 204–205
  strep throat (streptococcal pharyngitis), 205, 219–220, 219t, 220b, 429–430
  streptobacilli, 118
  streptomycetes, 132, 132t
  strepto- prefix, 117–118
streptomycetes, 132, 132t
strobila, 176
stroma layer, 54–55, 55f
stromatolites, 9
structural characteristics/arrangements
  algae, 46
  amino acids, 32f
  antibodies, 366–367
  atomic structure, 20–22, 21f
  bacteria, 42–57, 90–95, 116–118, 116f, 118t
  bacteriophages (phages), 143, 143f
  cellular, 31, 45–46, 75–78
  chemical molecular structure (CMS), 19b–20b

structural characteristics/arrangements (*Continued*)
  DNA (deoxyribonucleic acid), 37f
  enzymes, 62f
  eukaryotes, 42–57
  fluid-mosaic membrane structure, 42–43
  fungi, 46, 166f
  macroscopic, 41b–42b
  microscopic, 41b–42b
  molecular (*See* molecular structure)
  naked/enveloped viruses, 141f–142f
  peptidoglycans, 45f, 406f
  prokaryotes, 42–57
  proteins, 33, 33f
  surface structures, 47–49, 48f
  viruses, 141f–142f
structure-activity relationship (SAR) studies, 405b
struvite stones, 303b
subcutaneous administration of drugs, 394–395
subcutaneous layer (skin), 202
subcutaneous mycoses (fungal skin infections), 211, 213–214. *See also* fungal infections/diseases
sublingual drug administration, 394–395
submicroscopic particles, 136b
substrate(s), 61, 62f, 63
subviral agents, 155
sucrose, 31
sudden infant death syndrome (SIDS), 424b
sugars. *See* carbohydrates (sugars)
sulfa drugs (sulfonamides), 63b, 405b, 414
sulfur, 68–69, 122, 440–441, 441f
superbugs, 412–413
superficial mycoses, 163b
superinfections, 408, 410
superscripts in chemical notations, 27b
superweeds (Roundup Ready), 473, 473b
suppressed immune system. *See* compromised/suppressed immune system *under* immune system response; immune system response
suppressor T cells, 380
surface appendages, 47–49, 48f, 75–78
surfactants, 355t
Swammerdam, Jan, 41b–42b
swine flu (H1N1), 337b
symbiosis, 128b, 182, 182t, 439–440, 442
symbols (chemical notations), 20t, 27b
symptoms of infections. *See specific infection or disease*
synaptic vesicles, 57
synergism, 12, 409
synthesis, 25, 406
synthetic azoles, 418
synthetic chemistry, 400–401
synthetic drugs, 414, 416–417
  antiviral agents, 416–417
  quinolones (fluoroquinolones), 414, 415t
  sulfa drugs (sulfonamides), 414
  trimethoprim, 414
syphilis, 127t, 186t, 203t, 320–321, 320t, 324t, 325b, 426–427, 430
systemic infections, 276b. *See also* circulatory system
  definition, 190
  fungal, 289, 289t
  gonorrhea, 319

systemic infections (*Continued*)
  rat-bite fever, 283
  septicemia, 190, 196, 203–204, 203t, 280–281, 407
  septicemic plague, 284t
  sexually transmitted, 329
  skin manifestations of, 202
  urinary tract infections (UTIs) from, 297–298
systemic lupus erythematosus (SLE), 386t, 387

T

taeniasis, 253
tapeworms, 176, 177f
targets (receptors), 412
tastes, five basic, 28
taxis, 48
taxonomy, 11. *See also Bergey's Manual of Systematic Bacteriology;* kingdoms of life; morphology/morphological identification
  algae, 167–169
  antigens, 364–365
  antimicrobial agents, 420–421
  archaea, 10–11, 125–133
  bacteria, 10–11, 95, 125–133 (*See also Bergey's Manual of Systematic Bacteriology; Bergey's Manual of Systematic Bacteriology*)
  Baltimore classification system, 137, 138b (*See also Bergey's Manual of Systematic Bacteriology*)
  chemical bonds and forces, 23–25
  chemical classification of culture media, 85
  ciliates, 172
  criteria for, 125–126
  definition, 11
  by DNA (deoxyribonucleic acid), 95
  DNA viruses, 138b
  enzymes, 62
  eukaryotes, 10–11
  fungi, 164–166
  helminths, 176–178
  immunoglobulins, 367–368
  International Committee on Taxonomy of Viruses (ICTV), 137
  microorganisms, 10–11
  by mobility/locomotion, 171
  mutations, 124–125, 133
  NIH classification of pathogenic agents, 101
  organic, 11
  prions, 11
  prokaryotes versus eukaryotes, 10
  protozoans, 171–173
  retroviruses, 154
  RNA (ribonucleic acid), 95, 144
  RNA viruses, 138b
  taxa, 11
  toxic effects of drugs, 399–400
  viroids, 11, 155t
  viruses, 11, 137
T cells, 324, 375, 380–381, 387
TDP (thermal death point), 349
TDT (thermal death time), 349
technology/industry, 334–335. *See also* biotechnology

teeth. *See* oral cavity
temperate (lysogenic) phages, 146–147
temperature (of environment)
  antimicrobial effectiveness and, 353
  for bacteria growth, 122, 122t, 133
  cryofixation, 90
  for dry/moist heat sterilization, 83t
  incubation of cultures, 86
  LTLT (long temperature, long time), 348t
  for pasteurization, 357–358
  rates of chemical reactions according to, 63
  refrigeration/freezing, 107–108, 351
  soil, 441–442
  for sterilization methods, 348t, 349f
  ultrahigh, 348t
temperature (body), fever/pyrexia, 379, 379b, 431
temporal arteritis, 384t–385t
terminator sequence, 71
terrorism. *See* bioterrorism/bioweapons
tetanus (lockjaw), 264–265, 265b, 272–273
tetracyclines, 416
therapeutic class of drugs, 393, 393t
therapeutic index (drug safety), 397f, 410
thermal death time/point, 349
thermoacidophiles, 123
thermodynamics, 61
thermogenesis, 217b
thermophiles, 122t, 125, 131–133, 444
thimerosal, 400b
Thiobacillus, 348t
threats to public health. *See* control methods; global concerns; public health
thrush *(Candida albicans)*, 251f
thylakoid membrane, 54–55, 68–69, 68f
thymus gland, 371–372, 372f, 387, 430
thyroid
  Graves' disease (Graves' hyperthyroidism), 386–387, 386t
  Hashimoto's thyroiditis, 386t
TIGRIS DTS, 322b
time effects (drug administration), 398–399
time-response curve (drug administration), 398f
Tinea species (ringworm), 211–212, 211t, 212b, 212f, 328
tissue plasminogen activator (tPA), 471
titer test, 94–95
TNF (tumor necrosis factor), 257b
tobacco mosaic virus, 136b, 142f
togaviruses, 154
tolerogens, 364–365
tongue, 220, 220f
tonicity, 31f
tonoplast membrane, 56–57
tonsillitis, 369t
tonsils, 368–369
toxemia, 190, 254
toxicity, drug. *See* drug toxicity
toxicology, 392–393, 399
toxic shock syndrome (TSS), 203t, 276b, 307b, 309, 312t, 323b
toxins/toxic compounds
  aerosolized, 257b, 452, 455
  antidotes, 399
  antitoxin effectiveness, 452

toxins/toxic compounds (*Continued*)
  bacterial, 188
  bioremediation for, 15
  disinfectants, 83
  endotoxins, 43, 188–189, 189f, 190t
  endotoxin shock, 44b
  epsilon toxin, 454–455
  exotoxins, 188, 189f, 189t–190t, 264
  insecticidal, 473
  plant, 257b, 456t
  pyrogenic, 379
  Registry of Toxic Effects of Chemical Substances (RTECS), 103–105
  ricin, 454–455, 456t
  saxitoxin, 159b–160b
  species-specific, 188
  synthesis of, 162
  tetanus, 188, 447
  toxigenic organisms, 188
  toxin-producing organisms, 57t, 159b–160b, 202
  virulence/pathogenicity of, 187–188
Toxoplasma gondii (toxoplasmosis), 186t, 271, 290t, 292, 292f, 425f, 427, 427b, 428f
trace elements (micronutrients), 84t
trade (proprietary/brand) names of drugs, 393t
transcellular fluids, 58
transcription, 71–72, 148–149
transdermal drug administration, 394–395
transferases, 62
transforming infections, 149
transfusions, blood, 276b, 366
transgenic animals, 473–474
translation, 72, 73f, 407f
transmissible spongiform encephalopathies/prion diseases (TSEs), 11b, 155, 257b, 272–273, 358
  bovine spongiform encephalopathy (BSE), 11b, 155, 272, 358
  chronic wasting disease, 272
  feline spongiform encephalopathy, 272
  human prion diseases, 156t, 272
  kuru, 272
  prions, 11, 155
  scrapie, 272
  transmissible mink encephalopathy, 272
  ungulate spongiform encephalopathy, 272
transmission of infections, 100b. *See also* portals of entry; specific infection or disease
  after floods, 445
  airborne, 14t
  animal-related (*See* zoonoses)
  bacterial, 338t
  contact mode, 195–196
  emerging/reemerging, 336–337
  fecal-oral route, 176, 249–252, 268
  to fetuses, 321, 425–426
  first understanding of, 8, 249b
  by fomites, 82, 195–196, 207, 210, 212
  foodborne (*See* foodborne diseases/infections)
  future concerns about, 181b
  hand, 201b
  HIV, 336f
  human demographics and behavior, 333

transmission of infections (*Continued*)
 index cases, 191–192
 industrial effects on, 334–335
 inhalation/ingestion, 455
 modes of transmission, 194–195
 nosocomial infections, 196–198
 in nursing homes, 111
 parasitic, 253
 person-to-person, 101b
 respiratory, 220–221, 233, 262b
 during therapeutic procedures, 196
 vector-related (*See* vector-transmitted
  infections/diseases)
 vehicle mode, 195
 viral infections, 268
 waterborne (*See* waterborne diseases/
  infections)
 zoonotic infections, 194t
transplants. *See* organ transplants
transport mechanisms
 active, 59–61, 75–78
  cellular energy, 59
  endocytosis, 60
  exocytosis, 60–61
  pump transport, 59–60
 biotransport of drugs, 395
 bulk, 60
 carrier-mediated, 58, 60f
 cellular, 57
 membrane, 57–61
 passive, 58–59, 75–78
  diffusion, 58
  facilitated diffusion, 58
  filtration, 59
  osmosis, 58–59
 through blood-brain barrier, 406
transport vesicles, 57
transposons (jumping genes), 125
trauma, 204, 371t
travel-related diseases, 334
 cholera, 249
 dysentery, 245–246
 paratyphoid fever, 245
 traveler's diarrhea, 154
 tuberculosis, 224b
 typhoid fever, 245
 viral hemorrhagic fevers (VHFs), 289
treatment. *See* drugs of choice;
  pharmacology; specific infections/
  diseases; specific infection or disease
trematodes (flukes), 176f
Trichomonas vaginalis/trichomoniasis, 298,
  304, 311, 311f, 312t, 314–315, 315t,
  329, 427–428
triglycerides, 34, 34f, 38
trimethoprim, 414
trophozoite state, 169, 172, 251–252
Trypanosoma, 172f, 271–272
 African trypanosomiasis (sleeping
  sickness), 271
 blood infections, 172f
 T. cruzi (Chagas' disease/American
  trypanosomiasis), 271–272, 290t,
  292
TSEs. *See* transmissible spongiform
  encephalopathies/prion diseases
  (TSEs)
tsunamis, 447, 447t. *See also* natural
  disasters

tuberculin PPD test, 223–224
tuberculosis (TB), 14t, 219t, 223–224, 245b,
  325b
 aerosol transmission, 446–447
 multidrug-resistant tuberculosis
  (MDR-TB), 224b
 transmission during air travel, 224b
tubulin, 51
tularemia (rabbit fever), 282t, 283, 287t,
  451, 451b, 455t
tumor (swelling), 378b
tumor necrosis factor (TNF), 257b
turbidity, 8f, 93, 121
Tyndal, John, 8
tyndallization, 348t
Typhi serotype, 244–245
typhoid, 245b
typhoid fever, 244–245
Typhoid Mary (Mallon, Mary), 236b, 244,
  245b
typhus, 203t, 284t, 286–287, 454–455, 456t

U

unassigned viruses, 138b
uncoating, 147
uncoating stage of viral multiplication, 147
uncomplicated malaria, 291
undulant fever (brucellosis), 282–283, 282t,
  454–455, 456t
ungulate spongiform encephalopathy, 272
UNICEF, 268–269
unicellular organisms, 57, 75–78
United Nations (UN), 99b
universal donor group, 366
urbanization and infectious diseases,
  333–334
ureaplasmas, 130
urease, 303b
urethritis, 304
urinalysis, 299, 304, 325–326
urinary tract infections (UTIs)
 adenoviruses, 250
 alleviation of discomfort during, 303b
 anatomy/organs of, 297
 bacterial, 302–303, 302t
 causative organisms, 297–299
 cystitis, 298, 302t
 diagnosis of, 299
 Escherichia coli, 297–298
 female-specific, 297b, 299–301, 304
 fungal, 304
 glomerulonephritis, 299
 hemolytic uremic syndrome (HUS),
  128b, 247b
 hemorrhagic cystitis, 303–304
 iatrogenic, 314–315
 kidney stones, 303b
 leptospirosis, 299, 302t
 mental difficulties/dementia and,
  302–303
 nephritis, 303–304
 nongonococcal urethritis (NGU),
  321–322
 in older adults/elderly, 431–432
 parasitic, 304
 during pregnancy, 425t
 prevention of, 300–301, 301b
 pyelonephritis (kidney infection),
  298–299, 302t

urinary tract infections (UTIs) (*Continued*)
 recurrent, 301
 risk factors for, 299–300
 sites of infection, 304
 treatment of, 301, 302t, 304
 types of, 297–298
 urethritis, 298, 304, 321–322
 viral, 303–304
urinary/urogenital tract. *See also*
  reproductive tract infections (RTIs)
 abnormalities, 299–301
 anatomy, 297, 298f, 391b–392b, 397f
 normal flora of, 184t
 as portal of entry, 183–185
 protozoan parasites, 170t
urination, 299–303, 376
urine, 59, 297, 303b, 304
U.S. Department of Agriculture (USDA),
  391b–392b. *See also* agriculture;
  Food and Drug Administration
  (FDA)
 Biotechnology Regulatory Services,
  472–473
 diagnosis of chlamydia and gonorrhea,
  322b
 food monitoring/recalls, 247
 raw milk products, 358b
U.S. Department of Health and Human
  Services (HHS). *See* Health and
  Human Services (HHS)
U.S. Food and Drug Administration
  (FDA). *See* Food and Drug
  Administration (FDA)
use-dilution test, 354
uterus, 368
UTIs. *See* urinary tract infections (UTIs)

V

vaccinations (immunization), 335, 400b.
  See also immune system response
 Advisory Committee on Immunization
  Practices (ACIP), 229–230
 antigenic shift and drift, 335b
 autism and, 400b
 booster shots, 381
 childhood diseases, 430
 first, 9
 future approaches, 136b
 global smallpox vaccination program,
  452–453
 hepatitis B virus (HBV), 326–327
 human papillomavirus (HPV), 327b
 influenza, 224, 229–230, 230b, 407, 430
 measles/mumps, 154
 meningitis, 262, 262b
 National Immunization Program, 339
 plague, 284
 pneumonias, 217b, 222
 polio, 268–269
 preexposure/postexposure prophylaxis,
  382b
 rabies, 154, 269
 rotavirus, 250
 sexually transmitted infections, 318b
 smallpox, 152b, 210, 332b, 453
 swine flu (H1N1), 337b
 tetanus, 447
 tuberculosis, 223
 urinary tract infections (UTIs), 301b

vaccine development, 86b, 472
  clinical trials for, 382b
  development/production, 86b
  disease eradication and, 99b
  DNA, 472, 474
  egg culture, 362b–363b
  Global Alliance for Vaccines and
    Immunization, 250
  inactivated poliovirus vaccine (IPV),
    268–269
  live virus, 152
  mutations and, 362b–363b
  Sabin vaccine, 257b, 268–269
  Salk vaccine, 257b, 410
  subunit vaccines, 472
  thimerosal use, 356b
vaccine-preventable diseases, 429–430
Vaccine Research Center (VCR), 382b
vaccinia virus, 151
vacuoles, 56–57, 56f
vaginal infections, 307b, 427
  candidiasis, 251f, 328, 371, 428
  normal flora of vagina, 309
  pH of vagina, 307b
  in pregnancy, 427–428
  Streptococcus agalactiae, 310b
  Trichomonas vaginalis, 311f, 427–428
  trichomoniasis, 328–329
  vaginitis, 308–309, 312t
valence electrons, 21
van der Waals forces, 23, 25, 49
van Leeuwenhoek, Antonie, 2b–3b, 3, 5t, 7,
    41b–42b, 43t, 115b, 240, 276b
variability (drug administration), 399
Varicella. See under herpes viruses
varicella-zoster virus (VZV), 151, 429–430
  chickenpox, 151, 207, 208t, 209, 429–430
  shingles, 207, 208t, 209, 209f
variola virus. See smallpox
VCR (Vaccine Research Center), 382b
vectors, 173, 194t, 195, 195b, 283–287, 334,
    337b. See also zoonoses; main entries
    for specific infections
  animal, 210–211, 283–284, 287t, 290t,
    291–292, 446
  arthropod, 195b, 269–270, 288–289
  biological, 195, 195b
  in biotechnology, 467–468, 468f, 474
  control of, 339
  criteria for biotechnology use, 467
  definition, 280, 293
  DNA molecules as, 467
  insects, 337b, 339
    fleas, 283, 286
    lice, 286–287
    mosquitos, 270–271, 337b, 339 (See
      also malaria)
    sandflies, 290t, 293, 293b
    ticks, 175f, 195b, 287t
  mechanical, 195, 195b
  microarthropods, 441
  phage, 468, 469f
vector-transmitted infections/diseases
  babesiosis, 291–292
  of circulatory system, 283–287, 284t
  ehrlichiosis, 285–286
  epidemiology of, 195
  flood-related, 446, 448
  foodborne, 334

vector-transmitted infections/diseases
    (Continued)
  Lyme disease, 285–286, 285f–286f
  malaria, 159b–160b, 173, 174f, 336f, 425t
  plague (Yersinia pestis), 283–284, 284t
  relapsing fever, 287
  Rocky Mountain spotted fever, 284–285
  typhus, 286–287
  West Nile virus, 337b, 339
venereal disease. See sexually transmitted
    infections (STIs)
vesicles, 57
veterinary medicine, 147b
Vibrio cholerae, 454–455. See also cholera
vibrios, 117f, 118t
viral, 226–230
viral agents of bioterrorism, 452–454, 456t
viral envelopes, 133, 141
viral gastroenteritis, 254
viral infections/diseases, 99b, 149–150, 154,
    226–230. See also antivirals; main
    entries for specific infections
  abortive infections, 149
  circulatory system
    cytomegalovirus (CMV), 288
    infectious mononucleosis, 287–288
    viral hemorrhagic fevers (VHFs),
      288–289
  circulatory system diseases, 293
  disease-causing organisms (summary),
    237t–239t
  emerging/reemerging, 338t
  gastrointestinal (GI) tract, 249–250
    adenoviruses, 250
    astroviruses and caliciviruses, 250
    hepatitis viruses, 250
    noroviruses, 250
    rotaviruses, 250
  host cell damage, 149–150
    biochemical effects, 150
    genotoxic effects, 150
    morphological effects, 149–150
    physiological effects, 150
  nervous system, 268–273
    arboviral encephalitis, 269–271
    poliomyelitis, 268–269
    rabies, 269
    viral meningitis, 268
  opportunistic infections related to AIDS,
    325b
  plague, 159b–160b
  pneumonia, 227t–228t, 432
  respiratory tract, 154, 226–230, 228t
    common cold, 226–228
    hantavirus pulmonary syndrome
      (HPS), 230
    influenza (See influenza)
    pneumonia, 230
    severe acute respiratory syndrome
      (SARS), 230
  sexually transmitted, 318b, 324–328
    genital herpes, 327
    hepatitis B, C, and D, 326–327
    HIV and AIDS, 324–326
    human papillomavirus (HPV), 327
    molluscum contagiosum, 328
  skin, 207–210, 208t
    herpes simplex virus (HSV), 208–209
    molluscum contagiosum, 209

viral infections/diseases (Continued)
    portals of entry, 213–214
    roseola infantum, 209
    smallpox, 209–210
    varicella-zoster virus (VZV), 209
    warts, 207–208
  tonsillitis, 369t
  transmission of, 338t
  viral hemorrhagic fevers (VHFs), 111t,
    288t
    as biological weapons, 453, 455t
    families of RNA viruses causing, 453
    features of, 288
    study of, 289b
  zoonotic, 194t
viral isolation, 453
viral multiplication, 145–150, 146f
  adsorption, 145
  assembly, 145–147
  definition, 137
  penetration, 145
viremia, 190, 268
virions, 137
viroids, 11, 155, 155t
virucides. See antivirals
virulence and pathogenicity, 186–189
  botulism, 265
  Category B biological weapons, 454–455
  endotoxins, 188–189
  etiology of infectious diseases, 189–191
  exotoxins, 188
  Koch's postulates, 190–191
  patterns of infection, 190
  portals of exit, 189
  toxins, 188
  virulence factors, 186–188
viruses (in general), 11, 136b. See also
    subviral agents
  antigenic drift/shift of, 335b
  bloodborne, 111t
  cytopathic effects of, 150t
  description, 137
  discovery of, 217b
  enveloped, 137, 142f, 144t, 148f
  filtration and, 352
  fusion of viral envelope, 147
  genome changes, 144–145
  global spread of, 334b
  medically important, 139t–140t
  morphology, 136b, 137–143
    complex, 137, 142–143
    enveloped, 137, 141–142
    helical, 137–140
    icosahedral, 137, 140–141
  multiplication of, 148f
    adsorption, 147
    assembly, 149
    host cell machinery/metabolism, 145
    penetration, 147
    release, 149
    replication, 148–149
    uncoating, 147
  taxonomy, 137
  use in genetic engineering, 463
  vaccine development/production, 86b
virus groups, 137, 138b, 143, 150–155. See
    also DNA viruses; kingdoms of life;
    RNA viruses
virusoids (satellites), 155

vitamins, 63, 84t
von Kölliker, Rudolph Albert, 43t
VZV. *See* varicella-zoster virus (VZV)

W

war/famine, 335. *See also* bioterrorism/
    bioweapons
warts, 207–208, 208f, 208t
    genital, 207, 327–328
    skin, 207
waste, industrial, 442–443
waste product elimination, 60–61
wastewater treatment, 50, 440b
water. *See also* aquatic microbiology
    boiling point of, 29, 348t
    Coliform Index (purity rating),
        129b
    coliform index/testing, 129b
    freezing/boiling points, 29
    freezing point of, 29
    gas state of (steam), 29
    molecular structure of, 29
    osmotic diffusion, 58–59
    oxidation, 68–69
    pollution, 446
water (human body), 38, 58, 58f
waterborne diseases/infections, 13t, 334.
        See also gastrointestinal (GI) tract;
        main entries for specific infections
    amebiasis, 252
    Balamuthia, 172
    cholera, 249, 249b
    cryptosporidiosis, 252
    description, 13–14
    during/after floods, 445–447
    E. coli, 128b
    flood-associated, 446, 448
    gastroenteritis, 243
    Giardia lamblia, 171b
    giardiasis, 251
    harmful algal blooms (HABs), 167b
    mold-related, 165b
    poliomyelitis, 268
    prevention of, 13–14
    Staphylococcus enterotoxin B, 455
    symptoms of infections, 13t
    toxic algae, 166
    toxoplasmosis, 292
    transmission of, 195
water insects, 29b
water purity assays, 15
water supply treatment, 2b–3b, 15–16
WBCs. *See* white blood cells (WBCs)
weakened immune system. *See under*
    immune system response

Web sites
    AIDS-related opportunistic infections,
        325b
    blood doping, 472b
    BSL-3 facilities, 103
    CDC "Fight the Bite", 337b
    CDC immunization programs, 339
    emergency response standards/
        procedures, 457
    EPA, 438
    infections in children (CDC), 429–430
    level 4 biosafety laboratories in U.S., 104t
    Material Safety Data Sheet (MSDS), 105
    Morbidity and Mortality Weekly Report
        (MMWR), 192
    National Center for Environmental
        Health (NECH), 167b
    OSHA's Biosafety Program, 101b
    vaccinations (immunization), 400b
    WHO updates, 145b
Wesley, John, 217b
Western blot test, 325–326
West Nile virus (WNV), 270, 337b, 339
white blood cells (WBCs), 49, 372, 471
whooping cough (pertussis), 219t,
        222–223, 222f
World Health Organization (WHO), 99b,
        250
    avian influenza in humans, 145b
    emerging/reemerging diseases, 332b
    Global Strategy for Containment of
        Antimicrobial Resistance, 413
    leprosy, 206, 206b, 267
    malaria eradication program, 159b–
        160b, 291b
    overuse of antibiotics, 413b
    polio vaccination program, 268–269
    reproductive tract infections, 308
    shared information with CDC, 192
    smallpox eradication, 136b, 152b, 181b,
        210, 436b–437b, 452–453
    tuberculosis, 223
    "Tuberculosis and Air Travel" guidelines,
        224b
worm infections. *See* helminths/helminthic
    infections
wounds, 213, 247, 264, 265b, 344b

X

xenografts, 365–366
xenotransplants, 473–474

Y

yeast infections. *See under* fungal
    infections/diseases

yeasts. *See under* fungi
yellow fever, 453
Yersinia pestis. See plague
yersiniosis, 246
young adults. *See* adolescents/young
    adults

Z

Zernike, Frits, 6
zone of inhibition, 354f, 409
zoonoses, 229b, 310b, 334. *See also*
    main entries *for specific infections/*
    diseases
    animal reservoirs, 192, 252
    avian influenza, 145b, 229b, 337b,
        341t
    bacterial, 194t
    Balantidium coli, 252
    as biological weapons, 454–455
    bird-related, 194t (*See also* zoonoses)
        avian influenza (influenza A/H5N1),
            145b, 229b, 337b, 341t
        psittacosis, 14t, 219t, 225–226,
            454–455, 456t
        West Nile virus (WNV), 270, 337b,
            339
    brucellosis (undulant fever), 282–283,
        282t
    cat scratch disease, 282t, 283
    cowpox, 9, 152b
    definition, 12, 293
    emerging/reemerging, 337
    fungal, 194t
    glanders, 454–455
    hantavirus pulmonary syndrome (HPS),
        230, 339
    helminthic, 194t
    histoplasmosis, 231
    leptospirosis, 299
    mastitis (dairy cows), 310b
    paramyxoviruses, 154
    protozoan, 194t
    psittacosis, 219t, 225–226
    rabies, 150t, 154, 269, 272–273
    rat-bite fever, 282t, 283
    swine flu, 337b
    toxoplasmosis, 427
    transmissible spongiform
        encephalopathies/prion diseases
        (TSEs), 11b, 155
    transmission of, 335
    tularemia (rabbit fever), 282t, 283
    vector-borne, 194t
    viral, 194t, 337b
Zygomycota, 165–166